AMERICAN ACADEMY
OF OPHTHALMOLOGY®
美国眼科学会®

3

Clinical Optics
临床光学

2018–2019

BCSC

Basic and Clinical
Science Course™

基础与临床科学教程™

美国眼科学会　编

石一宁　方　严　主译

Protecting Sight. Empowering Lives.®
保护视力，享有生活。®

陕西新华出版传媒集团
陕西科学技术出版社
Shaanxi Science And Technology Press

著作权登记号 25-2019-85

图书在版编目（CIP）数据

临床光学：2018-2019 基础与临床科学教程 / 美国眼科学会编；石一宁，方严主译．— 西安：陕西科学技术出版社 2019.7

书名原文：Clinical Optics:2018-2019 Basic and Clinical Science Course™

ISBN 978-7-5369-7578-1

Ⅰ．①临… Ⅱ．①美… ②石… ③方… Ⅲ．①眼病—影像诊断—教 材 Ⅳ．① R770.43

中国版本图书馆 CIP 数据核字 (2019) 第 140233 号

临床光学

美国眼科学会　编

石一宁　方　严　主译

责任编辑　付　琨

封面设计　曾　珂

出 版 者　陕西新华出版传媒集团　陕西科学技术出版社
西安市曲江新区登高路1388号陕西新华出版传媒产业大厦B座
电话（029）81205187　传真（029）81205155　邮编710061
http://www.snstp.com

发 行 者　陕西新华出版传媒集团　陕西科学技术出版社
电话（029）81205180 81206809

印　　刷　西安牵井印务有限公司

规　　格　889mm × 1194mm　16开本

印　　张　45.5

字　　数　1000千字

版　　次　2019年7月第1版
2019年7月第1次印刷

书　　号　ISBN 978-7-5369-7578-1

定　　价　580.00元

This publication is a translation of a publication of the American Academy of Ophthalmology entitled Basic and Clinical Science Course™, Section 3: *Clinical Optics* published in 2016. This translation reflects current practice in the United States of America as of the date of its original publication by the Academy. The American Academy of Ophthalmology did not translate this publication into the language used in this publication and disclaims any responsibility for any errors, omissions or other possible fault in the translation.

本书为美国眼科学会系列教程“基础与临床科学教程”第3册《*临床光学*》的出版物译本，于2016年出版。这一译本的内容为美国眼科学会在出版时美国最新的临床实践。美国眼科学会没有将本出版物翻译成此书中所用的语言，声明对翻译中的任何错误、遗漏或其他可能的错误不承担任何责任。

The American Academy of Ophthalmology is the world's largest association of eye physicians and surgeons. A global community of 32,000 medical doctors, we protect sight and empower lives by setting the standards for ophthalmic education and advocating for our patients and the public. We innovate to advance our profession and to ensure the delivery of the highest-quality eye care. Learn more at www.aao.org.

美国眼科学会是全球最大的眼科内外科医师协会。作为一个拥有32 000名医生的全球组织，为了保护视力，使患者享有生活，我们制定眼科教育的准则，并向我们的患者和公众普及知识。我们不断进取以提升我们的专业水平，确保提供最高质量的眼健康服务。如需了解更多信息请访问网站 www.aao.org。

For information on becoming a member of the Academy or attending the Academy's Annual Meeting, call +1 (415) 561 8500, visit aao.org, or write to us at 655 Beach Street, San Francisco, CA 94109, USA.

有关加入本学会或参加学会年会的信息，请致电 +1（415）561 8500，或访问网站 aao.org，或致信美国加利福尼亚州旧金山海滩街 655 号。

“2018-2019 基础与临床科学教程”《临床光学》一书由美国眼科学会（AAO）组织编写。是国际眼科联盟（WOC）和中国医学考试网推荐图书，是国家医学考试的 ICO 考试点的第二步必考科目和必考书。现我们组织石一宁、方严等专家翻译。本书从光线的传播、单透镜的折射、多透镜组合成像过程、什么是可见光、光的波粒二重性、量子电力学等几何光学、物理光学基础出发，并在此基础上，讲授人类眼球的光学基础，进而对眼球的光学缺陷的问题、检查和处理进行讲解。且本书每一章节后还会配以相关的知识问题，读者通过做题和回答问题能进一步巩固前面所学的知识点，加深理解和记忆。本书结合临床实践延伸至多学科融合的眼视光学内容，指导我们的临床工作，并为眼视觉成像提供更好的理解和帮助。为眼科医师从惯有思路中开辟出新的思路并注入更丰富的内容，为眼健康的保障方法从单纯的临床方案拓展至更佳的光学方案，也为给视光师解决临床的困惑，从而使其从单一而机械的验配检查思路中跳脱出来，更好地结合患者的需求与临床状况来灵活应对提供了科学的方法。这样通过翻译和传播国际上的教学经验的综合学习模式，将眼科人的视野拓宽到更广阔的层级。本书的出版对于视光学专业人才的教育和培养有重要的作用，对于我国培养合格的视光学医师服务于社会有很积极的推动作用。

中文版翻译组

翻译组

扉　页　何　媛　张纯涛//审　校　陈研明　石一宁

导　言　何　媛　张纯涛　伊恩晖　许志强　姚　森　贺金刚　袁立飞//审　校　陈研明　石一宁

第一章　杨亚军　朱　丹　张　宁　孙西宇//审　校　石一宁//章节审校　魏瑞华

第二章　叶　璐　王景慧　王　岐　魏瑞华//审　校　石一宁//章节审校　魏瑞华

第三章　冯　坤　代秋楠　李　易//审　校　李　易　石一宁

第四章　石　蕊　杨　乐　谭　薇　王　涛　张　乐　肖　勇//审　校　肖　勇　石一宁

第五章　唐志萍　梅　颖　杨嘉嵩　姚春艳　郑　玲//审　校　石一宁　吴　捷//章节审校　郑　玲

第六章　卢淑杰　汪晓倩//审　校　汪晓倩　石一宁//章节审校　杨亚军

第七章　吴　捷　王文军//审　校　石一宁　吴　捷//章节审校　白　继

第八章　胡　箭　王西欧//审　校　石一宁　李　易//章节审校　朱　丹

第九章　刘　念　龚　慧//审　校　石一宁//章节审校　魏瑞华

测试练习　刘凤阳　许　军//审　校　石一宁　李　易

审校组

魏瑞华　郑　玲　杨亚军　白　继　朱　丹

专业总审校

高祥璐

英文总审校

陈研明　陈　卓

主译主审

石一宁　方　严

名誉主审

石广礼

翻译组译者简介

翻译组（以翻译章节为序）

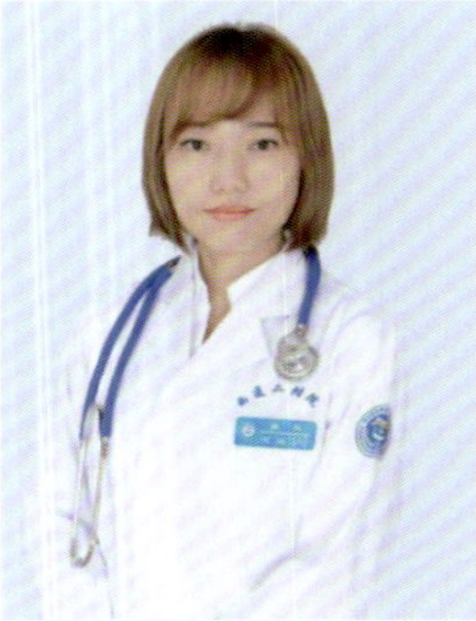

何媛，主任医师，教授，留美博士后。西安交通大学医学院和中山大学中山眼科中心硕士及博士。西安医学院第二附属医院眼科主任。陕西省防盲办公室副主任，西安市眼科学会常务委员，陕西省妇幼保健协会儿童眼病专委会常务委员。陕西省眼科学优势学科带头人，主持国家自然科学基金 2 项、省科技厅社发攻关项目 5 项。临床方面擅长白内障超声乳化手术及各类青光眼的诊治。发表论文 50 余篇，其中，以第一作者或者通讯作者身份发表的论文被 SCI 收录 20 余篇。指导博士后研究、博士生及硕士生 23 人（美国）。

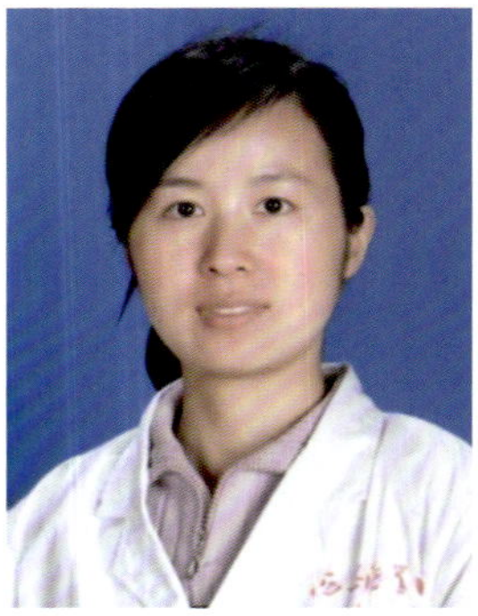

张纯涛，副主任医师。西安交通大学医学院硕士。在西安医学院第二附属医院眼科工作，从事眼科临床、科研和教学多年，遵章守纪，勤恳敬业，临床经验丰富，受到了患者及家属的一致好评。参加第 33 批援苏丹医疗队进行医疗援助 1 年。发表论文数篇。

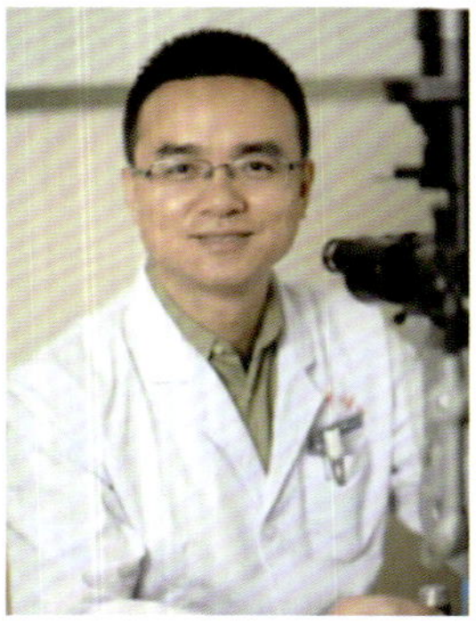

伊恩晖，副主任医师，硕士学位，2000 年毕业于西安交通大学医学院。陕西省保健协会防盲专业委员会常务委员，陕西省医学会眼科分会第七届委员，西安医学会眼科分会委员、白内障分会委员，西安市医疗事故鉴定专家库成员。曾赴苏丹参加中国医疗队进行援外工作 2 年。发表 SCI 收录论文 3 篇，中文核心期刊论文 10 篇。主持及参与省级课题 2 项、市级课题 1 项，市级课题获西安市科技进步二等奖，参与著书 3 部。擅长白内障和屈光性白内障手术治疗，屈光不正的矫治，斜视手术治疗，眼底病、青光眼和泪道疾病的激光治疗。对糖尿病视网膜病变防治，青少年近视防控、弱视规范治疗、视功能检查及训练有深入的研究。

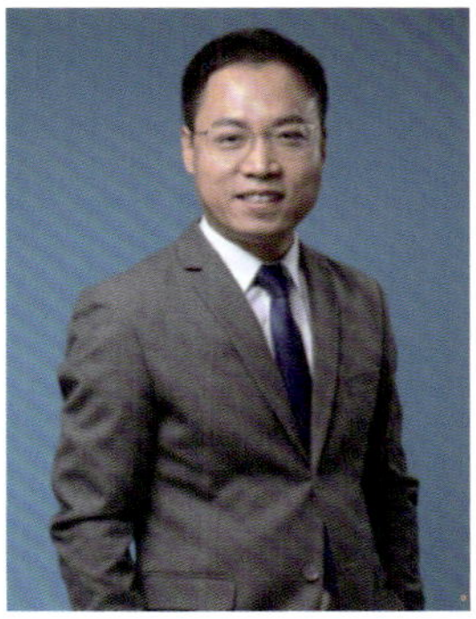

许志强，医师，验光技师，曾就读于山西医科大学临床医学专业及湖北科技学院眼视光专业。从事小儿眼科及视光行业 10 余年。师从我国知名眼科专家石一宁教授学习儿童青少年近视预测预警及防控、高度近视眼底病预防及治疗方面等内容。擅长儿童青少年斜视弱视康复、儿童青少年近视防控、角膜塑形镜及 RGP 镜验配、视功能检测分析及训练。

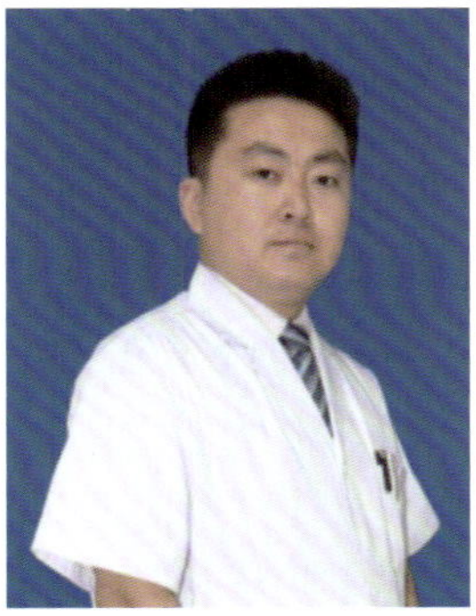

姚森，医学学士，医师，IAOA 会员，毕业于河北工程大学医学部，美国新英格兰视光学院和纽约州立大学视光学院访问学者。曾于河北省眼科医院（邢台眼科医院）完成 3 年眼科各亚专业进修学习，于天津医科大学早稻田培训学校进行眼视光学的相关培训学习，目前主要从事小儿眼科斜弱视及近视防治工作。

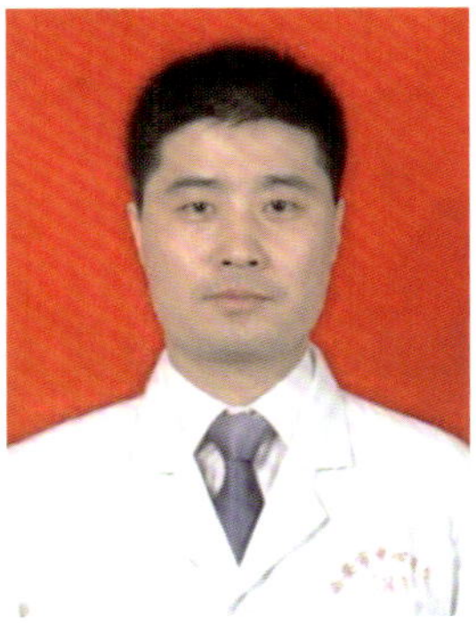

贺金刚，主治医生，西安市中心医院眼科。毕业于延安大学医学院，从事眼科临床工作 10 余年。擅长屈光不正、斜视及弱视的诊断及治疗，对眼底病的诊治和激光治疗积累了丰富的经验。

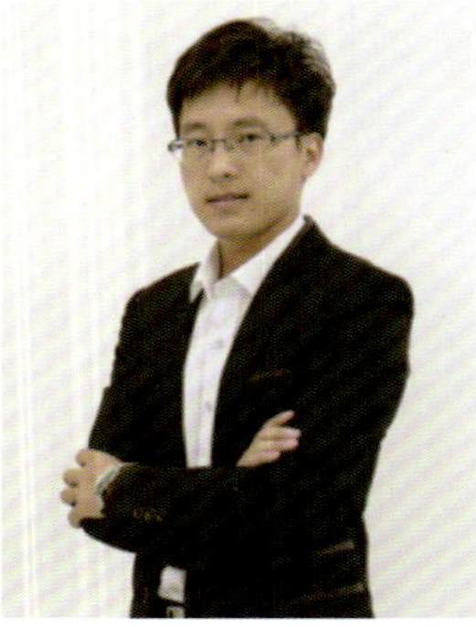

袁立飞，河北省眼科医院主治医师，眼科学硕士，毕业于天津医科大学，主要从事角膜病诊断治疗、眼底影像诊断与激光治疗和临床医疗管理工作。参与省市级科研项目 3 项，国家自然基金项目 1 项，发表临床和科研论文 8 篇，其中 SCI 论文 3 篇。获河北省医学科技进步一等奖 1 项。连续 5 年参加全国眼科年会并做发言交流。任中国民族医药学会眼科分会理事，河北省中西医结合学会眼科分会常务委员兼秘书，邢台市医学会眼科分会委员。

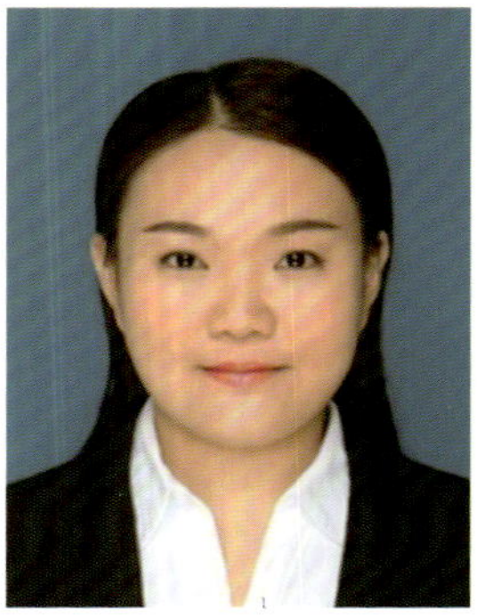

张宁，现就职于西安交通大学第一附属医院。2017 年四川大学眼视光专业博士毕业，为香港理工大学眼视光学和四川大学联合培养博士。共发表 SCI 论文 2 篇。临床主要研究方向是弱视、近视及双眼视。

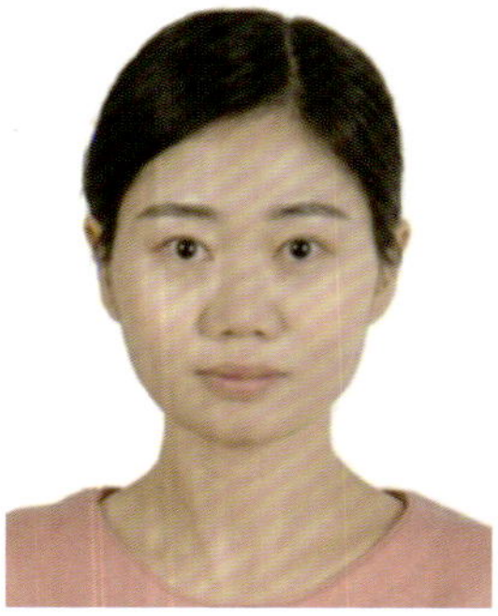

孙西宇，眼科学硕士，毕业于温州医科大学附属眼视光学院。主要从事角膜屈光手术的相关研究，近视、远视及散光的矫正与治疗，角膜塑形镜及硬性透氧性接触镜（RGP）的验配，以及常见眼表疾病的诊断及治疗。

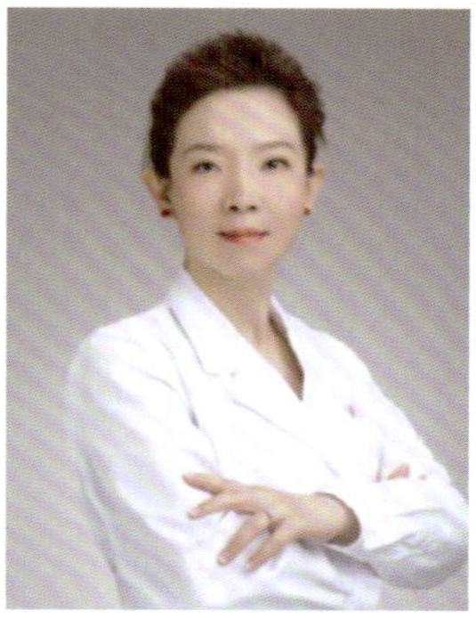

叶璐，主任医师，眼科学硕士，毕业于温州医学院眼视光学院。西安市医学会视光学分会副主任委员，陕西省保健协会青少年视力保健与视光学专业委员会委员，陕西省医学会眼科学分会第八届委员会视光学与屈光手术学组委员，国际角膜塑形镜学会亚洲分会（IAOA）会员，中华医学会眼科学分会会员。主持及承担10余项陕西省及西安市科技攻关项目，5次获得陕西省西安市科技进步奖。

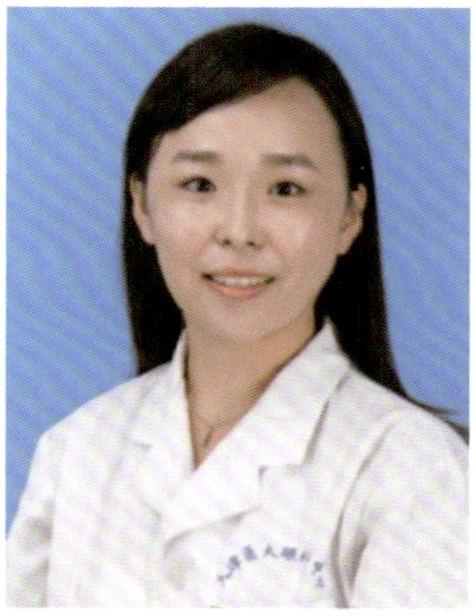

王景慧，眼视光学硕士，毕业于天津医科大学。美国Nova东南大学访问学者、IACLE会员，国际CORD会员。曾赴美国纽约州立大学眼视光学院、新英格兰视光学院、休斯顿州立大学眼视光学院、Bascom Palmer眼科中心、Wilmer眼科中心、Texas医学中心等多地进行交流学习。主要从事眼视光学教育与临床工作，擅长青少年近视防控、角膜塑形镜验配、双眼视异常诊断。在国内外发表多篇论文。

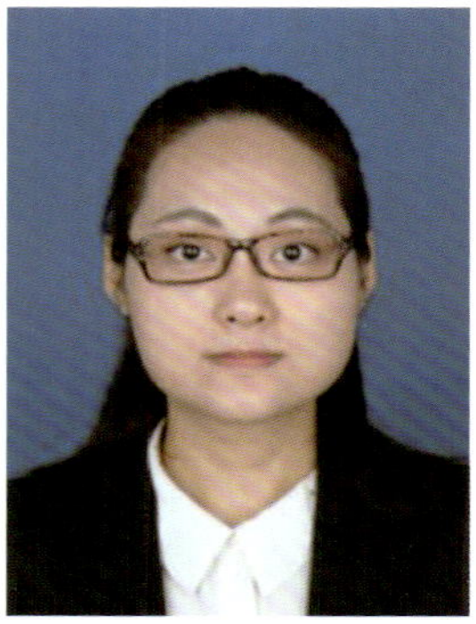

王頔，眼视光学博士，就读于天津医科大学。本科毕业于天津大学机械工程学院工程力学专业，硕士毕业于美国太平洋大学视觉科学专业。主要参与近视控制与视功能异常等的研究。硕士就读期间工作于美国太平洋大学视觉表现研究所，曾参与模拟光学离焦信号对视觉系统影响的研究、阅读疲劳研究及频闪对阅读效率影响等研究项目。

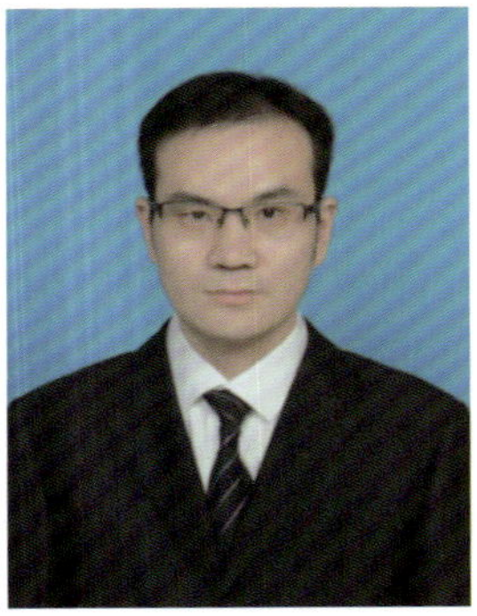

冯坤，北京中医药大学枣庄医院主治医师，医学硕士，师从广东省近视防控专家王幼生教授。目前主要从事中西医结合治疗青少年近视、弱视、眼科疾病的激光治疗等工作。

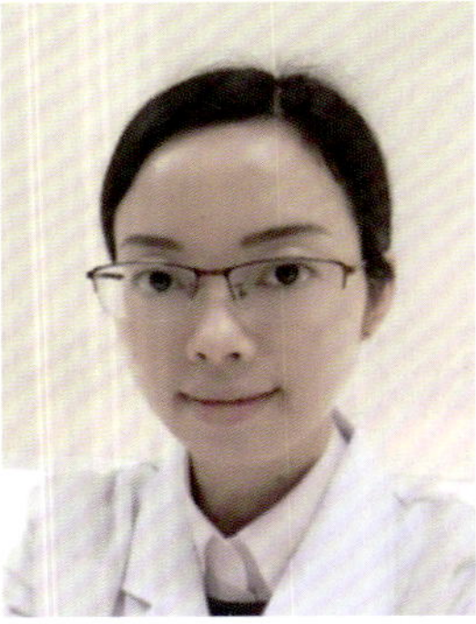

代秋楠，医学硕士，眼科主治医师、眼视光学教师。师从著名视光学专家王幼生教授，一直从事学生近视及儿童弱视的防治及视光学人才的培养工作。曾参与省教育厅工作课题“广东省中小学近视眼防控工作的对策性研究”的工作；曾在中山大学眼视光学系进修学习角膜塑形等接触镜技术，有丰富的视光教学工作经验及临床视光经验。专长于角膜塑形、RGP镜验配，视疲劳诊断、视功能分析和视觉训练。

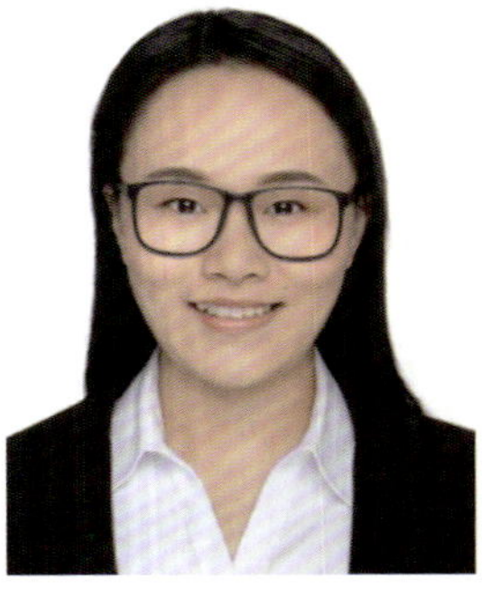

李易，主治医师，医学博士，就职于天津医科大学眼科医院，美国德克萨斯大学医学院访问学者。本科就读于中国医科大学临床医学专业。主要研究方向是眼科与视光学，硕博连读于中国医科大学。主要致力于青光眼视网膜神经节细胞凋亡机制及层粘连蛋白对视神经保护作用的研究。参与翻译多部眼科论著。

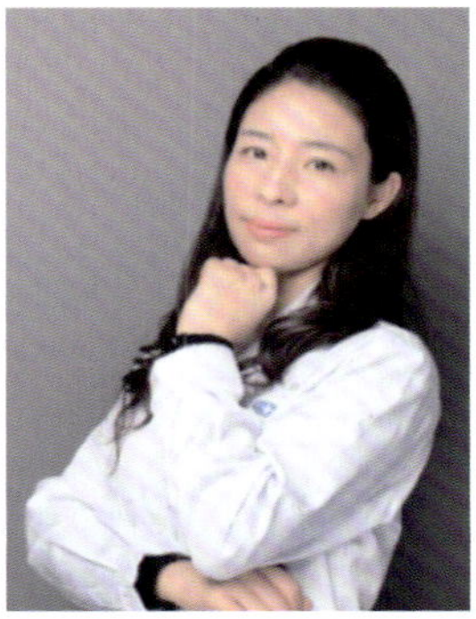

石蕊，眼科学副主任医师，副教授，在读博士。陕西省人民医院眼科教学秘书，陕西省保健协会防盲委员会委员，中华医学会陕西省眼科学会会员，《临床医学研究与实践杂志》编委、《国际眼科杂志》审稿专家。专业从事眼科临床、教学及科研工作10年，主要致力于玻璃体视网膜疾病、青少年近视防控的诊断和治疗。主持省级科研课题2项，参加国家自然科学基金1项及省市级科研项目5项，参编青少年近视相关论著4部。以第一作者身份发表文章14篇，其中3篇被SCI收录。

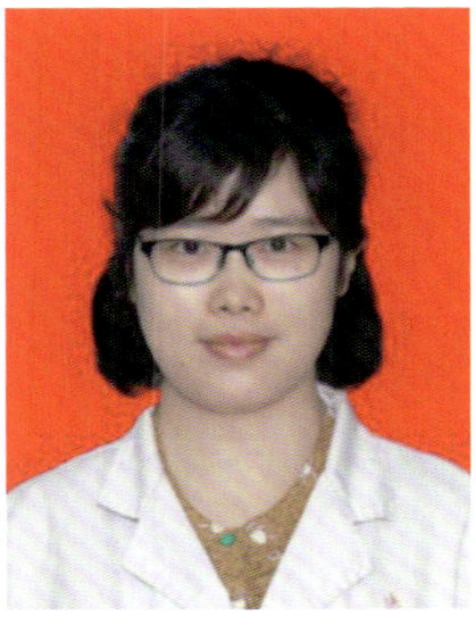

杨乐，2009年毕业于山东大学医学院，硕士，主治医师。擅长各类青光眼、白内障、眼底病及葡萄膜炎的诊断及治疗，尤其在糖尿病视网膜病变及多种视网膜病变的激光治疗方面积累了丰富的临床经验。主持并参与省级科研课题2项，在国内核心期刊发表科研论文10余篇。

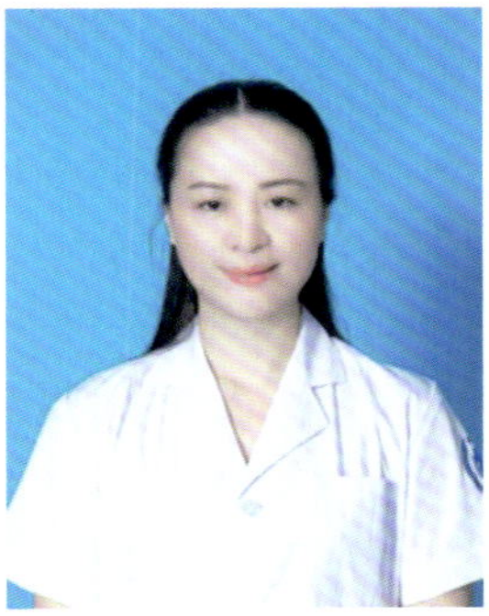

谭薇，医学博士，主任医师，教授，硕士生导师。遵义医学院第三临床学院副院长，遵义市第一人民医院眼科主任。中华医学会贵州省分会眼科学专委会常委，贵州省遵义市高级职称评审专家。从事眼科临床、教学、科研工作20余年，主要从事白内障和视光学的临床治疗和基础研究。擅长各种复杂、外伤、并发性白内障的手术治疗及角膜屈光手术。主持国家自然科学基金1项、省部级课题2项、地厅级课题3项，发表论文30余篇，其中被SCI收录5篇。

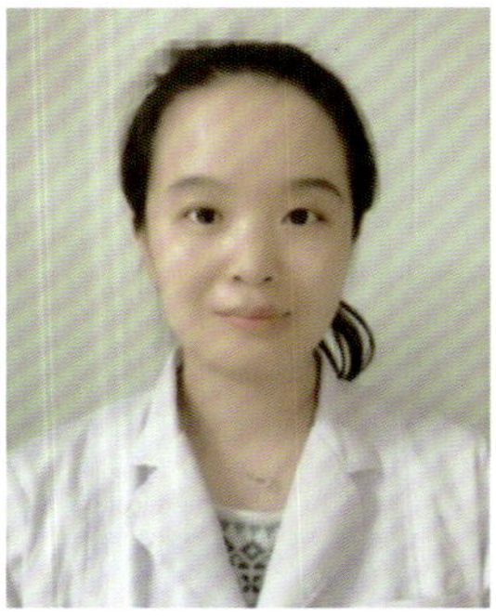

王涛，主治医师，中华医学会贵州省分会眼科学专委会委员。从事眼科临床、教学、科研工作 10 年，具有扎实的眼科专业理论知识和丰富的眼科临床诊疗经验。主要从事视光学和小儿眼科的临床治疗和基础研究。擅长各种小儿斜视手术及角膜屈光手术，在眼科常见病和疑难病的诊治方面具有丰富的临床经验。

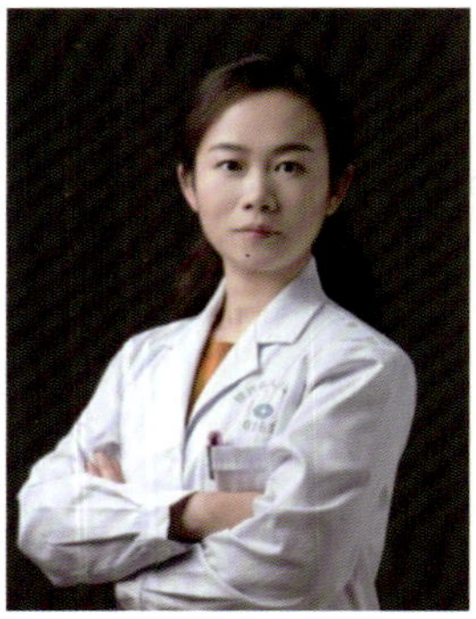

张乐，陕西省人民医院眼科副主任医师，医学博士。2014 年及 2018 年分别赴北京协和医院及天津眼科医院进修学习。国际角膜塑形术协会亚洲分会会员，陕西省保健协会青少年视力保健与视光学专业委员会委员，由英国格鲁斯特大学颁发“国际糖网阅片师”资格证书。主要专业方向为斜弱视及小儿眼科，儿童视觉发育及复杂眼底疾病的诊治。主持省厅级自然科学基金及社会发展基金 2 项，参与完成国家自然科学基金 3 项。发表 SCI 及中文核心期刊论文 10 余篇。

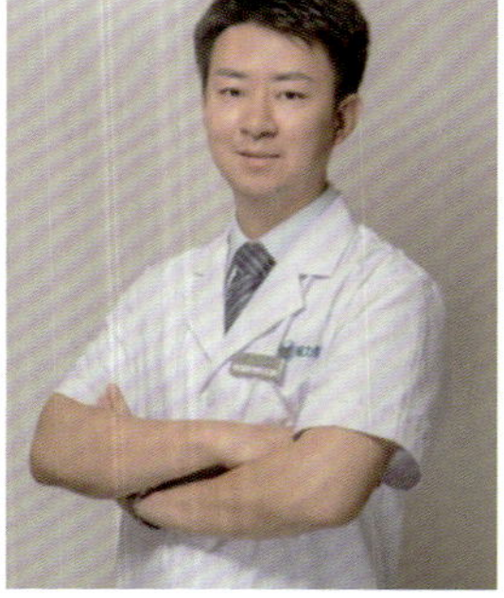

肖勇，国家高级（一级）技师，毕业于川北医学院眼视光学。曾先后就职于川北医学院附属医院眼科、成都精益眼镜有限公司，现任四川眼力健有限公司技术总监、成都眼力健眼科诊所视光主任。致力于近视防控、双眼视觉的研究工作。

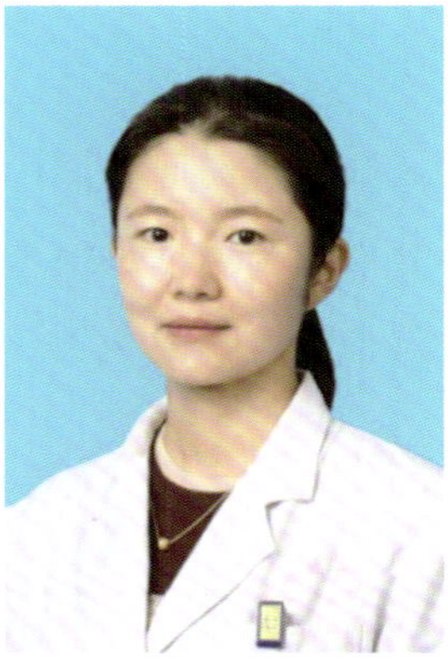

唐志萍，上海普瑞眼科医院，副主任医师，眼科学博士。现任云南省女医师协会眼科专业分会委员、上海非公医疗眼科分委会委员。从事眼科临床近20年，并对视网膜、视神经的损伤及保护进行了大量的研究工作。主持云南省科技厅自然科学基金面上项目、昆明医科大学创新基金项目，并参与多项国家自然基金的研究工作。2015年荣获云南省科技厅科技一等奖，2016年荣获云南省科技进步一等奖。主编人民卫生出版社出版书籍4部，参译书籍1部。在国内外期刊发表多篇文章。

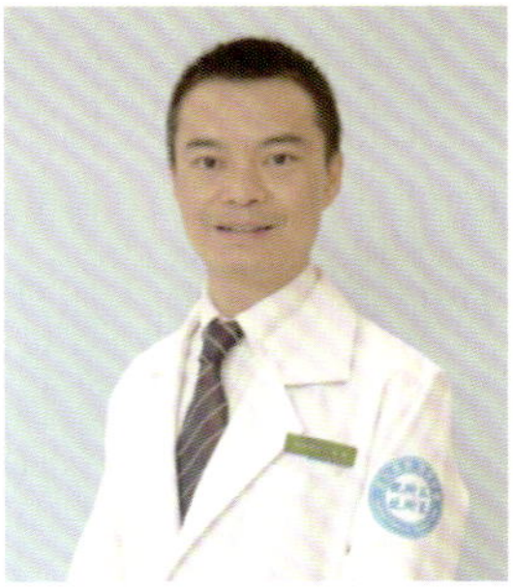

梅颖，上海新虹桥国际医学园区美视美景眼科中心业务院长，副主任医师，眼视光英才计划“明日之星”成员，中国妇幼保健协会儿童眼保健分会委员，上海眼视光学研究中心学术委员，中山眼科中心技术培训中心客座讲师，中国卫生信息与健康医疗大数据学会委员，《中国眼镜科技杂志》专栏作者。出版专著有《硬性接触镜验配案例图解》《硬性接触镜验配跟我学》等。

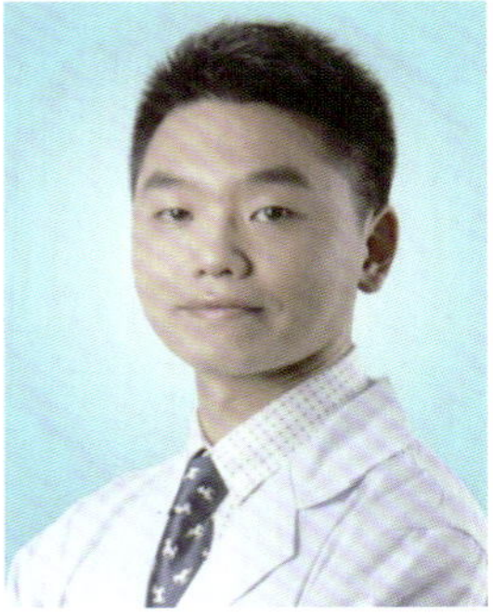

杨嘉嵩，师从河南省眼科研究所院长宋宗明教授、四川大学华西医院胡玉章教授。可熟练开展各类玻璃体视网膜手术、白内障手术。多次应邀在全国会议发言交流，在国内外发表多篇专业论文。创办杨嘉嵩眼底病工作室，服务于全国的眼科医师和患者。

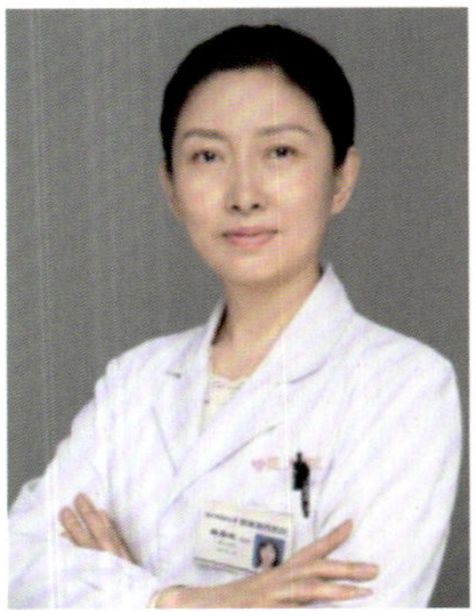

姚春艳，哈尔滨医科大学附属第四医院眼视光学门诊副主任，黑龙江省视光技术协会常务副会长兼秘书长，黑龙江省青少年学生近视眼防控指导中心指导组组长，哈尔滨城市职业学院眼视光学院教研室主任，教授，国家一级验光师。

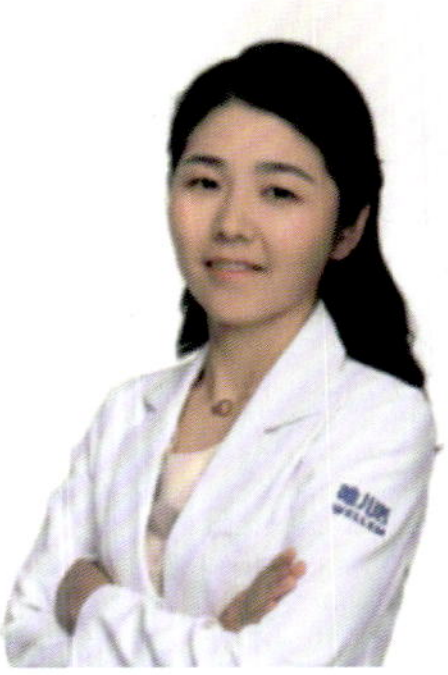

汪晓倩，硕士研究生，主治医师。上海唯宜儿科诊所副院长、唯儿诺眼视光负责人，江阴市中小学生近视眼防控中心主任，复旦大学眼科学硕士。专业方向为近视防控、斜弱视非手术治疗。师从褚仁远、瞿小妹教授，作为秘书协助褚仁远教授编写完成《眼病学》。

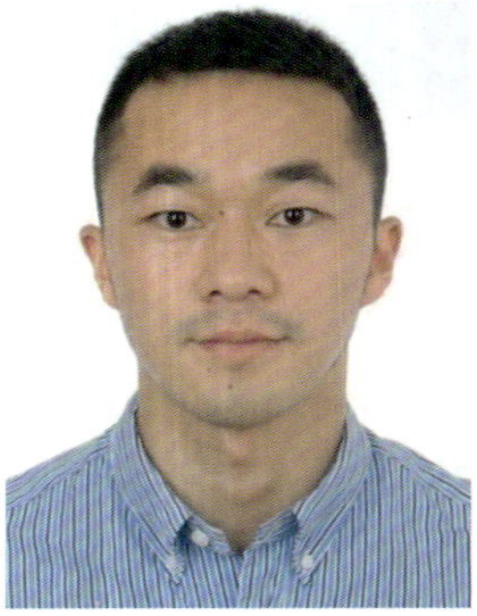

卢淑杰，江阴光明眼科医院主治医师。复旦大学眼科学硕士，师从瞿小妹教授，曾供职于复旦大学附属儿科医院。参与多项科研项目，完成了“视黄酸合成酶及核受体表达上调引发近视”的研究等。

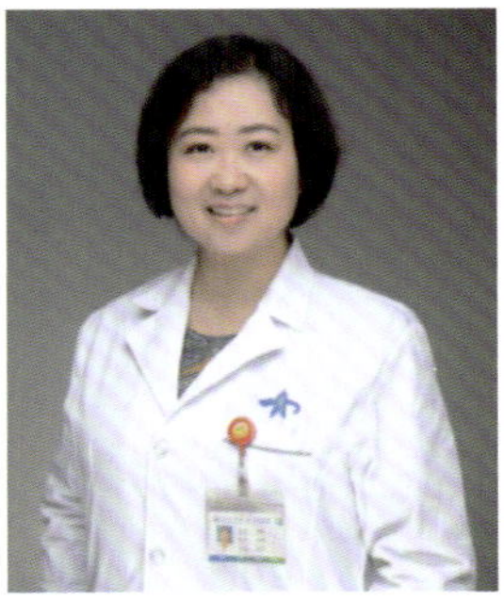

吴捷，眼科学博士，毕业于中山大学中山眼科中心。主要从事青少年近视眼防治、准分子激光屈光手术、硬性接触镜、角膜塑形镜和弱视等视光学方面研究。主持参与国家级、省市级、院校级科技攻关项目8项，发表SCI文章4篇、核心期刊文章8篇，开展“硬性接触镜及角膜塑形镜”新医疗新技术2项，获得发明专利1项。现为西安医学会第一届眼视光学分会常务委员，陕西省医学会眼科分会视光学与屈光手术学组委员，陕西省医学会激光医学分会青年委员，陕西省保健协会青少年视力保健与视光学专业委员会常务委员，国际角膜塑形学会（FIAO）资深会员，国际角膜塑形学会亚洲分会（SIAOA）资深会员。

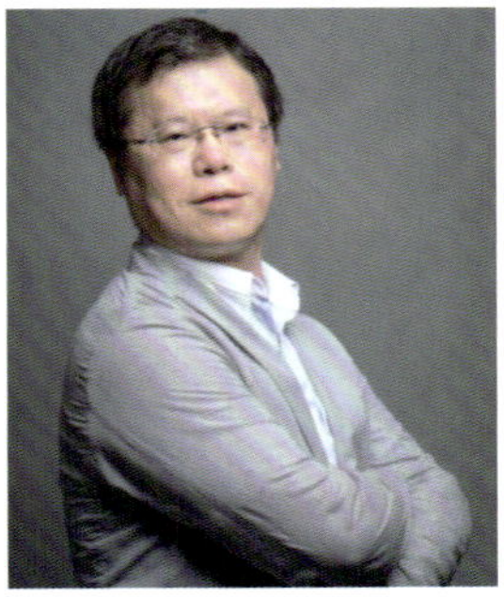

王文军，医学博士，儿童眼科专家，专治各类儿童斜弱视、屈光不正。特长为早产儿视网膜病变筛查、诊断及治疗，青少年近视防控。曾获得陕西省科技进步二等奖，主持省、市科技研究项目3项，参编专著2部，获得国家实用新型专利2项。西安医学院视光学专业特邀讲师。曾赴法国短期进修，参加国际眼科学术大会并就自研课题做大会发言。兼任国际角膜塑形镜学会亚洲分会资深会员，陕西省医学会新生儿分会早产儿学组委员，陕西省保健协会防盲专业委员会委员，陕西省妇幼保健与优生优育协会儿童眼保健专业委员会委员，西安医学会眼科学分会常委。

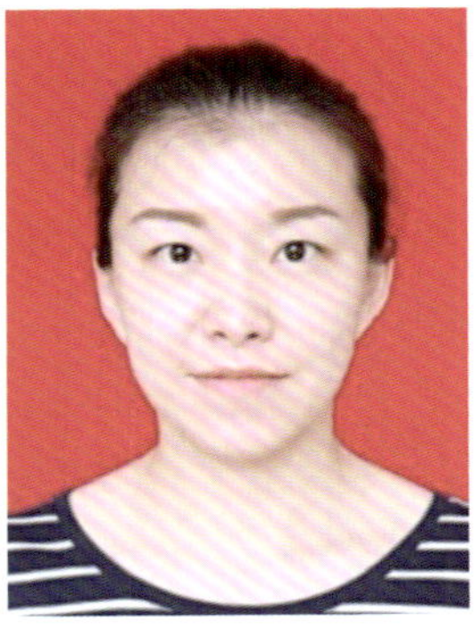

胡笳，本科毕业于四川大学华西临床医学院，硕士研究生毕业于西安交通大学医学院眼科学专业，师从石一宁教授。主要研究方向为家族性玻璃体淀粉样变性的临床及基因分析，以及近视的防治。现任职于西安交通大学第二附属医院眼科，主治医师。临床研究方向为玻璃体及视网膜病的激光及手术治疗。

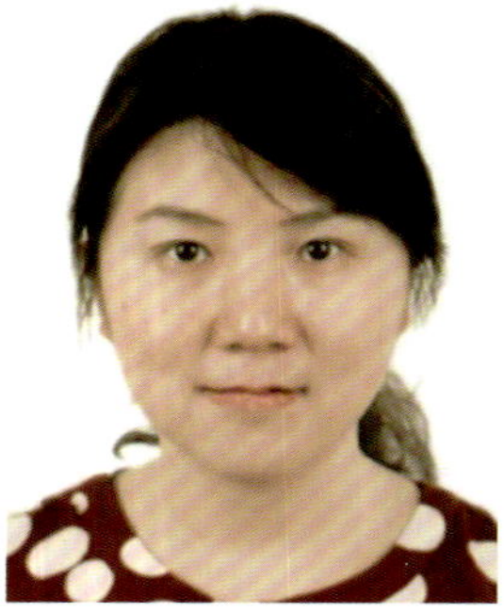

王西欧，2008 年毕业于澳大利亚悉尼大学斜弱视专业，在澳州从事斜弱视工作。2013 年回国。在陕西中医药大学仝警安教授的指导下于 2016 年获得中医眼科硕士学位。2017 年至今，在西安交通大学康前雁教授的指导下进行博士研究生的学习。

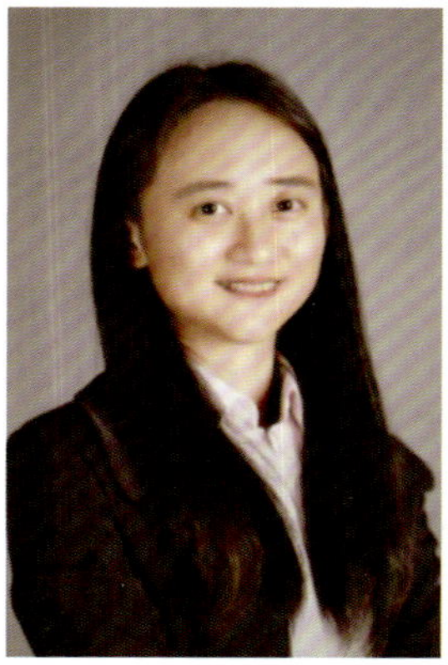

刘念，中山医科大学眼科视光学系首届毕业生，宾西法尼亚视光学院临床视光学硕士，全国验光与配镜职业教育教学指导委员会委员，中国视光学发展教育计划教师，全国高职高专教材评审委员会委员，全国中职教材评审委员会主任委员，广东省视光学会屈光专业委员会和低视力专业委员会常务委员，中山眼科培训中心客座讲师，IACLE 会员。现为广州市商贸职业学校眼视光与配镜专业带头人，高级讲师。主编全国中职“十二五”规划教材《验光技术》，主持全国中职眼视光与配镜专业教学标准的制定，负责全国中职专业目录的修订，主要研究“工作过程系统化一体化”课程的改革与开发。

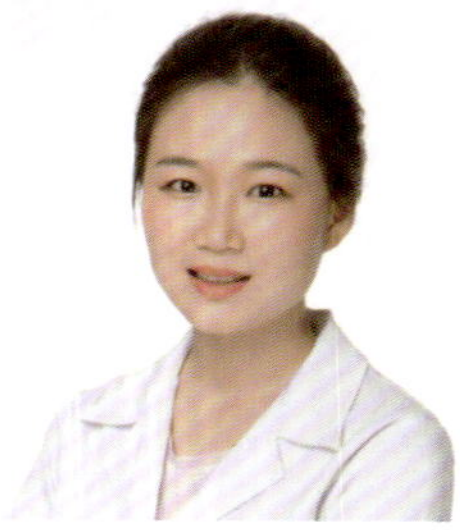

龚慧，中医眼科学硕士研究生。2017 年 6 月毕业于广州中医药大学，研究方向为眼视光学。目前工作于希玛林顺潮眼科医院。临床工作以小儿斜弱视、青少年近视防控、视功能训练为主。

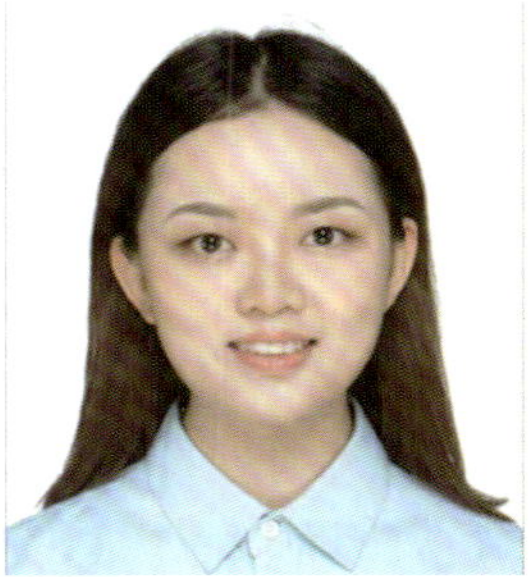

刘凤阳，就职于重庆医科大学附属第一医院。2018年四川大学眼视光学专业硕士毕业，发表SCI论文1篇。临床研究方向为近视、双眼视、接触镜。

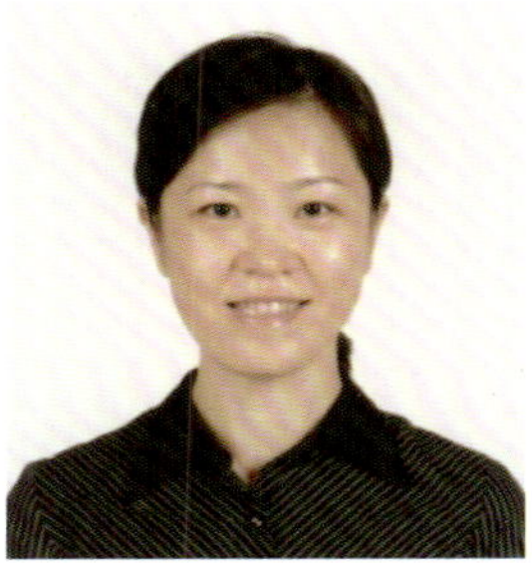

许军，眼科博士，副教授，副主任医师，硕士生导师。中国医科大学附属第四医院眼科视光中心主任。中华医学会眼科学分会眼视光学组委员，中国医师协会眼科医师分会眼视光学专业委员会委员，中国女医师协会视光学专委会委员，中国卫生信息与健康医疗大数据学会眼视光专业委员会委员；辽宁省医学会激光医学分会常委，辽宁省医学会眼科分会角膜病学组委员，辽宁省生命科学学会眼视光与屈光手术专业委员会副主任委员，辽宁省中小学生近视眼防控工作专家咨询委员会成员，美国加州大学伯克利分校访问学者。主持辽宁省科技厅课题3项、辽宁省教育厅课题1项、沈阳市科技计划项目4项，参与国家自然科学基金项目4项，获沈阳市科学技术进步三等奖1项。在国际及国内核心期刊发表相关论著30余篇。

审校组

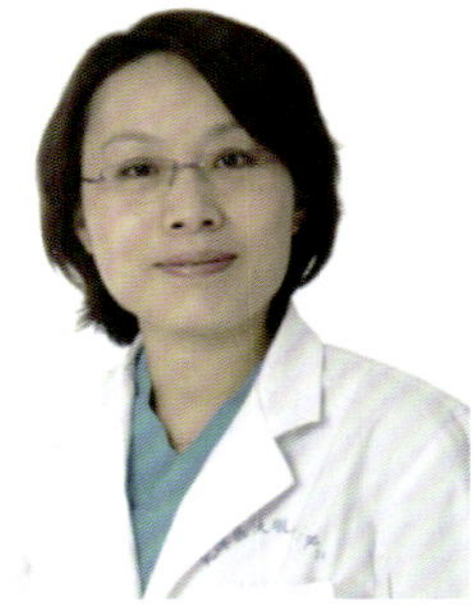

魏瑞华，教授，主任医师，医学博士，眼科学博、硕士生导师，眼视光学博硕士研究生导师。天津市“津门医学英才”人选，天津市高校“中青年骨干创新人才培养计划”人选，天津医科大学新世纪人才，中华医学会眼科学分会青年委员，中华医学会眼科学分会视光学组委员。从事眼科学工作 20 余年，擅长角膜病、屈光不正、白内障的诊治，致力于青少年近视防控和高度近视并发症诊治，同时擅长各种接触镜验配及并发症处理。

现任天津医科大学眼科医院和眼视光学院党委书记，同时承担天津医科大学眼视光学院的教学管理工作。参与完成多项国际课题，包括近视眼研究、屈光手术、角膜地形图研究、圆锥角膜研究、常见眼病流行病调查及干眼病研究。主持承担国家自然科学基金 2 项、天津市自然科学课题 1 项、天津市科技计划项目课题 2 项、天津市教委重点课题 2 项。发表专业论文 50 余篇，其中，以第一作者及通讯作者身份发表的论文被 SCI 收录 20 余篇。参编眼科论著 5 部。

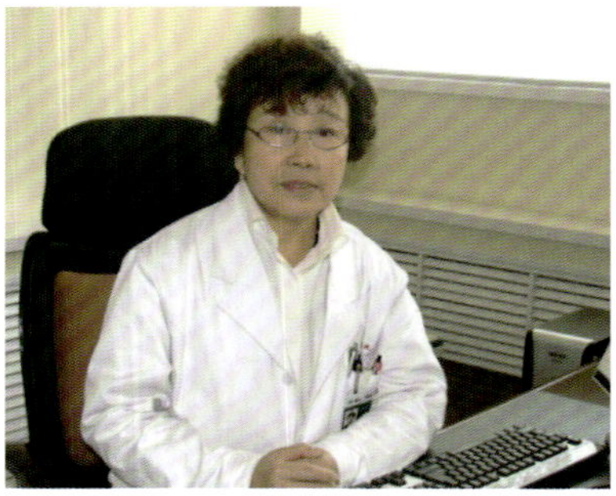

郑玲，哈医大四院眼视光门诊主任、教授、硕士生导师，全国角膜塑形镜安全监控联席会会员，全国卫生产业企业管理协会视光产业分会会员，黑龙江省视光技术协会会长，黑龙江省青少年近视防控指导中心领导小组主任，黑龙江省城市职业技术学院视光学院长，黑龙江医大四视光学职业培训学校校长。从事眼视光临床工作和小儿斜视弱视近 30 年。

1998 年创建了黑龙江省视光学中心； 1999 年申办了哈尔滨医科大学视光医学专业；2002 年创建了哈医大一院眼科医院；2006 年创建了哈医大四院视光门诊，组建了黑龙江医大四视光学职业培训学校；2008 年创建黑龙江省视光技术协会，最先将视光学理念引入黑龙江省。专注于准分子激光及有晶体眼人工晶体植入术（ICL 手术）、屈光不正眼的医学验光、渐进多焦点眼镜的医学验配、小儿斜视弱视的诊断治疗、圆锥角膜的诊断治疗、角膜塑形镜和高透氧性硬性接触镜（RGP）的医学验配等。

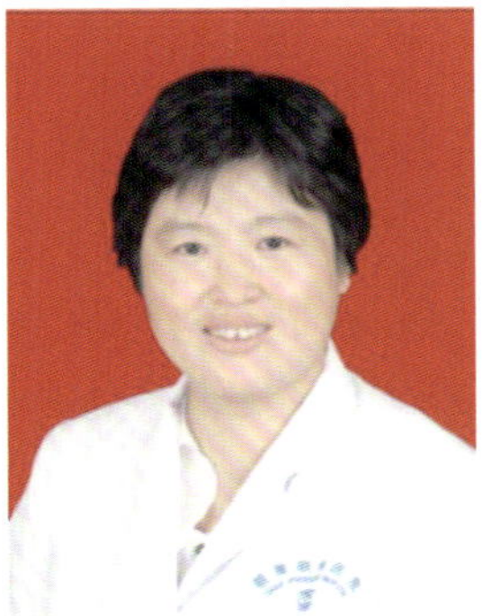

杨亚军，主任医师，朝聚眼科集团首席医务官。擅长角膜病、青光眼、白内障、眼内屈光手术。现任内蒙古自治区红十字眼角膜库主任、内蒙古医学会眼科专科分会委员，内蒙古医师协会眼科分会常委、非公医院协会眼科管理分会委员、中国研究型医院眼神经眼科学组委员。在中国科技核心期刊发表论文 10 余篇。为《超广角眼底照相图谱》一书的副主编，《OCT 血管造影》一书的译者。被评为“亚洲防盲协会白内障扶贫手术先进个人”。

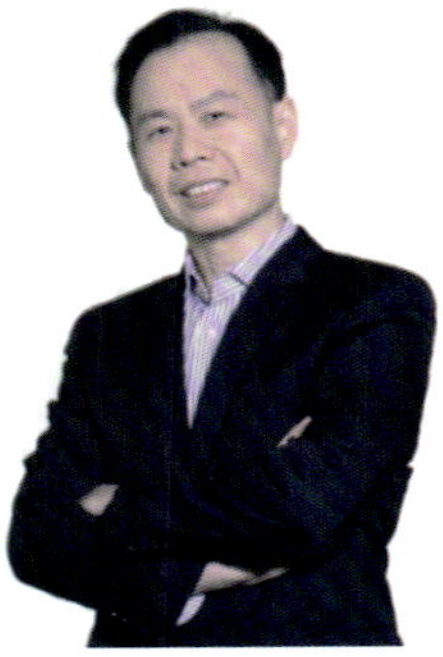

白继，教授，主任医师。全国著名眼视光及屈光手术专家，中华医学会激光医学分会委员兼任重庆市主任委员，《中华眼视光学与视觉科学杂志》等多个专科杂志编委。荣获国家科技进步二等奖、军队科技进步二等奖、国家教育教学大奖赛一等奖、国家级精品视频公开课优质课程奖、中国人民解放军育才银奖。

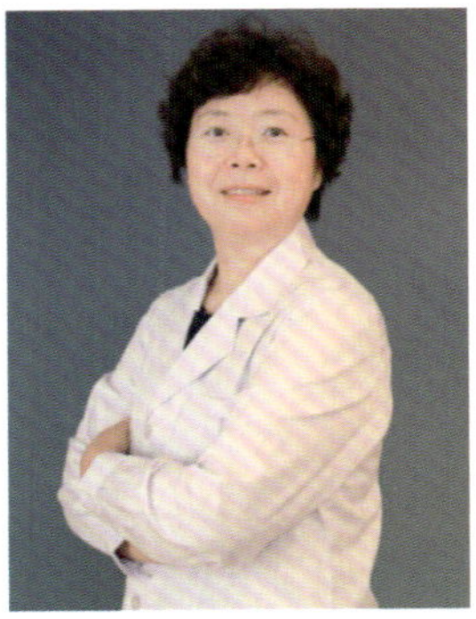

朱丹，内蒙古医科大学附属医院眼科主任，教授、主任医师，硕士生导师。擅长眼底病诊治，精于复杂白内障手术，开展玻璃体视网膜手术 10 年，年手术量为 200~300 台。先后在北京大学第一医院攻读硕士学位，在北京大学人民医院攻读博士学位。美国 TUFTS 大学医学院博士后，日本山梨大学医学院访问学者。任中华医学会眼科分会第十届、第十一届、第十二届全国委员，眼底病学组委员，中国医师协会眼科学分会常委；内蒙古自治区眼科质量控制中心主任，内蒙古自治区防盲指导组组长。内蒙古医学会眼科学会第十届、第十一届、第十二届主任委员。内蒙古医师协会眼科学分会第一届会长。任《中华眼科杂志》通讯编委，《中华眼底病杂志》《中华实验眼科杂志》《中华眼外伤职业眼病杂志》《中华眼科医学杂志》编委。承担国家自然科学基金项目 2 项，国家精准医学重大项目子课题 1 项，省部级科研项目 7 项。近 3 年发表 SCI 论文 9 篇，参编眼科学教材 3 部。为“中华医学会奖”“草原英才”获得者。

专业总审校

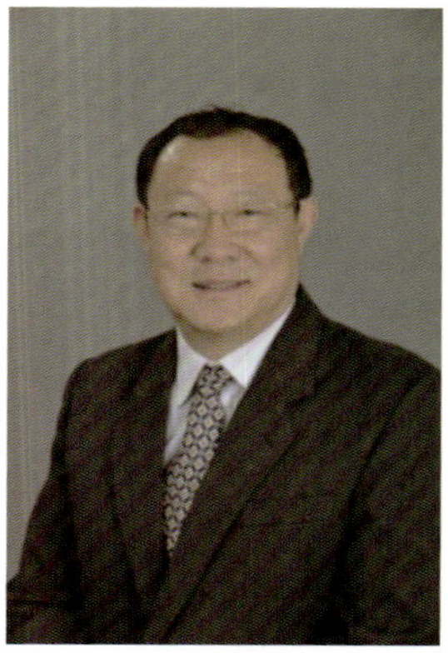

高祥璐，天津医科大学教授。退休前为天津医科大学眼视光学院硕士生导师，眼视光教研室主任。1990 年开始参与天津医学院早稻田眼镜专门学校暨天津医科大学眼验光制镜专业的组建工作；1991 年建立学校和专业后，开始从事眼视光教学和教学管理工作至退休。先后承担“眼应用光学”等多门课程的教学工作。近 3 年，任“十三五”规划教材《眼镜学》和《渐变焦眼镜验配技巧》的副主编，以通讯作者身份指导研究生发表论文 5 篇。

名誉主审

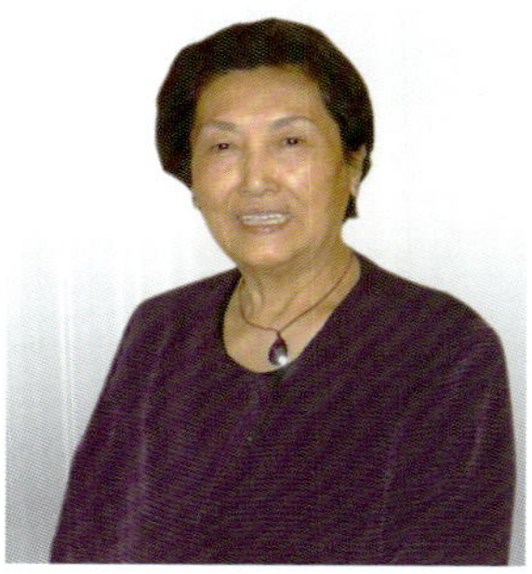

石广礼，眼科主任医师。1953 年毕业于西北医学院，从事医疗、教学、科研工作已 56 年。曾任第四届、第五届及第六届中华医学会眼科学会常务委员，陕西医学会理事，陕西医学会眼科学会主任委员。20 世纪 80 年代初，率先在国内开展儿童弱视研究，提出分娩产式对弱视的作用观点，并研制红闪增视仪、光刷治疗仪及实体镜，制定了儿童弱视治疗的三部曲，研发接触镜，均获省、市科技成果奖。1972 年举办眼科医生培训班，亲自编辑眼科学教材，撰写眼科科普书籍 10 本；发表论文 70 余篇，其中获国内、省、市图书论文奖 12 项。对儿童弱视治疗有丰富经验，疗程短、治愈率高；对眼底病、近视眼底病变及顽固性角膜炎、干眼等主张联合中药治疗；对显微青光眼减压术、斜视矫正术及眼部美容手术等有独特方法。作为“刘石氏饮”的研发人，数十年来，与刘光汉、石一宁一起研发可用于临床的中药散剂，探讨出中药治疗眼底病及近视眼底改变的治疗组方，与陈卓、陈研明一起研发出无添加辅料的药食同源的中药新剂型。

英文总审校

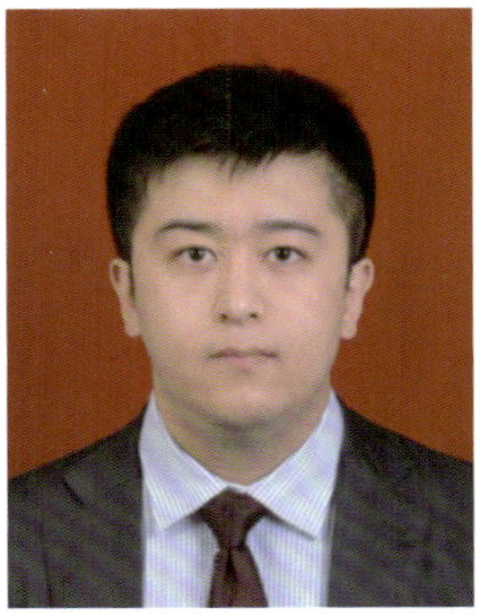

陈研明，2012 年毕业于西安交通大学医学院，2015 年毕业于中国医科大学眼科学研究院。2015 年作为美国纽黑文耶鲁大学医学院视觉科学交流访问学者进行临床研究至今，主要研究青光眼的分子和细胞学发病机制（视神经损伤机制、遗传学机制），以及视盘星形胶质细胞蛋白组学分析。参与了 5 项省级自然基金项目的研究。发表论文 11 篇，参与 4 部专著的撰写及翻译。

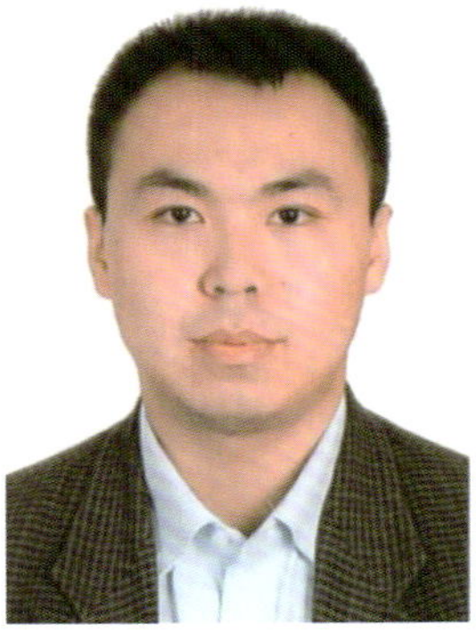

陈卓，副教授，西安医学院药物化学教研室主任。2010 年毕业于四川大学华西药学院药物化学专业。为药学专业学生主讲“药物化学”课程，并新开设了“药物合成工艺学”与“药物设计学”2 门课程。主要从事眼科新药的开发研究及药物合成工艺研究，主持完成多项自然科学基础研究项目。在头孢类抗生素关键侧链及天然活性产物辛弗林的合成工艺开发中，获得了具有突出市场价值的药物合成工艺。在抗翼状胬肉药物的研究中，获得的系列新颖化合物表现出良好的翼状胬肉抑制活性及相对现有药物较低的毒性。

主译主审

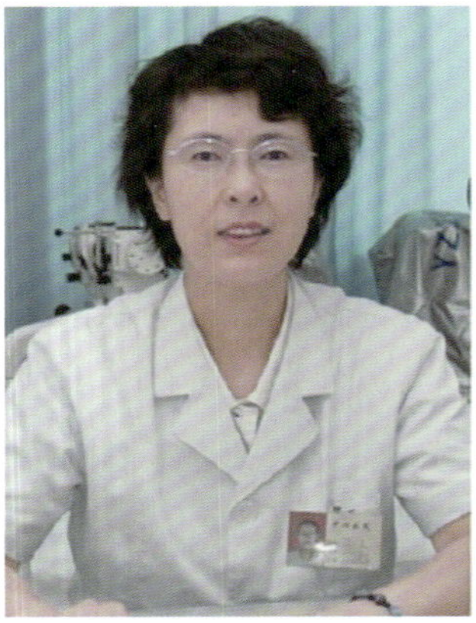

石一宁，西安交通大学硕士生导师。陕西省有突出贡献专家，享受国务院特殊津贴专家，第十届、第十一届、第十二届政协西安市常委。40 多年来，一直从事眼科临床、科研及教学工作。20 多年来，主要在儿童青少年近视的预测预警防控和高度近视及其严重并发症的防治 2 个方面进行了深入研究，并致力于中国近视防控的科普宣传。提出了中国儿童青少年近视形成机制的再认知——学前 3~6 岁的过度正视化过程的“二次发育理论”，以及眼球过长的“眼内扩张理论”；近视控制关键点；近视早发现、早控制、早治疗的创新性概念——“隐性近视”；量化描述近视常见眼底改变，建立了临床上简易可行的眼底观察指标；根据眼生物参数，提出了进展预测系统和预警机制（眼健康的三级监测和近视防控的三级预警），并提出要建立七级眼健康档案和及时发布中国眼健康年度蓝皮书；提出一揽子计划——近视防控体系：①近视的连续性防控思想；②近视的个性化防控设计；③近视的综合性防控理念。

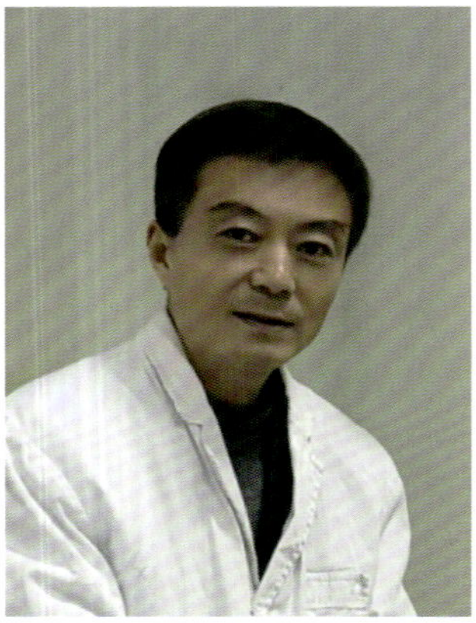

方严，安徽理工大学第一附属医院、第一临床学院名誉院长，安徽理工大学眼科研究所所长、研究员、教授，淮南市第一人民医院眼科主任、主任医师，为安徽医科大学主办的《临床眼科杂志》的执行主编，研究生导师。安徽省眼科学会主任委员，中华医学会眼科学分会青光眼学组委员，中国医师协会眼科医师分会委员。第十四届“九三学社”中央委员。主编《病理性近视眼眼底改变》(国家科学技术学术著作出版基金资助)等学术专著8部。曾获“中华眼科学会奖”，曾被评为“中国职业教育先进个人”。

序一

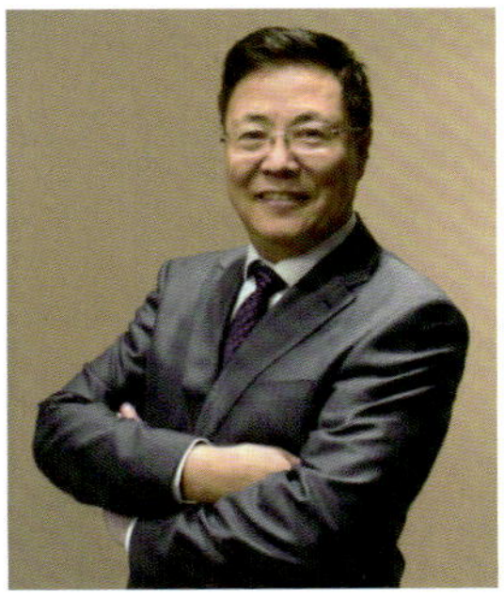

从生物学角度看，眼睛是人体诸多器官之一；从视觉科学角度看，眼睛又是以光作为适宜刺激的视觉光学器官。人类获得视觉信息的重要前提是外界物体反射的光线经过眼的屈光系统后成像在视网膜上。眼睛屈光系统的构造如同精密的光学仪器，同样包含着复杂的光学原理，屈光系统中的任何成分出现问题都有可能影响视力。

临床中，眼的光学系统出现问题可能会引发诸多眼疾，如近视、远视、散光等。目前近视已成为影响我国儿童青少年眼健康的重要公共卫生问题，调查显示，2018 年全国儿童青少年的总体近视率已达 53.5%。而屈光不正的矫正也直接依赖光学设计，如框架眼镜片、接触镜等。临床上许多眼科诊疗中的问题及其解决，也涉及眼球的光学特性，如白内障人工晶状体厚度的计算、准分子激光矫治屈光不正的角膜切削厚度等。因此，作为视光师和临床眼科医师，学习和掌握临床光学的知识，将为更好地开展眼科临床和研究工作打下基础。

鉴于眼的光学系统问题相关的眼疾趋于增多，就非常需要出版一本包括光学基础知识及从光学角度出发讲解其临床矫治方式的专著，以加强视光师的培养，指导临床医师从光学系统的角度进行相关眼科疾病的诊治。

石一宁教授组织翻译的这本《临床光学》是由美国眼科学会（AAO）编写的视光教材，内容涵盖广，包含从基础光学知识到临床眼科中所能遇到的光学、屈光以及接触镜、人工晶体、屈光手术等各类问题，这将极大促进我国视光师和眼科医师获得系统的眼科临床光学知识。同时，此书作为国际眼科医师考试（ICO）必考的视光教材，一直没有中文版，此译作将为我国视光师和眼科医师参加考试带来极大的帮助和指导。更难能可贵的是这本《临床光学》采用中英双语对照的形式进行排版，这不仅可以使读者学习其中的临床光学知识，还有助于其专业英语水平的提高，为拓展更多的相关英文专著的学习及以后参与国际学术交流打下坚实的基础。

国内众多的教授和视光学学者参与了本书的翻译和审校工作。从开始翻译到最终出版历时半年有余，经过反复的打磨，保证了准确、原汁原味地翻译出这本国际通用视光教材，相信这本译作的出版会对我国视光学教育及视光学的发展起到积极的推动作用。

在此对译作的顺利出版，表示衷心的祝贺。

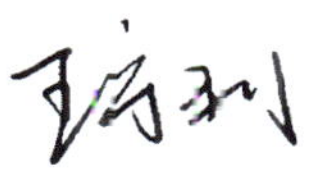

北京同仁医院眼科中心主任，全国防盲技术指导组组长

2019 年 5 月 22 日于北京

序二

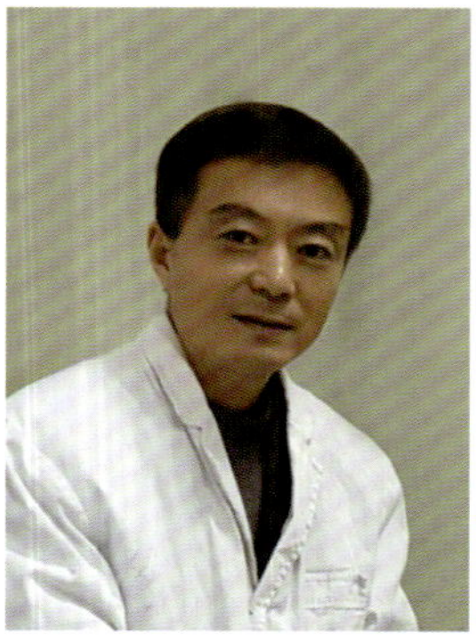

视光学是现代光学技术和现代眼科学两大学科的有机整合，是运用现代光学的原理和技术解决视觉障碍的新兴交叉学科，是一类隶属于医学科学范畴、实践性强的应用型医疗职业。

视光学专业技能的培养既需要有扎实的医学相关专业知识及光学专业知识，也要有良好的人际交流能力，可通过学习视光学的基础理论、基本知识，来掌握眼科学、视光学理论知识及眼病诊断、预防与治疗的基本技能。视光学专业在我国具有非常广阔的服务市场和发展前景。

由于历史的原因，我国视光学发展起步较晚。目前国内已有数十家医学院校开展了视光学医学高等教育。在视光学专业人才培养方面，除了要让学生学习基础学眼科学，尤其要求学生在视光学专业方面要具有较全面的专业知识和实践能力。因此，对视光学专业的教材编写与教程设计安排显得十分重要。

我和石一宁教授前 10 年主要从事儿童青少年近视的流行病学、发病机制及近视防控等方面的探索和研究，现在由衷地感到视光学专业人才的教育和培养的意义更加重大，中国需要更多合格的视光学医师服务于社会。

此书的意义在于以下三个方面：第一，“2018–2019 基础与临床科学教程”《临床光学》一书由美国眼科学会（AAO）编写。国际眼科联盟（WOC）推荐全世界的眼科医生参加国际眼科医师考试（ICO），其中必考的视光教材就是我们组织翻译出版的这本书。第二，此书还是国家医学考试 ICO 考试点的第二步必考科目和必考书，一直没有中文版。此次的翻译将对中国眼科医生和视光医生的培训有很大的帮助。第三，尤为重要的是，我们一直在做健康快车中国眼科医生的国际化培训，期待更多的年轻医生走向世界，希望中国眼科医生和视光医生能够阅读到原版国际眼科医生培养的基础教材，在这本翻译版中保留了英文原文，以提升读者的专业英语水平，有助于读者进行国际交流。这次在陕西科学技术出版社进行校版，希望这本书能够成为国内眼科学及视光学专业培养学生的参考书。

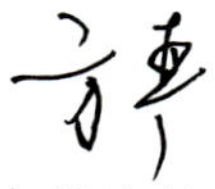

安徽理工大学第一附属医院、第一临床学院名誉院长

2019 年 1 月 1 日

序三

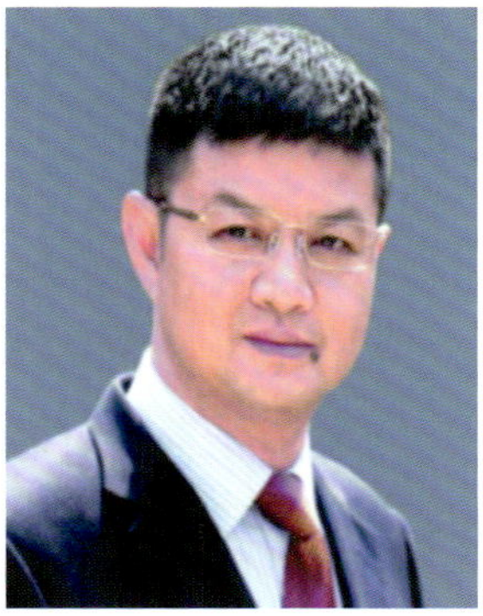

如今，在获取爆炸的信息量的同时，我们的视觉系统也面临着越来越大的压力，甚至连我们的视觉健康也受到了威胁。面对如此严峻的形势，国际考核中对眼科医生的要求也不断提升，眼科医生的责任从眼部疾患的诊治过渡到视觉健康的维护，从单纯的看得见走向看得更清晰、更舒适、更持久。

他山之石，可以攻玉。美国眼科学会的《临床光学》教材从光线的传播、单透镜的折射、多透镜组合成像过程，可见光的定义、光的波粒二重性、量子电力学等几何光学、物理光学基础出发，讲授人类眼球光学基础，进而对眼球的光学缺陷的问题、检查和处理进行讲解。该教材结合临床实践，延伸至多学科融合的临床光学内容，指导我们在临床中更好地理解视觉成像；为眼科医师在惯有思路中开辟和注入更丰富的内容，使得眼健康保障从单纯的临床方案拓展至更佳的光学方案；也为视光师解决了临床的困惑，使他们能够从单一而机械的验配检查思路中跳脱出来，结合患者需求与临床状况灵活应对。通过这样的综合学习模式，通过翻译和传播国际上的教学经验，将眼科人的视野拓宽到了更广阔的层级。在当今时代下，每一个眼科人都应该与国际接轨、与人文接轨，从单纯解决患者眼部疾患提升到为患者提供更加清晰舒适的视觉体验。

我们要披荆斩棘、砥砺前行。与美国等国家将视光教育体系与眼科医生培养体系明确区分不同，我国在发展过程中形成了较为复杂和多样的学科交叉的新局面。眼科医生在本身的临床工作基础上，需要掌握系统的视光学知识，结合患者病情，使其更好地提升视觉成像质量；视光医生在其本职工作经验的基础上，同样需要结合临床，帮助患者解决视觉问题。当前，我国近视率居高不下，青少年近视率更是控制不力，总体公共视觉健康任务繁重。学习本书可以为多元学科融合、个人综合发展，以及更快更好地解决我国乃至世界眼健康问题提供有力的帮助。

尽管我国对于眼科学术方面的探索从未停止，但很多亚学科却止步于传统眼科。虽然眼科学中的视光学教育在我国仍处于起步阶段，但正如一轮新升起的朝阳，在我们不断摸索和发展过程中，照亮了前进的路途。视光学的理论和实践基础都是眼科新发展中的最重要的支撑和辅助，其中本书后面的章节提到了视觉重建，正是目前眼科追求的新方向，我们的目光不能止步于解决眼部病变，单纯关注视力（高对比度下），而是要通过更多的新思路、新方法提升视觉质量乃至重建视觉。江山代有才人出，才要登高，方能望远！谨愿此书为更多放眼国际、放眼未来的眼科人提供最好的帮助和指导，也愿每一个视觉健康的捍卫者为我们视觉的未来点亮一份光明。

刘陇黔

四川大学华西临床医学院眼视光学系主任兼眼科副主任

2018 年 12 月 31 日

序四

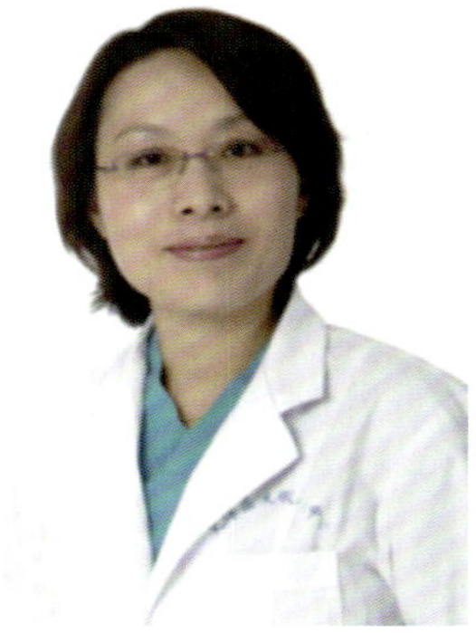

在中国改革开放 40 年之际，华西医科大学视光专业紧随改革开放的脚步孕育而生。天津医科大学、温州医科大学、原中山医科大学分别在 20 世纪 90 年代先后开展了眼视光专业的高等教育，至今已近 30 年。随着我国经济发展及国民生活水平的提高，人民对基础眼保健服务的需求日益增加，触动和引领着视光行业的蓬勃发展。同时，我国儿童青少年近视发病率迅猛增加，也警醒着所有的医护人员，要不断提升眼视光专业水平，提高社区和临床服务水平，加强研究的深度和广度。

光学是眼科学和视光学的一门主要的基础课，是眼科学和视光学学习的根基，但是单纯的光学知识并不能满足视光的专业需求。我在对于视光学本科生及研究生的教学工作中发现，很多视光专业的学生认为光学课程的内容过于公式化，不容易在临床中找到相应的应用，从而不能很好地在学习和工作中理解光学、应用光学、研究光学。而本书从几何光学和物理光学入手，结合人视光学与眼科临床中光学部分的应用，系统地剖析视光学中的“光学”特点，梳理逻辑，找到眼视光临床应用中光学的切入点，如人工晶体、接触镜、视觉质量等，深入地分析与解读光学，使读者能够切实感受到学可以致用。

本书的英文原版已经在国际上得以广泛的认可、使用，被作为国际眼科理事会（WOC）国际眼科医师考试推荐用书，也成为中国国家医学考试中心承担的国际眼科医师相关考核的推荐用书。国际眼科医师考试是由国际认可、国家认可的，在旨在推动我国眼科的视光学继续教育及临床应用的重要考试——ICO 考试中，试卷使用英文原版，但为了满足基层医生的需求，现已将基础和视光 2 部分中所有的试题配上中文翻译，而目前所有的复习资料均为英文版本，语言的差异给基层的眼科医生及视光医生带来了极大的不便。本书的翻译和解读，为国内眼科医生和视光医生提供了更多的有利于临床工作的知识，也为眼科和视光的学生以及从业人员的专业学习及临床工作提供了有力的帮助。

随着社会对初级眼保健需求的增长，视光医生的需求也将是巨大的，相信眼视光的未来是光明的，这是一个甜蜜的“负担”。社会对视光服务需要不断加大的同时，对我们业务水平的要求也在不断地提升，激励着所有从业人员时刻保持满腔热情，对社会有担当、对知识有渴望、对科研有钻研。希望通过石一宁教授等专家和团队的力量，集全球的精华，汇聚成中国的语言、中国的模式，发展我们中国的眼科与视光行业，推动我们中国的基础眼健康保健事业不断发展。

魏瑞华

天津医科大学眼科医院和眼视光学院党委书记

2019 年 1 月 2 日

序五

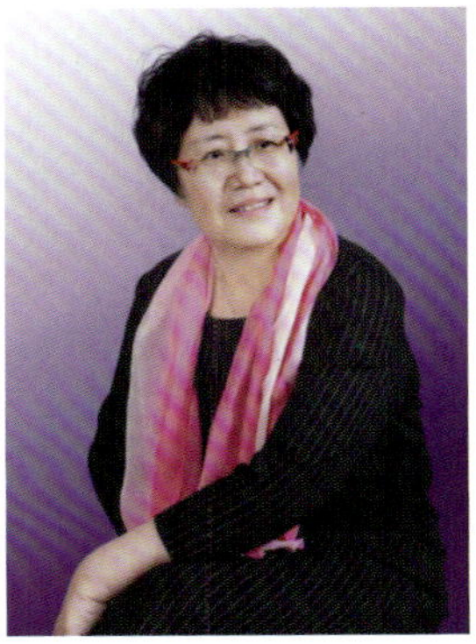

2018 年 9 月 3 日，国家卫生健康委员会在北京召开了儿童青少年近视防治有关工作会议，会议列出了医疗机构内设视光中心的标准和规范、2018 年我国近视情况基线调查、眼健康档案的建设和细则、眼健康科普知识的标准化及规范化（科普书等）、协助学校设置眼保健课程的方案（内容、课时等）、视光师的培养及培训方案等主要工作重点。我国的眼视光学体系有待完善。

国际眼科联盟（International Council of Ophthalmology，ICO）是代表和服务于世界范围内眼科专业协会的国际组织。ICO 的主要任务是将眼科组织及相关机构联合起来，加强教育，共同改善高质量眼保健工作，以达到世界范围内最大限度地保护视力、维持现有视力状态、提高视力的目标，共促眼健康。国际眼科医师考试（International Basic Science and Clinical Sciences Assessment for Ophthalmologists）是中华医学会眼科分会和国家医学考试中心于 2005 年引进的一项国际性的考试，是由 ICO 统一组织，可用于眼科住院医师的培养，并对考生本人提供他们是否获得世界统一标准的眼科知识的评价。国际眼科联盟 WOC 和中国医学考试网都推荐参加考试，这是中国眼科医师融入国际化的途径之一。临床光学是 ICO 考试点的第二步必考科目必考书，教材一直没有中文版。

与石一宁教授相识 20 多年，她在甘肃省开展玻璃体视网膜手术时给予过我们很多的帮助和支持，一直是我的良师益友。多年来我们一起有感于近视的高发、高度近视并发症的危害，痛惜面对许多患者时的束手无策。2008 年我们又一起开始做健康快车中国眼科医生的国际化培训。令人敬佩的是她作为主任医师参加 ICO 考试的坚定和执着，她是我们学习的榜样！10 多年前她利用著书、讲学、研究、网络、开设工作室等多种形式，踏上了专职防控近视之路。2018 年 12 月，我作为国家近视防控组专家成员，参加国家卫健委组织的近视基线调查抽查工作，与石一宁教授有了为时 1 周的深层次交流。我们为近视防控春天的到来欢呼不已，相互交流，一起为有效落实近视防控献计献策。了解到她在翻译 ICO 视光学教材《临床光学》一书，欣然接受了为这本书作序的邀请。因为我们一直在期待更多的年轻医生走向世界，希望这本书能够作为我们视光学专业学生的参考书，对中国眼科医生和视光中心提供帮助。更重要的是，希望中国的眼科医生和视光医生能够看到原版的国际眼科医生培养基础教材，同时，通过阅读原文，提升专业英语水平，以便日后进行国际交流。

由陕西科学技术出版社出版的《临床光学》（双语版）是非常实用的双语教材，必将对我国视光学科发展起到积极的推动作用。衷心希望《临床光学》（双语版）的出版取得圆满成功！

兰州大学第二医院副院长

2018 年 12 月 31 日于兰州

序六

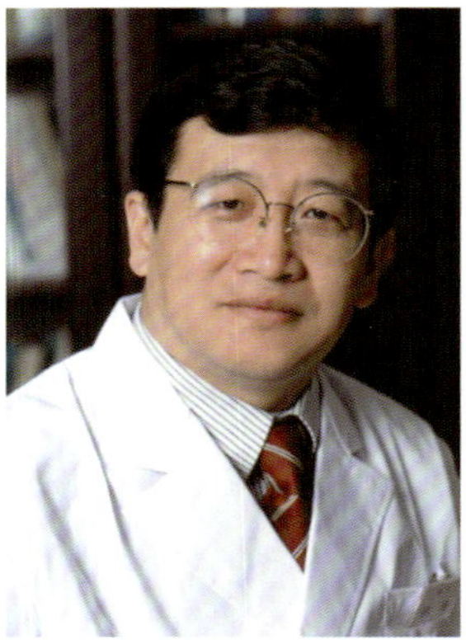

中国拥有世界上最多的眼病患者和眼部亚健康人群，但中国的眼健康医疗资源却严重不足，尤其是眼科医生和视光医生严重缺乏。其中，视光医生的缺乏主要因为我国医学院校中视光学专业起步与发展都比较晚，到目前为止，在现有的眼科教育体系中，眼视光的相关知识依然欠缺严重。

视光学是眼科诊疗工作的起点，对每一位眼病患者的筛查都是从基础的视力检查开始的；同时视光学也是眼科诊疗工作的终点，眼科诊疗不仅包含药物和手术治疗，还包括视觉功能康复训练、屈光不正的矫正及功能性眼病的诊疗。当前我国的青少年近视防控工作和老年视觉康复保健工作，更是要求眼科医生掌握全面系统的视光学知识体系。

从某种程度上来说，一本好的视光学教育类图书，可以推进中国专业视光人才培养的标准化，有利于推进青少年眼健康事业的发展。我作为一位从事眼科诊疗工作 30 余年的医生，很欣慰能看到美国眼科学会（AAO）的“基础与临床科学教程 ”BCSC 第 3 册 *Clinical Optics* 的译作《临床光学》的出版。

作为视光教学参考书籍，本书填补了中国视光学教科书的空白，它的出版对国内视光教育教学将起到积极的推动作用，为中国未来眼科和视光教学注入新鲜血液。

一部眼科学，半部屈光史。作为国际眼科医师考试（ICO）必考科目的指定教材，本书从视光理论知识和临床实践需求的角度，详尽介绍了眼科医生必须掌握的知识要点。内容涵盖了精准物理光学、几何光学、生物光学器官、眼科仪器设备设计、眼科手术材料设计等相关知识，为眼科医生提供了完整的视光学知识架构，填补了国内眼科医生的视光系统学习空白。

采用中英文对照的形式是本书的一大亮点，它使国内的视光专用词汇更加规范化。相信系统学习本书，将对未来眼科国际学术交流大有帮助。

我相信在这本书的帮助下，会有更多的有国际视角的视光人才与我们携手未来，共同推进中国视光学的发展。

何伟

辽宁何氏医学院院长，何氏眼科医院院长

2018 年 12 月 18 日于沈阳

序七

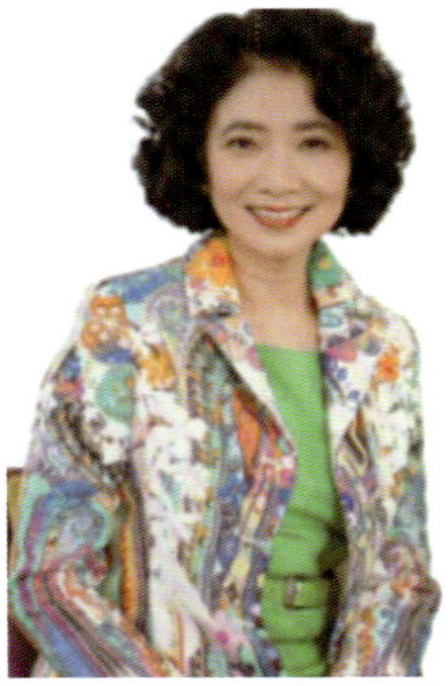

本书是美国眼科学会（AAO）的教材之一，同时也是国际眼科医师（ICO）视光学和器械学考试部分的参考书之一。2009年，“健康快车”引入ICO考试的中文试卷，使英文欠佳的医生也可以参加这一国际考试。然而，由于考试的所有参考书目均为英文版，国内医生普遍反映备考存在很大的困难。本书的中文翻译出版对视光学和器械学考生们来说无疑是一个大好消息。阅读本书，中国的眼科医生不仅能阅读基础教材的原文，提升专业英文水平，更能看到翻译版的内容，从而增进知识。感谢石一宁教授的倾力翻译。

自1997年成立以来，“健康快车”一直致力于中国内地的扶贫治盲及眼科医生的培训工作。石一宁教授曾担任“健康快车”陕西西安眼科中心（陕西省人民医院眼科）主任，且一直热心于眼科医生的培训与相关知识技能的分享，“健康快车”对石一宁教授深存敬意。

方黄吉雯
中华健康快车创会主席
2018年12月31日

序八

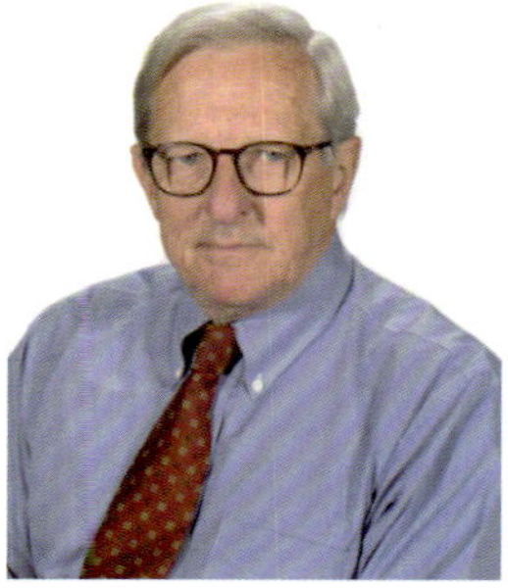

This book is a brilliant concept! The original book in English is a classic and it is wonderful that Prof Shi Yining has created this bilingual version which is not just translated from English to Chinese but it has the two languages side-by-side: English on the left and Chinese on the right. This is a book that will clearly help Chinese doctors to learn the vital basis of their practise. It will also help them to better their English and do we even dare hope that some English ophthalmologists will learn some Chinese!

这本书真是十分的精彩！英文原版自是一部经典，另外石一宁教授更是创造性地做出了一个双语版本。这不仅仅是从英文翻译为汉语，而是两种语言并排显示：左边英文右边汉语。毫无疑问，这本书将帮助中国医生认识并提高其行医中的重要理念。这也将有助于他们提升英语水平，甚至也能帮助一些使用英语的眼科医生学习一点汉语！

Professor Shi has had extensive experience in residency education, she has published a hundred scientific papers and 5 ophthalmic books, including other bilingual interpretations. This new bilingual version is poised to become a very significant part of Chinese ophthalmology's rapid advances in learning and ultimately in improving patient care based on the scientific foundations of our profession.

石教授在培训住院医师方面有着丰富的经验，她已发表了 100 余篇论文和 5 本眼科书籍，还有其他双语版本书籍。这一新的双语版书籍必将成为快速发展的中国眼科学的重要组成部分，并且在我们的科学研究基础之上最终更好地服务患者。

Prof David Taylor, FRCOphth. FRCPCH, DSc (Med)

Professor Emeritus, Paediatric Ophthalmology, Great Ormond Street Institute of Child Health, University College London. Previously, Director(Honorary), International Council of Ophthalmology Examinations

大卫泰勒教授，皇家眼科学院会员，皇家儿科与儿童健康学院会员，理学博士（医学），小儿眼科荣誉教授，大奥蒙德街儿童健康研究所，伦敦大学学院。国际眼科考试委员会前荣誉主任。

BCSC® volumes are designed to increase the physician's ophthalmic knowledge through study and review. Users of this activity are encouraged to read the text and then answer the study questions provided at the back of the book.

The Academy provides this material for educational purposes only. It is not intended to represent the only or best method or procedure in every case, nor to replace a physician's own judgment or give specific advice for case management. Including all indications, contraindications, side effects, and alternative agents for each drug or treatment is beyond the scope of this material. All information and recommendations should be verified, prior to use, with current information included in the manufacturers' package inserts or other independent sources, and considered in light of the patient's condition and history. Reference to certain drugs, instruments, and other products in this course is made for illustrative purposes only and is not intended to constitute an endorsement of such. Some material may include information on applications that are not considered community standard, that reflect indications not included in approved FDA labeling, or that are approved for use only in restricted research settings. **The FDA has stated that it is the responsibility of the physician to determine the FDA status of each drug or device he or she wishes to use, and to use them with appropriate, informed patient consent in compliance with applicable law.** The Academy specifically disclaims any and all liability for injury or other damages of any kind, from negligence or otherwise, for any and all claims that may arise from the use of any recommendations or other information contained herein.

Cover image: From BCSC Section 12, Retina and Vitreous. End-stage chorioretinal atrophy in pathologic myopia. (Courtesy of Richard F. Spaide, MD.)

BCSC 卷旨在通过研究与回顾来增加医生的眼科知识。鼓励学者阅读课文，然后回答书后提出的问题。

封面图片来自 BCSC 第 12 册《视网膜与玻璃体》中的“病理性近视的终末期脉络膜萎缩”。（由 Richard F. Spaide 医学博士提供。）

Basic and Clinical Science Course

Section 3

Faculty

Scott E. Brodie, MD, PhD, *Chair*, New York, New York
Pankaj C. Gupta, MD, Cleveland, Ohio
Kristina Irsch, PhD, Baltimore, Maryland, and Paris, France
Mary Lou Jackson, MD, Vancouver, Canada
Thomas F. Mauger, MD, Columbus, Ohio
Leon Strauss, MD, PhD, Baltimore, Maryland
Edmond H. Thall, MD, Highland Heights, Ohio
Joshua A. Young, MD, New York, New York

The Academy wishes to acknowledge the following committees for review of this edition:
Vision Rehabilitation Committee: Joseph L. Fontenot, MD, Mobile, Alabama
Practicing Ophthalmologists Advisory Committee for Education: Bradley D. Fouraker, MD, *Primary Reviewer*, Tampa, Florida; Edward K. Isbey III, MD, *Chair*, Asheville, North Carolina; Alice Bashinsky, MD, Asheville, North Carolina; David J. Browning, MD, PhD, Charlotte, North Carolina; Steven J. Grosser, MD, Golden Valley, Minnesota; Stephen R. Klapper, MD, Carmel, Indiana; James A. Savage, MD, Memphis, Tennessee; Michelle S. Ying, MD, Ladson, South Carolina

EBO

European Board of Ophthalmology: Tero T. Kivelä, MD, EBO *Chair*, Helsinki, Finland; Peter J. Ringens, MD, PhD, EBO *Liaison*, Maastricht, Netherlands; Jorge L. Alio, MD, PhD, Alicante, Spain; Vytautas Jasinskas, MD, Kaunas, Lithuania; Eija T. Vesti, MD, Turku, Finland

基础与临床科学教程

Louis B. Cantor, 医学博士，印第安纳波利斯市，印第安纳州，*高级临床教育秘书*
Christopher J. Rapuano，医学博士，费城，宾夕法尼亚州，*终身学习与评估秘书*
George A. Cioffi，医学博士，纽约市　纽约州，*BCSC 教程主席*

第三册

教师

Scott E. Brodie，医学博士，哲学博士，*大学教授*，纽约市，纽约州
Pankaj C. Gupta，医学博士，克利夫兰市，俄亥俄州
Kristina Irsch，哲学博士，巴尔的摩市，马里兰州，及巴黎，法国
Mary Lou Jackson，医学博士，温哥华，加拿大
Thomas F. Mauger，医学博士，哥伦布市，俄亥俄州
Leon Strauss，医学博士，哲学博士，巴尔的摩市，马里兰州
Edmond H. Thall，医学博士，高地，俄亥俄州
Joshua A. Young，医学博士，纽约市，纽约州

学会致谢的评审委员会：
视觉康复委员会：Joseph L. Fontenot，医学博士，莫比尔，亚拉巴马州
专业教育委员会：Bradley D. Fouraker，医学博士，*主审查员*，坦帕市佛罗里达州；Edward K. Isbey Ⅲ，医学博士，*大学教授*，阿什维尔，北卡罗来纳州；Alice Bashinsky，医学博士，阿什维尔，北卡罗来纳州；David J. Browning，医学博士，哲学博士，夏洛特市，北卡罗来纳州；Steven J. Grosser，医学博士，黄金谷，明尼苏达州；Stephen R. Klapper，医学博士，卡梅尔镇，印第安纳州；James A. Savage，医学博士，孟菲斯市，田纳西州；Michelle S. Ying，医学博士，莱德森，南卡罗来纳州。

欧洲眼科委员会：Tero T. Kivelä，医学博士，EBO 主席，*大学教授*赫尔辛基，芬兰；Peter J. Ringens，医学博士，哲学博士，EBO *联络员*，马斯特里赫特，荷兰；Jorge L. Alio，医学博士，哲学博士，阿利坎特，西班牙；Vytautas Jasinskas，医学博士，考纳斯，立陶宛；Eija T. Vesti，医学博士，图尔库，芬兰。

Financial Disclosures

Academy staff members who contributed to the development of this product state that within the 12 months prior to their contributions to this CME activity and for the duration of development, they have had no financial interest in or other relationship with any entity discussed in this course that produces, markets, resells, or distributes ophthalmic health care goods or services consumed by or used in patients, or with any competing commercial product or service.

The authors and reviewers state that within the 12 months prior to their contributions to this CME activity and for the duration of development, they have had the following financial relationships:*

Dr Alio: Akkolens (C, S), Bloss Group (L), Bluegreen Medical (O), Carevision (C, S), Carl Zeiss Meditec (S), CSO Costruzione Strumenti Oftalmici (C), Dompé (S), Hanita Lenses (C), International Ophthalmolgy Consulting (O), Jaypee Brothers (P), KeraMed (C, S), Magrabi Hospital (C), Mediphacos (C), Novagali Pharmaceuticals (S), Oculentis (C, S), Oftalcare Nutravision (O), Omeros (C), OPHTEC (L), Presbia (C), Schwind Eye Tech Solutions (L, S), Tekia (P), Topcon (C)

Dr Brodie: Sanofi (L)

Dr Browning: Aerpio Therapeutics(S), Alcon Laboratories (S), Alimera Sciences(C), Genentech (S), Novartis Pharmaceuticals(S), Ohr Pharmaceuticals(S), Pfizer(S), Regeneron Pharmaceuticals (S), Zeiss (O)

Dr Fouraker: Addition Technology (C, L), Alcon Laboratories (C, L), KeraVision (C, L), OASIS Medical (C, L)

Dr Grosser: Injectsense (O), Ivantis (O)

Dr Isbey: Alcon Laboratories (S), Allscripts (C), Bausch + Lomb (S), Medflow (C), Oculos Clinical Research (S)

Dr Jackson: Advanced Cell Technology (C), Astellas (C), Novartis Pharmaceuticals (C, L), Visus Technology (C)

Dr Jasinskas: Alcon Laboratories (C)

Dr Vesti: Allergan (L), Santen (L), Thea (L)

The other authors and reviewers state that within the past 12 months prior to their contri-butions to this CME activity and for the duration of development, they have had no financial interest in or other relationship with any entity discussed in this course that produces, markets, resells, or distributes ophthalmic health care goods or services consumed by or used in patients, or with any competing commercial product or service.

财务信息

参与开发此产品的学会工作人员声明，在对发布此次 CME 活动 12 个月之前和开发该产品期间，他们与该教程中涉及的任何产品没有经济利益和其他关系，没有将其使用或应用于患者，包括产品的生产、市场出售、推广眼科医疗保健商品或服务中，没有与任何实体或金融机构产生关系，没有与任何产品或服务进行商业竞争。

作者和评审人员声明，在发布 CME 活动之前的 12 个月以及开发期间，他们拥有以下财务关系。

Alio 博士 : Akkolens (C, S), Bloss Group (L), Bluegreen Medical (O), Carevision (C, S), Carl Zeiss Meditec (S), CSO Costruzione Strumenti Oftalmici (C), Dompé (S), Hanita Lenses (C), International Ophthalmolgy Consulting (O), Jaypee Brothers (P), KeraMed (C, S), Magrabi Hospital (C), Mediphacos (C), Novagali Pharmaceuticals (S), Oculentis (C, S), Oftalcare Nutravision (O), Omeros (C), OPHTEC (L), Presbia (C), Schwind Eye Tech Solutions (L, S), Tekia (P), Topcon (C)

Brodie 博士 : Sanofi (L)

Browning 博士 : Aerpio Therapeutics(S), Alcon Laboratories (S), Alimera Sciences(C), Genentech (S), Novartis Pharmaceuticals(S), Ohr Pharmaceuticals(S), Pfizer(S), Regeneron Pharmaceuticals (S), Zeiss (O)

Fouraker 博士 : Addition Technology (C, L), Alcon Laboratories (C, L), KeraVision (C, L), OASIS Medical (C, L)

Grosser 博士 : Injectsense (O), Ivantis (O)

Isbey 博士 : Alcon Laboratories (S), Allscripts (C), Bausch + Lomb (S), Medflow (C), Oculos Clinical Research (S)

Jackson 博士 : Advanced Cell Technology (C), Astellas (C), Novartis Pharmaceuticals (C, L), Visus Technology (C)

Jasinskas 博士 : Alcon Laboratories (C)

Vesti 博士 : Allergan (L), Santen (L), Thea (L)

其他作者和审稿人声明：在发布 CME 活动之前 12 个月内及在此开发期间，他们与本教程中讨论的生产、营销、转售或所消费或使用的眼科保健产品或服务的任何实体，或与任何竞争性商业产品或服务没有任何财务利益或其他关系。

*C = consultant fees, paid advisory boards, or fees for attending a meeting; L = lecture fees (honoraria), travel fees, or reimbursements when speaking at the invitation of a commercial sponsor; O = equity own-ership/stock options of publicly or privately traded firms (excluding mutual funds) with manufacturers of commercial ophthalmic products or commercial ophthalmic services; P = patents and/or royalties that might be viewed as creating a potential conflict of interest; S = grant support for the past year (all sources) and all sources used for a specific talk or manuscript with no time limitation

Recent Past Faculty

Dimitri T. Azar, MD
Nathalie F. Azar, MD
Kenneth J. Hoffer, MD
Tommy S. Korn, MD

In addition, the Academy gratefully acknowledges the contributions of numerous past faculty and advisory committee members who have played an important role in the devel opment of previous editions of the Basic and Clinical Science Course.

American Academy of Ophthalmology Staff

Dale E. Fajardo, EdD, MBA, *Vice President, Education*
Beth Wilson, *Director, Continuing Professional Development*
Ann McGuire, *Acquisitions and Development Manager*
Stephanie Tanaka, *Publications Manager*
D. Jean Ray, *Production Manager*
Susan Malloy, *Acquisitions Editor and Program Manager*
Jasmine Chen, *Manager of E-Learning*
Beth Collins, *Medical Editor*
Eric Gerdes, *Interactive Designer*
Naomi Ruiz, *Publications Specialist*

*C= 顾问费，支付给顾问委员会或出席会议的费用；L= 应商业赞助商邀请发言时的演讲费（酬金）、差旅费或报销费用；O= 公开或私营贸易公司（不包括共同基金）与商业眼科产品制造商的股权 / 股票期权或商业眼科服务的费用；P= 可能被视为造成潜在利益冲突的专利和（或）版税；S= 过去 1 年（所有来源）的资助以及无时间限制的特定谈话或手稿的所有财务来源。

近年卸任的教师

Dimitri T. Azar，医学博士
Nathalie F. Azar，医学博士
Kenneth J. Hoffer，医学博士
Tommy S. Korn，医学博士

此外，学院衷心感谢以往的许多教员和咨询委员会成员，他们在"基础与临床科学教程"前几版的发展中发挥着重要的作用。

美国眼科学会工作人员

Dale E. Fajardo，*教育部副总裁*
Beth Wilson，*持续专业发展总监*
Ann McGuine,*采购和开发经理*
Stephanie Tanaka，*出版社经理*
D. Jean Ray，*生产部经理*
Susan Malloy，*采购编辑和项目经理*
Jasmine Chen，*电子学习经理*
Beth Collins，*医学编辑*
Eric Gerdes，*互动设计师*
Naomi Ruiz，*出版专家*

（翻译 何媛 张纯涛 // 审校 陈研明 石一宁）

CONTENTS

目录

General Introduction

The Basic and Clinical Science Course (BCSC) is designed to meet the needs of residents and practitioners for a comprehensive yet concise curriculum of the field of ophthalmology. The BCSC has developed from its original brief outline format, which relied heavily on outside readings, to a more convenient and educationally useful self-contained text. The Academy updates and revises the course annually, with the goals of integrating the basic science and clinical practice of ophthalmology and of keeping ophthalmologists current with new developments in the various subspecialties.

The BCSC incorporates the effort and expertise of more than 90 ophthalmologists, organized into 13 Section faculties, working with Academy editorial staff. In addition, the course continues to benefit from many lasting contributions made by the faculties of previous editions. Members of the Academy Practicing Ophthalmologists Advisory Committee for Education, Committee on Aging, and Vision Rehabilitation Committee review every volume before major revisions. Members of the European Board of Ophthalmology, organized into Section faculties, also review each volume before major revisions, focusing primarily on differences between American and European ophthalmology practice.

Organization of the Course

The Basic and Clinical Science Course comprises 13 volumes, incorporating fundamental ophthalmic knowledge, subspecialty areas, and special topics:

1 Update on General Medicine
2 Fundamentals and Principles of Ophthalmology
3 Clinical Optics
4 Ophthalmic Pathology and Intraocular Tumors
5 Neuro-Ophthalmology
6 Pediatric Ophthalmology and Strabismus
7 Orbit, Eyelids, and Lacrimal System
8 External Disease and Cornea
9 Intraocular Inflammation and Uveitis
10 Glaucoma
11 Lens and Cataract
12 Retina and Vitreous
13 Refractive Surgery

In addition, a comprehensive Master Index allows the reader to easily locate subjects throughout the entire series.

References

Readers who wish to explore specific topics in greater detail may consult the references cited within each chapter and listed in the Basic Texts section at the back of the book. These references are intended to be selective rather than exhaustive, chosen by the BCSC faculty as being important, current, and readily available to residents and practitioners.

概述

“基础与临床科学教程”（BCSC）旨在满足住院医师和执业医师对眼科领域全面而简明课程设置的要求。BCSC 已经从最初的大纲格式（主要依赖于课外阅读）发展成为一种更方便、教育上更为有用的独立教材。学会每年对教程进行更新和修订，目标是将眼科基础科学与临床实践相结合，使眼科医生与各专科的新进展保持同步。

BCSC 凝聚了 13 个科系的 90 多名眼科医生的努力和专业知识，以及眼科学会编辑人员的共同努力工作。此外，本教程还得益于前几任学会人员所作的多年贡献，学会执业眼科医师教育咨询委员会、老龄委员会以及视力康复委员会都会在重大修订之前，审查每一册。欧洲眼科委员会也组成分册编委会，审查每一册，然后进行重大修订，主要集中于美国和欧洲眼科实践之间的差异。

教程编制

“基础与临床科学教程”包括 13 册，包含基本的眼科知识、亚专业领域和专题：

1 医学的新进展
2 眼科基础与原理
3 临床光学
4 眼病理与眼肿瘤
5 神经眼科学
6 小儿眼科与斜视
7 眼眶、眼睑与泪腺系统
8 外眼疾病与角膜
9 眼内炎症与葡萄膜炎
10 青光眼
11 晶状体与白内障
12 视网膜与玻璃体
13 屈光手术

此外，一个全面的主索引使得读者易于在整个教程中寻找到主题。

参考文献

读者欲更详细地探讨特定主题，可参考书中每一章所引用的参考文献，以及书后的基础书籍一节列出的书籍。这些参考资料是有选择性的，并不详尽，由 BCSC 编委会选择重要的、最新进展的，并可以提供给住院医师和医生。

Multimedia

This edition of Section 3, Clinical Optics, includes videos related to topics covered in the book. The videos were selected by members of the BCSC faculty and are available to readers of the print and electronic versions of Section 3 (www.aao.org/bcscvideo_section03). Mobile-device users can scan the QR code below (a QR-code reader must already be installed on the device) to access the video content.

Self-Assessment

Each volume of the BCSC is designed as an independent study activity for ophthalmology residents and practitioners. The learning objectives for this volume are given on page 6. The text, illustrations, and references provide the information necessary to achieve the objectives; the study questions allow readers to test their understanding of the material and their mastery of the objectives.

Conclusion

The Basic and Clinical Science Course has expanded greatly over the years, with the addition of much new text, numerous illustrations, and video content. Recent editions have sought to place greater emphasis on clinical applicability while maintaining a solid foundation in basic science. As with any educational program, it reflects the experience of its authors. As its faculties change and medicine progresses, new viewpoints emerge on controversial subjects and techniques. Not all alternate approaches can be included in this series; as with any educational endeavor, the learner should seek additional sources, including Academy Preferred Practice Pattern Guidelines.

The BCSC faculty and staff continually strive to improve the educational usefulness of the course; you, the reader, can contribute to this ongoing process. If you have any suggestions or questions about the series, please do not hesitate to contact the faculty or the editors.

The authors, editors, and reviewers hope that your study of the BCSC will be of lasting value and that each Section will serve as a practical resource for quality patient care.

多媒体

这一版的第 3 册,《临床光学》包括与书中主题相关的视频。这些视频由 BCSC 编委会挑选出来，可供读者阅读第 3 册的印刷版和电子版（www.aao.org/bcscvideo section 3）。移动设备用户可以扫描下面的二维码来访问视频内容。

自我评价

每册 BCSC 都是为眼科住院医师和执业医师设计的独立研究活动。本册的学习目标见第 7 页。教材、插图和参考文献提供了实现目标所需的信息，研究问题旨在让读者测试他们对教材的理解和对目标的掌握程度。

结论

近年来,“基础与临床科学教程”有了很大的扩展,具有大量的新内容、大量的插图和视频内容。最近的版本试图在保持基础科学坚实基础的同时，更强调临床的适用性。与任何教育项目一样，它体现了作者的经验。随着学会的更换和医学的进步，对有争议的学科和技术产生了新的观点。不是所有的替代方法都可以包含在这个系列中；与任何教育努力一样，学习者应该寻求更多的资源，包括眼科学会的眼科临床指南 PPP。

BCSC 编委会不断努力提高教程的教育作用。作为读者，您可以为进行中的教程作一些贡献。如果您对该系列有任何疑问或不解，请立即与教师或编辑联系。

作者、编辑和评审者希望您的 BCSC 学习有持续的价值，并希望每个部分能够为患者高质量保健提供实用资源。

（李甸　译）

Objectives

Upon completion of BCSC Section 3, *Clinical Optics*, the reader should be able to

- explain the principles of light propagation and image formation and work through some of the fundamental equations that describe or measure such properties as refraction, reflection, magnification, and vergence
- explain how these principles can be applied diagnostically and therapeutically
- describe the clinical application of Snell's law and the lensmaker's equation
- describe the relationship between physical optics and geometric optics
- describe the clinical and technical relevance of such optical phenomena as interference, coherence, polarization, diffraction, and scattering
- explain the basic properties of laser light and how they affect laser– tissue interaction
- identify optical models of the human eyes and describe how to apply them
- describe various aspects of visual performance, including visual acuity, brightness sensitivity,
- summarize the steps for performing streak retinoscopy
- identify the steps for performing a manifest refraction using a phoropter or trial lenses
- describe the use of the Jackson cross cylinder
- describe the indications for prescribing bifocal and progressive lenses and common difficulties encountered in their use
- identify the materials and fitting parameters of both soft and rigid contact lenses
- discuss the basic methods of calculating intraocular lens (IOL) powers and the advantages and disadvantages of the different methods
- explain the conceptual basis of multifocal IOLs and how the correction of presbyopia differs between IOLs and spectacles
- explain the optical principles underlying various modalities of refractive correction: spectacles, contact lenses, intraocular lenses, and refractive surgery
- describe the operating principles of various optical instruments in order to use them effectively
- appraise the visual needs of low vision patients and determine how to address these needs through use of optical and nonoptical devices and/or appropriate referrals

目　标

完成 BCSC 第 3 册《*临床光学*》的学习，读者应该可以了解到以下知识：

- 通过描述或测量一些基本方程的特性，诸如折射、反射、放大和聚散等，来解释光传播和成像的原理；
- 解释这些原则如何在诊断和治疗上应用；
- 描述 Snell 定律和透镜制作商方程的临床应用；
- 描述物理光学和几何光学之间的关系；
- 描述干涉、相干、偏振、衍射和散射等光学现象的临床和技术相关性；
- 解释激光的基本属性以及它们如何影响激光 – 组织相互作用；
- 认识人眼的光学模型，并描述其如何应用；
- 描述视觉的各个方面，包括视力、亮度敏感度、色觉和对比敏感度；
- 总结实施带状光检影的步骤；
- 确定使用综合验光仪或试镜进行显性验光；
- 描述 Jackson 交叉圆柱镜的使用；
- 描述双焦镜和渐进镜的配镜处方适应症，以及在使用中常见的问题；
- 确定软性和硬性接触镜的材料和验配参数；
- 讨论人工晶体（IOL）焦度的基本计算方法，以及不同方法的优缺点；
- 解释多焦点人工晶体的基本概念，以及人工晶体和眼镜对老视的矫正有何不同；
- 解释各种屈光矫正方法的光学原理：眼镜、接触镜、人工晶体和屈光手术；
- 描述各种光学仪器的工作原理，以便有效地使用它们；
- 评估低视力患者的视觉需求，并确定如何通过使用光学和非光学设备和（或）适当的方法来满足这些需求。

Quick-Start Guide to Optics and How to Refract

Part 1: Introductory Optics

Highlights

- pinhole optics and the role of lenses
- convex (spherical) lenses: imaging distant objects, focal length, and power
- adjacent lenses taken together: addition of lens powers
- imaging nearby objects: vergence and the vergence equation
- concave (spherical) lenses
- imaging in air and denser media: correction for index of refraction
- axial refractive errors: myopia and hyperopia
- astigmatism and cylindrical lenses

Glossary

Astigmatism The imagery formed by a toric lens, with power that varies according to meridian.

Camera obscura A small light- tight room or box in which a pinhole aperture forms an inverted image.

Focal length The distance between a lens and the image it forms of an object at great distance (*optical infinity*).

Hyperopia A refractive error in which distant objects are imaged behind the retina.

Image distance The distance from a lens to the image it forms of an object. Distances to the left of a lens are considered as negative numbers; distances to the right of a lens are considered as positive numbers.

Meridian The orientation of a plane passing through the optic axis of a lens, or of the intersection curve of such a plane with a lens surface. This orientation is usually specified in degrees, increasing counterclockwise from the horizontal as viewed from in front of the lens. The horizontal meridian is by convention designated as 180° (not 0°); the vertical meridian is at 90°.

Myopia A refractive error in which distant objects are imaged in front of the retina.

光学快速入门指南和如何验光

第 1 部分：光学介绍

重点

- 针孔光学和透镜的作用。
- 凸面（球面）镜：对远距离物体成像、焦距和焦度。
- 密接镜片叠加：透镜焦度相加。
- 对近距物体成像：聚散度和聚散度方程。
- 凹面（球面）镜。
- 在空气和光密介质中的成像：矫正折射率。
- 轴性屈光不正：近视和远视。
- 散光和柱镜。

术语

散光 由复曲面镜形成的图像，其屈光力根据子午线而变化。

相机暗箱 一个小的不透光的空间或盒子，通过其中的针孔形成倒像。

焦距 透镜与远距离物体的成像之间的距离（*光学无限远*）。

远视 一种屈光不正，远处的物体成像在视网膜之后。

像距 透镜到物体成像的距离。透镜左侧的距离被视为负数，透镜右侧的距离被视为正数。

子午线 穿过透镜光轴平面的方向，或该平面与透镜表面相交曲线的方向。该方向通常以度（°）为单位，从透镜前方观察时按水平方向逆时针增加。按照惯例，水平子午线指定为 180°（不是 0°），垂直子午线是 90°。

近视 一种屈光不正，远处的物体成像在视网膜之前。

Object distance The distance from a source object to the lens, in meters. The sign conventions are the same as for image distance.

Power (of a lens) The reciprocal of the focal length. Measured in m^{-1}, referred to as *diopters* (D).

Power cross A diagrammatic representation of the action of a toric lens, showing the power and orientation of the 2 (perpendicular) principal meridians.

Principal meridian The flattest or steepest meridian of a toric lens. The principal meridians are in general perpendicular to each other.

Refractive index The speed of light in air (or a vacuum) divided by the speed of light in a different medium. As light always travels more slowly through a material medium (sometimes referred to as a *denser* medium) than in a vacuum, the refractive index is always greater than 1.00.

Toric lens A lens with a surface resembling the outer rim of a torus, such as an automobile tire or the side of a rugby ball or an American football.

Vergence (in air) The reciprocal of the object distance (*object vergence*) or image distance(*image vergence*).

Vergence (in media other than air or a vacuum) The refractive index of the medium in which light travels divided by the object distance or image distance. Sometimes referred to as *reduced vergence*, even though this is numerically greater than the vergence in air, as refractive indices of denser media are always greater than 1.00.

Vergence equation The formula relating object vergence, lens power, and image vergence.

Introduction

The term *optics* refers to the properties and manipulation of light. In this part of the Quick- Start Guide, we introduce the basic ideas of optics—sufficient to understand the essence of clinical refraction, as presented in Part 2, "How to Refract." Readers already familiar with this material are welcome to turn immediately to Part 2.

The Tale of the Camera Obscura

The term *camera obscura* (Latin for "dark chamber") was introduced in the 17th century to describe the use (already known to the ancients) of a small light- tight room or box fitted with a small hole on 1 side. The hole allowed the inverted image of a bright scene or bright object to be projected onto the opposite wall or side of the box, where it might be conveniently viewed or studied. The earliest known drawing of such a device is shown in Figure I-1, where it is being used to view a solar eclipse.

Experience with such devices leads to 3 important observations:

1. The projected image is inverted.
2. The "depth of field" of the projected image is superb: objects are simultaneously in focus at all distances, from foreground objects to distant hills and even astronomical objects (Figure I-2).
3. The image is very dim.

物距 从发光物体到透镜的距离，以 m 为单位。符号规则与像距相同。

（透镜的）焦度 焦距的倒数。以 m^{-1} 为单位，称为*屈光度*（D）。

屈光力十字 复曲面作用的示意图，显示了 2 条主子午线（相垂直）的屈光力和方向。

主子午线 复曲面透镜最平坦或最陡的子午线。主子午线通常相互垂直。

折射率 以空气（或真空）中的光速除以不同介质中的光速即为折射率。由于光在普通介质（有时为*光密*介质）比在真空中通过的速度更慢，因此折射率总是大于 1.00。

复曲透镜 具有类似于复曲面外缘表面的透镜，例如汽车轮胎、橄榄球、美式橄榄球的侧面。

聚散度（在空气中） 物距的倒数（*物的聚散度*）或像距的倒数（*像的聚散度*）。

聚散度（在空气或真空以外的介质中） 光传播介质的折射率除以物距或像距。即使其在数值上大于空气中的聚散度，有时也称为*简化聚散度*，因为光密介质的折射率总是大于 1.00。

聚散度方程 关于物的聚散度、镜片焦度和像的聚散度的公式。

引言

术语*光学*是指光的特性和处理。在《快速入门指南》的这一部分，我们介绍了光学的基本概念——这有助于大家理解临床验光的本质，如第 2 部分“如何验光”中所述。已熟悉此部分的读者可以直接进入第 2 部分的学习。

暗箱的故事

术语*暗箱*（拉丁语为“暗室”）始于 17 世纪，用于描述一侧有 1 个小洞且小而不透光的房间或盒子（古人已知）。该孔将明亮物体的倒置图像投射到盒子内壁，以利于观察或研究。已知最早的这种装置见图 I–1 所示，其用于观察日食。

使用此类设备可得出 3 个重要观察结果：

1. 投影像是倒立的。
2. 投影像的“景深”特别好：不同距离的物体同时聚焦，从眼前的物体到远处的山丘，甚至是天文物体（图 I–2）。
3. 像非常暗淡。

The inverted image clearly arises from the straight- line propagation of light rays originating from each point in the original object, with the pinhole acting like a sort of fulcrum (Figure I-3).

The great depth of field is due to the small aperture, which allows light rays from each object to reach only a very small region in the image plane.

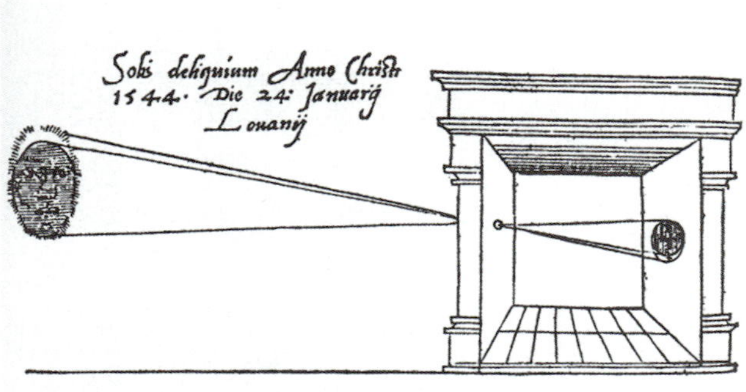

Figure I-1 Earliest known depiction of a camera obscura. *(From De Radio Astronomica et Geometrica;1545.)*

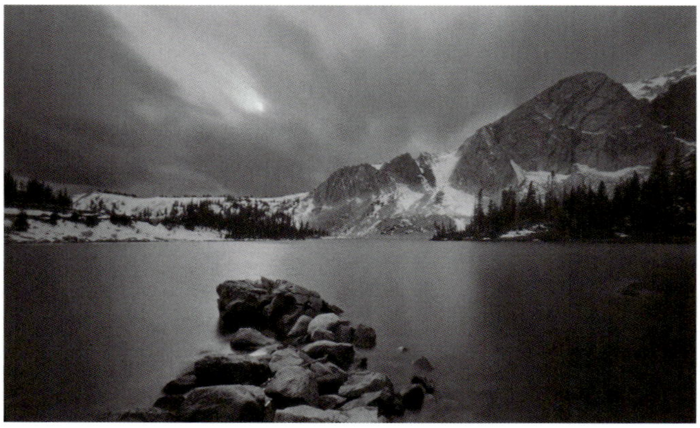

Figure I-2 Camera obscura (pinhole camera) image. Notice the great depth of field, with both the rocks on the foreground and the mountains in the background simultaneously in sharp focus. *(Courtesy of Mark James.)*

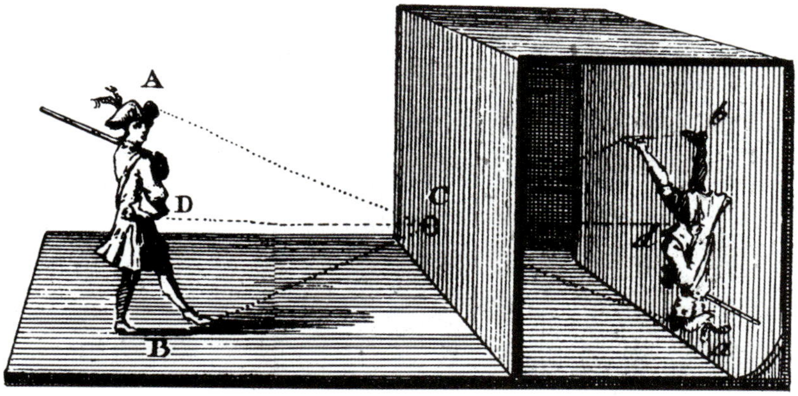

Figure I-3 Image formation in a camera obscura. An inverted image forms when rays of light from points of the original object (eg, **A, D, B**) follow straight paths through the pinhole (**C**) to the corresponding points (eg, **a, d, b**) in the image on the far wall.

倒像清晰是由于原物体中的每个点的光线沿直线传播，而针孔就像是它的支点（图 I–3）。

大景深源自小光圈，这使得每个物体的光线仅到达像平面中的非常小的区域。

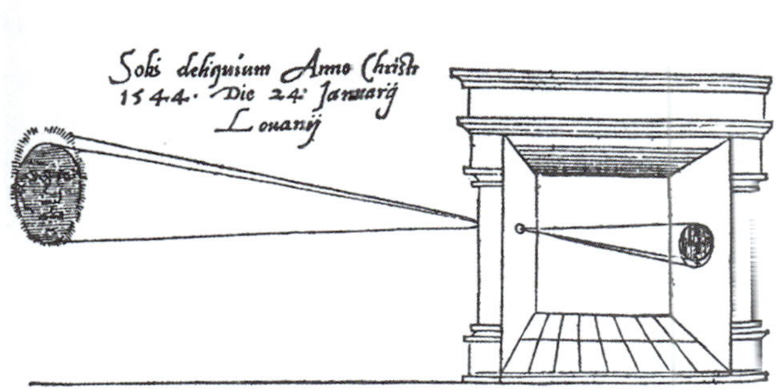

图 I–1　已知最早的暗箱描述。*（译者注：资料来源见前页原文。）*

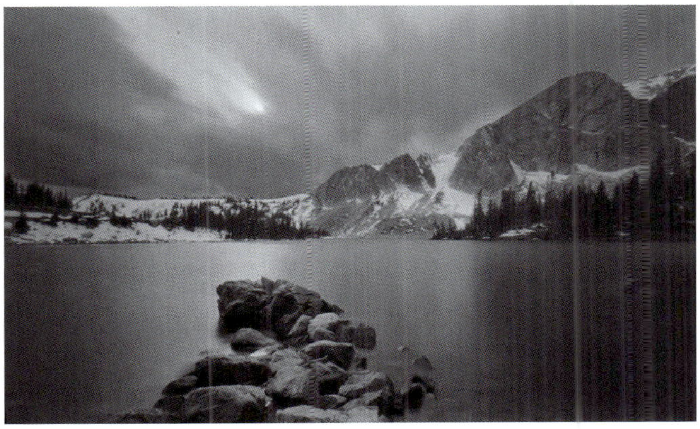

图 I–2　暗箱（针孔相机）像。其景深很大，前面的岩石和背景中的山脉同时处于清晰的焦点处。*（译者注：资料来源见前页原文。）*

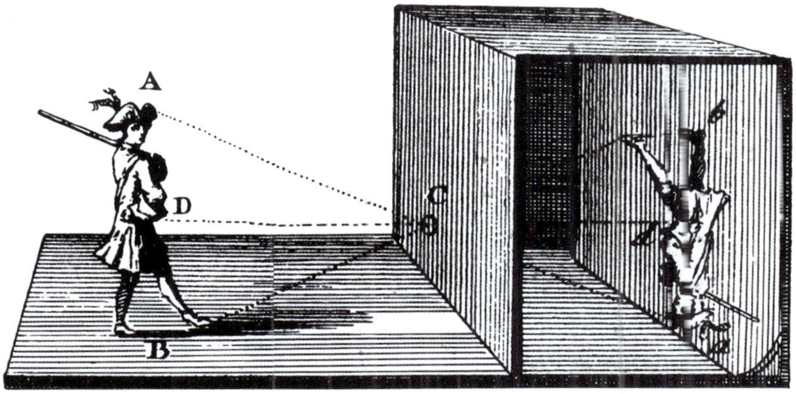

图 I–3　暗箱中的像形成。光线从原物体的点（如 A、D、B）经过针孔（C），以直线路径到达远处壁上的对应点（如 a、d、b），形成倒像。

Of course, the small aperture also greatly limits the amount of light that is available to form the image, which explains why it is so dim.

To obtain a brighter image, suitable for the activation of a detector (such as a photographic plate, a CCD chip, or the retina), it is necessary to enlarge the pinhole aperture to admit more light. Unfortunately, enlarging the aperture also allows the rays of light emanating from each point of the source object to form a cone of light, which illuminates a proportionally larger disc on the image plane. These "blur circles" (or perhaps more generally, "blur ellipses") smear out the image, resulting in substantial blurring (Figures I-4, I-5).

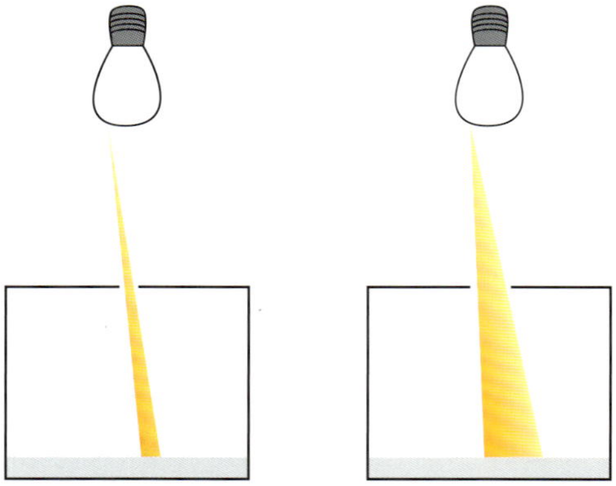

Figure I-4 Enlarging the pinhole in a camera obscura results in larger blur-circle images of each point of the original object.

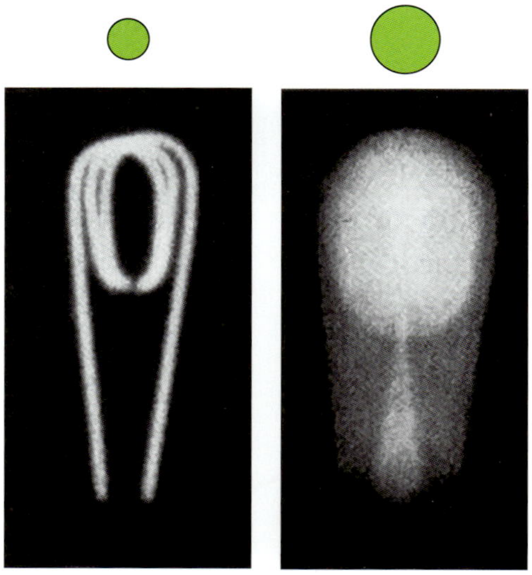

Figure I-5 Effect of pinhole size (as indicated schematically by the circles at the top) on image sharpness in a camera obscura.

To recover a sharp image while retaining the image intensity afforded by a larger aperture, it is necessary to recombine the light rays that originate from each point of the source object so that they will converge on a single image point. This can be accomplished by placing a suitable lens in the aperture (Figure I-6).

而小光圈也极大地限制了可用于形成像的曝光量，这就解释了为什么它会很暗淡。

为了得到更亮的图像，必须扩大针孔，使更多的光进入，这也适合于激活检测器（例如照相板、CCD 芯片或视网膜）。但是，放大孔径也使得发光物体的每个点发出的光线形成一个光锥，其在照射像平面上形成更大的圆盘。这些“模糊圆圈”（或者常见的“模糊椭圆”）会弄混形成的像，导致其更为模糊（图 I–4、图 I–5）。

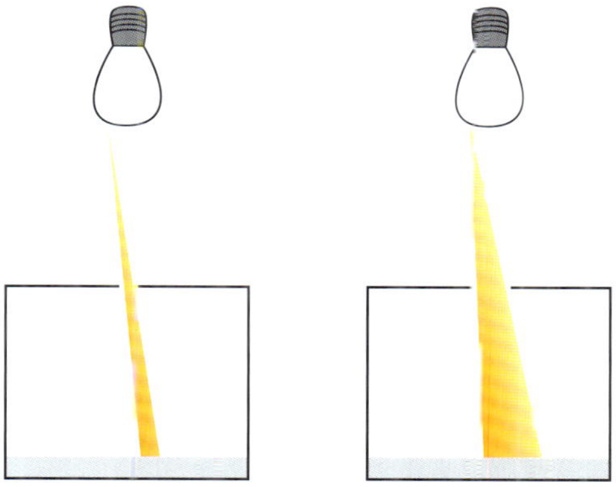

图 I–4 放大暗箱的针孔孔径，会导致发光物体上每个点的模糊像变大。

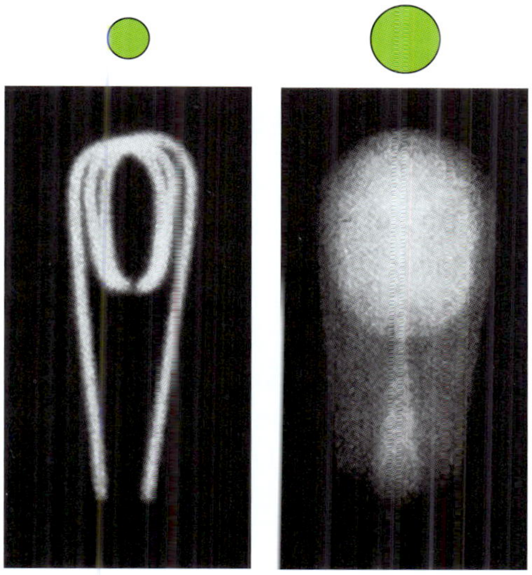

图 I–5 针孔孔径大小（由顶部圆圈示意）对暗箱中像清晰度的影响。

为了在保持较大光圈下像亮度的同时恢复像的清晰度，需要重新组合发光物体每个点发出的光线，使它们会聚在单个图像点上，这可以通过在光圈中放置合适的透镜来实现（图 I–6）。

However, the strategy of using a lens to recover the sharpness of images by enlarging the aperture necessarily sacrifices the depth of field obtained with the simple pinhole. Though the lens will simultaneously bring to focus rays of light from different points in the source object, it can do so only for source points at the same distance from the lens(Figure I-7).

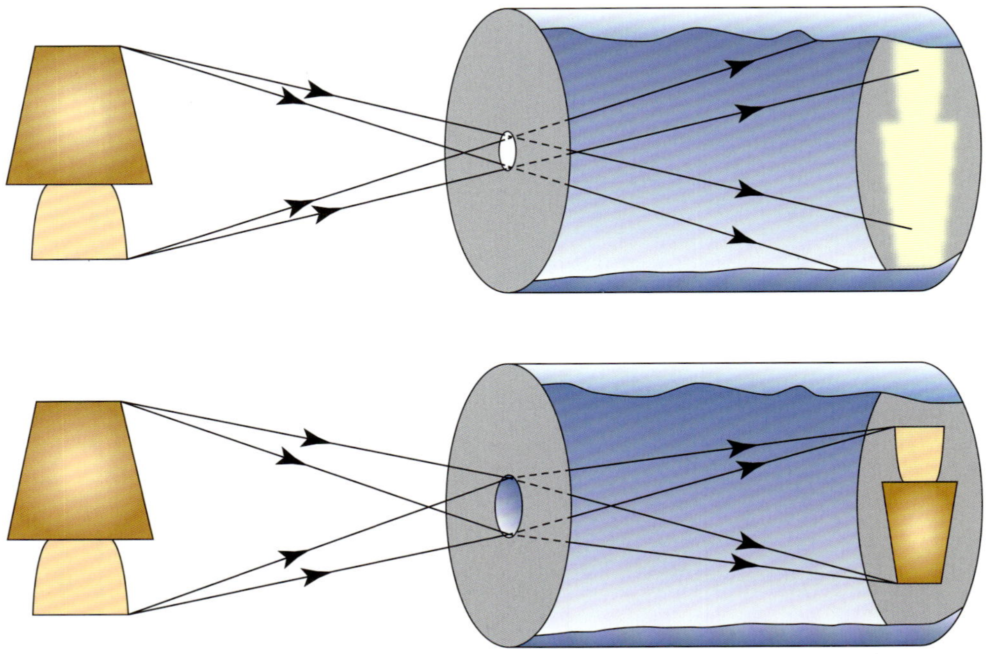

Figure I-6 Recovering a sharp image by placing a lens in the aperture of a camera obscura after the aperture has been enlarged. The same lens simultaneously recombines the rays of light from each point of the source object to land at a single point in the image plane.

These observations about image formation in simple cameras essentially summarize the entire challenge of basic optics: to form sharp images from beams of light defined by apertures of finite size to provide sufficient brightness for the application at hand. The rules for the proper selection of lenses for this purpose are discussed in the next section.

然而，通过扩大孔径、使用透镜恢复图像清晰度的策略，必然会损失简单针孔获得的景深。虽然透镜同时聚焦来自发光物体中不同点的光，但也只能是与透镜相同距离的光源点（图I–7）。

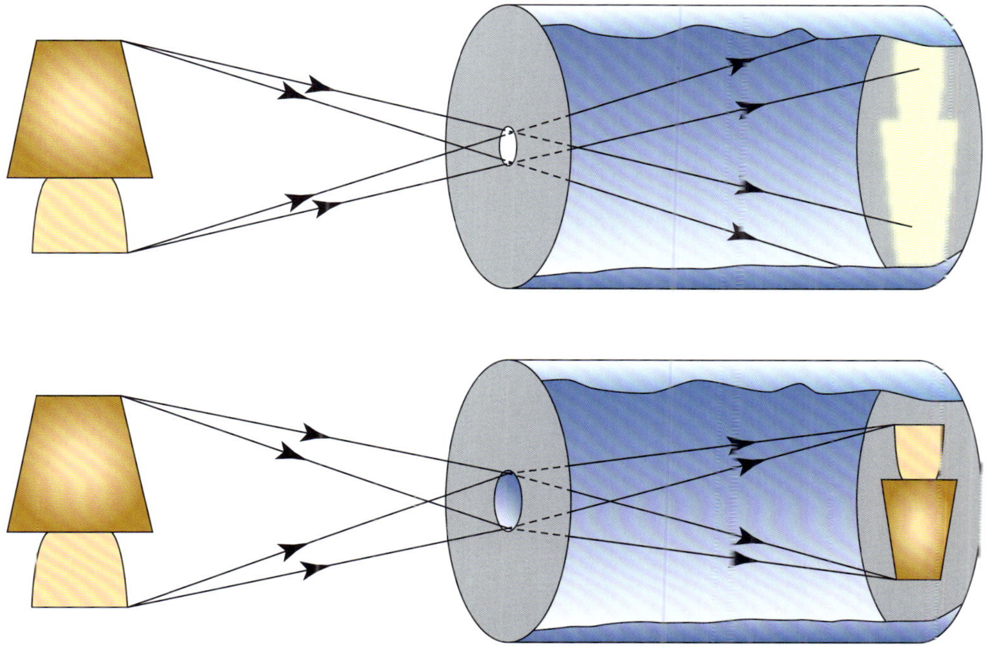

图 I–6 放大光圈后，将透镜放入暗箱，图像恢复清晰度。同时，透镜重新组合了发光物体每个点发出的光线，使其可以到达像平面中的每个点。

这些关于简单相机成像的研究基本上总结了基本光学的全部问题：从有限大小的针孔中经过的限定光束形成清晰像，并提供足够的亮度。下一节将讨论正确选择透镜的原则。

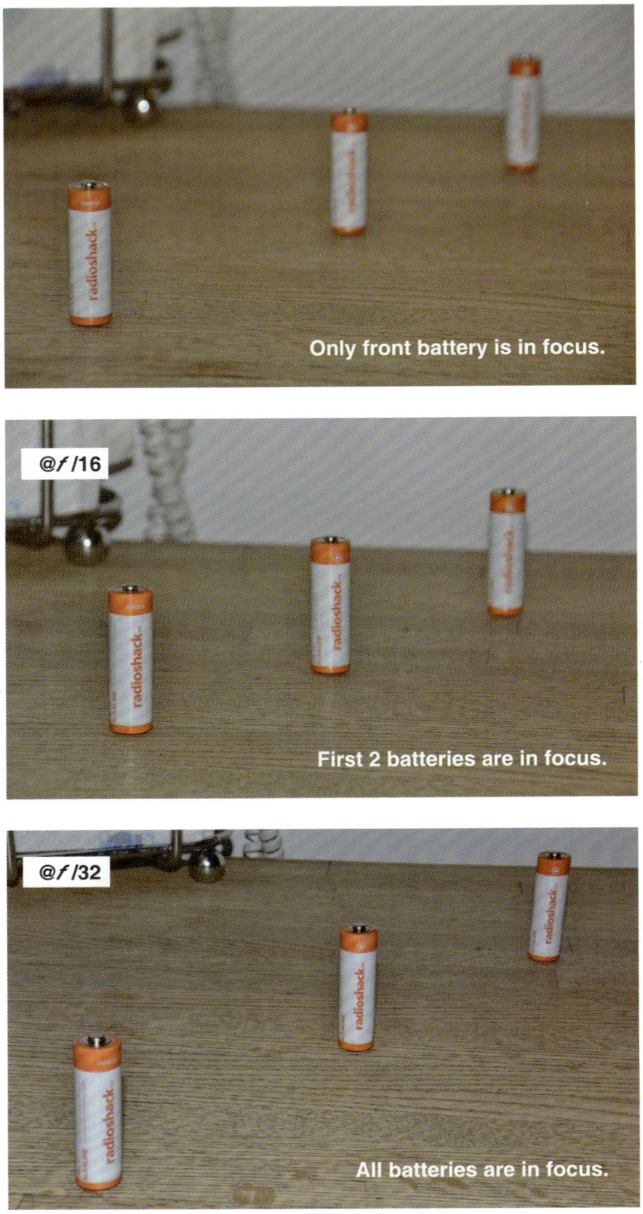

Figure I-7 Reduced depth of field in images obtained with lenticular optics. Even in this case, smaller aperture (larger f/ numbers) result in greater depth of field. *(Courtesy of Scott E. Brodie, MD, PhD.)*

Convex Lenses

Consider a thin (spherical) convex lens intended to form an image of an object at "optical infinity"—that is, very far away (say, a star)—located to the left of the lens. The image will be formed to the right of the lens—say, at a distance f, measured in meters. This distance is referred to as the *focal length* of the lens. The *power* of the lens is then $P = 1/f$, where the unit for P is reciprocal meters, which is referred to as the "diopter" (abbreviated "D").For example, a lens that images starlight 0.5 m to its right has a power of $P = 1/0.5\text{ m} = 2.0\text{D}$(FigureI-8).

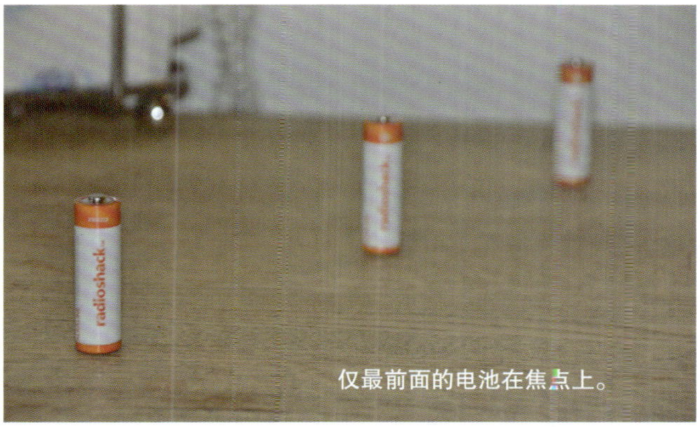

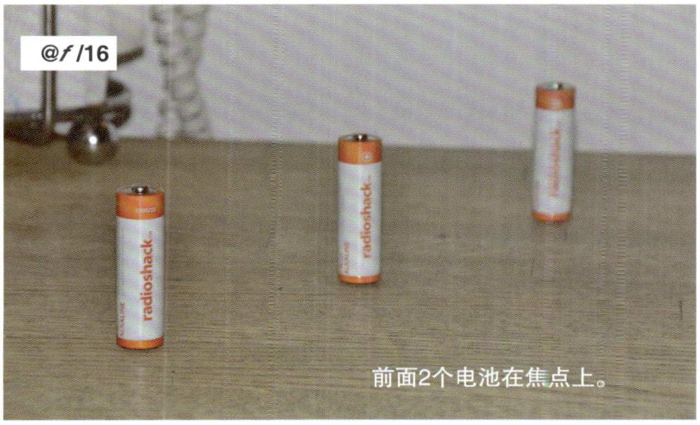

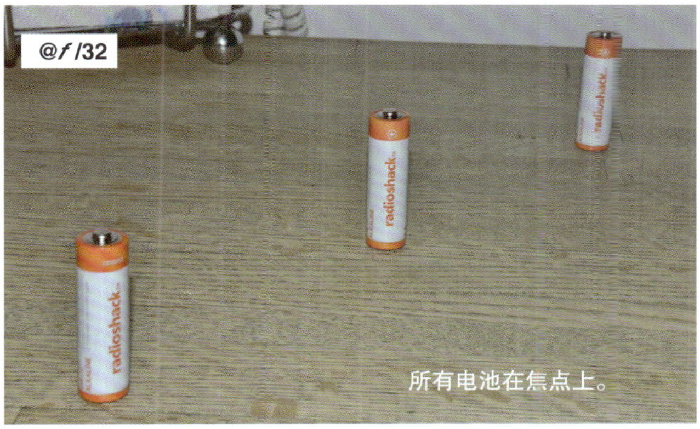

图 I–7 透镜获得的景深减少，而即使在这种情况下，也会是光圈越小（f/n 越大），景深越大。*（译者注：资料来源见前页原文。）*

凸透镜

考虑一个薄（球形）凸透镜成像，在“光学无穷远”，即非常远（如恒星）时，如果物体位于透镜左侧，则像成于透镜右侧。距离 f，以 m 为单位，被称为透镜的*焦距*。此时透镜的*焦度*为 $P = 1/f$，其中 P 的单位是 m^{-1}，称为“屈光度”（缩写为“D”）。例如，对于一个右侧焦距为 0.5m 的星光成像的透镜来说，其具有 P =1/0.5 m =2.0D 的焦度（图 I–8）。

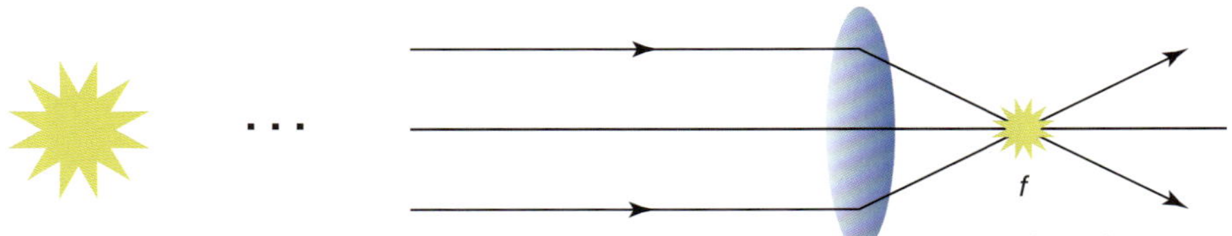

Figure I-8 Image formation for an object at infinite distance (such as a star) by a simple convexlens.The distance from the lens to the image is f, the focal length of the lens; the power of the lens is given by $P = 1/f$, where P is given units of diopters (D), equivalent to reciprocal meters.

Combining Lenses

If 2 (thin) lenses—say, of powers P_1 and P_2—are placed in contact immediately adjacent to one another, and we consider them together as a single compound lens system, the power of the 2 lenses taken together is given, to an excellent approximation, by the sum of the powers of the constituent lenses: $P = P_1 + P_2$. This summation is the utility of the reciprocal description of lens power.

EXAMPLE I-1

If 2 convex lenses of power P_1 = 1.0D and power P_2 = 4.0D are combined and treated as a single unit, where does this combination lens form the image of a distant star?

$$P = P_1 + P_2 = 1.0\text{D} + 4.0\text{D} = 5.0\text{D} = 1/f$$

Thus, $f = 1/P$ = 0.20 m, or 20 cm to the right of the lens, which is the location of the image of the distant star.

EXAMPLE I-2

Moving an image closer to the lenses: the image in Example I-1 must be moved 2.0 cm = 0.02 m closer to the compound lens. We may do so by adding a third convex lens: since we wish to have a result of f = 0.18 m, $P = 1/f$ = 1/0.18 m = 5.55 D = $P_1 + P_2 + P_3$. Thus, P_3 = 0.55 D. This is an example of a general method: adding a convex lens to a system of lenses will generally shift an image that is located to the right of the lens closer to the lens system.

Imaging Nearby Objects: Vergence and the Vergence Equation

If the source object is located only a finite distance to the left of a convex lens, but at greater distance than the focal length, f, the image will be farther to the right of the lens than the image of an object that is infinitely far away, such as a star. The distance from the source object to the lens is referred to as the *object distance*; the distance from the lens to the image is known as the *image distance*. Assuming both the source object and the image are in air, the formula for locating the image is

$$U + P = V$$

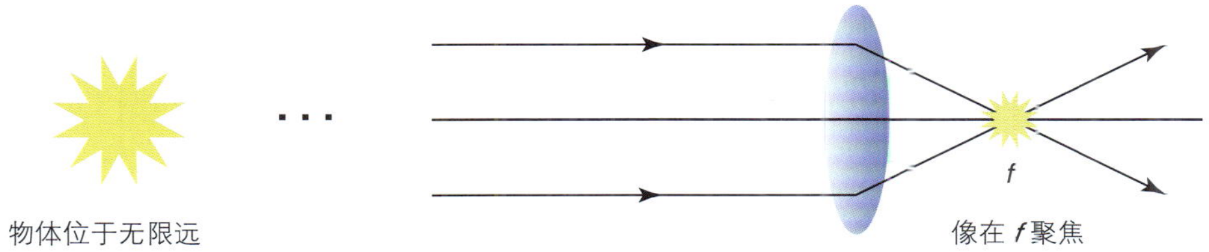

图 I–8 通过简单的凸透镜对无限远的物体（如恒星）进行成像。从透镜到像的距离为 f，即透镜的焦距；透镜的焦度 $P = 1/f$，其中 P 的单位是屈光度（D），相当于 m^{-1}。

组合透镜

如果 2 个（薄）透镜（如焦度为 P_1 和 P_2）彼此紧邻放置，将它们视为单个复合透镜系统，则 2 个透镜的总焦度近似于组成透镜的焦度之和：$P = P_1 + P_2$。这个总和是对透镜焦度倒数描述的结果。

例 I –1

如果 2 个凸透镜的焦度为 $P_1 = 1.0D$，$P_2 = 4.0D$，将其组合并视为一个单元，那么这个组合透镜将遥远恒星的图像形成在哪里？

$$P = P_1 + P_2 = 1.0D + 4.0D = 5.0D = 1/f$$

因此，$f = 1 / P = 0.20$ m，即透镜右侧 20 cm 处是遥远恒星像的位置。

例 I –2

将图像移近透镜，若将例 I–1 中的像移近 2.0 cm = 0.02 m，使其更靠近复合透镜，可以通过增加第 3 个凸透镜来实现。因为我们希望得到 $f = 0.18$ m 的结果，$P = 1/f = 1/0.18$ m = 5.55 D = $P_1 + P_2 + P_3$。因此，$P_3 = 0.55D$。这是一般方法的示例：将凸透镜增加到透镜系统中，通常会使位于透镜右侧的像更靠近透镜系统。

近物体成像：聚散度和聚散度方程

如果发光物体位于凸透镜左侧、为有限但大于焦距 f 的距离时，则所成像将比无限远的物体所成的像更靠近透镜的右侧，如恒星。从透镜到发光物体的距离被称为*物距*；从透镜到像的距离被称为*像距*。假设发光物体和像都是在空气中，则像位置的公式是

$$U + P = V$$

where $U = 1/u$ is the *vergence* of the object at a distance u to the left of the lens, P is the power of the lens, and $V = 1/v$ is the vergence of the light emerging from the lens to form the image at distance v to the right of the lens (Figure I-9). Note: In this *vergence equation*, distances to the LEFT of the lens are treated as *negative numbers* (so, in this situation, $u< 0$). The vergence, $U = 1/u$, of an object to the left of a lens is likewise a negative number. Distances to the RIGHT of a lens, and thus, in this case, the image vergence $V = 1/v$, are considered positive. In this context, it is important to keep track of the *sign* of the power of a convex lens as a *positive number* as well. Objects infinitely far from the lens generate beams of light that reach the lens with a vergence of $V = 1/\infty=0$.

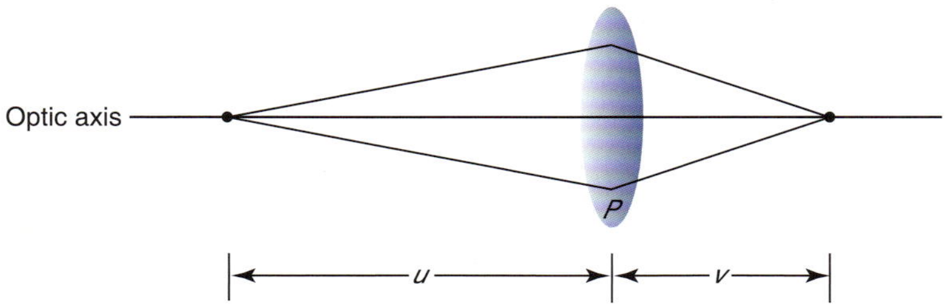

Figure I-9 The vergence equation: the object distance is u, the image distance is v, and the power of the lens is P.

EXAMPLE I-3

A lens of power P = +3.0D images an object at position u = –1.0 m to the left of the lens as follows:

$U + P = V$: 1/(–1.0 m) + (+3.0D) = + 2.0D = V, so v = 1/V = +0.50 m =50 cm,

measured to the right of the lens.

EXAMPLE I-4

Moving the source object closer to the lens: if the object in Example I-3 is moved closer to the lens (but not closer than the focal length f = 1/P)— say, to a location –0.50 m to the left of the lens—then

$U + P = V$: 1/(–0.50 m) + (+3.0D) = –2.0D + 3.0D= +1.00, so v = 1/V =+1.0 m.

That is, moving the source object closer to the lens shifts the image away from the lens on the other side.This, too, is a general method. What happens if you move the source object farther to the left of the lens?

其中，$U = 1/u$是在透镜左侧距离为u处的物的聚散度，P是透镜的焦度，$V = 1/v$是像的聚散度，像成在透镜右侧时，像距为v（图 I–9）。注：在聚散度方程中，将透镜**左侧**的距离视为负数（因此，$u<0$）。透镜左侧物体的聚散度 $U = 1/u$ 同样是负数。将透镜**右侧**的距离视为正数，像的聚散度 $V = 1/v$。在这种情况下，重要的是将凸透镜焦度的*符号*保持为*正数*。距透镜无限远的物体形成的光束到达透镜时，其聚散度为 $V = 1/\infty = 0$。

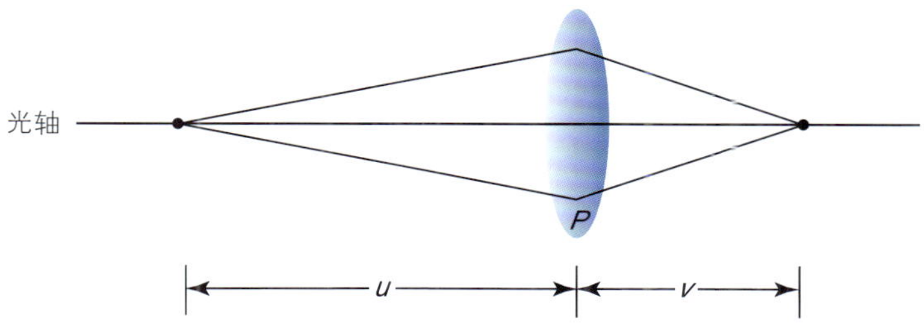

图 I–9　聚散度方程：物距为 u，像距为 v，透镜焦度为 P。

例 I –3

透镜焦度 $P = +3.0$D 的透镜，对透镜左侧 $u = -1.0$ m 处的物体进行成像，如下所示：

$U + P = V$: 1/(–1.0 m) + (+3.0D) = + 2.0D = V, 所以 v = 1/V = +0.50 m =50 cm，

测量到透镜右侧。

例 I –4

将发光物体移近透镜，如果将例 I–3 中的物体移近透镜（但不要超过焦距 $f = 1/P$）——距离透镜左侧 –0.50m 处，则

$U + P = V$: 1/(–0.50 m) + (+3.0D) = –2.0D + 3.0D= +1.00, 所以 v = 1/V =+1.0 m。

也就是说，将发光物体移近透镜会使像远离透镜。这也是一种通用的方法。如果将发光物体移动到透镜左侧，将会发生什么?

Concave Lenses

Concave lenses do not by themselves form images, but they can be used to shift an image away (to the right) from an existing lens or lens system.

A (spherical) concave lens will cause light from an infinitely distant object to diverge. If these divergent rays are extended back toward the light source (eg, to the left of the lens for a source object to the left), they will intersect at a "virtual" focal point—say, at a distance f to the left of the lens (Figure I-10). In keeping with the sign conventions above, the power of this lens is given by $P = 1/f$ (with f in meters). Here, f is a *negative* number, and the power of the concave lens is likewise a *negative* number.

Concave lenses can be combined with other immediately adjacent lenses. The power of such a lens system follows the same simple addition formula that we introduced for convex lenses:

$$P = P_1 + P_2$$

where, now, we must track the algebraic signs carefully.

EXAMPLE I-5

A lens of power $P1$ = + 4.0D will form the image of a source object at location u = –0.5 m as follows: the object vergence is U = –2.0; the image vergence is –2.0D + 4.0D = +2.0D, so the image location is v = 1/(+2.0D)=+0.50 m to the right of the lens. If a concave lens of power P_2 = –1.0D is placed adjacent to the +4.0D lens, the combination has a power of P =+4.0D + (–1.0D) = +3.0D.The image vergence is then V = –2.0D + 3.0D =+1.0D, so the image location is v = 1/(+1.0D) = +1.0 m.That is, adding the "minus" lens to the optical system has shifted the image from +0.50 m to the right of the lens to a new location, +1.0 m to the right of the lens.This example illustrates a common method.

Summary Thus Far

Starting with an object a finite distance to the left of a convex lens that is strong enough to form an image to the right of the lens (that is, with a focal length f shorter than the object distance), there are 2 ways to move the image to the left (closer to the lens): by moving the object to the LEFT or by adding an additional convex lens to the lens system. Similarly, there are 2 ways to move the image to the right (farther from the lens): by moving the object to the RIGHT (so long as it remains farther from the lens than the focal length) or by adding a concave lens to the system.

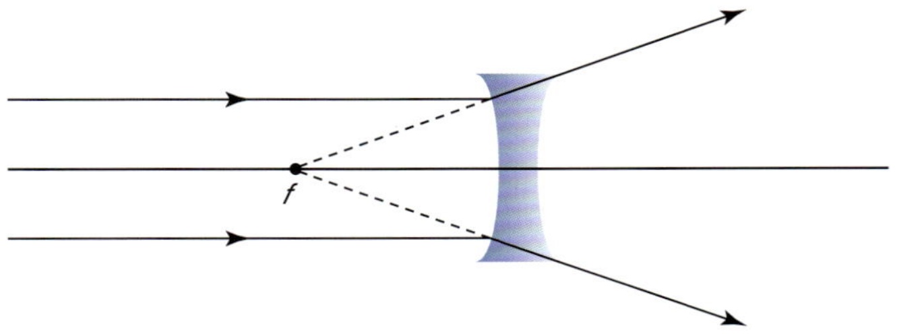

Figure I-10 Formation of a virtual image of an object infinitely far away to the left of the lens by a concave lens. The focal point is to the left of the lens; the focal length is a negative number, and the power of the lens $P = 1/f$ is likewise negative.

凹透镜

凹透镜本身不成像，但可将像从透镜或透镜系统中移开（向右）。

凹透镜（球形）会使无限远处物体的光发散。如果这些发散光线向后朝光源的方向延伸（如发光物体向左延伸到透镜的左侧），它们将在“虚”焦点处相交，即在透镜左侧距离 f 处相交（图 I–10）。根据上述符号约定，该透镜的焦度 $P= 1/f$（以 m 为单位）。这里的 f 是负数，凹透镜的焦度同样也是负数。

凹透镜可与其直接相邻的镜片组合。这种透镜系统的焦度与凸透镜的公式相同：

$P = P_1 + P_2$

须注意代数符号。

例 I –5

焦度 P_1 = + 4.0D 的透镜，在位置 u = –0.5m 处形成发光物体的像如下：物体的聚散度为 U = –2.0，像的聚散度为 –2.0D + 4.0D = + 2.0D，因此像的位置为 v=1 /（ + 2.0D ）= 透镜右侧 +0.50m。如果焦度 P_2 = –1.0D 的凹透镜与 + 4.0D 的透镜相邻放置，则该组合的焦度为 P =– 4.0D +（ –1.0D ）= + 3.0D，像的聚散度则为 V = –2.0D + 3.0D =–1.0D，因此像的位置为 v = 1 /（ + 1.0D ）= +1.0 m。也就是说，将“负”透镜添加到光学系统已将像从 +0.50 m 移动到透镜右侧的一个新的位置——透镜右侧 +1.0m 处。这个例子说明了一种常用的方法。

小结

凸透镜左侧有限距离的物体，在透镜右侧成像（即焦距 f 小于物距），有 2 种方式移动左侧的像（靠近透镜）：将物体移向**左侧**，或通过在透镜系统中添加额外的凸透镜。同样的，有 2 种方法可以将像向右移动（远离透镜）：将物体移动到**右侧**（只要离透镜的距离远于焦距），或者向系统添加凹透镜。

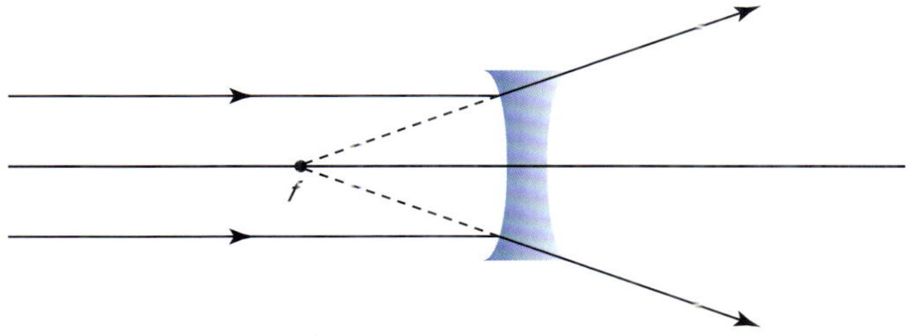

图 I–10 透镜左侧无限远的物体通过凹透镜形成的虚像。焦点位于透镜的左侧，焦距是负数，透镜的焦度 P = 1 / f 同样也是负的。

Images in Denser Media

If the light leaving a lens travels in a medium in which the speed of light is less than its speed in air, such as a watery tissue like the aqueous or vitreous humor of the eye, we must modify the image vergence term in the vergence equation. Here

$$V = \eta/v$$

where η is the *refractive index* of the denser medium: the ratio of the speed of light in a vacuum (or air—they are nearly the same) to the speed of light in the "denser" medium. The refractive index is always a number greater than 1.00, as light travels more slowly in dense media than in air. For the watery tissues in the eye, the value $\eta = 1.33$ is a useful approximation. (This casual use of the term "denser" has nothing to do with the specific gravity of the medium!)

EXAMPLE I-6

A nominal value for the power of the human cornea is $P = 44$ D. We can calculate the location of the image of a distant star formed by such a cornea in an aphakic eye (an eye with no lens): $U + P = V$, so 0 + 44 D = 1.33/v, or v = 1.33/44 m = 0.0302 m = 30.2 mm. (Since the typical human eye has an axial length of about 24 mm, the need for additional refracting power after removal of the crystalline lens is evident!)

A Very Much Simplified Model Eye

We now have in hand the tools to illustrate the correction of simple axial refractive errors, which arise from a mismatch between the optical power of the anterior segment (cornea and crystalline lens) and the axial length of the eye.

Emmetropia

Suppose that all the refracting power of the eye is concentrated at a single plane, at the apex of the cornea, and assume the typical axial length of 24.0 mm. If this ultra-simplified model eye is to focus light from distant objects on the retina (Figure I–11A)—the power at the corneal apex must be given by the vergence equation: $0 + P = 1.33/0.024$ m = 55.42 D. [The actual total nominal power of the human eye is in fact about 60D, so our simplistic model is off by only about 10%.]

Myopia

Now suppose that our eye has the standard anterior segment with optical power 55.42 D but is 1.0 mm longer than normal—so the axial length is 25.0 mm. In such an eye, which is said to be *myopic*, light from a distant point source comes to a focus where the retina "should have been" (Figure I-11B); then the rays cross and continue for another millimeter before they form an (annoying) blur-circle on the retina. To correct the refractive error, we must shift the image location 1.0 mm toward the back of the eye. This can be done, say, with a concave (diverging, "minus" power) contact lens of power P placed adjacent to the corneal apex according to the vergence equation: $0 + (P + 55.42$ D) = 1.33/0.025 D =+53.20D. Thus, the power of the required contact lens is P = 53.20D – 55.42 D = –2.22 D.[In a more precise calculation, the correction would be about –3 D for each millimeter of excess axial length.]

光密介质中的像

如果离开透镜的光在一种介质，如眼睛的房水或玻璃体的水状组织中传播，光在其中的速度小于在空气中的速度，则聚散度方程中的像聚散度为

$V = \eta / v$。

其中 η 是光密介质的*折射率*：真空（或空气——几乎与真空相同）中的光速与“光密”介质中的光速之比。折射率总是大于 1.00，因为光在光密介质中的传播比在空气中更慢。眼睛中的水样组织，η= 1.33 是一个近似值。（“光密”一词与介质的比重无关！）

例 I –6

人的角膜屈光力是 P = 44 D。计算远处恒星经过无晶状体眼（没有晶状体的眼睛）的角膜形成的像位置：$U + P = V$，所以 0 + 44 D = 1.33 / v，或 v = 1.33 / 44 m = 0.0302 m = 30.2 mm。（由于人眼的轴向长度约为 24 mm，因此在去除晶状体后需要有额外的屈光力！）

简化模型眼

我们现在有工具，用于阐明单纯轴性屈光不正的矫正，屈光不正是由于前段（角膜和晶状体）的光学屈光力与眼睛的轴向长度不匹配引起的。

正视

假设眼睛的所有屈光力都集中在角膜顶点的单一平面上，轴向长度为 24.0 mm。如果这个简化模型眼将远处物体的光线聚焦在视网膜上（图 I–11A）——角膜顶点的屈光力须由聚散度方程给出：0 + P = 1.33 / 0.024 m = 55.42 D。人眼的实际总体屈光力约为 60D，因此我们的简化模型仅减少了约 10%。

近视

假设我们的眼睛有标准的前段，屈光力为 55.42 D，但比正常长度长 1.0 mm——轴长为 25.0 mm。在这种被认为是*近视*的眼睛中，来自远点的光进入“应该”在视网膜的焦点（图 I–11B），然后光线交叉，并继续前行 1mm，在视网膜上形成一个（恼人的）模糊圈。要矫正这种屈光不正，必须将像的位置移向眼睛后方的 1.0mm 处。例如，根据聚散度方程式，可以使用邻近角膜顶点放置的屈光力 P 的凹透镜接触镜（发散，“负的”）：0 +（F + 55.42 D）= 1.33 /0.025 D =+53.20D。因此，所需接触镜的屈光力为 P = 53.20D – 55.42 D = –2.22 D。在更精确的计算中，当轴向长度每超出 1mm 时，矫正量大约为 –3D。

Hyperopia

Similarly, if the axial length of our ultra-simplified model eye were reduced by 1.0 mm, distant objects would form an image behind the retina (Figure I-11C). Such an eye is *hyperopic*. The required contact lens power would be given by the vergence equation: 0 + (P + 55.42 D] = 1.33/0.023 m = +57.83 D, or P = +57.83 D – 55.42 D = +2.41 D, a convex"plus" lens.

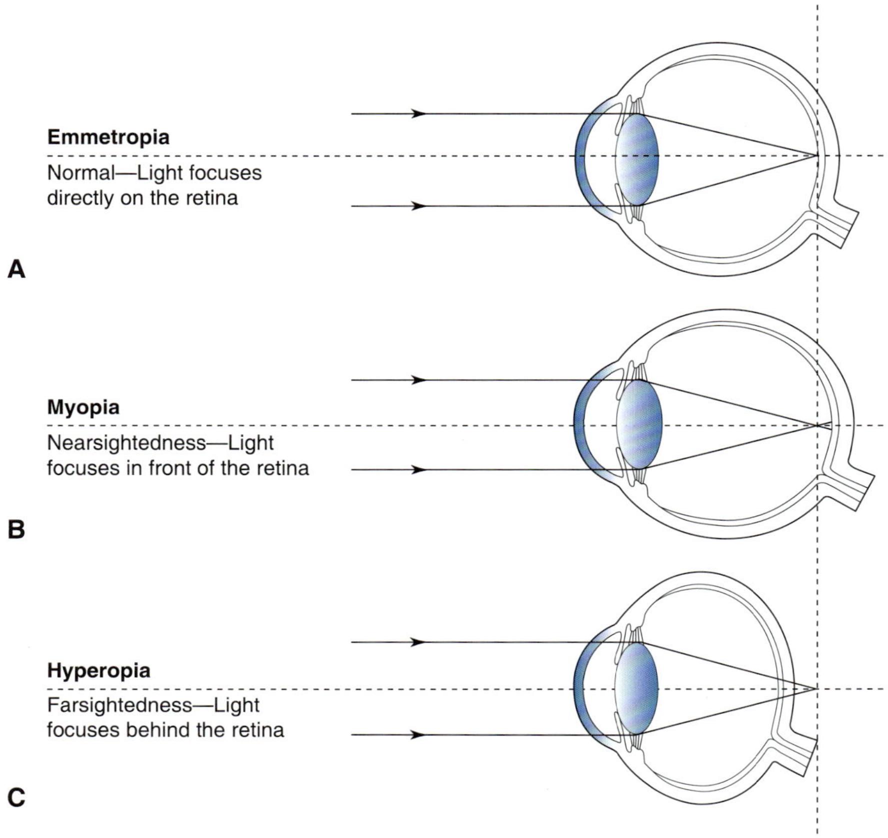

Figure I-11 The position of light rays focusing. **A**, The normal eye. **B**, A myopic eye. **C**, A hyperopic eye. (Illustration developed by Scott E. Brodie, MD.)

> *Thus, correction of axial refractive errors requires only the determination of the optimal spherical lens power needed to re-focus the light from a distant source on the retina.*

Astigmatism

In addition to the axial refractive errors discussed previously, it is necessary to deal with refracting surfaces that lack circular symmetry, which allows spherical lenses to focus all the light emerging from a point source in a single image point. Consider a "toroidal" surface, such as the side of a rugby ball, an (American) football, or the outer rim of automobile tire inner tube (a torus), as in Figure I-13.

To envision the effect of such a refracting surface, called a *toric lens*, consider the curvature of the intersection of the surface with a plane that rotates about the line perpendicular to the surface at the apex (the "normal" line; see Figure I-14). The orientation of such a plane, or the intersection curve itself, is referred to as a *meridian* of the lens.

远视

同样，如果将简化模型眼的轴向长度减少 1.0mm，远处的物体会在视网膜后面成像（图 I–11C）。这样的眼睛是*远视的*。所需的接触镜屈光力将由聚散度方程给出：0 +（P + 55.42 D）= 1.33 / 0.023 m = +57.83 D，或 P = +57.83 D – 55.42 D = +2.41 D，即为“正的”凸透镜。

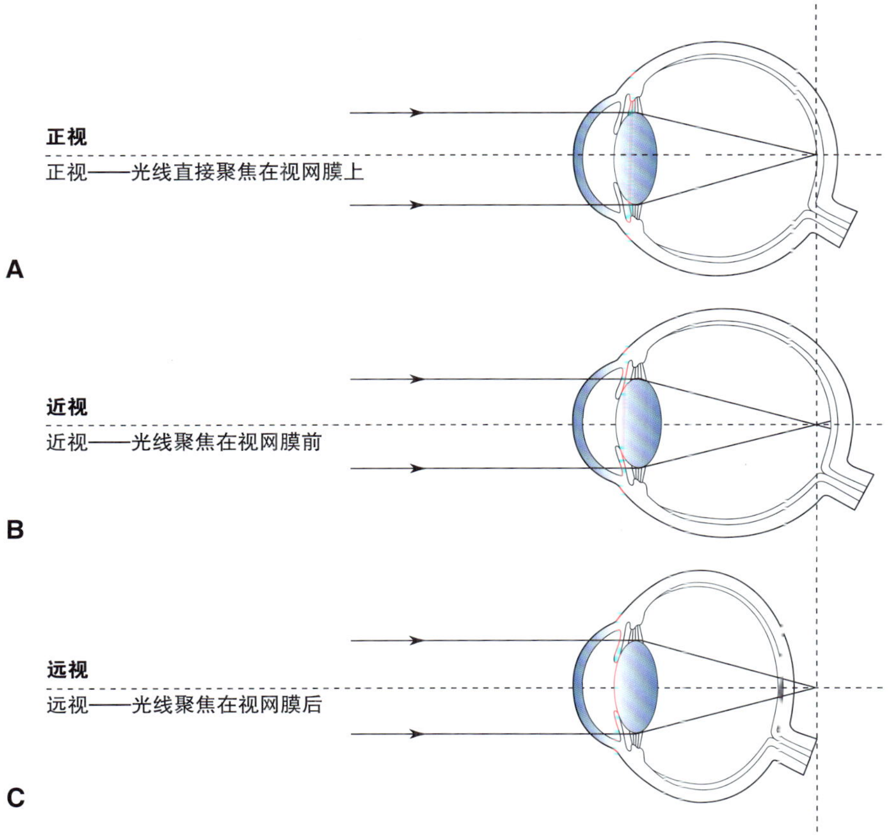

图 I–11 光线聚焦的位置。A. 正常的眼睛。B. 近视眼。C. 远视眼。*（译者注：资料来源见前页原文。）*

> *因此，对于轴向屈光不正的矫正仅需要确定将远处光源的光重新聚焦在视网膜上所需的最佳球面透镜的屈光力。*

散光

除了前面讨论的轴性屈光不正之外，还必须研究非圆形对称的屈光面，使球镜将点光源发出的所有光聚焦在单个像点中。假想一个“环形”表面，例如橄榄球（美式足球）的一侧，或汽车轮胎内胎（圆环）的外缘，如图 I–13 所示。

为了理解这种称为*复曲面镜*的屈光面效果，我们设想一个与平面相交的弯曲面，该平面围绕垂直于顶点表面的直线（“法线”，见图 I–14）旋转。将这种平面的方向或交叉曲线本身称为透镜的*子午线*。

Try It Yourself! I-1

1. Find a "trial lens set" with an assortment of + and – spherical lenses. (The signs of the lenses will be indicated on the handles or by the color of the lens frames). Work in groups of 3: 1 person should hold up a small light source (a penlight or the Finoff transilluminator on your instrument stand will work well); a second person should hold the lens or lenses at least 2 or 3 meters away; the third person should hold a small white card, which will serve as a screen to catch the images of the light formed by the lenses (Figure I-12). Start with, say, a +2.0D sphere lens, and find the image (a small, round dot of light) about 66 cm farther away from the light source than the lens. (Why is the image not exactly 50 cm from the lens? Because your colleague holding the penlight is not infinitely far away!)
2. Move the light source closer to the lens, and find the new image: it will be farther away from the lens.
3. If you have the room, move the light source farther away from the lens than in step 1, and locate the new image: it will be closer to the lens than when you started.
4. Returning to the set-up in step 1, add a second + sphere lens (say, +1.0D) and hold the lenses together to act as a single lens system. Locate the image: it will be closer to the lenses than when you started.
5. Remove the additional +1.0D lens, and replace it with a –1.0D lens. Now locate the image: it will be farther away from the lenses than when you started.
6. Compare the location of the image formed by your +2.0D and +1.0D lens combination with the location of the image formed by the actual +3.0D lens from the trial set. They should agree closely.
7. Try comparing the +2.0D and –1.0D combination with an actual +1.0 lens.
8. Verify this "lens arithmetic" with other combinations of +and/or – lenses.

A net minus lens will not form an image; the white card will show only a dimmer circle of light inside the shadow of the frame than outside it. Why? (Because the minus lens diverges light, reducing the intensity of the illumination/cm^2 of the light that passes through it.)

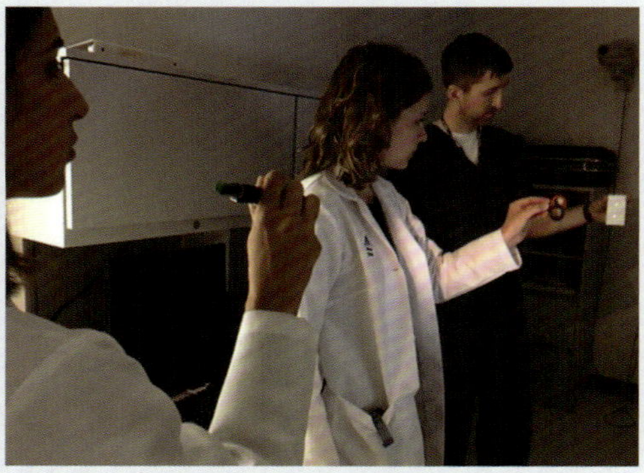

Figure I-12 Three residents forming a "human optical bench." One holds a penlight, the second compares a +3.00D sphere with a +4.00D sphere held together with a –1.00D sphere, and the third holds a small white card. Notice that the images on the white card are the same. *(Courtesy of Scott E. Brodie, MD, PhD.)*

试一试！ I–1

1. 按顺序排列的 + 球镜片和 – 球镜片的 “试镜箱”。（在手柄上或通过透镜框的颜色即可分类。）3 个人一组：第 1 个人举起 1 个小光源（笔灯或工作台的 Finoff 透照灯）；第 2 个人站在 2~3m 处持 1 个透镜；第 3 个人拿 1 张白色卡片，作为屏幕来获得经透镜成的像（图 I–12）。先从一个 +2.0D 球镜开始，找到离光源比透镜更远，距透镜 66c m 处的像，（一个小的圆形光点）。（为什么像距离透镜不到 50cm？因为手里拿着的笔灯不在无限远处！）

2. 将光源移近透镜，找到新像：它将离透镜更远。

3. 如果有空间，将光源移到离透镜更远的地方，比步骤 1 更远，并定位新像：它将比开始时更靠近透镜。
4. 返回步骤 1 中的设置，添加第 2 个 + 透镜（如 + 1.0D），并将透镜固定在一起，作为单透镜系统。定位像：它比开始时更接近透镜。

5. 取出添加的 +1.0D 透镜，并用 –1.0D 透镜更换。定位像：它将比开始时离透镜更远。
6. 将 + 2 .0D 和 +1.0D 透镜组合所形成的像位置与 +3.0D 透镜形成的像位置进行比较，两者应该一致。

7. 尝试将 +2.00D 透镜和 –1.0D 透镜组合，并与实际的 +1.0D 透镜进行比较。
8. 用 + 透镜和（或）– 透镜等其他组合验证这个‘透镜算数法”。

单纯的负透镜不会成像。白色卡片将会形成一个比外面更暗的光圈。（为什么？因为负透镜可以使光发散，降低了通过它的单位面积（/cm²）上的光照强度。）

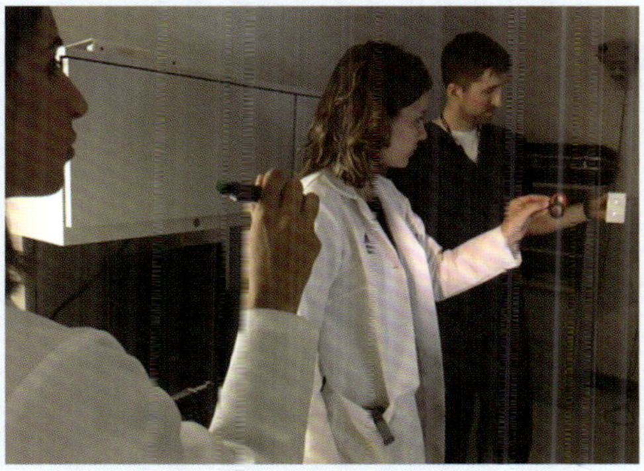

图 I–12 3 个人组成一个“人类光学工作站”。1 个人拿着笔灯，第 2 个人比较 +3.00D 球镜和 +4.00D 球镜联合 –1.00D 球镜，第 3 个人拿着白色卡片。请注意，白色卡片上的图像是相同的。*（由 Scott E. Brodie 医学博士，哲学博士提供。）*

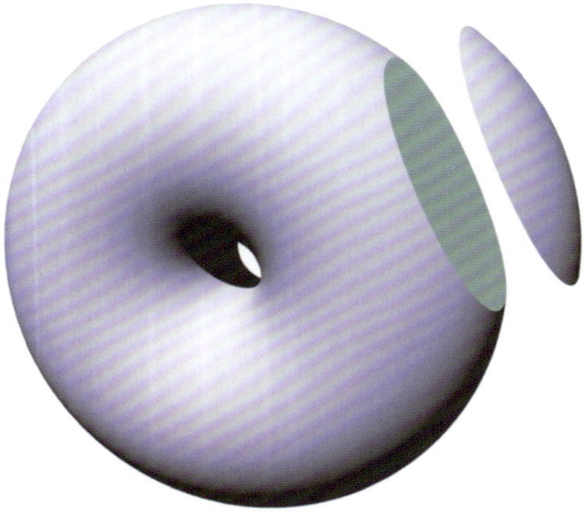

Figure I-13 The outer rim of a torus forms a toric surface. *(Illustration by Ir. H. Hahn, from Creative Commons.)*

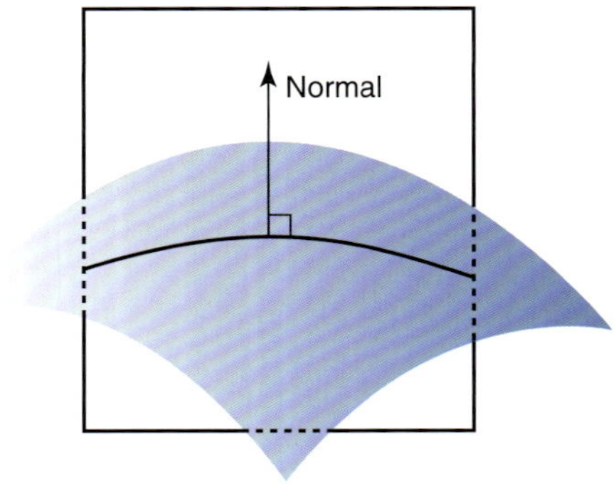

Figure I-14 A normal plane intersecting a toric surface. The curvature of the curve where the plane intersects the surface will vary with the orientation of the plane about the perpendicular to the apex. Each such curve is a meridian of the surface at that point.

As this normal plane rotates, the curvature of the intersection varies, from a flattest meridian to a steepest meridian, 90° away (Figure I-15).

Light rays from a distant point source that land on the steepest meridian are refracted as if they encountered a spherical lens of the same curvature. Light rays that land on the flattest meridian are refracted as if they encountered a spherical lens with less dioptric power. Thus, the focal length varies with the choice of meridian, and the toroidal surface does not image the light from a single point source at a single image point. This situation is referred to as *astigmatism*, from the Latin for "absence" of a (single) point, or focus (Figure I-16).

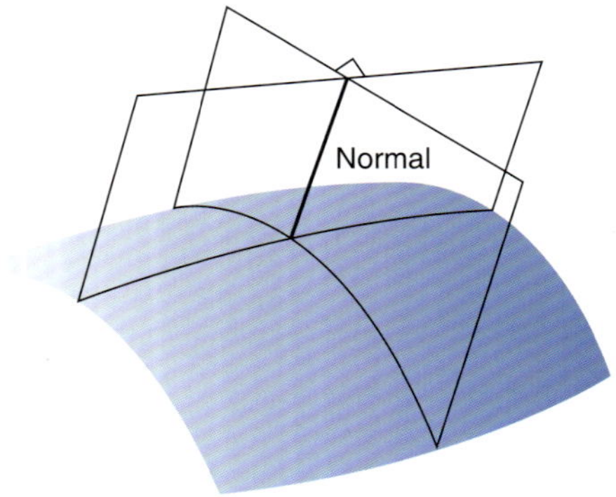

Figure I-15 Variation of the curvature of a toric surface along 2 different meridians. The meridians for which the curvature is minimal or maximal are 90° apart.

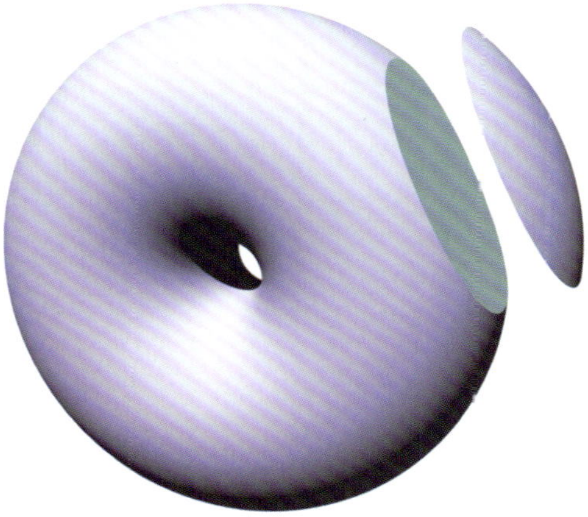

图 I–13 圆环的外缘形成复曲面。*（译者注：资料来源见前页原文。）*

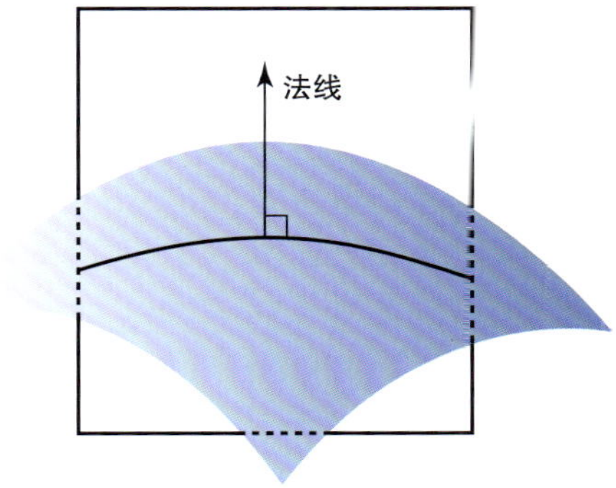

图 I–14 与复曲面相交的法线平面。平面与表面相交，曲线的曲率将随着平面围绕与顶点垂直的方向而变化。每条这样的曲线都是该点表面的子午线。

当这个法线平面旋转时，交叉点的曲率从最平坦的子午线到最陡的子午线，变化 90°（图 I–15）。

光从远处的点光源发出，在最陡子的午线上被折射时，就好像它们遇到相同曲率的球面透镜一样。在最平坦的子午线上的被折射时，就像它们遇到具有较小屈光力的球面透镜一样。因此，焦距随子午线的不同而变化，不能聚集于一点（焦点），也就不能形成清晰的物像。这种情况被称为*散光*，来自拉丁语的“缺席”（单一）或焦点（图 I–16）。

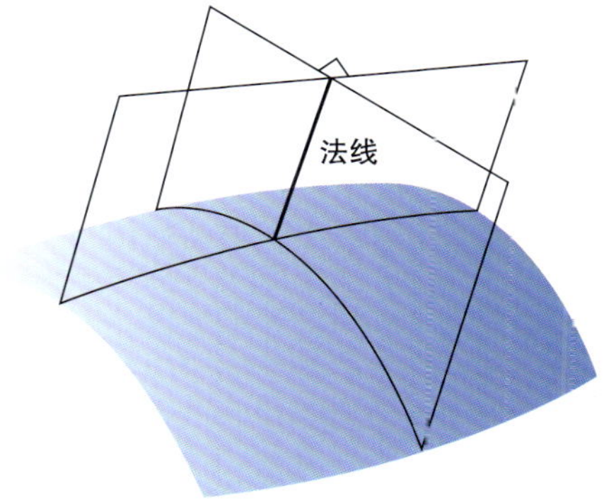

图 I–15 沿 2 个不同子午线的复曲面曲率的变化。曲率最小或最大的子午线相差 90°。

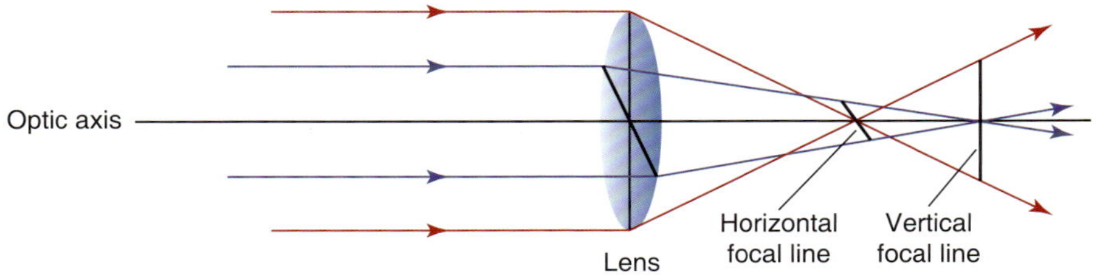

Figure I-16 Astigmatic image formation by a toric surface. In this example, light rays that land on the horizontal meridian (ie, rays shown in blue) reach a focus farther from the lens than rays that land on the vertical meridian (ie, rays shown in red).

The flattest and steepest meridians lie 90° apart from each other; they are known as *principal meridians*. We can keep track of this situation by drawing a *power cross*, which shows the orientation of the steepest and flattest meridians, and indicates their respective refractive powers (Figure I-17).

In practice, it is often convenient to emphasize the *difference* in the refractive powers of the principal meridians. In this case, we can interpret the refracting surface as the combination of a spherical refracting surface, which refracts equally in all directions, and a purely "cylindrical" refracting surface, with maximal power corresponding to one of the directions indicated in the power cross (and no refracting power in the orthogonal direction). Thus, for example, a lens with a power of +1.00D horizontally and + 2.00D vertically could be described as the combination of a spherical lens with power +1.00D and a cylindrical lens with power +1.00D in the vertical direction. This is notated +1.00 ⊂ +1.00 @ 90°. Alternatively, the same refracting surface could be described as a spherical lens with power +2.00D combined with a cylindrical lens with power -1.00D acting in the 180° meridian, notated +2.00 ⊂ −1.00 @ 180°.

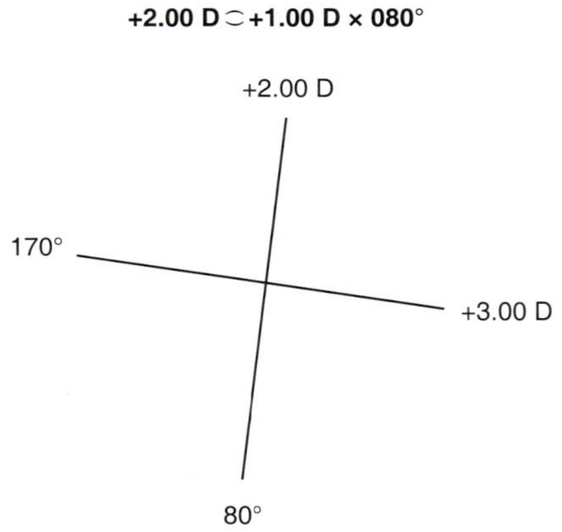

Figure I-17 Power–cross representation of a toric lens with slightly oblique axes. The meridians with maximal and minimal power are shown.

Indeed, we can realize such lenses in practice by combining spherical lenses with actual lenses with cylindrical surfaces, either convex ("plus cylinders") or concave ("minus cylinders); see Figure I-18. These can be found in standard trial lens sets.

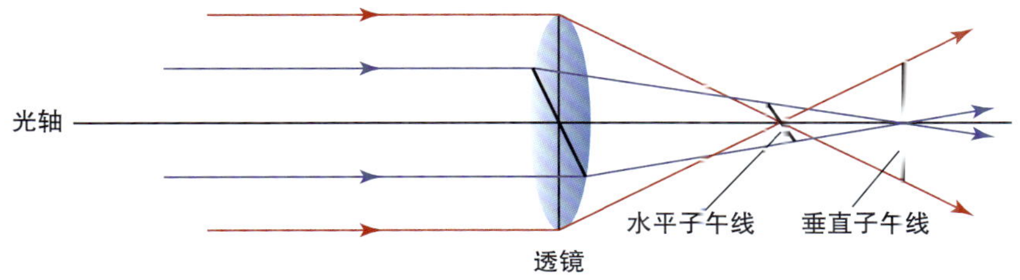

图 I–16 由复曲面表面形成的散光像。在该示例中，落在水平子午线上的光线（即以蓝色表示的光线）比落在垂直子午线上的光线（即以红色表示的光线）能到达更远离透镜的焦点。

最平坦与最陡的子午线相互垂直，称为*主子午线*。我们可以通过绘制一个*焦度十字*来示意这种情况：标出最陡和最平坦的子午线的方向，并给出各自的焦度（图 I–17）。

在实践中，通常以主子午线的焦度表示这种焦度的*差异*。在这种情况下，可以将折射表面理解为在所有方向上均匀折射的球状屈光面和纯粹的"柱形"屈光表面的组合，后者对应了焦度十字方向上的最大焦度（并且在正交方向上没有屈光力）。例如，水平 +1.00D、垂直 + 2.00D 的透镜可被描述为垂直方向焦度为 +1.00D 的球镜和垂直方向焦度为 +1.00D 的柱镜，可记录为 +1.00 ⊃ +1.00 @ 90°。或者相同的折射表面可描述为在 180° 子午线方向 –2.00D 的球镜联合 –1.00D 的柱镜，记录为 +2.00 ⊃ –1.00 @ 180°。

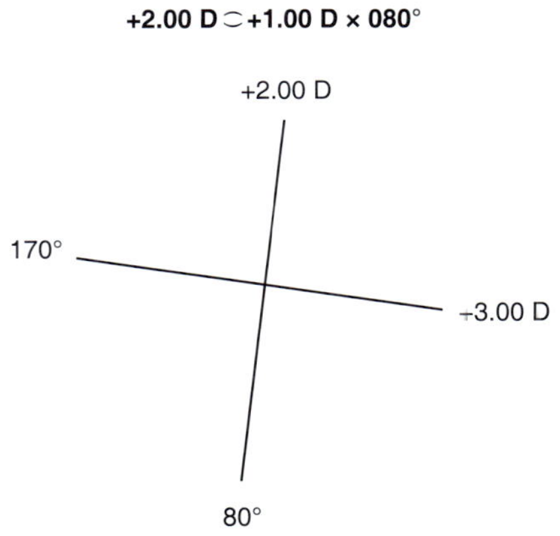

图 I–17 伴有轻微倾斜轴的复曲面透镜的焦度十字表达方法。子午线显示出了最大和最小焦度。

实际上，在实践中可以通过将球镜与具有圆柱形表面的透镜相结合来形成这种透镜，这里所述的圆柱形表面是凸面（正圆柱体）或凹面（负圆柱体）的，见图 I–18。这些可以在标准试镜箱中找到。

These cylindrical lenses are marked to indicate the orientation of the original axis of the glass cylinder from which the cylindrical surface was derived. The refracting power of such a cylindrical lens acts in the direction *perpendicular* to the orientation of the cylinder axis. For example, we obtain a plus cylinder lens with power +1.00D along the horizontal meridian by slicing the surface from a glass cylinder with axis vertical. Such a glass cylinder lens is denoted +1.00 × 90°. The notation for combinations of spherical and cylindrical lenses uses the "×" symbol ("x" for "axis"). Thus, the lens described in the preceding paragraph can be realized with either a plus cylinder or minus cylinder combination: +2.00 ⊂ −1.00 × 90° or +1.00 ⊂ +1.00 × 180°.

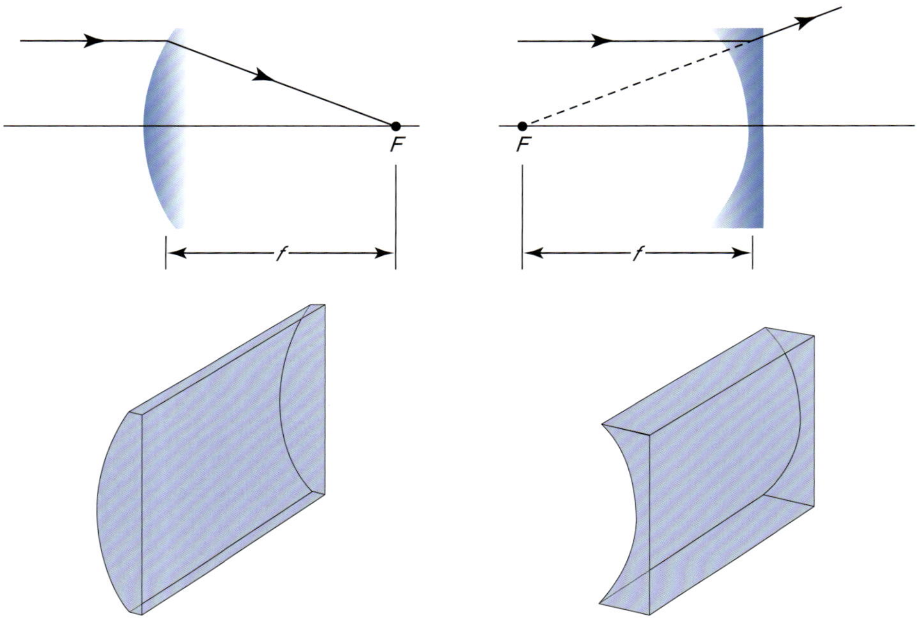

Plus cylinder lens **Minus cylinder lens**

Figure I-18 Convex (plus cylinder) and concave (minus cylinder) glass lenses.

Notice that we use the notation "@" (read "at") to denote the meridian (direction) in which a cylindrical lens exerts refractive power. That contrasts with the "×" notation (read "axis"), which indicates the orientation axis of the cylindrical lens, which will exert its refractive power 90° away from the orientation of the axis.

There are always 2 choices to describe the same toric refractive surface: (1) start with the maximal sphere power and describe the minus cylinder that provides the difference between the powers of the strongest and weakest meridians, or (2) start with the minimal sphere power and describe the plus cylinder that provides the difference between the weakest and strongest meridians. To convert from one description to the other, simply add the sphere and cylinder (keeping track of + and − signs) to determine the new sphere power, change the sign of the cylinder, and add or subtract 90° to the axis (to keep the final axis between 0° and 180°). The process of converting between the plus cylinder and minus cylinder descriptions of a toric lens is referred to as *transposition*. This duality occurs in every context where we consider toric lenses.

标记这些柱镜，可以提示玻璃圆柱体的原始轴线方向，而圆柱形表面就是从该原始轴线导出的。这种柱镜的屈光力作用在*垂直于*圆柱轴向的方向。例如，我们通过垂直轴向切割圆柱体来获得水平子午线具有 +1.00D 屈光力的正柱镜。将这种柱镜记录为 +1.00 × 90° 。球面和柱面透镜组合的符号使用“×”符号（“x”表示“轴”）。因此，前一节中描述的透镜可以用正圆柱或负圆柱联合来表示：+2.00⊃ −1.00 × 90° 或 +1.00⊃ +1.00 × 180° .

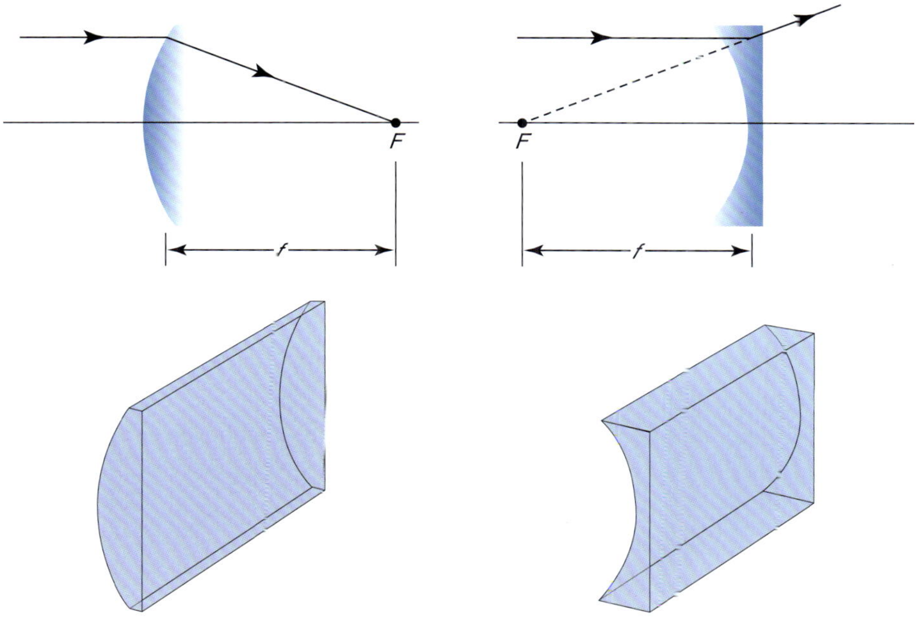

图 I–18 凸面（正圆柱体）和凹面（负圆柱体）玻璃透镜。

请注意，我们使用符号“@”（读作“at”）来表示柱镜屈光力的子午线（方向）。这与符号“×”（读作“轴”）相反，后者表示柱镜的轴向，使其折射力与轴的方向形成 90° 。

描述相同的复曲面有 2 种方法：用最大球镜联合最强和最弱屈光力子午线之差的负柱镜来描述，或者用最小球镜联合最弱和最强屈光力子午线之差的正柱镜来描述。要将一种记录方法转换为另一种记录方法述，只需增加球镜和柱镜（改变 + 和 – 符号）并确定新的球镜度数，更改圆柱体的符号，轴向增加或减去 90° （以保持最终轴在 0° 和 180° 之间）。在复曲面镜的正柱镜和负柱镜之间进行转换的过程被称为*换应*。这和二元性发生在复曲面透镜的每个环节中。

Try It Yourself! I-2

Set up a "human optical bench" as before:

1. Start with a +3.00D sphere lens and locate the image, perhaps about 40 cm from the lens.
2. Add to this a +1.00D cylinder lens, with the axis marks placed horizontally. Observe that this added lens distorts the focal point located in the previous step into a vertical focal line.
3. Gradually move the card closer to the lenses. Observe that the focal line continuously deforms into an ellipse, further rounds up into a circle (the "circle of least confusion"), then gradually deforms into an ellipse (with horizontal major axis) and ultimately into a horizontal focal line.
4. Compare the location of this horizontal focal line to the location of the point image formed by a +4.00D sphere lens. (They should agree.)
5. Starting again with the +3.00D sphere lens of step 1, now add a −1.00D cylinder, again with axis horizontal. The original focal point will again be distorted into a vertical focal line, but now the circle of least confusion will lie farther from the lenses, and the horizontal focal line will be found even farther still.
6. Verify that this horizontal focal line coincides with the location of the point image formed by a +2.00D sphere lens.
7. Compare the focal lines formed by a +4.00D sphere together with a −1.00D cylinder, axis horizontal, to those formed by a +3.00D sphere together with a +1.00D cylinder, axis vertical. (They should agree— these 2 spherocylinder combinations are transpositions of each other.)
8. Compare the image formed by combining 2 +3.00D cylinders, 1 with axis horizontal and the other with axis vertical, to the image formed by a +3.00D sphere. (Be careful—you may have to hold the handles of the trial lenses slightly apart to get the axes precisely perpendicular.)

Astigmatic Refractive Errors

Astigmatic refractive errors of the human eye are not uncommon. Corneal astigmatism is most common, but lenticular astigmatism is also found. In each case, we can consider the net refractive surface as equivalent to a spherical component with a concurrent plus cylinder astigmatic component (corresponding to the forward bulging of the cornea into the surrounding air). For example, the most common pattern of corneal astigmatism seen in younger patients, known as "with-the-rule" astigmatism, suggests a compression of the cornea by the pressure of the eyelids. This compression deforms the cornea, steepening the vertical meridian and flattening the horizontal meridian. This acts as a plus cylinder lens with axis horizontal (Figure I-19).

The net astigmatic error is corrected by placing a cylinder of equal power and opposite sign over the eye, with the same axis as the intrinsic cylindrical error. For example, with- the-rule astigmatism can be corrected with a minus cylinder correcting lens placed with axis horizontal (Figure I-20).

Equivalently, such a refractive error can be corrected by placing a plus cylinder lens with axis vertical, and then compensating with a corresponding reduction in the power of the spherical component.

试一试！ I–2

像以前一样建立一个“人类光学工作台”：

1. 从 +3.00D 球面透镜开始，找到距离透镜大约 40cm 的像。

2. 再添加一个 +1.00D 圆柱透镜，轴标记在水平位置。观察到这个添加的透镜将步骤 1 中的焦点变成了垂直焦线。

3. 逐渐将卡纸移近透镜。观察到焦线连续变形成为椭圆状，再过一步向上变为圆圈（“最小弥散圆”），接着再逐渐变形成为椭圆状（具有水平长轴），并最终变成水平焦线。

4. 将该水平焦线的位置与由 +4.00D 球面透镜形成的点像的位置进行比较。（应该一致。）

5. 再次使用步骤 1 中的 +3.00D 球面透镜，现在再添加 1 个 –1.00D 圆柱体，同样是水平轴线。原始焦点将再次变成垂直焦线，但现在的最小弥散圆将远离透镜，并且水平焦线将在更远的地方被发现。

6. 确认此水平焦线与由 +2.00D 球面透镜形成的点像的位置一致。

7. 将由 +4.00D 球镜和 –1.00D 柱镜在水平轴向形成的焦线与由 + 3.00D 球镜和 +1.00D 柱镜在垂直轴向形成的焦线进行比较。（它们应该一致——这 2 个球柱镜组合可以彼此转换。）

8. 将由 2 个 + 3.00D 柱镜（一个为观察水平轴，另一个为观察垂直轴）成像，与由 1 个 +3.00D 球镜形成的像进行比较。（注意，可能需要将试镜的手柄稍微分开一些，以使轴向相互垂直。）

散光性屈光不正

散光在人群中并不少见。其中角膜散光是最常见的，但也有晶状体散光。在这种情况下，净屈光面相当于伴有正柱散光成分的球面（相当于角膜向前凸出到空气中）。例如，在年轻患者中最常见的角膜散光，为“顺规”散光，为眼睑对角膜的压力。这个压力使角膜变形，使角膜垂直子午线变陡、水平子午线变平，呈现出水平轴向的正柱镜状态（图 I–19）。

可以通过在眼前放置具有相同度数、相反符号的柱镜来矫正散光，其轴位应相同。例如，可以使用放置轴向水平的负柱镜矫正顺规散光（图 I–20）。

同样，可以通过放置具有垂直轴向的正柱镜来矫正这种屈光不正，然后通过相应地减小球镜度数来进行补偿。

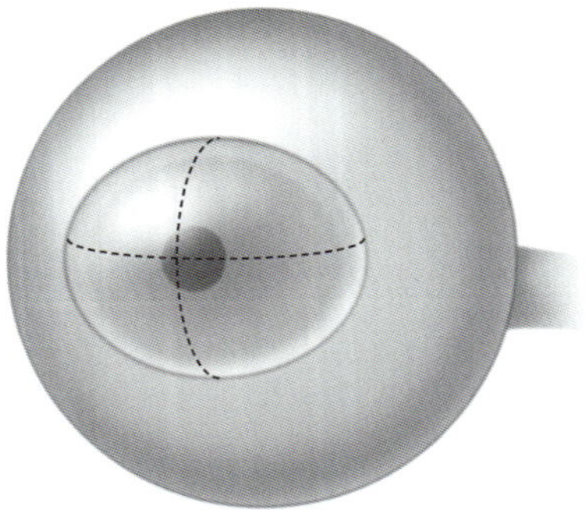

Figure I-19 Schematic drawing of an eye that has "with-the-rule" astigmatism, with horizontal flattest corneal meridian. *(Illustration developed by Scott E. Brodie, MD, PhD; original illustration by Mark Miller.)*

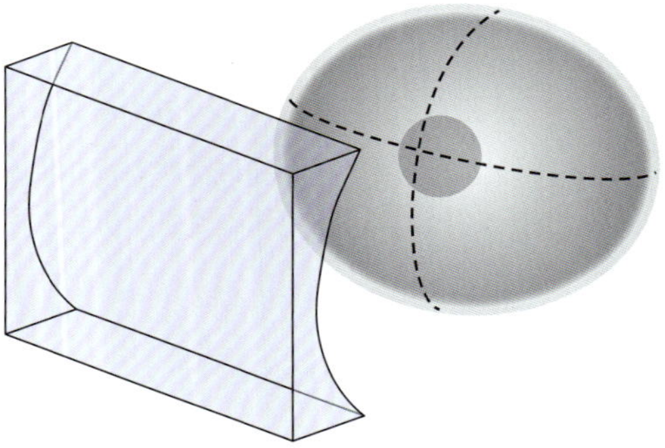

Figure I-20 Schematic illustration of correction of with the rule astigmatism with a minus cylinder lens placed with axis horizontal, to compensate for excess forward bulging of cornea with steepest axis vertical. *(Illustration developed by Scott E. Brodie, MD.)*

Thus, correction of an eye with an astigmatic refractive error requires the determination of 3 quantities: the power and axis of the correcting cylindrical component, and the power of the remaining spherical component. In practice, this task is accomplished as follows:

- Attempt to correct the eye with spherical lenses only, or at least to determine the optimal purely spherical correction.
- Determine whether there is an astigmatic component to the refractive error.
- If astigmatism is present, determine the correcting cylinder axis. This can be done even when the optimal cylindrical correcting power is not yet known.
- Determine the optimal cylindrical correcting power.
- Determine the optimal power to correct any residual spherical error.

Step-by-step instructions for this process are provided in Part 2 of this Quick-Start Guide.

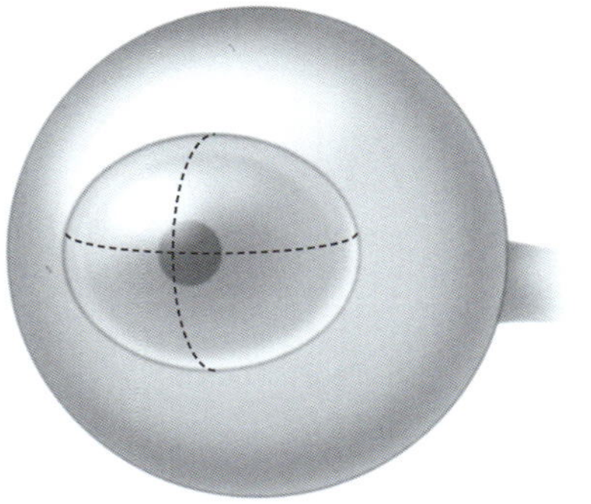

图 I–19 具有“顺规”散光的眼睛的示意图，具有水平方向最平坦的角膜子午线。*（译者注：资料来源见前页原文。）*

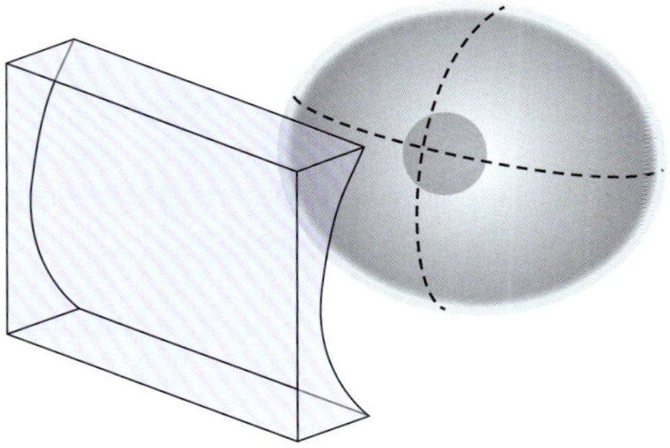

图 I–20 将负柱镜放置在水平轴位置，以补偿角膜垂直方向过度向前凸的状况，从而矫正顺规散光的示意图 *（译者注：资料来源见前页原文。）*

因此，矫正散光需要确定 3 个量：柱镜的度数、轴向以及球镜度数。实际操作步骤如下：

- 尽量用球镜矫正，或者至少要通过确定最佳的球镜度数的方法来矫正。

- 确定屈光不正是否存在散光成分。
- 如果存在散光，则应先确定柱镜轴向，即使尚不能确定最佳的柱镜度数。

- 确定最佳的柱镜度数。
- 确定纠正残余球镜的最佳度数。

本《快速入门指南》的第 2 部分提供了此过程的逐步说明。

Part 2: How to Refract

Highlights

- steps of clinical refraction
- visual acuity
- estimating refractive correction
- spherical lenses: optimal correction
- detecting astigmatism
- cylindrical lenses: optimal correction
- accommodative control and binocular balance

Glossary

Accommodation The ability of the eye to increase the optical power of the crystalline lens, allowing adjustment of focus for near objects and self-correction of hyperopic refractive errors.

Accommodative control Refraction techniques that suppress accommodation and allow determination of the refractive state with accommodation relaxed.

Asthenopic complaints Symptoms due to persistent or excessive accommodative effort.

Binary comparison Asking a patient to perform a 2-alternative forced-choice comparison of the clarity of vision with alternative lens choices; for example, ***"Which is better, '1' or '2'?"***.

Binocular balance Verification that a clinical refraction equally relaxes the accommodation of the 2 eyes.

Clinical refraction The process of measuring the refractive status of the eyes of a patient.

Fogging The use of plus lens power to blur the vision in 1 or both eyes, encouraging relaxation of accommodation; a method of accommodative control.

Jackson cross cylinder A lens with cylinders of equal and opposite power, with axes perpendicular to each other, useful for determination of optimal correcting cylinder axis and power.

Manifest refraction The measurement of refractive errors through patients' subjective descriptions of how well they can see.

Phoropter (generic: refractor) An instrument containing geared spherical and cylindrical lenses for each eye to facilitate subjective refraction.

Pinhole (or pinhole occluder) A device with a small aperture, or an array of small apertures, allowing a patient to reduce the effective aperture of the eye. If pinhole viewing clarifies a patient's vision, this suggests the presence of an uncorrected refractive error.

第 2 部分：如何验光

重点

- 临床验光的步骤。
- 视力。
- 评估屈光矫正。
- 球镜：最佳矫正。
- 检测散光。
- 柱镜：最佳矫正。
- 调节控制和双眼平衡。

术语

调节 增加晶状体的屈光力，并通过改变焦点看清近距离物体，自行矫正远视。

调节控制 通过抑制调节，使眼睛在调节放松的状态下确定其屈光状态的验光技术。

视疲劳 持续或过度的调节产生的症状。

二元比较 要求患者对配戴哪个眼镜更清晰的感受进行强制性比较，例如，*“哪个更好，‘1’或‘2’？”*

双眼平衡 确定验光使双眼调节同时达到了放松的状态。

临床验光 检测患者眼屈光状态的过程。

雾视 一种调节控制的方法，是用正透镜使单眼或双眼视物模糊，尽量放松眼睛调节的方法。

Jackson 交叉柱镜 由 2 个度数相等、符号相反的柱镜组成，其轴线彼此垂直，可用于确定矫正的最佳柱镜轴及度数。

显然 / 主观验光 是通过患者对其看到的主观描述进行屈光不正检测的方法。

综合验光仪（通常被称为验光仪）是含双眼球镜和柱镜的轮盘透镜的验光仪器，多用于主观验光。

针孔（或针孔遮光板） 具有 1 个小孔径或 1 排小孔径的装置，可以有效地减少患者瞳孔的有效孔径。如果通过针孔观察可以提高患者的视力，这就表明存在未矫正的屈光不正。

Introduction

Clinical refraction is the process of measuring the refractive status of the eyes of a patient. It is an essential tool in a great many eye examinations: refractive errors are present in nearly half of all adults and children. In most settings, "best-corrected visual acuity" is the gold standard for measuring visual performance. In this section of the Quick-Start Guide, we outline the basic technique of *manifest refraction*—the measurement of refractive errors through patients' subjective descriptions of how well they can see.

Do not confuse manifest refraction with the prescribing of eyeglasses. The latter is a clinical art, for which refraction is only a first step. Guidelines for prescribing glasses are presented in Chapter 4.

Manifest refraction is a subjective process. Success is based on the ability to elicit the cooperation of the patient as much as the knowledge and skill of the examiner

The steps in the process of manifest refraction follow this sequence:

1.Perform the preliminaries (check visual acuity, obtain a visual history).
   a.Indications for refraction: which patients should be refracted?
2.Occlude 1 eye.
3.Make an initial estimate of the refractive error:
   a.Determine the best initial estimate of the refraction, if available, from prior records, old glasses, retinoscopy, or the auto-refractor, and place it in the phoropter or trial frame. If there is any known cylindrical correction, go to step 4; if not, go to step 5.
   OR
   b.If there is no prior refraction information, retinoscopy, or auto-refractor data, begin by refracting only with spherical lenses to obtain the best-possible refraction using only spheres. Go to step 3c.
   c.Check for astigmatism by inserting a cylinder lens, adjusting the sphere to pre-serve the spherical equivalent, and rotating the cylinder—if this affects image clarity, you have detected some astigmatism. Leave the cylinder in the optimal position (this becomes the starting point for cross cylinder refinement—go to step 4); if rotating the cylinder has no effect on image clarity, assume there is no astigmatism. Remove the cylinder, restore the original sphere, and go directly to step 5.
4.Refine the cylinder using the Jackson cross cylinder, first in the "axis position" to identify the correct cylinder axis, then in the "power position" to determine the optimal cylinder power. Preserve spherical equivalent when adjusting cylinder power by adjusting sphere power 1 click (0.25 D) in the opposite direction for every 2 click (0.50D) change in cylinder power. Go to step 5.
5.Refine the sphere power, first using a 0.50D difference between the alterna-tive, bracketing the previous selection, then using 0.25 D difference between the alternatives.
6.Reverse the occlusion, and repeat for the fellow eye.
7.Check for binocular balance.

Additional comments, set off in boxes, are interspersed between the step-by-step instructions. Most of the step-by-step instructions that we discuss here describe refraction performed with minus cylinder equipment. Equivalent instructions for plus cylinder equipment are labeled as directions and marked with a tinted background. Recommended language to use with patients is printed in ***boldface italics***.

引言

*临床验光*是测量患者眼睛屈光状态的过程。它是许多眼科检查中必不可少的工具：近一半的成人和儿童都有屈光不正。在大多数情况下，“最佳矫正视力”是测量视功能的黄金标准。在《快速入门指南》的这一部分中，我们概述了*显然验光*的基本技术——通过患者对其能够看到的物体清晰度的主观描述来测量屈光不正的程度。

不要将显然验光与眼镜处方混为一谈。后者是一种临床艺术，而验光只是其中的第一步。眼镜处方指南见第 4 章。

显然验光是一个主观过程，它以检查者的知识和技巧及启发引导患者的合作作为验光成功的基础。

显然验光过程中的步骤顺序如下：

1. 第 1 步是检查视力、记录视力。
   a. 验光的适应证：哪些患者应该验光？
2. 遮住 1 只眼睛。
3. 初步估计屈光不正：
   a. 可通过先前的记录、旧眼镜、检影镜或自动验光仪来确定屈光最佳初始估值，并将其输入综合屈光仪或试镜器。如果有已知圆柱矫正值，则直接进入操作步骤 4；如果没有，则进入步骤 5。

   b. 如果没有先前的屈光信息、检影镜或自动验光仪数据，仅使用球镜开始屈光，就可以获得仅使用球镜的最好的屈光值。进入步骤 3c。

   c. 插入柱镜，调整球镜以保持球镜等值，并旋转柱镜透镜来检查散光——如果该做法影响图像的清晰度，则表明已检测到了散光现象。将柱镜调至最佳位置（该位置是交叉圆柱镜精度的初始点），然后进入步骤 4；如果旋转柱镜对图像的清晰度没有影响，则可能无散光现象。移走柱镜，恢复原始球镜状态，然后直接进入步骤 5。

4. 利用 Jackson 交叉柱镜调整柱镜的精准度，首先在“轴的位置”确定准确柱镜轴，然后在“屈光力的位置”确定最佳柱镜屈光力值。再以反方向将柱镜度 1 键（0.25 D）调至 2 键（0.50D）以保持球镜等值。

5. 首先使用 0.50D 等差值，用括号标注之前的选择，再使用 0.25D 等差值来进行柱镜度的精准化。
6. 调换遮眼，另一只眼重复此法。
7. 检查双眼平衡。

在框内附加的说明穿插于上述步骤指令中。我们在此讨论的大多数步骤指令均用负柱镜设备描述验光。正柱镜设备的说明加有颜色背景标注的指令。推荐用于患者的语言是用***黑体字斜体印刷的***。

Step 1: Perform the Preliminaries

Check Visual Acuity

We use eye charts consisting of optotypes (letters or pictures) to test visual acuity. If a patient's visual acuity is known from a prior examination, start at that line of the eye chart. Otherwise, first cover the left eye, and ask the patient to read the 20/40 line on the eye chart with the right eye (Figure I-21A). Go up or down the eye chart to find the line your patient can just barely read. Then cover the right eye and repeat the process to measure the acuity of the left eye.

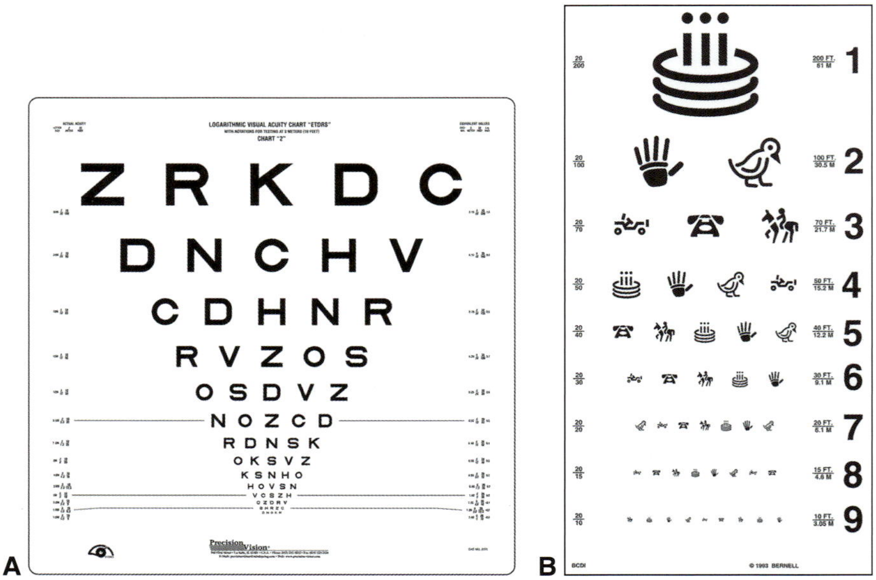

Figure I-21 Eye charts for testing visual acuity. **A**, ETDRS-type chart with Sloan letters; **B**, Allen Symbols (not recommended). *(Part A Courtesy of Precision Vision; part B courtesy of Vision Training Products.)*

> *Many patients will balk if asked to "**Read the smallest line you can.**" You may get the response "But Doctor, I can't read the smallest line." Expect patients to slow down as they reach the line(s) they can just barely see. Checking visual acuity well takes more time than you would imagine. Think of it as an opportunity to observe your patient's vision, much as a neurologist carefully watches a patient walk into the exam room. Encourage patients to guess at letters they can barely see.*
>
> *It is traditional to perform ophthalmology examinations first for the right eye, then for the left eye. Get into this habit to minimize confusion as to which findings go with which eye. Notice systematic errors at the beginning or end of the lines of the eye chart, which might suggest a visual field defect. Craning of the neck may indicate an attempt to cheat in cases of amblyopia ("lazy eye"). "Searching" may suggest a central scotoma (blind spot). Discourage squinting!*

> *Modern picture optotypes, such as the LEA symbols (circle, square, apple, and house) or the "HOTV" character set (see Figure 3-6D, E) are preferred over traditional picture optotypes (Allen symbols: telephone, hand, bird, car, birthday cake, and horse and rider); the latter remain distinguishable even with a great deal of blur and may be confusing (Figure I-21B). Few children recognize a dial telephone these days!*

第 1 步：准备工作

检查视力

我们使用由视标（字母或图片）构成的视力表测试视力。如果可以知道患者以前检查的视力情况，请从对应的那一行开始检查。否则应该首先遮盖患者的左眼，用右眼指认视力表的 20/40 行（0.5 行）（图 I–21A）。在视力表上上上下下地移动，以确定患者无法看清的是哪一行。然后遮盖右眼，重复上诉过程以测量左眼的视力。

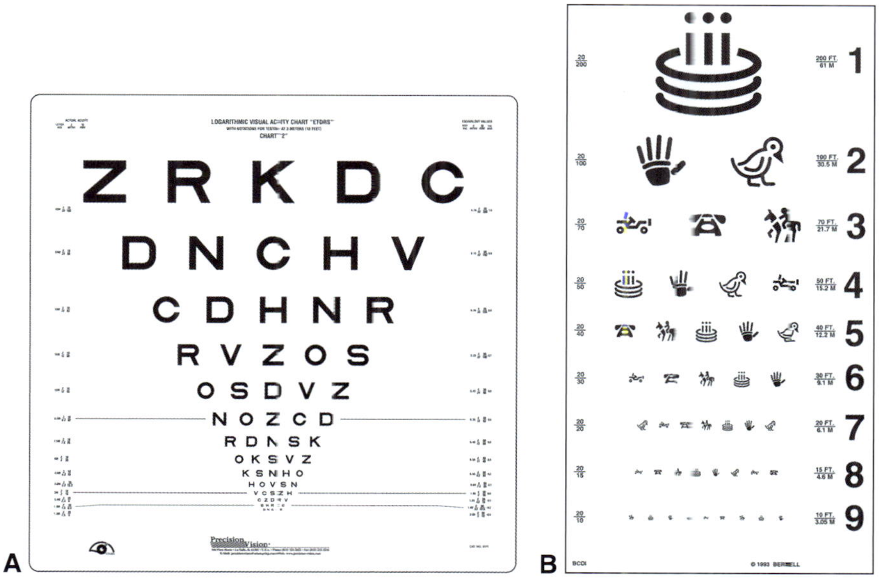

图 I–21 测试视力的视力表。A. Sloan 字母的 ETDRS 型视力表；B. Allen 符号（不推荐）。（A 是精确视觉，B 是视觉培训产品。）

> *如果要求“**读出你能读到的最小一行**”，就会有许多患者犹豫不决。患者可能会说“医生，我看不清最小的一行”。应让患者在读到看不清的那一行时放慢速度。检查视力会比预期的时间更长，就像神经科医生会仔细观察患者走进测试室的状态一样，将此视为观察患者视力的机会，鼓励患者猜一猜他们几乎看不见的字母。*
>
> *传统的眼科检查是先进行右眼检查，然后再进行左眼检查。养成这一习惯会减少将 2 只眼睛的检查结果相互混淆的情况。要注意视力表行首或行末的系统性错误，这意味着可能存在视野缺陷。伸长脖子可能是弱视（“懒惰眼”）患者在作弊。“寻找”则提示可能有一个中央盲点。不能眯眼！*

> *现代视力图标，如 LEA 符号（圆形、方形、苹果和房子）或“HOTV”字符（见图 3–6D、E）优于传统的视力图标 [Allen 符号（图 I–21B）：电话、手、鸟、车、生日蛋糕、马匹和骑手]；后者视力图标即使可以区分，但也可能引起困惑，因为现在已经很少有孩子认识拨号电话了！*

If visual acuity is subnormal, try a *pinhole occluder*, a device with 1 or more small apertures used to reduce the eye's effective aperture (Figure I-22). Note: Best-refracted vision may be better than, worse than, or the same as pinhole corrected vision! Failure to improve with a pinhole does not exclude refractive error and does not justify omitting the refraction.

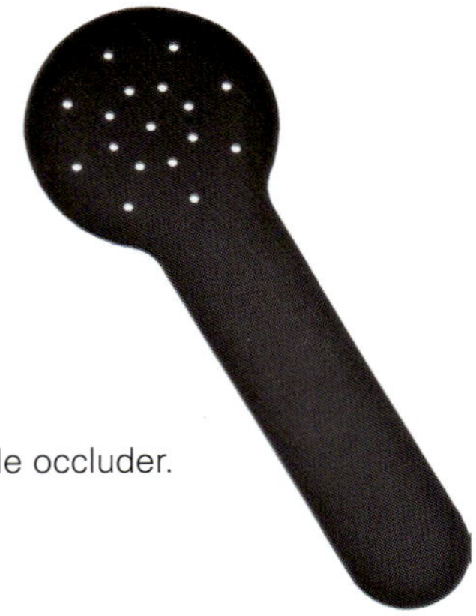

Figure I-22 Pinhole occluder.

For example, pinhole vision is typically worse than best-corrected vision in cases of dense cataracts and in many cases of macular degeneration. Conversely, when looking through a pinhole occluder, patients with early, inhomogeneous cataracts may improve dramatically but may fail to achieve this acuity with spectacles. Using the single pinhole that is provided in the phoropter accessory wheel, a patient may have difficulty finding the eye chart.

If the patient has distance glasses, there is rarely any reason to check the visual acuity without them, unless the patient requests it or acuity with the existing glasses is very poor. A patient may inadvertently use reading glasses while attempting to see at distance!

Check visual acuity at near (ie, reading vision) routinely only in the following cases: potential presbyopes (with age-related loss of near vision), latent hyperopia suspects, patients (especially children) suspected of amblyopia, and patients with a near-vision or an asthenopic complaint.

Asthenopic complaints are various symptoms associated with accommodative effort— that is, with the ability of the eye to increase the optical power of the crystalline lens.

Asthenopic symptoms include fatigue, headache, "eyestrain," double vision, fluctuating visual acuity, and lengthening of the clearest reading distance. They suggest hyperopic refractive errors, presbyopia, "accommodative spasm," or the possibility that the patient's existing glasses contain a stronger myopic correction (or a weaker hyperopic correction) than is necessary. These topics are discussed in greater detail in Chapter 4.

In amblyopia, near vision may be better than distance vision. However, many patients, especially children, seem to see better at near only because they are permitted to hold the near-vision testing card closer than the calibrated distance (typically 14 inches, or 40 cm). Such compensations are impossible at distance.

如果视力低于正常水平，可以尝试使用*针孔遮眼板*，这是带有 1 个或多个可减少瞳孔有效孔径的小孔的装置（图 I–22）。注：最佳屈光视力可能优于、低于或与针孔矫正视力相同！当用针孔遮眼板并没有提升视力的时候，也不能排除屈光不正。

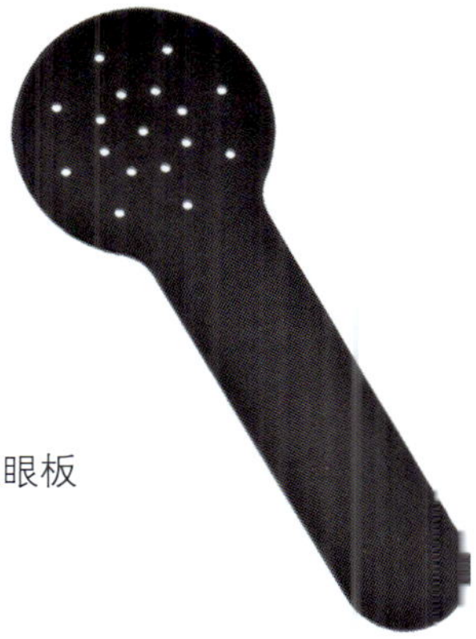

Figure I-22 针孔遮眼板

例如，对于白内障和许多黄斑变性的患者，其针孔视力通常比最佳矫正视力差。相反，当通过针孔遮眼板观察时，早期不均匀性白内障患者可能会有很大的改善，但戴镜时可能无法达到这种视力。使用综合屈光仪附件中的单个针孔，患者可能很难找到视标。

如果患者有远用眼镜，几乎没有理由不用它们来检查矫正视力，除非患者提出要求，或者现有眼镜的矫正视力很差。因为患者可能无意中在看远处的时候使用了近用阅读眼镜！

仅在以下情况下才会进行近处视力（即阅读视力）的检查：老视（与年龄相关的近视力丧失）、怀疑隐性远视、弱视（特别是儿童），以及有近视眼或视疲劳的患者。

*视疲劳症状*是与调节力有关的各种症状，即眼增加晶状体屈光力的能力。

视疲劳症状包括疲劳、头痛、"眼睛疲劳"、重影、视力模糊和阅读距离增加。这提示远视屈光不正、老视、"调节性痉挛"，或患者现有的近视眼镜过矫（或远视低矫）的可能性。这些问题将在第 4 章中详细讨论。

在弱视患者中，近视力可能比远视力好。然而，许多患者，特别是儿童，似乎在近处看得更清楚，只是因为他们持近视测试卡的距离比标准距离更近（通常为 14in，或 40cm）。这种补偿在远距离检测时是不可能实现的。

Patients over the age of 40 or so should routinely be checked for presbyopia. It is better to allow such patients to hold the near-card at their own preferred reading distance (with or without reading glasses, according to the patient's typical reading habits), and record the smallest legible line, and the distance at which the patient chose to hold the near-card, than to enforce the standard reading distance. Use "Jaeger notation," optotype size in "points," or both to record the patient's near vision.

Obtain a Visual History

As in any other patient care encounter, obtaining an accurate history is a vital initial step in clinical refraction. Understanding the patient's visual complaints, if any, is often critical to providing a satisfactory refractive solution. For example, the patient may benefit from glasses suitable for specific activities, such as using a computer, playing a musical instrument, or going shopping. Prescribing glasses for a patient without visual complaints is rarely helpful.

Seek the following items if they are not volunteered:

- decreased visual acuity: At distance? At near? Both?
- eyestrain
- headaches
- presbyopia (difficulty reading at comfortable distance)
- age
- occupation (computer work, in particular)
- hobbies (eg, music, sewing)
- other ocular history (eg, amblyopia, trauma, glaucoma, prior eye surgery)

Refractive errors are only rarely the cause of headaches. Headaches that wake a patient from sleep, or occur early in the morning, are almost never due to refractive error.
You may be called on to design spectacles for an occupational or recreational application.
Beware of ophthalmic disorders that might limit best-corrected visual acuity.

Review Indications for Refraction

Which patients need to be refracted?

- those with subnormal visual acuity. Remember, 20/25 is not normal visual acuity. Patients with acuity of 20/25 or worse should generally be refracted, unless a credible refraction documenting a stable best-corrected visual acuity of 20/25 or worse is already present in the medical record. Patients with acuity of 20/30 or worse should be refracted routinely
- those with asthenopic symptoms
- those with decreased visual acuity since their previous visit
- postoperative patients (especially after cataract surgery)

Some cataract surgeons delay postoperative refractions until there has been sufficient healing to ensure a good visual result. This delay may prevent the detection of an early, vision-threatening complication.

40 岁左右的患者应该定期检查是否有老视。最好是让患者按自己喜欢的阅读距离拿着近视力检测卡（是否戴老视镜，要根据阅读习惯），并记录辨认的最小文字行以及检测距离，而不要强制采用标准阅读距离。使用“Jaeger 法”或以“点数”记录的视标，或两者同时使用来记录患者的近视力。

获取患者的视觉病史

与任何其他患者的护理经历一样，获得准确的病史是临床验光非常重要的第一步。了解患者视觉方面的主诉，对获得满意的验光结果至关重要。例如，适合的眼镜可以使患者的生活活动便利，如使用电脑、演奏乐器或购物。没有视觉症状的患者则配镜的帮助不大。

如果患者不愿意验光，请考虑以下几项内容：

- 视力下降：视远？视近？两者都有？
- 眼睛疲劳。
- 头痛。
- 老花眼（在舒适的距离难以阅读）。
- 年龄。
- 职业（特别是计算机工作）。
- 爱好（如音乐、缝纫）。
- 其他眼病史（如弱视、外伤、青光眼、接受过眼科手术）。

> *屈光不正很少是引起头痛的原因。屈光不正从不会使患者从睡眠中醒来或导致清晨的头痛。*
>
> *患者可能要求使用职业或娱乐用途的眼镜。*
>
> *要注意眼科疾病可能会导致患者达不到最佳矫正视力。*

复习验光适应证

哪些患者需要验光？

- 视力低于正常人的人。记住，20/25（0.8）不是正常的视力。视力为 20/25（0.8）或更低的患者应该进行验光，除非病历中的屈光记录说明 20/25 或更低的视力是其最佳矫正视力。视力为 20/30（0.7）或以下的患者应进行常规验光。

- 有视疲劳症状的人。
- 自上次问诊以来视力下降的人。
- 术后患者（特别是白内障手术后）。

> *一些白内障手术医生会推迟术后验光，直到患者充分愈合，以确保良好的视觉结果。这可能会妨碍早期发现视觉威胁的并发症。*

Step 2: Occlude 1 Eye

Occlude the Left Eye, Refract the Right Eye First

- The next step is to occlude 1 eye in order to refract the patient's other eye.
- Barring exceptional circumstances, begin by occluding the *left* eye, so as to do the initial refraction in the *right* eye.
- If you are using a phoropter, you may dial an opaque occluder into place using the accessory wheel (Figure I-23A).
- If the patient is cooperative and will not find it too distracting, it is often preferable to occlude the nonrefracting eye with a plus lens, such as the +1.50D retinoscopy lens (marked "R") in the accessory wheel of the phoropter (Figure I-23B). This practice often better relaxes the accommodation of the eye you *are* refracting than occlusion of the fellow eye with an opaque occluder. However, this method will not work well on patients with latent hyperopia—first verify that the +1.50D lens really does reduce the visual acuity. Dial in extra plus lens power if needed. This process is known as *fogging*. If you suspect hyperopia, attempt to relax accommodation by gradually dialing in plus sphere power, 1 click (0.25 D) every 15–20 seconds while talking amiably with the patient, until the visual acuity is substantially reduced.

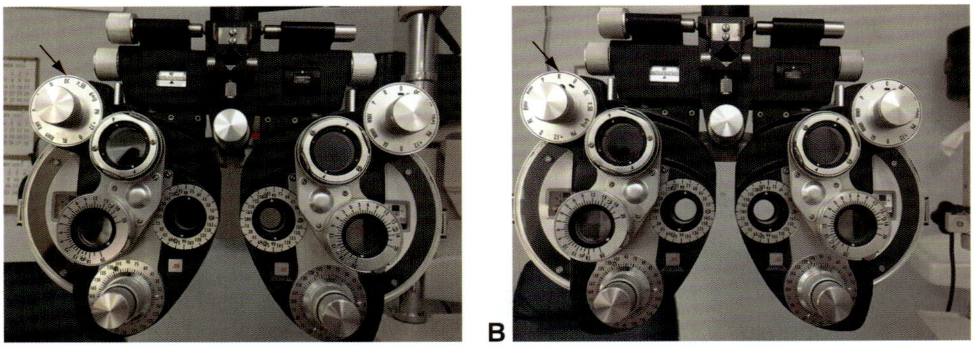

A B

Figure I-23 Occluding the right side of the phoropter: **A**, opaque occluder. **B**, +1.50D "R" accessory lens. Notice the settings of the accessory wheel for the right eye, at the top left of the photos.

> *Some patients develop nystagmus (rapid involuntary eye movements) when 1 eye is completely occluded. You can sometimes avoid that by using an adequate plus lens, rather than an opaque occluder, to occlude the fellow eye.*

Step 3: Obtain Initial Estimate of the Refractive Error

Having established that a patient needs to be refracted, obtain the best-available initial estimate of the refractive correction (if any) and dial it into the phoropter or place it in a trial frame.

第 2 步：遮蔽一只眼睛

遮住左眼，先给右眼验光

- 下一步是遮住一只眼，以使患者的另一只眼睛接受验光。
- 除特殊情况外，一般先遮盖住*左眼*，从*右眼*进行初始验光。

- 如果使用综合屈光仪，可以调拨一个不透明的遮眼片（图 I-23A）。

- 如果患者配合良好，而且注意力不太分散，通常是用正透镜来遮蔽非验光眼，如辅助轮中的 +1.50D 视网膜检影片（标记为“R”）（图 I-23B）。这种做法比用不透明遮眼片能更好地放松*正在*验光的眼睛的调节。但这种做法对隐性远视不能起效——首先要验证 +1.50D 透镜确实降低了视力。如有需要，增加正透镜，而这一过程被称为*雾视*。如果患者有远视，应逐步增加正镜从而放松眼睛的调节度。与患者交谈时，每隔 15~20s 调拨 1 个刻度（0.25 D）球镜，直到视力开始降低为止。

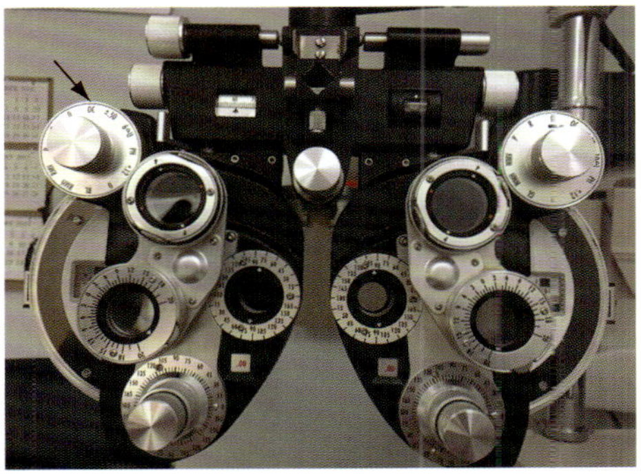

A

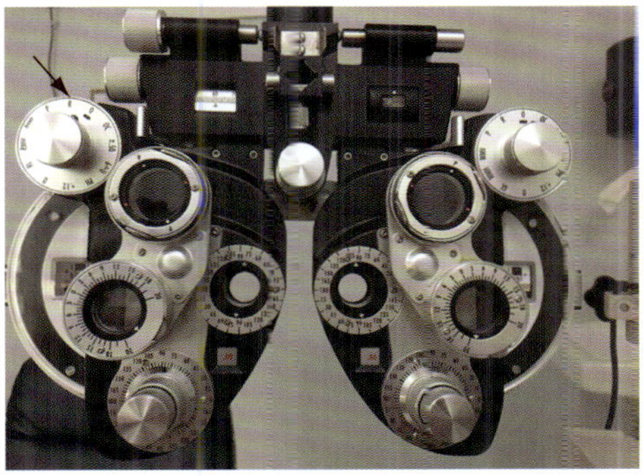

B

图 I-23 遮盖综合屈光仪右侧: A. 不透明遮盖片。B.+1.50D“R”辅助透镜。注意右眼副轮的设置，在照片的左上。

> *当一只眼睛被遮挡时，有些患者会出现眼球震颤（快速的非自主性眼运动）。有时可以使用适当的正透镜，而不是用不透明的遮盖片遮住另一只眼睛，以此来避免眼球震颤的现象。*

第 3 步：获得屈光不正的初始估计值

在确定患者需要验光后，获得屈光矫正的最佳初始估计值（如果有的话），并将其输入验光仪或放在试镜架中。

The phoropter is a device that holds trial lenses on geared wheels to facilitate exchanging lenses in front of the patient's eyes during a manifest refraction (Figure I-24A). An alternate term is refractor; the term Phoroptor is a trademark of Reichert Technologies (Depew, NY). Each side of the phoropter holds lenses for a large range of plus sphere and minus sphere power. The "cylinder battery," or array of cylindrical lenses, contains cylinders of only 1 sign, either plus or minus, depending on the individual instrument. Before beginning a refraction, you must determine whether the phoropter in front of you is a plus cylinder or minus cylinder instrument. Note: On American-made instruments and their knock-offs, minus cylinders are indicated with red numbers (Fig I-24); plus cylinders are indicated with black numbers.

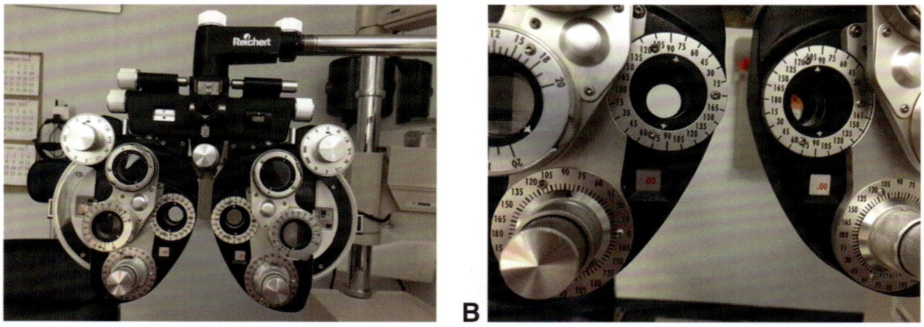

A B

Figure I-24 Phoropter. **A**, A minus cylinder phoropter. **B**, The red numbers indicate the cylinder power.

Perform Either Step 3a or Steps 3b and 3c

Step 3a. Use prior information to obtain initial estimate of refractive error

- Measure the patient's current eyeglasses, if available, and dial these values into the phoropter. (Use of the lensmeter to measure—"neutralize"—glasses is described in Chapter 8.) Use the result of a previous refraction, such as a previous prescription for glasses as provided by the patient, or as recorded in the patient's medical record.
- Perform retinoscopy (see Chapter 4).
  - If lenses in the phoropter are clean, retinoscopy may be performed through the phoropter, so that the results of the retinoscopy will be immediately available as the phoropter settings to serve as the starting point for subjective refraction. It is a good habit to write down the retinoscopic findings for comparison with the final refraction.
- Use an autorefractor or a photorefractor.
  - This procedure seldom saves time if you have to take the patient to a different room. Autorefractors are essentially automated retinoscopes. They work well on eyes with clear media and adequate pupils in patients with steady, central fixation. In patients with media opacities, small pupils, or an inability to sit still—just the pa-tients with whom you could appreciate some automated help—they generally fail.
- If there is no known astigmatic correction, proceed directly to step 5; if there is an astigmatic correction, go to step 4.

综合验光仪是一种在齿轮传动轮上运行的试镜装置，在明显的屈光状态下，方便在患者眼睛内调换镜片（图 I–24A）。另一个术语是验光仪，术语 Phoroptor（综合验光仪）是徕卡公司的商标（徕卡科技，迪普，纽约）。

综合验光仪的每侧都有一组调节范围很大的正球镜和负球镜。“徕卡科技柱镜组”或柱镜列，各种不同的仪器只包含 1 个标记柱镜（或正号或负号的柱镜）。在验光前，必须确定镜片的正负。注：在美国制造的仪器及其仿制品上，用红色数字表示负柱镜（图 I–24），用黑色数字表示正柱镜。

A
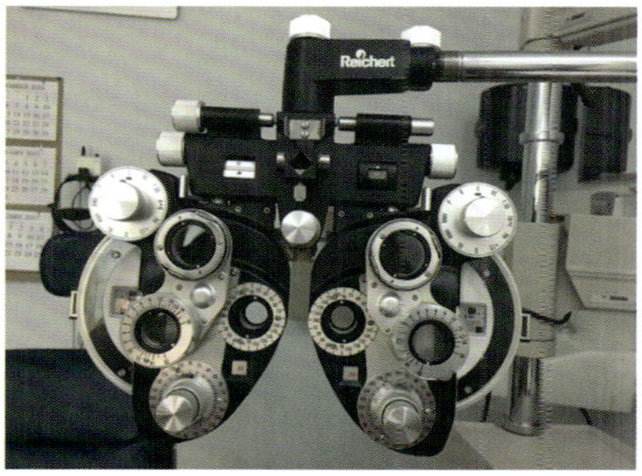

B
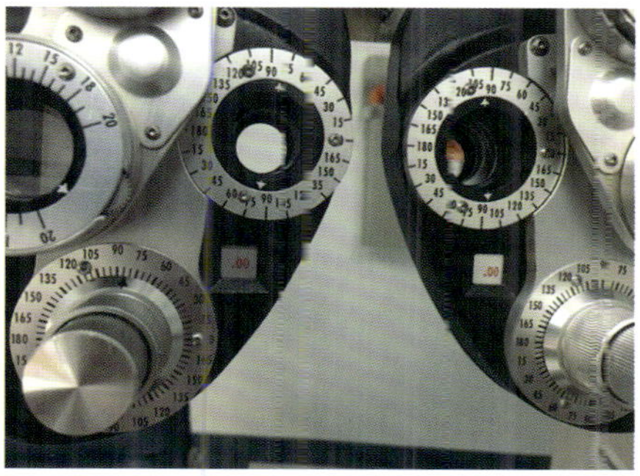

图 I–24 综合验光仪。**A**. 负柱验光仪。**B**. 红色数字表示柱镜屈光力。

执行步骤 3a 或步骤 3b 和 3c

第 3 步 a. 利用先期信息获得屈光不正的初步估计值

- 测量患者正在使用的眼镜，并将这些数值输入综合验光仪。（用焦度计测量——“中和”眼镜，见第 8 章。）可以使用以前的验光结果，如以前的眼镜处方或病历记录。

- 进行检影（见第 4 章）。

如果综合屈光仪上的镜片是干净的，可以通过该仪器进行检影，这样，检影结果将显示在综合屈光仪的设置中，以此作为主观验光的起始点。将检影结果记录下来，并比较最后的验光结果是一个很好的习惯。

- 使用自动验光仪或摄影验光仪。

如果你不得不带患者去另一个房间，这个程序很少能节省时间。自动验光仪本质上是自动检影镜。它们对间质清晰、瞳孔完整、视中稳定集中的患者有极好的效果。对于间质混浊、瞳孔小或不能静坐的患者（尤其是那些你认为需要机械辅助的患者）通常没有作用。

- 如果没有已知的散光矫正的记录，直接进行第 5 步；如果有散光矫正的记录，则转到第 4 步。

Step 3b. Make direct initial measurement of spherical refractive error

- If no preliminary estimate is available from old glasses, the medical record, retinoscopy or autorefraction, determine the best spherical correction by offering the patient successive choices of alternative spherical corrections. Starting with the spherical power at 0.00, use the low-power sphere lens wheel on the phoropter (or hand-held lenses if using a trial frame), offer the patient a choice between a spherical lens power of +0.25 D or −0.25 D. This gives the patient a choice between spherical lenses that differ by 0.50D. (If the patient's visual acuity is very poor, offer a greater difference between the 2 choices of sphere power.) Use the language ***"Which is better, 1 or 2?"*** This "forced choice" is referred to as a *binary comparison*.
  - Make certain the patient is referring to your choice between *lens 1* or *lens 2*, not line 1 or line 2 of the eye chart. If necessary, mask off all but 1 line of the chart.
  - If the patient's acuity is very poor, it may be preferable to offer binary comparisons with choices that differ by 1.00D.
- Advance the sphere setting 0.25 D toward the preferred alternative, and then offer the next binary comparison to bracket the patient's most recent choice of sphere power setting, again with a 0.50D difference. (For example, if the patient's initial preference is for the -0.25 lens, the next choice offered should be between 0.00 and -0.50D lenses.)
- Repeat this process until the patient suggests that the 2 choices are about the same.
- Recheck this endpoint, using choices that differ by only 0.25 D.
- Generally, try to move most of the time from *more plus* to *less plus* (or from *less minus* to *more minus*). By offering the more plus or less minus choice first, you will stimulate accommodation only minimally.
  - Try to be sensitive to the patient's responses. As you near the endpoint, responses are typically slower. The patient may simply stop responding rather than volunteer that the choices are about the same. This is still useful information.
- Do not worry about making a mistake by going too far—the method is self-correcting.
- Once the best possible spherical correction has been determined, go to step 3c to determine if there is any astigmatic refractive error.

Step 3c. Detect astigmatism

Now that you have found the optimal correction by using only spheres, determine whether there is any astigmatism as follows.

(Directions for use with a *minus cylinder* phoropter)

A. Dial in −0.50D of the cylinder.

B. Increase the *sphere* power by +0.25 D.

C. Rotate the cylinder *axis* knob slowly once or twice around, and ask the patient to tell you to stop when he or she perceives the clearest vision. (Alternatively, you may ask the patient to turn the knob and leave it where his or her vision is best.)

D. If the patient reports that rotating the dial makes no difference to the visual clarity—even if the vision is rather poor—then you may *assume* that the patient has *no significant astigmatism*, and proceed to step 5. If the patient *can* select a preferred axis, you have detected an astigmatic refractive error. Leave the cylinder dial at the preferred *axis orientation*, and proceed to step 4.

第 3 步 b. 球性屈光不正的直接初始测量

- 如果没有从旧眼镜、医疗记录、检影或自动验光中得到初步估计值，则要通过给患者提供可供选择的球镜矫正方案来确定最佳的球镜矫正。从球镜屈光度数 0.00D 开始，在验光仪上使用低度数球镜轮（或使用试镜架上的手持镜片），让患者在 –0.25 D 或 –0.25 D 之间的球面镜片中做出选择。这可以使患者在相差 0.50D 的球镜中做出选择。（如果患者的视力很低，应给出更大差别的 2 种球镜让其做选择。）如问 ***"哪个更好，'1'或'2'？"***，这被称为*强制选择*的二元比较。

  - 确保患者是在*透镜 1* 或 *2* 之间的选择，而非对视力表第 1 行或第 2 行的选择。如有必要，除第 1 行以外，其他所有行的视标均应予以遮挡。
  - 如果患者的视力很差，最好使用相差 1.00D 的二元比较法。

- 将 0.25D 球镜调整至最佳，然后提供下一个二元比较法，标注出患者最近选择的球镜值，相差 0.50D。（例如，如果患者最初的偏好是 –0.25D，则下一个选择应该是在 0.00~0.50D 之间的透镜。）

- 重复这个过程，直到患者认为这 2 种选择大致相同。
- 重新检查此终点，选用相差 0.25D 的透镜。
- 通常，花一些时间试着把*较高正镜*调整到*较低正镜*（或从*较低负镜*移到*较高负镜*）上。先用*较高正镜*或*较低负镜*，把对眼的刺激调节到最小。

  - 尽可能地对患者的反应敏感。当接近终点时，患者的反应会变慢，可能只是停止反应，而不是说这些选择几乎是一样的。这些仍然是有用的信息。

- 不要担心出错——该方法具有自我纠正的功能。
- 确定了最佳可能的球镜矫正，进入第 3 步 c，确定是否存在散光。

第 3 步 c. 散光检测

现在仅通过球镜进行光学矫正，随后将确定是否有散光。

（*负柱镜*综合屈光仪使用规程）

A. 将柱镜度数拨至 –0.50D。

B. 以 +0.25D 的幅度增加*球镜*度数。

C. 慢慢旋转柱镜*轴位*旋钮 1 个或 2 个刻度，请患者在其视力最清晰时告知停止。或者请患者自己旋转柱镜旋钮，直至其获得最清晰的视力时停止。

D. 如果患者回应旋转轴位按钮对视觉的清晰度没有影响时，即使视力相当差——那么也可以*假设*该患者*没有明显的散光*，并进入第 5 步。如果患者*能够*选择合适的轴位，则表示检测到了散光，此时将柱镜轴位拨盘停留在合适的*轴位方向*，然后进入第 4 步。

(Directions for use with a *plus cylinder* phoropter)

A. Dial in +0.50D of the cylinder.

B. Decrease the *sphere* power by –0.25 D.

C. Rotate the cylinder *axis* knob slowly once or twice around, and ask the patient to tell you to stop when he or she perceives the clearest vision. (Alternatively, you may ask the patient to turn the knob and leave it where his or her vision is best.)

D. If the patient reports that rotating the dial makes no difference to the visual clarity—even if the vision is rather poor—then you may *assume* that the patient has *no significant astigmatism*, and proceed to step 5. If the patient *can* select a preferred axis, you have detected an astigmatic refractive error. Leave the cylinder dial *at the preferred axis orientation*, and proceed to step 4

If the visual acuity is very poor, especially if there is a very large astigmatic refractive error, the patient may be unable to appreciate a variation in visual acuity by rotating a cylinder lens as described above. If possible, check for astigmatism by retinoscopy, by keratometry, or by using the stenopeic slit (see Chapter 4).

Step 4: Refine Cylinder Axis and Power

Once you have confirmed that an astigmatic refractive error is present, refine the cylinder *axis* as follows.

(Directions for use with a *minus cylinder* phoropter)

With the initial estimate of the cylindrical correction dialed into the phoropter, place the *Jackson cross cylinder* device in the "axis" position; that is, with an imaginary line connecting the 2 small thumb-wheels aligned parallel to the axis of the cylinder battery (Figure I-25). That alignment is indicated by the arrows on the axis knob and by indicator lines or arrowheads near the aperture of the phoropter. The cross cylinder should click into place. Present a binary comparison between the 2 positions of the cross cylinder by rotating 1 of the thumb-wheels. Notice how this interchanges the indicator dots (red and white) on the cross cylinder lens. Continue the binary comparisons, and after each, turn the (minus) cylinder axis toward the orientation of the *red* dots on the cross cylinder lens in the position where the patient reports clearer vision. The endpoint is often vague ("about the same," "equally bad," and so on). Watch for increased hesitation by the patient, or a reversal of the progression of the axis as you make successive binary comparisons. The process is self-correcting—if you go too far in 1 direction, the patient's responses will indicate that the cylinder axis should be brought back to a previous position.

（*正柱镜*综合屈光仪使用规程）

A. 拨入柱镜度数 +0.50D。
B. 以 –0.25D 的幅度减少*球镜*度数。
C. 慢慢旋转柱镜*轴位*旋钮 1 个或 2 个刻度，请患者在其视力最清晰时告知停止。或者请患者自己旋转柱镜旋钮，直至其获得最清晰的视力时停止。

D. 如果患者回应旋转轴位旋钮对视觉的清晰度没有影响时，即使视力相当差，那么也可以假设该患者*没有明显的散光*，并进入第 5 步。如果患者选择了合适的轴位，则表示检测到了散光，此时将柱镜轴位拨盘停留*在合适的轴位方向*，然后进入第 4 步。

如果患者的视力非常差，特别是有非常大的散光时，可能无法通过上述旋转柱镜的方法检测到视力的变化，此时可以通过检影、角膜曲率计，或小孔裂隙来检查散光（参看第 4 章）。

第 4 步：精确柱镜轴位和度数

一旦确认存在散光，请按如下方法明确柱镜*轴*位。

（*负柱镜*综合屈光检查仪使用规程）

将散光轴位初始估计值拨入综合屈光检查仪的矫正柱镜上，将 *Jackson 交叉柱镜*装置置于“轴”位置，即连接 2 个小拇指轮的假想线与矫正柱镜的轴位平行（图 I–25）。轴位调整旋钮上的箭头应与综合屈光仪孔径附近的指示线或箭头对齐。交叉柱镜应该卡入到位。通过旋转 1 个转动手轮来实现交叉柱镜的 2 个位置转换，进行 2 面比较。请注意在交叉柱镜上如何交换指示点（红色和白色）。继续进行 2 面比较，旋转负柱镜轴位旋钮，向交叉柱镜的*红*点方向旋转，直至患者获得最清晰的视力。终点通常是含糊不清的（表述“差不多”、“同样糟糕”等）。通过观察患者犹豫的变化，或反转旋钮，来帮助你自己做出正确的 2 面比较。该过程是个自我纠正的过程，如果在 1 个方向上走得太远，患者的反应会提示你将柱镜轴恢复到先前的位置。

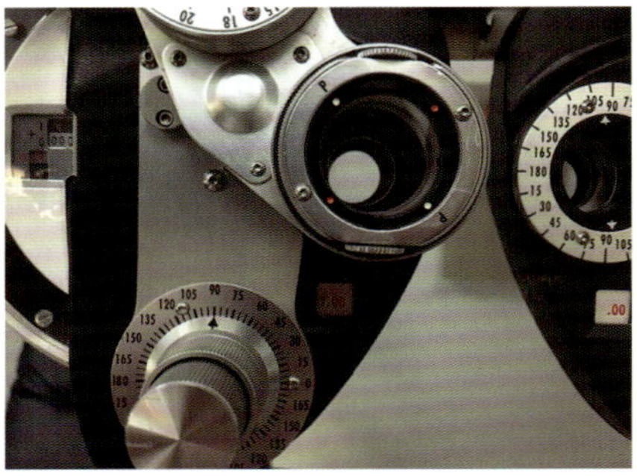

Figure I-25 Phoropter with Jackson cross cylinder in "axis" position. The cylinder battery has been set with the cylinder axis vertical

(Directions for use with a *plus cylinder* phoropter)

Place the Jackson cross cylinder device in the "axis" position; that is, with an imaginary line connecting the 2 small thumb-wheels aligned parallel to the axis of the cylinder battery (Figure I-25). That alignment is indicated by the arrows on the axis knob and by indicator lines or arrowheads near the aperture of the phoropter. The cross cylinder should click into place. Present a binary comparison between the 2 positions of the cross cylinder by rotating 1 of the thumb-wheels. Notice how this interchanges the indicator dots (red and white) on the cross cylinder lens. Continue the binary comparisons, and after each, turn the plus cylinder axis toward the orientation of the *white* dots on the cross cylinder lens in the position where the patient reports clearer vision. The endpoint is often vague ("about the same," "equally bad," and so on). Watch for increased hesitation by the patient, or a reversal of the progression of the axis as you make successive binary comparisons. The process is self-correcting—if you go too far in 1 direction, the patient's responses will indicate that the cylinder axis should be brought back to a previous direction.

Next, refine the cylinder *power*.

(Directions for use with a *minus cylinder* phoropter)

Turn the cross cylinder turret 45° to the "power" position, as indicated by an imaginary line connecting the "P" marks on the cross cylinder lens rim running parallel to the (newly determined) cylinder axis (Figure I-26). Flip the cross cylinder to provide a binary comparison. Notice how either the red dots or the white dots on the cross cylinder will line up along the cylinder axis. If the patient's preferred position of the cross cylinder places the *red* dots along the cylinder axis, *increase* the minus cylinder power. (If the preferred position of the cross cylinder places the line through the *red* dots *perpendicular* to the cylinder axis, so the line connecting the white dots lies parallel to the cylinder axis, *reduce* the minus cylinder power.) Repeat until you reach an endpoint, where the views through the alternate positions of the cross cylinder are "about the same." [At this stage, the view may still not be very good!] When in doubt, go with the numerically weaker choice of minus cylinder power.

KEY STEP: For each 0.5 D (2-click) *increase* in minus *cylinder* power as determined by these cross cylinder flips, *add* +0.25 D (1 click) of plus *sphere* power. After you have located the endpoint, remove the cross cylinder from the optical pathway. If all is well, the patient should experience a considerable improvement in visual acuity.

Once the optimal cylinder axis and power have been determined, proceed to step 5.

图 I–25 综合屈光仪与 Jackson 交叉柱镜“轴”的位置。柱镜组与柱镜轴位垂直。

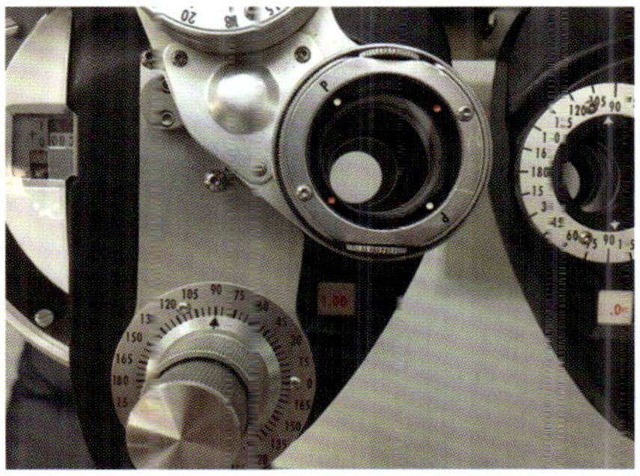

（*正柱镜*综合屈光检查仪使用规程）

将散光轴位初始估计值拨入综合屈光仪的矫正柱镜上，将 Jackson 交叉柱镜装置置于“轴”位置，即连接 2 个小拇指轮的假想线与矫正柱镜的轴位平行（图 I–25）。轴向调整旋钮上的箭头应与综合屈光仪孔径附近的指示线或箭头对齐。交叉柱镜应该卡入到位。通过旋转 1 个转动手轮来实现交叉柱镜的 2 个位置转换，进行 2 面比较。请注意在交叉柱镜上如何交换指示点（红色和白色）。继续进行 2 面比较，旋转正柱镜轴位旋钮，向交叉柱镜的*白点*方向旋转，直至患者获得最清晰的视力。终点通常是含糊不清的（表述“差不多”“同样糟糕”等）。通过观察患者犹豫的变化，或反转旋钮，来帮助你自己做出正确的 2 面比较。该过程是个自我纠正的过程，如果在 1 个方向上走得太远，患者的反应会提示你应将柱镜轴恢复到先前的位置。

接下来，确定柱镜*度数*。

（*负柱镜*综合屈光仪使用规程）

将交叉柱镜转盘以 45° 转向“度数”位置，使得交叉柱镜环上的 P 标记的假想连线与（新确定的）矫正柱镜轴位平行（图 I–26）。翻转交叉柱镜以提供 2 面比较。注意交叉柱镜上的红点或白点是如何沿柱镜轴排列的。如果患者优选的交叉柱镜的*红点*位置与柱镜轴一致时物像清晰，则应*增加*负柱镜度数。（如果交叉柱镜的优选位置连线*垂直*于柱镜轴的*红点*，而连接白点的线平行于柱镜轴，则应*减小*负柱镜度数。）重复上述操作直到到达终点，即通过交叉柱镜的交替位置的视力“大致相同”。（在这个阶段，视力可能仍然不是很好！）如有疑问，请选择数值较小的负柱镜度数。

关键步骤： *负柱镜*度数每*增加* 0.50D（旋转 2 个刻度），*球镜*度数需*增加* +0.25D（旋转 1 个刻度）。当达到终点后，将柱镜从视路中移开。如果一切顺利，患者的视力应该有相当大的改善。

一旦确定了柱镜轴位和度数，则继续第 5 步。

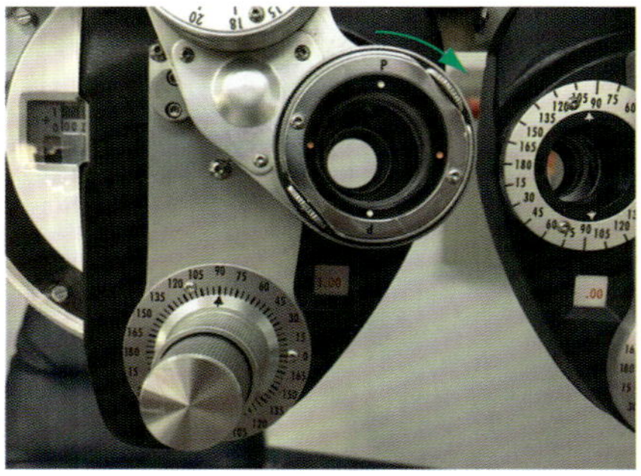

Figure I-26 Phoropter with Jackson cross cylinder in "power" position. The cylinder battery remains set with the cylinder axis vertical. *(Courtesy of Scott E. Brodie, MD.)*

(Directions for use with a *plus cylinder* phoropter)

Turn the cross cylinder turret 45° to the "power" position, as indicated by an imaginary line connecting the "P" marks on the lens rim running parallel to the ((newly determined) cylinder axis. Flip the cross cylinder to provide a binary comparison. Notice how either the red dots or the white dots on the cross cylinder will line up along the cylinder axis. If the patient's preferred position of the cross cylinder places the *white* dots along the cylinder axis, *increase* the plus cylinder power. (If the preferred position of the cross cylinder places the line through the *white* dots *perpendicular* to the cylinder axis, so the line connecting the red dots lies parallel to the cylinder axis, *reduce* the plus cylinder power.) Repeat until you reach an endpoint, where the views through the alternate positions of the cross cylinder are "about the same." [At this stage, the view may still not be very good!] When in doubt, go with the numerically weaker choice of plus cylinder power.

KEY STEP: For each 0.5 D (2-click) increase in plus *cylinder* power as determined by these cross cylinder flips, *reduce* the *sphere* power by 0.25 D (1 click). After you have located the endpoint, remove the cross cylinder from the optical pathway. If all is well, the patient should experience a considerable improvement in visual acuity.

Once the optimal cylinder axis and power have been determined, proceed to step 5

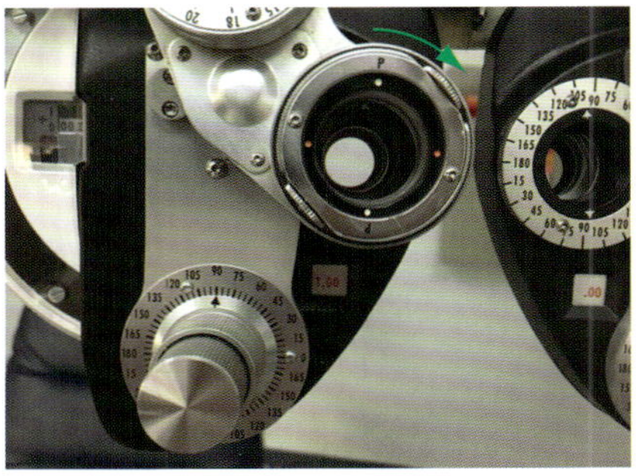

图 I–26 综合验光仪的 Jackson 交叉柱镜位于"度数"位置。柱镜组仍然与柱镜轴位垂直。*（译者注：资料来源见前页原文。）*

（*正柱镜*综合屈光检查仪使用规程）
将交叉柱镜转盘以 45° 转向"度数"位置，使交叉柱镜环上的 P 标记的假想连线与（新确定的）矫正柱镜轴位平行（图 I–26）。翻转交叉柱镜以提供 2 面比较。注意交叉柱镜上的红点或白点是如何沿柱镜轴排列的。如果患者优选的交叉柱镜的*白*点位置与柱镜轴一致时物像清晰，则*增加*正柱镜度数。如果交叉柱镜的优选位置连线*垂直*于柱镜轴的*白*点，而连接红点的线平行于柱镜轴，则*减小*正柱镜度数。重复上述操作直到通过交叉柱镜的交替位置的视力"大致相同"。（在这个阶段，视力可能仍然不是很好。）如有疑问，请选择数值较小的负柱镜度数。

关键步骤：正*柱镜*度数每增加 0.5D（旋转 2 个刻度），*球镜*度数需*减少* 0.25D（旋转 1 个刻度）。当达到终点后，将柱镜从视路中移开。如果一切顺利，患者应该在视敏度方面有相当大的改善。

一旦柱镜轴位和度数确定，则继续第 5 步。

As with sphere power, the determination of cylinder axis and cylinder power by means of binary comparisons of the view through the cross cylinder in its various positions is self-correcting. If you make an error in adjusting the lenses, the next comparison you offer the patient will create a contrast between views that is even clearer than the last.

If you are using loose trial lenses in a trial frame instead of a phoropter, you will have to align the hand-held Jackson cross cylinder (Figure I-27) with the tentative axis of the correcting cylinder in the trial frame by yourself. To refine the cylinder axis, hold the cross cylinder with the handle parallel to the correcting cylinder axis. After each binary comparison, rotate the cylinder axis toward the preferred position of the red (or white) dots on the cross cylinder, depending on whether you are working with minus cylinder or plus cylinder trial lenses, respectively. For the next binary comparison, you will have to adjust the orientation of the cross cylinder handle to align with the new position of the trial cylinder axis. (This realignment of the cross cylinder takes place automatically in the phoropter.) To refine the cylinder power, hold the handle of the cross cylinder 45° away from the axis of the trial cylinder. This will align the lines between the red and white dots on the cross cylinder either parallel or perpendicular to the axis of the trial cylinder; then proceed as above.

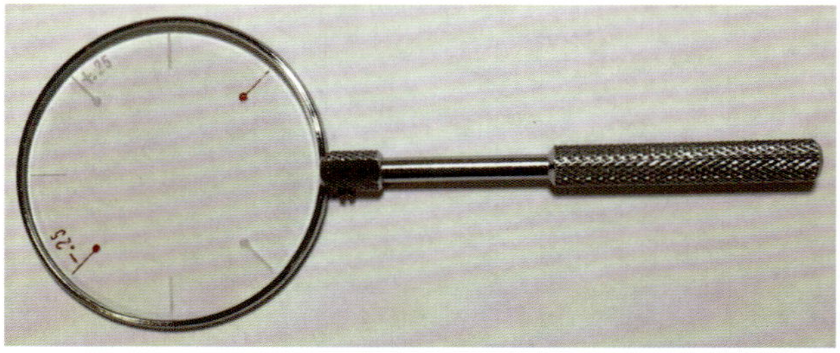

Figure I-27 Hand-held Jackson cross cylinder. Notice the red and white dots that straddle the axis of the handle. *(Courtesy of Scott E. Brodie, MD.)*

After optimizing the cylinder power, you may find it useful to recheck the cylinder axis. If the cylinder axis is substantially changed, recheck the cylinder power as well.

Step 5: Refine Sphere Power

Once you have achieved the optimal cylinder axis and power, recheck the sphere power, as in step 3b.

Step 6: Occlude the Right Eye—Refract the Left Eye

You have completed refraction of the right eye. To refract the patient's other eye, repeat the process of steps 3 through 5 for the fellow eye.

与球镜度数一样，柱镜轴位和度数需要通过交叉柱镜不同的位置转换所得到的图像的 2 面比较来确定，这个过程是个自我修正的过程。如果在调整镜片时出错，那么你为患者提供下一次比较时，将产生一个比上一次更清晰的图像。

如果在试镜架上使用插片检查，而不是综合屈光仪，则须将手持式 Jackson 交叉柱镜（图 I–27）与试镜框中的矫正柱镜的轴位对齐。在精确调整柱镜轴位时，需握住交叉柱镜，使其手柄平行于矫正柱镜轴。在每次 2 面比较之后，将柱镜轴旋转到交叉柱镜上的红色（或白色）点的首选位置，这取决于使用的是负柱镜还是正柱镜试镜。在下一次 2 面比较时，必须调整交叉柱镜手柄的方向使其与新的柱镜轴位对齐。（在综合屈光仪中交叉柱镜的这种重新对准是自动进行的。）在确定柱镜度数时，握住交叉柱镜的手柄使其保持在与试验柱镜轴线成 45° 的位置。这将使交叉柱镜上的红点和白点之间的线平行或垂直于试验柱镜的轴线；然后按上述步骤进行。

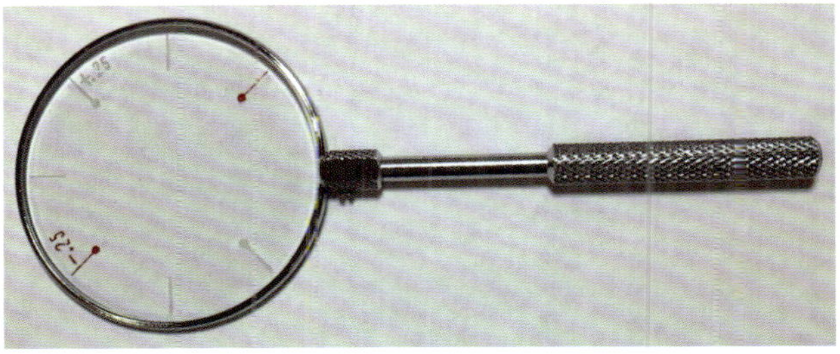

图 I–27 手持 Jackson 交叉柱镜。注意横跨手柄轴的红色和白色圆点。*（译者注：资料来源见前页原文。）*

在明确了柱镜度数后，可能会发现还需要重新检查柱镜轴位。如果柱镜轴位完全改变，还需要重新检查柱镜度数。

第 5 步：确定球镜度数

获得最佳柱镜轴位和度数后，重新检查球镜的度数，如第 3 步 b 所示。

第 6 步：遮住右眼，给左眼验光

完成了右眼的屈光检查以后，要检查患者另一只眼的屈光状态，重复第 3~5 步。

Try It Yourself! I-3

- **Refract the wall.** A good way to see how the logic of cross cylinder refraction works is to try this simple exercise. Position the phoropter parallel to a wall about 20 cm away. Occlude 1 side of the phoropter. Tape a random cylinder trial lens to the back of the other side; the metal clip will help hold it in place. (About 1.5 D works well. Start with a cylinder of sign opposite to the sign of the cylinders in your phoropter.) Ask a friend to hold a penlight or Finoff transilluminator several feet away, pointing it toward the open aperture of the phoropter. You should see a small elliptical spot projected on the wall behind the phoropter (Figure I-28).
- **Refract with spheres.** Using binary comparisons, find the optimal spherical "correction" for the wall. This will be a circular image (the circle of least confusion).

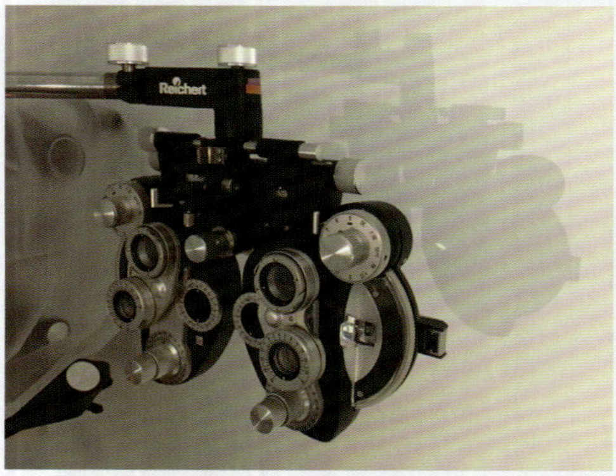

Figure I-28 Refracting the wall. Notice the elliptical image of a distant penlight on the wall behind the phoropter. *(Courtesy of Scott E. Brodie, MD.)*

- Is there astigmatism? Set the cylinder battery to 0.50D of cylinder power, and adjust the sphere power 0.25 D in the opposite direction. Now slowly rotate the cylinder axis knob, and observe the changes in the diameter of the blur circle on the wall. You should be able to set the axis to the optimal position (with the smallest, brightest image) within a few degrees or so. For practice, set it about 10° away from the optimal setting.
- Refine the cylinder axis. Swing the cross cylinder in place, in the "axis" position. Use binary comparisons to optimize the cylinder axis. You should be able to find the optimal axis within a degree or so.
- Refine the cylinder power. Rotate the cross cylinder turret 45° to the "power" position. Use binary comparisons to refine the cylinder power. Notice how the "Key Step" of adjusting the sphere power 0.25 D for each 0.5 D change in cylinder power is necessary to keep the image optimal.When you reach the endpoint, you may see the image flip between small elliptical spots—you are seeing the residual astigmatism that the cross cylinder itself introduces into the optical pathway.
- Remove the cross cylinder, and refine the sphere power to obtain the smallest, brightest image.

试一试！ I–3

- **墙面验光**。了解交叉柱镜工作原理的一个好方法是尝试这个简单的练习。将综合验光仪平行放置在距离墙面大约 20cm 处。挡住综合验光仪一侧的测试孔。随机选一柱镜粘贴到综合验光仪另一侧的背面；金属夹有助于将其固定。（大约在 1.5 D 时效果会很好。从一个与综合验光仪上的柱镜度数相反的柱镜开始。）请一位朋友拿着笔灯或 Finoff 透照仪站在几英尺（1ft=0.3048m）远的地方，指向综合验光仪光圈的开孔。你会看到在综合验光仪后面的墙上投射出一个小椭圆点（图 I–28）。

- **检测屈光球镜**。使用 2 面比较的方法，找到墙上的最佳球形"矫正"。这将是一个圆形图像（最小弥散圆）。

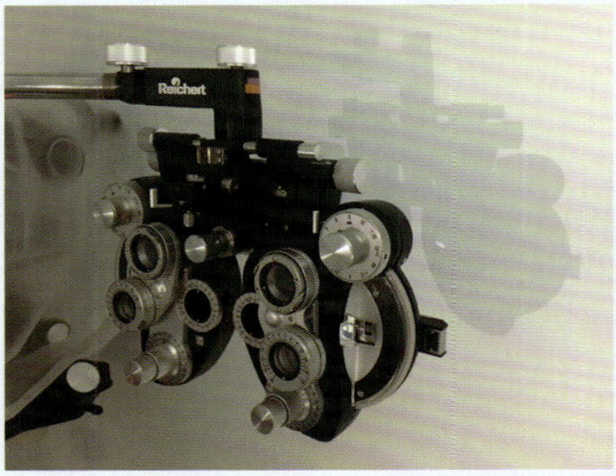

图 I–28 墙面验光。请注意，在综合验光仪后面的墙上有一个遥远的笔灯的椭圆图像。*（译者注：资料来源见前页原文。）*

- 有散光吗？将柱镜度数设置为 0.50D，向相反方向调整 0.25D 球镜度数。现在缓慢旋转柱镜轴位旋钮，并观察墙上模糊圆圈直径的变化。你应该能够在几度左右的范围内将轴设置为最佳位置（最小，最亮的图像）。练习时，请将其设定在 10° 左右，这是最佳距离。

- 精确柱镜轴位。将交叉柱镜摆动到"轴"的位置。使用 2 面比较方法来优化柱镜轴。应该在 1° 左右找到最佳轴。

- 精确柱镜度数。将交叉柱镜转盘从 45° 旋转至"度数"位置。使用 2 面比较方法来明确柱镜度数。为了保持图像的最佳呈现，请注意柱镜度数每改变 0.5D，球镜度数需向反方向调整 0.25D，这一"关键步骤"是非常必要的。在到达终点时，你可能会看到图像在小椭圆点之间翻转—— 你看到的正是交叉柱镜本身引入的光学路径的残余散光。

- 移除交叉柱镜，精确球镜度数，以获得最小、最亮的图像。

- Check your work. The final cylinder correction should closely approximate the power of the "error cylinder" you introduced at the start, with the same axis. (Be careful as you compare axes from the 2 sides of the phoropter!) The final sphere power should be slightly greater than the dioptric equivalent of the distance between the phoropter and the wall, because your light source is not infinitely far away.
- Try this exercise with another error cylinder of the same sign as your phoropter cylinders. The final correcting cylinder will be of nearly the same power, perpendicular to the error *cylinder*.

Step 7: Accommodative Control and Binocular Balance

Accommodation is the ability of the eye to increase the focusing power of the crystalline lens, mainly to allow clear vision for near objects. In general, the primary goal of clinical refraction is to determine the refractive error, if any, with the accommodation fully relaxed. That means the eyes are focused for distant targets; the patient has the full use of the accommodative amplitude to focus over as large a range of nearer objects as possible. In addition, accommodation should be equally relaxed for the 2 eyes—a state referred to as *binocular balance*.

In practice, this fully relaxed state of accommodation may not occur spontaneously as patients sit for refraction, complicating the task of the refractionist. Many factors, such as hyperopic refractive errors (which can often be corrected by a patient's own accommodative effort), awareness of near objects (including the refracting instruments and lenses), and "accommodative spasm," may induce an increase in accommodative tone, steering the refractive process toward undercorrection of a hyperopic error or overcorrection of a myopic error. In some cases, patients seem to prefer the high-contrast, minified image seen by accommodating to compensate for a myopic overcorrection. It is thus important to make every effort to use *accommodative control*—techniques that relax the accommodation during the refraction process and guard against inadvertent stimulation of accommodation and overminusing the patient as a result. The use of a plus lens occluder (instead of an opaque occluder), and biasing the binary comparisons to offer the more-plus choice first, will help prevent spurious accommodation.

It is good practice to double-check the accommodative control as the final step in a routine refraction to guard against these errors, at least in patients below the age of 50 or 60 years. (Accommodation is discussed more fully in Chapter 3.)

The "Rule-1" test is a quick and easy way to check accommodative control. You can perform this test for each eye separately or binocularly if the vision is comparable in the 2 eyes:

A. Dial in +1.00D sphere power above the final refractive correction. Visual acuity should fall at least 2 lines on the eye chart. (For example, if the final refraction brings the acuity to 20/20, adding +1.00D sphere to both eyes should reduce the acuity to 20/30 or worse.)

B. If the acuity does not drop 2 lines as expected, continue to increase the plus sphere power until the acuity is reduced by 2 lines.

- 检查你的工作。最后的柱镜矫正应该与你在开始时设置的“误差柱镜”的度数非常接近，并且是相同的轴。（比较综合验光仪两侧的轴时要小心！）最终的球镜度数应该略大于综合验光仪和墙壁之间距离的等效屈光度，这是因为你的光源不是无限远。

- 尝试使用与你的综合验光仪柱镜符号相同的另一个误差柱镜进行此练习。最终的矫正柱镜将具有几乎相同的度数，并且轴位垂直于误差柱镜。

第 7 步：调节控制和双眼平衡

*调节*是眼睛增加晶状体屈光力的能力，主要是为了让近距离物体有清晰的视觉。一般来说，临床验光的主要目的是确定屈光不正，并需要完全放松调节。这意味着眼睛要专注于远处的目标，患者要充分利用调节幅度来聚焦尽可能大范围的近距离物体。此外，2 只眼睛的调节也应该同样放松——这种状态称为*双眼平衡*。

在检查时，这种完全放松的调节状态不是自发的，因为患者是坐着进行屈光检查的，这使得验光师的任务较为复杂。许多因素，例如远视（通常可以通过患者自身的调节力来纠正）、近距离物体的影响（包括屈光设备和镜片）以及“调节性痉挛”都可能会导致调节张力的增加，使验光对远视矫正不足或对近视过度矫正。在某些情况下，患者通过调节看到高对比度、缩小的像，以此来补偿近视矫正过度。因此，使用*调节控制*——技术是很重要的，该技术在验光过程中要求要放松调节，并防止意外的刺激调节，从而避免导致对患者的过度负镜化。使用正镜片遮盖（而不是不透明的遮盖），并首先提供更多的正镜选择作为二元比较，将有助于防止出现假调节。

作为常规屈光检查的最后一步，最好再次检查调节控制，以防止这些错误发生，至少在 50 岁或 60 岁以下的患者中更要如此。（第 3 章将更全面地讨论调节问题。）

“规则 –1”测试是检查调节控制的一种快速简便的方法。如果 2 只眼睛的视力相当，你可以分别进行单眼测试或双眼同时测试：

A. 拨入大于最终屈光矫正度数 +1.00D 球镜度数。视力表上，视力应至少下降 2 行。（例如，如果最终的屈光度数使视力达到 20/20，那么在 2 只眼睛上加上 +1.00D 的球镜度会使视力降低到 20/30，甚至更差。）

B. 如果视力没有如预期那样下降 2 行，继续增加正球镜度数，直到视力下降 2 行为止。

C. Next, remove the excess added plus sphere power 1 click (0.25 D) at a time until the acuity returns to the optimal level. (Ask ***"Is this step definitely better, or are the letters just smaller and blacker?"***) The final endpoint should be the last step that permits the patient to read additional letters. Disregard the patient's enthusiasm for any additional minus sphere (or reduced plus sphere) power that does not allow more letters to be read.

If you perform this procedure for each eye separately, it also serves as a check of "binocular balance"—that is, assuring that the 2 eyes are accommodating to the same degree.

The Lancaster red-green ("duochrome") test is recommended for patients with 20/40 or better best-corrected acuity. It can be performed monocularly or binocularly. Performed for each eye separately, this test functions as an effective check of binocular balance:

A. Bring up the duochrome slide or filter on your chart projector. This will display 1 side of the chart against a bright red background, and the other side against a bright green background
B. Ask "***Which side of the chart has the clearer, crisper, blacker letters: the red side or the green side?***" (If the patient is confused by the intense colors, add "***Concentrate on the letters, not on the backgrounds. Look at the smallest letters you can read.***"
C. If the patient reports that the letters seen against the *red* background are clearer, more *minus* sphere power is needed; if the *green* side is preferred, more *plus* sphere power is indicated.
D. When in doubt, leave the patient with the more plus (or less minus) sphere choice (ie, with a slight preference for the seeing against the red background), which will better relax the accommodation.

Try It Yourself! I-4

Refract a friend or colleague to become familiar with the process:

- If he or she has little or no refractive error, introduce an error cylinder by taping a cylindrical trial lens to the back of the phoropter. Pay attention to how the ability to provide evaluations of the binary comparisons slows down as you approach the endpoints and the differences in appearance of the targets become subtler. This is an important clue for you as the refractionist. In turn, it is only fair to let him or her refract you.
- Try deliberately overminusing your subject. Notice how far beyond the real refractive endpoint you can go without blurring the vision. Ask your subject to say whether the optotypes start becoming "smaller and blacker."
- With your subject clearly overminused, slowly dial back the refraction toward the correct endpoint. Notice that the accommodative tone is "sticky"—you will likely return to optimal acuity before returning to the original endpoint. Beware: this can happen with your patients, too!
- Refract yourself. Sit behind the phoropter and reach around to operate the knobs in the front. Notice how easy or difficult are the various comparisons you will be asking your patient to make.

C. 接下来，去除额外添加的正球镜度数，每次拨动 1 次（0.25 D），直到视力恢复到最佳水平为止。（问 ***"这一步是否更好吗？或者字母是否更小、更黑？"*** 。）最后的终点应该是最后一步能使患者增加阅读字母。不能增加任何负球镜（或减少正球镜），增加的度数并不能让患者读取更多的字母。

如果你对每只眼睛分别进行了这个步骤，它也可以作为"双眼平衡"的检查——也就是说，确保 2 只眼睛调节的程度相同。

Lancaster 红绿（"双色"）试验用于 20/40（0.5）或更好矫正视力的患者。它可以单眼或双眼进行。该测试可以有效地检查双眼平衡：

A. 打开投影仪上的彩色幻灯片或滤镜。这将使图的一边显示亮红色背景，另一边显示亮绿色背景。

B. 问 ***"哪一侧图像显示更清晰、更黑的字母：红色的一侧还是绿色的一侧？"*** 。如果患者对浓重的颜色感到困惑，可以加上一句：***"把注意力集中在字母上，而不是背景上。看看你能读的最小的字母。"***

C. 如果患者报告在*红*色背景下看到的字母更清晰，则需要增加的*负*球镜度数。如果是在*绿*色背景下看到的字母清晰，则需要增加*正*球镜度数。

D. 当有疑问时，给患者更多的正球镜度数（或减少负球镜度数），即让患者对红色背景下的视觉略有偏好，这样会更好地放松调节。

试一试！ I–4

让朋友或同事验光，以帮助你熟悉这个过程：

- 如果他或她有很少的或没有屈光不正，请通过将试验柱镜粘贴到综合屈光验光检查仪的背面来引入散光屈光不正。请注意，当你接近终点时，研究对象提供 2 面比较评估的能力是如何降低的，目标的外观差异会变得更加微妙。作为验光师，这是一个重要的线索。反过来，让他或她来给你验光。

- 试着有意过度负镜化。请注意，在不模糊视力的情况下，你可以越过真实的屈光终点有多远。问你的研究对象，他们所见的视标是否开始变得"更小、更黑"。

- 当你的研究对象明显感觉到过度的负度数时，慢慢拨回至正确的终点。注意调节是"黏性的"——在回到最初的终点之前，即可恢复到最佳锐度。注：这也可能发生在你的患者身上！

- 给自己验光。坐在综合验光仪后面，伸手去操作前面的旋钮。注意体会你要求患者做的各种比较是简单还是困难。

The duochrome test is based on the chromatic aberration of the human eye. This test works just as well in color-blind patients as in patients with normal color vision, so long as you describe the alternatives as left versus right instead of red versus green.

Step 8: Refraction at Near

Refracting at near (ie, determining the optimal correction, if any, needed for near vision) is not routinely done on patients younger than 40 years of age unless they have a specific near-vision complaint:

A. Begin with the current distance correction in place in the phoropter or trial frame.If you do not know the distance refraction with confidence, perform a careful distance refraction even if the patient volunteered no complaints at distance.

> *This step is critical to detect latent hyperopia.*

Converge the phoropter, so that the optics point toward the near eye chart—use the 2 small levers just below the top of the instrument (Figure I-29). Install the near eye chart on the stick and holder provided for near work at a working distance of 40 cm (Figure I-30). (The multipanel "Rotochart" provided with the phoropter is excellent for near-vision testing. The "Rosenbaum card" also works well.) If this is not available, the patient can hold a near-vision testing card at the appropriate distance. Be sure to provide suitable illumination.

B. Add plus sphere power over the distance correction until near acuity is optimized, with the zone of clear vision centered at 40 cm, or at the patient's preferred reading distance. (Check this by sliding or moving the near card toward and away from the patient.)

Rough near- point "add" guidelines according to age are as follows: 40 years: +1.00D to +2.00D; 50 years: +1.50D to +2.50D; 60 years and older: +2.00D to +2.75 D.

> *Patients frequently prefer higher adds. Try to resist this bias-the higher adds not only require that text be held unnaturally close to the eyes but also decrease the range over which the material can be seen clearly. This decreased range of comfortable reading positions hastens fatigue during reading.*

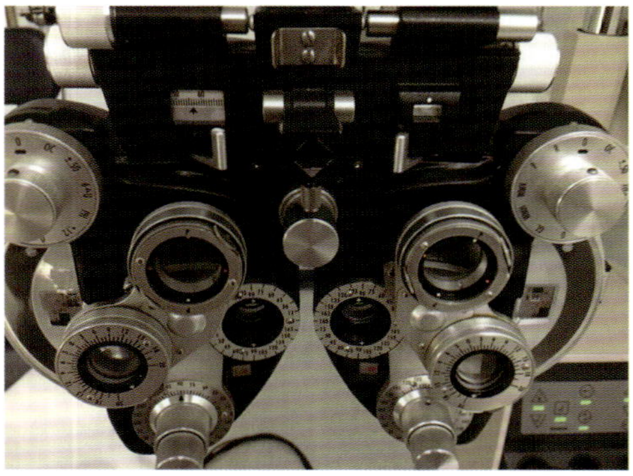

Figure I-29 Converging the phoropter. (Notice the position of the small vertical levers near the top; compare Figure I-23.) *(Courtesy of Scott E. Brodie, MD.)*

双色测试是根据人眼的色差进行的。这个测试在色盲患者和正常色觉患者中同样有效，只要你描述的选项是左或右，而不是红或绿。

第 8 步：近距离验光

一般不会对 40 岁以下的患者常规进行近距离验光（如果仅有近视觉需求，也应进行最佳矫正的测定），除非他们有特定的近视诉求。

A. 从综合验光仪或试镜架的当前距离矫正开始。如果你没有信心确定是否要进行视远验光，即使患者对距离没有诉求，也要小心地进行视远验光。

这一步对检测隐性远视非常重要。

收拢综合验光仪，使光学器件指向近视力表——使用仪器顶部下方的 2 个小杠杆（图 I–29）。在工作距离为 40cm 的工作棒和工作架上安装近视标卡（图 I–30）。（综合验光仪提供的多面板“旋转图表”非常适合近视力测试。“Rosen baum 卡”也很好用。）如果这些不可用，患者可以手持一个近视力测试卡在适当的距离。确保提供适当的照明。

B. 在距离矫正的基础上增加正球镜度数，直到近视力达到最佳状态，清晰视野的区域集中在 40cm 处，或者在患者选择的阅读距离处。（通过朝向和远离患者方向滑动或移动近视力测试卡来检查。）

根据年龄高低，近点粗略“添加”指南如下：40 岁：+1.0D 至 +2.0D；50 岁：+1.5D 至 +2.5D；60 岁：+2.0D 至 +2.75D。

患者通常喜欢更高的视近度数。尽量阻止这种偏离——视近度数越高不仅需要阅读文本不自然地靠近眼睛，而且还要减少清晰地看到文本的范围。这种舒适阅读位置的减少会加速阅读过程中疲劳的产生。

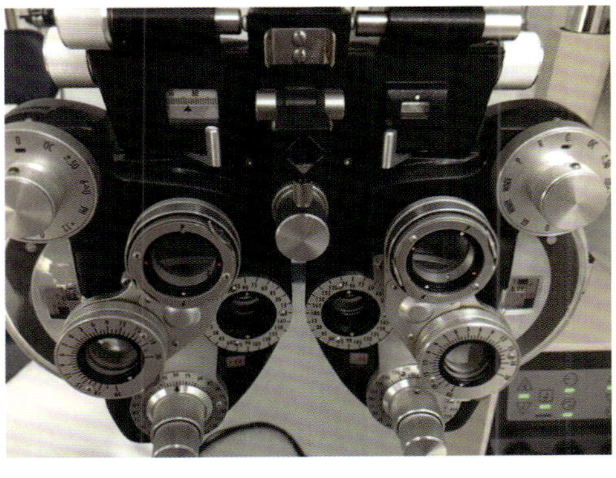

图 I–29 收拢综合验光仪。（注意靠近顶部的小垂直杠杆的位置；与图 I–23 比较。）*（译者注：资料来源见前页原文。）*

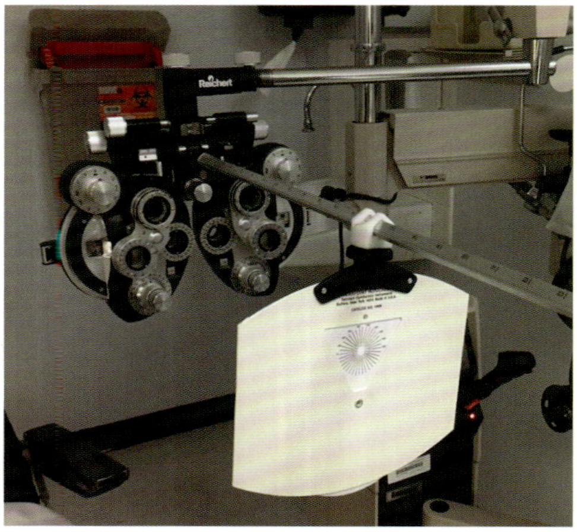

Figure I-30 Phoropter with near-point chart in place at distance 40 cm. *(Courtesy of Scott E. Brodie, MD.)*

When in doubt, chose the lesser add. It should rarely be necessary to use an add greater than +2.75 D, except as a low- vision aid.

> *Corrected acuity at near should roughly correspond to the same Snellen fraction as the distance acuity. (A significant discrepancy, in either direction, suggests the presence of ocular pathology.)*

Final Remarks

At the core of ophthalmic practice is the ability to assess a patient's visual function. To accomplish this, your capacity to perform an efficient, accurate refraction is critical. Subjective refraction is a clinical art—facility takes time to develop. Learn to refract well.

- There are many excuses to avoid refracting almost any patient you see. Refract every patient who needs it. Just because a refraction is not easy does not mean it is not important to the patient or that successful refraction would not greatly benefit the patient. Difficult refractions are an inevitable part of ophthalmology. If necessary, reschedule the difficult patient to allow the additional time.
- Carefully adjust the pace of the refraction to the ability of the patient to respond. The patient should not feel rushed, but offer the binary comparisons crisply to encourage the patient to respond based on his or her initial visual impression. The pace should discourage the patient from attempting to accommodate before deciding on the better lens choice.
- Cycloplegia (paralysis of accommodation with anticholinergic eyedrops) is indicated whenever there is uncertainty about the accommodative status. This technique should be routine for children below the age of 10 years. (See Chapter 4.)
- Many healthy young adults can see 20/15 if given the chance. Don't settle for 20/20, let alone 20/25. Children below the age of 6 or even 7 years are frequently uninterested in reading past the 20/30 line, even though more sophisticated testing methods have shown that they may possess 20/20 acuity. (That is why many "picture" eye charts stop at the 20/30 line.)

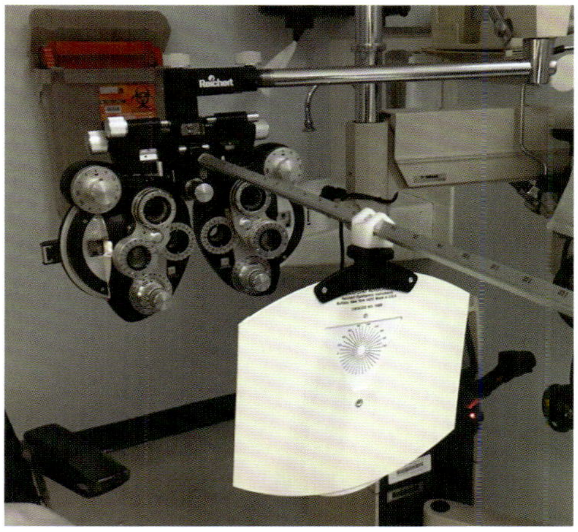

图 I–30 近视力测试卡在距离综合验光仪 40cm 的位置上。（*译者注：资料来源见前页原文。*）

如有疑问，请选择较小的附加度数。除了作为低视力辅助外，很少需要使用大于 +2.75 D 的附加度数。

> *近处的矫正视力应大致对应于 Snellen 分数的远视力（远近视力的显著差异表明存在眼病理学改变）。*

最后评论

眼科实践的核心是正确评估患者的视觉功能。要做到这一点，拥有进行有效、准确验光的能力至关重要。主观屈光检测是一种需要时间来发展的临床艺术。要学好验光技术。

- 许多患者（几乎你看到的所有患者）都有很多借口拒绝验光，仅仅是因为验光不容易，但这并不意味着验光对患者不重要，或者成功的验光不会给患者带来很大的好处。我们应为需要验光的患者验光。复杂性屈光不正是眼科学不可避免的一部分。如果有必要，重新安排那些比较难沟通的患者，以便留出额外的时间。

- 仔细调整验光的速度以适应患者的反应能力。患者不应感到匆忙，而应清晰地提供 2 面比较，要鼓励患者积极配合，并根据其最初的视觉印象作出反应。在决定选择更好的镜片之前，这种速度应该会阻止患者尝试适应。

- 当调节状态不确定时，应使用睫状肌麻痹剂（使用抗胆碱能眼药水麻痹调节）。对于 10 岁以下的儿童，这种技术应该是常规的。（见第 4 章。）

- 如果有机会，许多健康的年轻人可以看到 20/15。不要满足于 20/20，更不要满足于 20/25。6 岁或 7 岁以下的儿童通常对超过 20/30 行的阅读不感兴趣，尽管更复杂的测试方法可以显示出他们可能拥有 20/20 的敏锐度。这就是许多“图片”视力表停留在 20/30 线的原因。

- For children under the age of 6 or 7 years, use a chart with "tumbling" E's, Landolt Cs, or picture targets (see Figure 3-6). Do not rely on a parent's assurance that the child knows the letters.

There are few opportunities in clinical ophthalmology to improve your patient's visual function as convincingly as the chance to prescribe a good pair of glasses. Competent refraction is key tool toward developing a patient's confidence in you.

- 对于 6 岁或 7 岁以下的儿童，使用带有翻转 E、Landolt C 视标或图像目标的图表（见图 3–6）。不要指望父母能保证孩子知道这些字母。

在临床眼科中，几乎没有比像给患者开一副好眼镜那样更能令人信服地改善他们的视觉功能的机会了。有效的验光是让患者对你产生信任的关键工具。

（翻译 何媛 张纯涛 伊恩晖 许志强 姚森 贺金刚 袁立飞 // 审校 陈研明 石一宁）

CHAPTER 1

Geometric Optics

Highlights

- refractive index
- refraction at an interface: Snell's law
- Prisms
- refraction at a single curved interface: the lensmaker's equation
- two-sided lenses
- general refracting systems
- real and virtual objects and image
- transverse magnification; axial magnification
- ray tracing
- nodal points
- reduced or equivalent optical systems
- aberrations
- astigmatism
- mirrors
- telescopes

Glossary

Aberration Any deviation of an optical system from stigmatic imaging.

Angle of incidence The angle between a ray incident to a mirror and the surface normal at the point of incidence.

Angle of reflection The angle between a ray reflected off a mirror and the surface normal at the point of incidence.

Astigmatism The disparity in focal length for rays from a single object point that are incident at different meridians of the lens.

Axial magnification The ratio of the axial extent (depth) of the image of an extended source object to the depth of the object—measured along the optic axis.

Chromatic aberration A variation in the power of a lens system with the wavelength of incident light.

第 1 章

几何光学

重点

- 折射率。
- 界面折射：Snell 定律。
- 棱镜。
- 单曲界面的折射：透镜制作商方程。
- 双面透镜。
- 一般折射系统。
- 实和虚的物与像。
- 横向放大率；轴向放大率。
- 光线追踪。
- 节点。
- 简化或等效的光学系统。
- 像差。
- 像散。
- 面镜。
- 望远镜。

术语

像差 光学系统与共点成像的偏差。

入射角 在入射点处，入射光线与镜面或由面法线之间的夹角。

反射角 在入射点处，反射光线与镜面或由面法线之间的夹角。

像散 来自单个物点的光线，入射至透镜的不同子午线时，焦距的差异。

轴向放大率 当一个扩展发光物体形成一个具有一定大小的像时，这个像沿光轴的长度（深度）与沿光轴测量的物体深度的比。

色差 透镜系统屈光力随入射光波长的变化。

Coma A disparity in focal length for rays from a single off-axis object point that are refracted at different distances from the center of the lens.

Conjugate points Points that share an object–image relationship.

Conoid of Sturm A geometric figure traced by the refraction of a single point source object by an astigmatic lens.

Critical angle The angle at which a light ray passing from one medium to another with a lower refractive index undergoes total internal reflection.

Curvature of field A disparity in focal length for objects at different distances from the optic axis.

Defocus An aberration corresponding to an axial refractive error, a disparity between the power and the axial length of the eye.

Depth of field The range of locations of a source object for which an optical system forms acceptably sharp images.

Depth of focus The range of image locations over which an optical system forms acceptably sharp images of a fixed source object.

Diopter The reciprocal meter, the customary unit for vergence and the power of lenses.

Distortion A disparity in transverse magnification for objects at different distances from the optic axis.

Effectivity of lenses The adjustment in the power of a lens necessary to compensate for changes in the distance between the lens and the desired image location.

Fermat's principle Among alternative paths between 2 points, light rays travel along the path with the shortest total travel time.

Galilean telescope A telescope with a convex objective lens and a concave ocular lens.

Gaussian optics An efficient mathematical treatment for the paraxial optical regime by means of linear algebra.

Geometric optics Optical phenomena that are effectively described in terms of light rays, which travel along straight lines unless deviated by lenses or mirrors.

Jackson cross cylinder A lens superimposing cylindrical lenses of equal and opposite power, placed with axes perpendicular to each other.

Keplerian telescope A telescope with convex objective and ocular lenses.

Law of reflection The statement that the angle of incidence equals the angle of reflection.

Lensmaker's equation A mathematical formula for the power of a curved refracting surface.

Nodal points The conjugate points on the optic axis through which incident and exiting light rays form equal angles with the optic axis.

彗差　来自单个偏离轴物点的光线，在距离透镜中心不同距离处折射时，在焦距方面的差异。

共轭点　物－像点的关系。

Sturm 锥体　单个点发光物体的光线被像散透镜折射后，折射光线的几何踪迹图。

临界角　光线从一种介质射向另一种折射率较低的介质时，发生全反射时的入射角。

场曲　在距离光轴不同距离处的物体的焦距差异。

离焦　对应于轴性屈光不正的像差，眼的屈光力和眼轴长度之间的差异。

景深　一个光学系统呈可接受的清晰像的发光物体的位置范围。

焦深　一个固定位置的发光物体，其光线经光学系统后所形成的可接受的清晰像的位置范围。

屈光度　米的倒数，聚散度和透镜屈光力的常用单位。

畸变　物体在距光轴不同距离时横向放大率的差异。

透镜有效性　为补偿透镜与所需像位置之间距离的变化，对透镜屈光力的调整。

Fermat 原理　光线在 2 个点之间的多路径传播中，总是沿传播时间最短的路径传播。

Galileo 望远镜　由具有凸透镜的物镜和凹透镜的目镜组成的望远镜。

Gauss 光学　利用线性代数对近轴光学区域进行有效的数学计算。

几何光学　用光线特性描述的光学现象，除非被透镜或面镜偏离，否则光线沿直线传播。

Jackson 交叉圆柱镜　轴相互垂直，焦度大小相等、符号相反的 2 个柱镜叠加的透镜。

Kepler 望远镜　具有凸透镜物镜和目镜的望远镜。

反射定理　入射角等于反射角的陈述。

透镜制造商方程　计算曲面折射面屈光力的数学公式。

节点　入射光和出射光线与光轴形成的角相等时，在光轴上共轭点。

Paraxial (or paraxial ray) The optical regime in which light rays travel close to the optic axis and form only small angles with the optic axis. Rays conforming to this description are termed *paraxial rays*.

Point spread function The distribution of light from a point source in the image plane, which characterizes the aberration of an optical system.

Power cross A graphical depiction of the action of a toric lens, showing the orientation of the principal axes and the power along each axis.

Power-versus-meridian graph A graph showing the power of an astigmatic lens at each meridian.

Prentice position An orientation for an ophthalmic prism such that incoming light rays strike the anterior surface of the prism perpendicularly.

Principal plane One of 2 planes at which the refraction of a general lens system appears to take place.

Principal point The intersection of either principal plane with the optic axis.

Prism diopter A unit describing the deflection of light by an ophthalmic prism equal to 100 times the tangent of the angle of deflection.

Ray tracing The graphical localization of images by drawing rays of light from the source object through the focal points and nodal points of an optical system.

Real image An image formed by the actual convergence of light rays.

Real object An actual object that serves as the source of light rays in an optical system.

Reduced optical system A simplified optical system equivalent to a general multi-element optical system characterized by the power and the locations of the principal planes and the nodal points.

Reduced vergence The product of object or image vergence and the refractive index of the medium through which the light travels.

Reference sphere The hypothetical spherical wavefront surface that corresponds to a perfect point image.

Refractive index The ratio of the speed of light in a vacuum to the speed of light in a material medium.

Seidel aberrations A series of common aberrations of simple optical systems.

Snell's law A mathematical description of the deflection of light as it passes between media with different refractive indices.

Spherical aberration A disparity in focal length for rays from a single axial object point that are refracted at different distances from the center of the lens.

Spherical equivalent The power of a spherical lens approximately equivalent to the average power of an astigmatic lens.

Stigmatic imaging Imaging by a lens system that focuses the light from a point source at a single image point.

近轴（或近轴光线）　光线靠近光轴并且仅与光轴形成很小角度的光线区，符合这样的光线称为*近轴光线*。

点扩散函数　来自点光源的光在像平面的光强分布，表征光学系统的像差。

屈光力十字　复曲面镜作用的图示，显示了主轴的方向和沿每个轴的屈光力。

屈光力与子午线图　显示散光透镜在每个子午线屈光力的图表。

Prentice 方位　可以使入射光垂直地入射至棱镜前表面的眼用棱镜摆放方位。

主平面　一般透镜系统发生折射的 2 个平面之一。

主点　任意 1 个主平面与光轴的交点。

棱镜度　描述眼用棱镜的光偏向程度的单位，等于偏向角正切的 100 倍。

光线追踪　来自发光物体的光线，经光学系统的焦点和节点后所成像的定位图。

实像　由光线实际会聚形成的像。

实物　光学系统中发光的实际物体。

简化光学系统　一种简化的光学系统，相当于一般的多元件光学系统，以屈光力、主平面位置以及节点位置为特征。

简化聚散度　物或像的聚散度与光线所经过介质的折射率之积。

参考球　对应于理想点像的假想球面波前。

折射率　真空中光速与物质介质中光速的比率。

Seidel 像差　简单光学系统的一系列普通像差。

Snell 定律　光经过折射率不同的两种介质时发生的光的偏向的数学描述。

球面像差　来自轴上单一物点的光线，在距透镜中心不同距离处折射时的焦距差异。

等效球镜　近似等于散光透镜平均屈光力的球镜屈光力。

共点成像　通过透镜系统成像，将来自单个点光源的光聚焦成单个像点。

Surface normal A line perpendicular to a surface through a central point of interest.

Thin-lens approximation An approximate treatment appropriate for thin lenses that ignores the spacing between the front and back lens surfaces.

Tilt An aberration equivalent to the direction of light rays at an angle from the optic axis, as if deflected by a prism.

Toric surface A curved (spherocylindrical) surface resembling a portion of the outer curvature of a torus, such as an automobile tire inner tube.

Total internal reflection The reflection of a light beam directed from one medium to another with a lower refractive index when the angle of incidence exceeds the critical angle, and no emerging ray can satisfy Snell's law.

Transverse magnification The ratio of the height of an image to the height of the source object, measured perpendicular to the optic axis.

Vergence equation A mathematical relationship between object vergence, the power of a lens or mirror, and the resultant image vergence.

Vergence The reciprocal of the distance between a source object or image and a lens or mirror.

Virtual image An apparent image inferred as the source of a divergent bundle of light rays.

Virtual object An intermediate image formed by an optical system that serves as the apparent source of a bundle of light rays, which in turn is imaged by a subsequent optical element.

Wavefront A surface connecting the points of equal travel time for rays of light emerging from a single point source.

Zernike polynomials A standard mathematical system of polynomial functions used to describe the deviation of a wavefront from the reference sphere as a description of the aberration of an optical system.

Introduction

Geometric optics refers to those optical phenomena that are effectively described in terms of light rays, which travel along straight lines unless deviated by lenses or mirrors. Phenomena such as diffraction, polarization, and interference, which illustrate the wave properties of light, and fluorescence, phosphorescence, and amplification by stimulated emission (as in lasers), which illustrate quantum properties of light, are discussed in Chapter 2.

The basic principles of geometric optics can be summarized in 4 simple rules:

1. Light rays travel in straight lines through uniform media.
2. The paths of light rays can be altered only by reflection (when they encounter a smooth reflective surface, such as a mirror) or by refraction (when they travel at different speeds from one medium to another), according to the law of reflection and Snell's law, respectively.

曲面法线　通过目标中心点并垂直于表面的线。

薄透镜近似　适用于忽略前后表面之间间距的薄镜片的近似处理。

倾斜　与光轴成一定角度的光线方向上的等效像差，类似棱镜偏向。

复曲面　（球柱形）曲面，类似于圆环外曲面的一部分，如汽车轮胎内胎。

全内反射　光束从一种介质射向另一种低折射率介质，当入射角超过临界角时的反射，此时没有出现满足 Snell 定线的折射光线。

横向放大　垂直于光轴测量的像高与发光物体高度的比率。

聚散度方程　物的聚散度、透镜或面镜的屈光力与最终像的聚散度之间的数学关系式。

聚散度　发光物体或像和透镜或面镜之间距离的倒数。

虚像　看作是发散光束的光源时，所推测出的表观像。

虚物　它是光学系统所成的像，被看作后续光学元件的表观光源，可再次成像。

波前　连接从单点光源发出的光线、经过相等时间到达的点连成的面。

Zernike 多项式　用于描述波前与参考球镜的偏差的多项式函数的标准数学系统，描述光学系统的像差。

引言

*几何光学*是指根据光线特性描述的光学现象，光线沿着直线传播，除非遇到透镜或镜子才会发生偏离。在第 2 章中讨论衍射、偏振和干涉等现象来阐明光的波动特性，讨论荧光、磷光和受激辐射的放大（如激光）等现象来阐明光的量子特性。

几何光学的基本原理可以归纳为 4 个简单的规则：

1. 光线在均匀介质中以直线传播。
2. 根据反射定律和 Snell 定律，光线的路径分别只能通过反射（遇到光滑的反射表面，如面镜）或通过折射（当以不同的速度从一种介质传播到另一种介质）来改变。

3. When light rays pass through more than one refractive surface, the image formed at each surface in turn becomes the source object for the action of the next refracting surface the rays encounter.
4. The paths of light rays are reversible.

The basic ideas of refraction with lenses were introduced in Part 1 of the Quick-Start Guide. If you are not familiar with this material, it would be helpful to review that chapter now, before proceeding with the more detailed treatment provided here.

Refractive Index

The speed of light in a vacuum (299,792,458 m/s) is one of the fundamental constants of nature. The speed of light in air is essentially the same. It is convenient to refer to the speed of light in other ("denser") materials by comparison to the speed of light in a vacuum: the ratio of the speed of light in a vacuum to the speed of light in another medium is referred to as the refractive index of the medium. (This casual use of the term denser has nothing to do with the specific gravity of different materials.) We abbreviate the refractive index as n,

$$n = \frac{\text{Speed of light in a vacuum}}{\text{Speed of light in a medium}}$$

and use subscripts to designate different media as appropriate. Because the speed of light in a vacuum is always greater than its speed in any material medium, the refractive index of any material medium is always greater than 1.0.

A material's chemical composition, and sometimes other factors, strongly influence its refractive index. By incorporating small amounts of various additives, manufacturers can vary the refractive index (and other properties) of optical glass from less than 1.4 to more than 1.9. The refractive indices of various materials of interest are listed in Table 1-1.

Table 1-1 Refractive Indices of Some Clinically Important Media[a]

Medium	Refractive Index	Refractive Index (Approximate)
Vacuum	1.00000 (exactly)	
Air at STP	1.000277	1.000
Water at 25°C	1.3325	1.33, or 4/3
Aqueous and vitreous humors	1.336	1.33, or 4/3
Cornea	1.376	
PMMA	1.49	1.50, or 3/2
HEMA (monomer)	1.4505	

[a]The approximate values are used in this text. The values may depend on conditions. For instance, the refractive index of water varies with temperature. The refractive index of HEMA polymer depends on its water content and differs somewhat from that of HEMA monomer.

Although it is occasionally critical to determine the refractive index to several decimal places, approximate values are sufficiently accurate for most clinical purposes. For example, the refractive index of the vitreous humor is 1.336, but the approximate value of 4⁄3 is much easier to remember and introduces negligible error.

3. 当光线通过 1 个以上的折射表面时，在每个表面形成的像依次成为下一个折射面的发光物体。

4. 光路是可逆的。

《快速入门指南》第 1 部分介绍了透镜折射的基本概念，如果不熟悉这些材料，那么在继续本章的学习之前，请复习前一章。

折射率

真空中的光速（299 792 458 m / s）是自然界的基本常数之一。空气中的光速本质上基本相同。通过与真空中的光速进行比较，可以方便地参考其他（“密度”）材料的光速：真空中的光速与另一种介质中的光速的比率称为介质的折射率（这使用术语“密度”一词与不同材料的比重无关），此折射率缩写为 n，

$$折射率 = \frac{真空中的光速}{介质中的光速}$$

并使用下标来指定不同的媒体。因为真空中的光速总是大于其在任何材料介质中的速度，所以任何材料介质的折射率总是大于 1.0。

材料的化学成分和其他因素会影响其折射率。通过少量加入各种添加剂，制造商可以将折射率小于 1.4 的光学玻璃（和其他性能）改变到 1.9。各种材料的折射率列于表 1–1 中。

表1–1　一些临床重要介质[a]的屈光指数

介质	折射率	折射率（近似）
真空	1.00000（准确的）	
在STP的空气中	1.000277	1.000
在 25℃水中	1.3325	1.33 或 4/3
房水和玻璃体	1.336	1.33 或 4/3
角膜	1.376	
PMMA	1.49	1.50 或 3/2
HEMA（单体）	1.4505	

[a] 本文中用近似值。条件不同，屈光指数值也不同。例如，水中折射率随温度变化 HEMA单体取决于水的含量，不同水含量的HEMA单体的折射率也不同。

虽然有时候将折射率精确到小数点后几位是很重要的，但近似值也可以满足大多数临床要求。例如，玻璃体的折射率是 1.336，但是 4/3 的近似值更容易被记住，且可以忽略误差。

Flat Refracting Surfaces—Snell 's Law

The optics of a flat refracting interface, such as the surface of a still pool of water or a flat slab of glass, are easy to describe. As light passes from a "less dense" medium (lower refractive index, greater speed of light) to a denser medium (higher refractive index, lesser speed of light), light rays bend toward the line perpendicular to the interface at the point of entry (the *surface normal*, or just the "normal line"), according to *Snell's law* (Figure 1-1):

$$n_1 \sin \theta_1 = n_2 \sin \theta_2$$

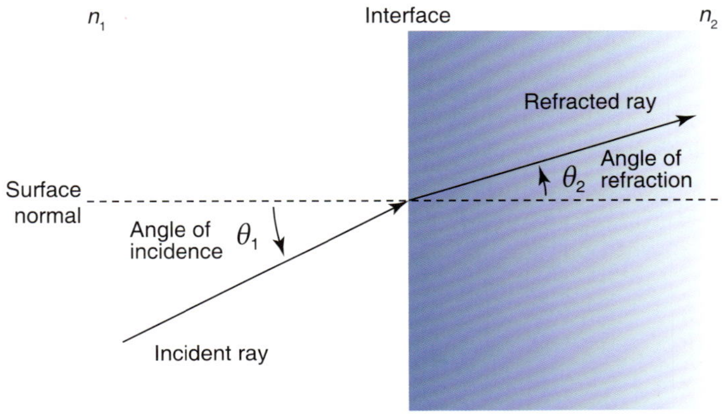

Figure 1-1 Snell's law. The angle of incidence θ_1 is defined by the incident ray and the sur face normal (dashed line). The angle of refraction θ_2 is defined by the refracted ray and the surface normal. The 4 variables n_1, n_2, θ_1, and θ_2 are related by Snell's law, $n_1 \sin \theta_1 = n_2 \sin \theta_2$. When $n_1 < n_2$ (ie, the speed of light is reduced when rays cross the interface from left to right), the refracted ray bends toward the surface normal; when $n_1 > n_2$, the refracted ray bends away from the normal. *(Illustration developed by Edmond H. Thall, MD.)*

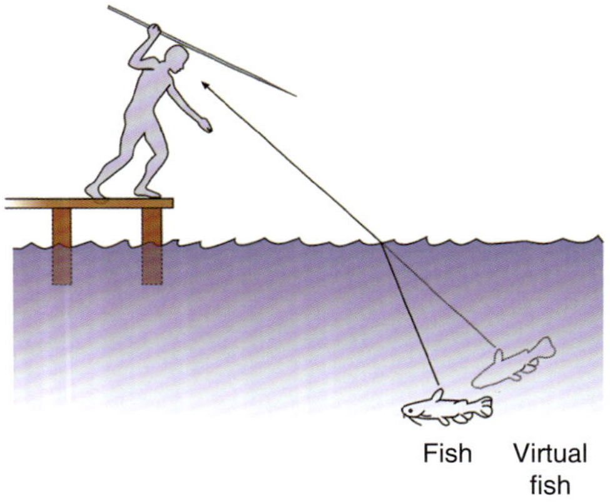

Figure 1-2 The fisherman must throw the spear in front of the virtual fish to hit the actual fish. *(Illustration developed by Kevin M. Miller, MD, rendered by Jonathan Clark, and modified by Neal H. Atebara, MD.)*

If light travels from a denser medium to a less dense medium, light rays bend *away* from the surface normal.

This redirection of light at a flat interface produces an apparent object displacement, such as that seen when you look into a body of water (Figure 1-2) or that provided by an ophthalmic prism.

平面折射面——Snell 定律

平面折射面的光学系统，例如静水池或平板玻璃的表面，是很容易描述的。当光从“低密度”介质（较低的折射率，较高的光速）传递到更密集的介质（更高的折射率，更低的光速）时，根据 *Snell 定律*，光线偏向入射点，且垂直于分界面（*面法线或法线*）一侧：

$$n_1 \sin\theta_1 = n_2 \sin\theta_2$$

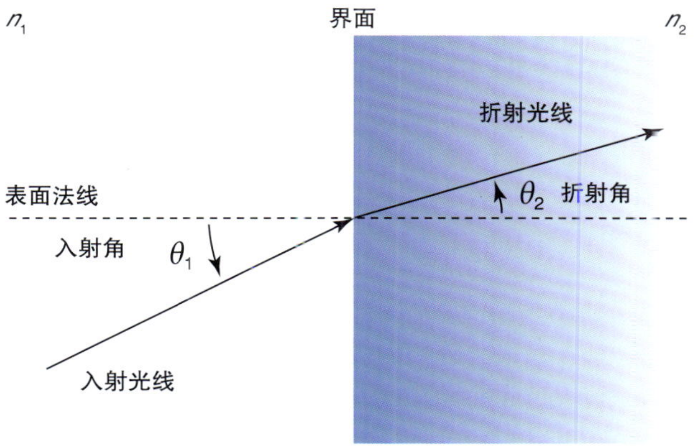

图 1–1　Snell 定律。入射角 θ_1 由入射光线和表面法线（虚线）组成。折射角 θ_2 由折射光线和表面法线组成。4 个变量 n_1，n_2，θ_1 和 θ_2 与 Snell 定律相关，$n_1\sin\theta_1=n_2\sin\theta_2$。当 $n_1<n_2$ 时（即当光线从左向右穿过界面时光速减小），折射光线向表面法线弯曲；当 $n_1>n_2$ 时，折射光线偏离法线。*（译者注：资料来源见前页原文。）*

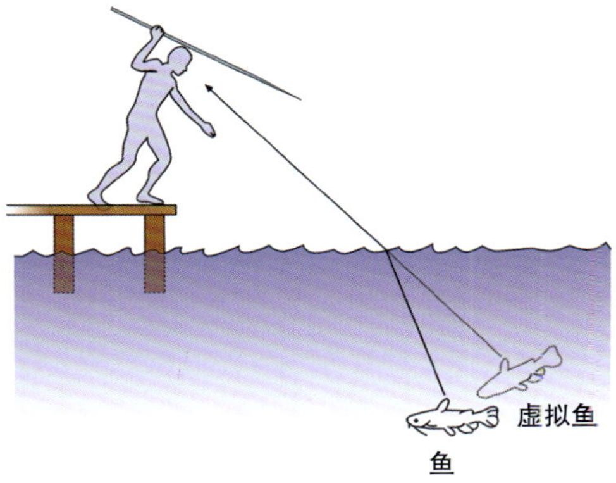

图 1–2　渔民必须将矛投在虚拟鱼的前面才能击中真实鱼。*（译者注：资料来源见前页原文。）*

如果光从光密介质传播到光疏介质时，光线就会*偏离*表面法线。

在这种平面界面上，光会重新会聚产生明显的物体位移，例如当我们观察水中物体（图 1–2）或用眼经棱镜观察物体时所看到的位移。

Prisms

You are probably already familiar with dispersing prisms that produce rainbows or spectra. Refractive index varies with frequency (or wavelength) of light, a phenomenon known as *dispersion* (discussed in Chapter 2). When light containing a mixture of frequencies traverses a dispersing prism, each frequency is deviated by a different amount, producing a spectrum. Ophthalmic prisms help minimize the separation of colors by using materials that have nearly the same refractive index for all frequencies so that all the light is deviated by essentially the same amount.

When a ray traverses a prism, the ray is deviated in accordance with Snell's law. The same prism can produce a range of deviations. The angle of deviation is greatest when the ray strikes one face of the prism at normal incidence (the Prentice position, Figure 1-3A). The angle of deviation is least when light passes through the prism symmetrically (the minimum deviation position, MAD; Figure 1-3B).

Prism Power

Prisms are labeled with a prism power—its strength, or amount of deviation produced as a light ray traverses the prism. That labeled power is correct only if the prism is positioned in front of the patient in a manner consistent with its labeling. Glass prisms should be held in the Prentice position and plastic prisms or plastic prism bars in the MAD position. You can approximate the latter by holding the prism with its back surface perpendicular to the direction of the fixation object, which for distant objects corresponds to the frontal plane position (Figure 1-3C).

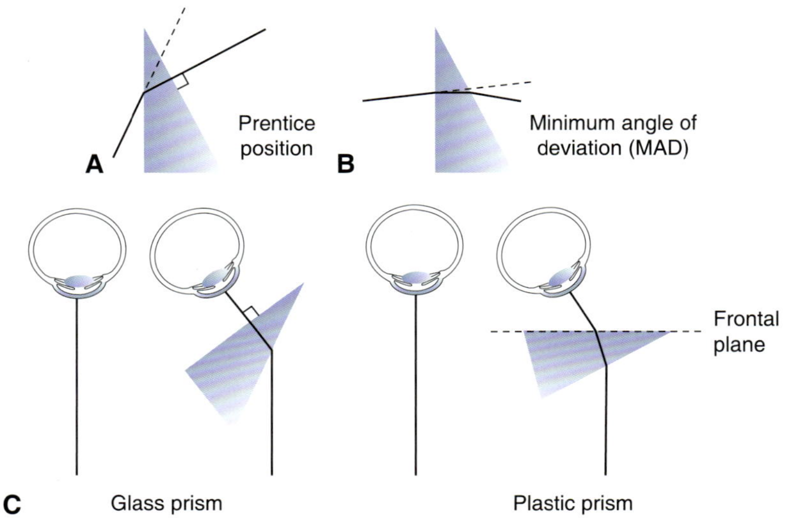

Figure 1-3 Positioning of prisms. **A**, Prentice position. The prism is held with its back surface perpendicular to the line of sight. Use this position for glass prisms. **B**, Minimum deviation position, MAD. The prism is held such that the line of sight makes an equal angle with 2 faces of the prism. **C**, Left: glass prisms should be used in the Prentice position; Right: Plastic prisms should be held in the frontal plane position. The prism is held with its rear surface in the frontal plane (perpendicular to the direction of the fixation object). This position approximates the minimum deviation position, which is difficult to estimate. *(Parts A and B are courtesy of Edmond H. Thall, MD; part C is an illustration developed by Edmond H. Thall, MD, and Kevin M. Miller, MD, and rendered by C. H. Wooley.)*

棱镜

我们已经熟悉会产生彩虹或光谱的色散棱镜。折射率会随光的频率（或波长）而变化，这种现象称为*色散*（在第 2 章中讨论）。当混合频率的光穿过色散棱镜时，每个频率都会发生不同程度的偏离，从而产生光谱。眼用棱镜通过使用对于所有频率具有相同折射率的材料，使所有光偏离量相同，来减小色光分开。

当光线穿过棱镜时，会根据 Snell 定律发生偏离。相同的棱镜可以产生一系列偏差。当光线在法线垂直入射（Prentice 方位，图 1–3A）到棱镜的 1 个面时，偏差角最大。当光线对称通过棱镜时，偏差角最小（最小偏差位置，MAD; 图 1–3B）。

棱镜焦度

棱镜用棱镜焦度标记——即棱镜强度或光线穿过棱镜时产生的偏差量。只有当棱镜以与其标记一致的方式置于患者前方时，标记的屈光力才是正确的。玻璃棱镜在 Prentice 方位，而塑料棱镜或塑料棱镜杆应在最小偏向角（MAD）方位，后者的近似值通过将棱镜的背面垂直于固视物体的方向获得，对于远处物体，该棱镜对应于前平面位置（图 1–3C）。

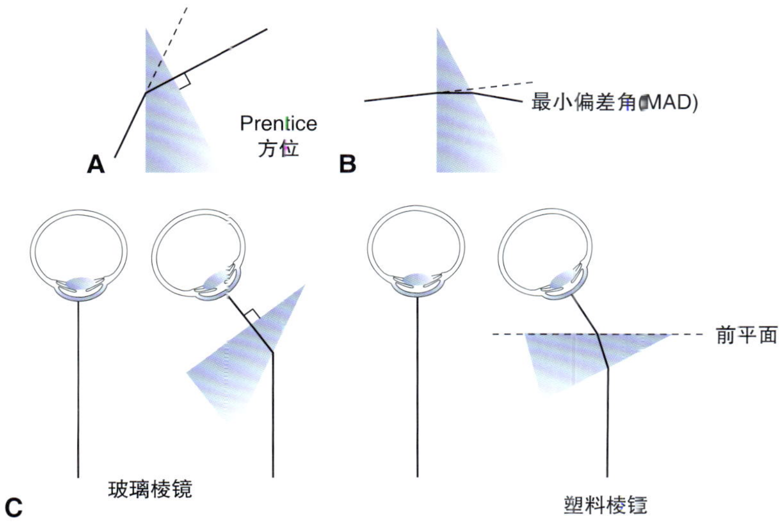

图 1–3　棱镜的方位。**A**.Prentice 方位。棱镜被抬起到后表面垂直于视线。将此位置用于玻璃棱镜。**B**. 最小偏向角，MAD。使视线与棱镜的 2 个面形成相等的角度。**C**. 左：玻璃棱镜应在 Prentice 方位使用；右：塑料棱镜应保持在前平面位置。棱镜的后表面位于前平面（垂直于固视物体的方向）。该位置近似于最小偏向角，这很难估计。*（译者注：资料来源见前页原文。）*

The power of prisms combined with surfaces adjacent is *not* additive (Figure 1-4A). To verify this, look at the interface between 2 such combined prisms (Figure 1-4B). Notice, however, that the net effect of 2 prisms placed over the 2 eyes separately is additive. It is thus preferable to split the prisms between the 2 eyes when you measure large strabismic deviations.

The angular deviation a prism produces is measured not in degrees or radians but in prism diopters. A *prism diopter* is the number of centimeters of deviation at 100 cm from the prism (Figure 1-5). This is equal to 100 times the tangent of the angle of deviation. The prism diopter is indicated by a delta symbol (Δ). Thus, 15Δ is a deviation of 15 cm at 1 m.

A prism deviates light toward its base. Therefore, the virtual image that the eye sees is shifted toward the apex of the prism (Figure 1-6).

The orientation of a prism is designated by its base, as base up, base down, base in, or base out. A patient may have both a vertical and a horizontal deviation, in which case prism power adds as vectors. For instance, a 4Δ base-out prism combined with a 3Δ base-up prism in front of the right eye produces a net 5Δ base at the 143° meridian, base up-and-out. (Meridians are discussed in the Quick-Start Guide.) Clinically, it is rarely necessary to be concerned with this detail. You can prescribe the prism by specifying the individual base-up and base-down powers; the optician will perform the calculation. However, be aware that the lens will be ground with a single prism at an orientation that is neither base up nor base down.

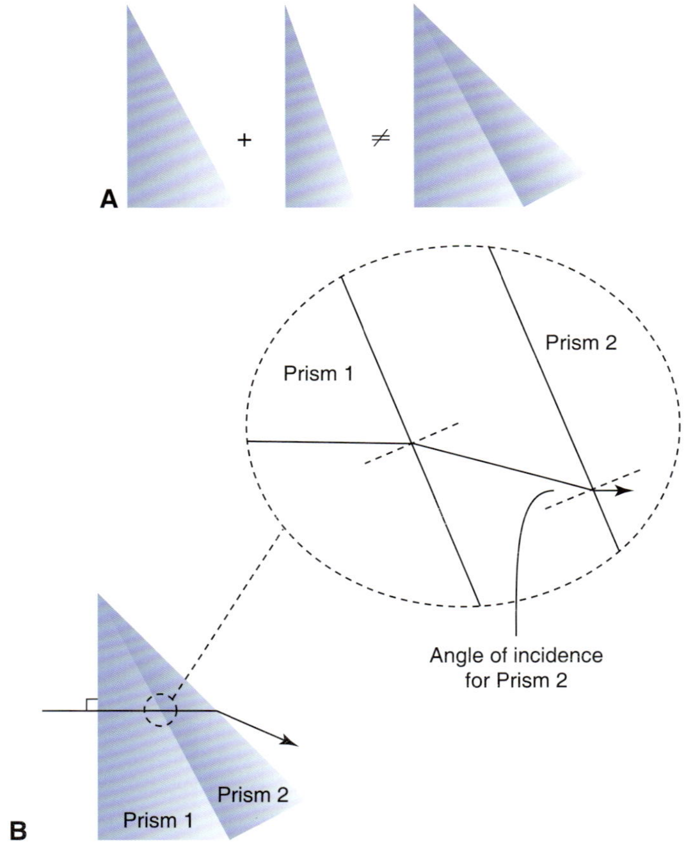

Figure 1-4 Prism power is not additive. **A**, The power of 2 prisms in contact is not equal to the sum of the powers of the individual prisms. The resulting deviation is much larger. Prisms should never be combined in this way. Look at the interface between 2 stacked glass prisms: **B**, with prism 1 in the Prentice position, the light ray is perpendicular to the first surface of prism 1; with prism 2 nowhere near the Prentice position, the light ray enters at an angle far from perpendicular. *(Part A developed by Edmond H. Thall, MD. Part B from Irsch K. Optical issues in measuring strabismus. Middle East African Journal of Ophthalmology. 2015;22:265–270.)*

相邻棱镜间的屈光力*不是*相加的（图 1–4A）。这一点可以通过 2 个组合棱镜之间的界面得到验证（图 1–4B）。但是，分别放在 2 只眼睛上的 2 个棱镜的净效应是相加的。因此，当测量较大的斜视偏差时，可以将棱镜拆分后放在 2 只眼睛上。

棱镜产生的角偏差不是以度或弧度计算的，而是以棱镜度计算的。*棱镜度*（图 1–5）是距离棱镜 100cm 处的偏差值（以 cm 为单位）。这等于 100 倍的角度正切的偏离。该棱镜度用符号 Δ 表示。因此，15Δ 是 1m 处的 15cm 的偏差。

棱镜将光偏向棱镜底部。因此，眼睛看到的虚像向棱镜的顶点移动（图 1–6）。

棱镜的方向由其基底部决定，如底向上、底向下底向内或底向外，可同时具有垂直偏差和水平偏差。在这种情况下，棱镜屈光力为矢量和。例如，4Δ 底向外的棱镜联合 3Δ 底向上的棱镜放置在右眼前，产生净 5Δ 底向 143° 子午线，底向上外。（《快速入门指南》中讨论了子午线。）临床上，很少需要关注这个细节。可以给出单独的底向上和底向下棱镜屈光力，让配镜师进行计算。但是，请注意镜片中的棱镜是单独磨制的，其方向既不是底向上也不是底向下。

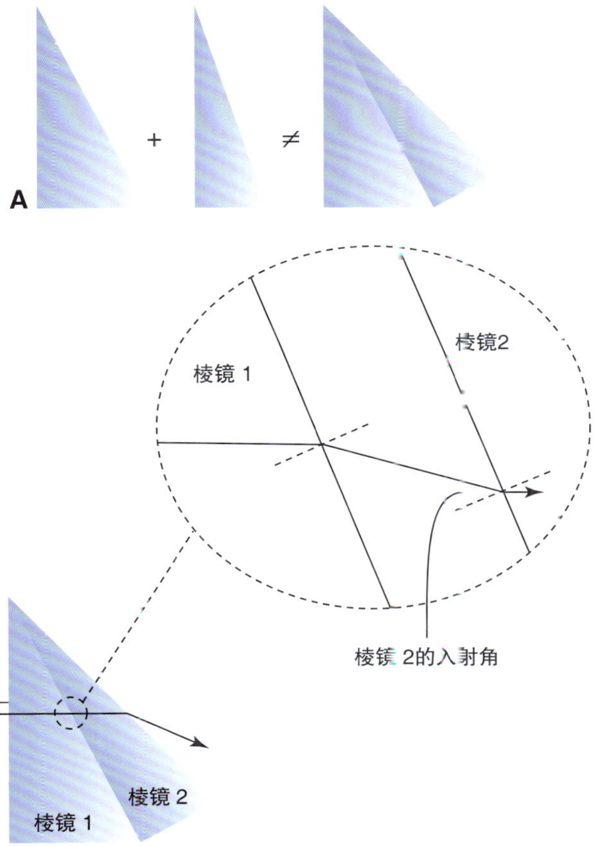

图 1–4　棱镜屈光力不是相加。**A.** 2 个接触的棱镜屈光力不等于各个棱镜屈光力之和，会产生很大的偏差。不能以这种方式组合棱镜。观察 2 个叠加的玻璃棱镜界面：**B.** 棱镜 1 在 Prentice 方位，光线垂直于棱镜 1 的第一表面；棱镜 2 远离 Prentice 方位，光线也不是以垂直的角度进入的。*（译者注：资料来源见前页原文。）*

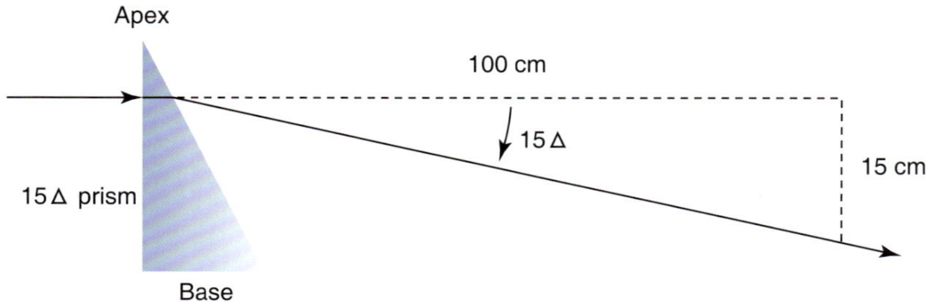

Figure 1-5 Definition of a prism diopter. One prism diopter is a deviation of 1 cm at a distance of 1 m from a prism. This prism is a 15Δ prism, so light is deviated 15 cm toward the base, measured 100 cm away from the prism. *(Courtesy of Kristina Irsch, PhD.)*

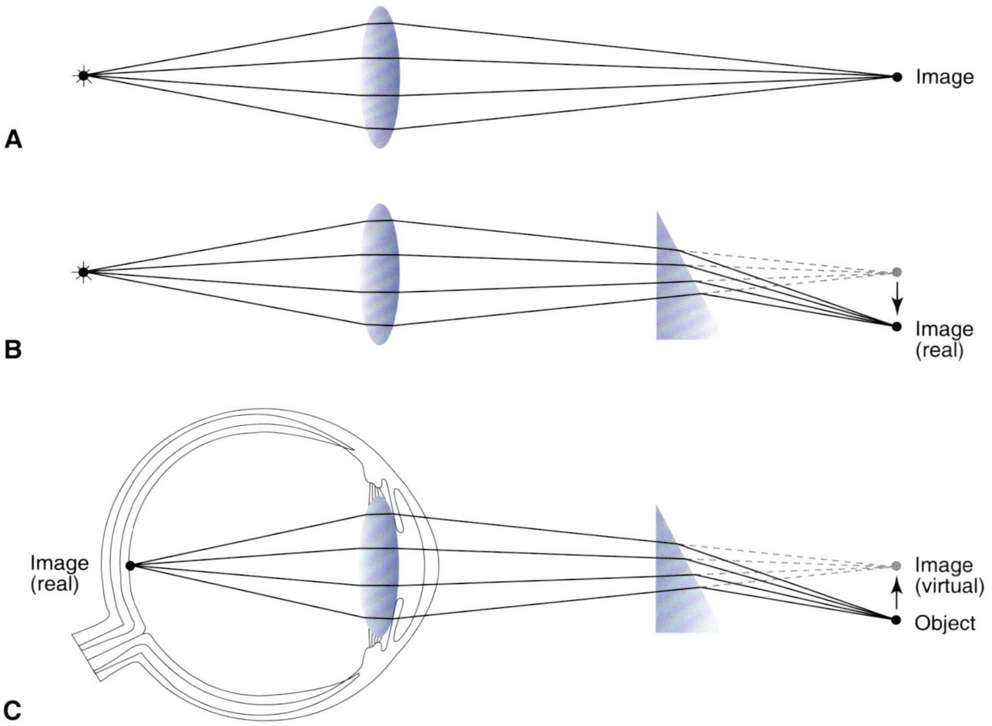

Figure 1-6 Effect of prisms on image position. **A**, Original real image formed by a lens. **B**, Base-down prism added. Because light passing through a prism is always refracted toward the prism's base, the original real image is also displaced toward the base, in this case down- ward. **C**, By turning the light around, we see that a virtual image viewed through a prism is always shifted toward the apex of the prism. *(Reproduced from Guyton DL et al. Ophthalmic Optics and Clinical Refraction. Baltimore: Prism Press; 1999.)*

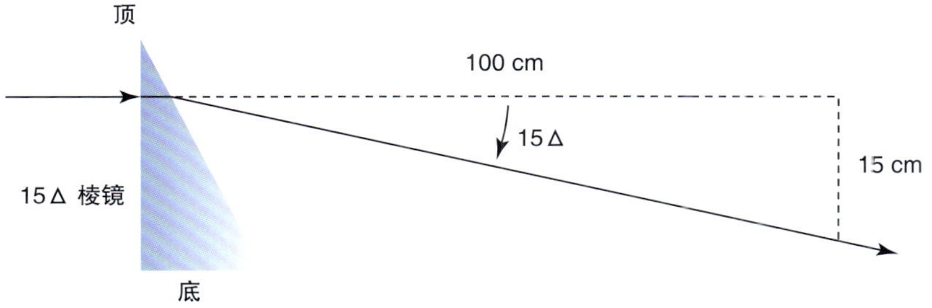

图 1-5　棱镜度的定义。1 个棱镜度是距棱镜 1m 距离的 1cm 偏差。这是 15Δ 棱镜，所以距离棱镜 100cm 处，光线偏向 15cm。*（译者注：资料来源见前页原文。）*

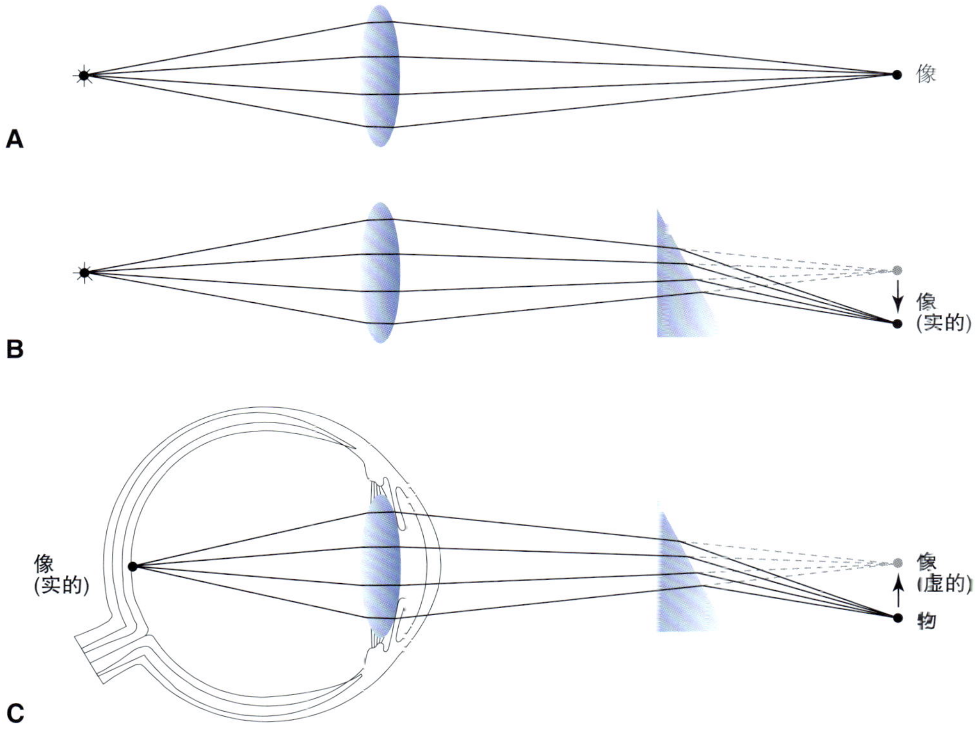

图 1-6　棱镜对成像位置的影响。**A**. 透镜形成原始实像。**B**. 加底向下棱镜。因为穿过棱镜的光总是向棱镜底部折射，所以原始实像也向底部移动，在这种情况下看到的物体就会向下移动。**C**. 把光线转过来，通过棱镜观察的虚像总是朝向棱镜的顶点移动。*（译者注：资料来源见前页原文。）*

EXAMPLE 1-1

Apply Snell's law to calculate the power of a prism in Prentice position.

The prism is oriented such that the incident ray (A) is perpendicular to the first surface of the prism and parallel with the normal (N) of that surface. The ray (B) is not deviated by this surface and is transmitted to the second surface. It is not perpendicular to this surface or parallel with its normal (E) (Figure 1-E1). The ray is therefore deviated away from the normal because it is traveling from a medium of greater index of refraction (n_1 = 1.5) to air (n_2 = 1.0). The amount of the deviation is defined by Snell's law, $n_1 \sin \theta_1 = n_2 \sin \theta_2$.

For example, for a prism vertex angle θ_1 of 30°, Snell's law gives (1.5) (0.5) = (1.0) (sin θ_2), so sin θ_2 = 0.75, or θ_2 = 48.6°. Thus, the angle between the incoming ray and the deviated ray exiting the prism is $\theta_2 - \theta_1$ = 18.6°. Because tan (18.6) = 0.3365, the strength of the prism is 33.65 prism diopters.

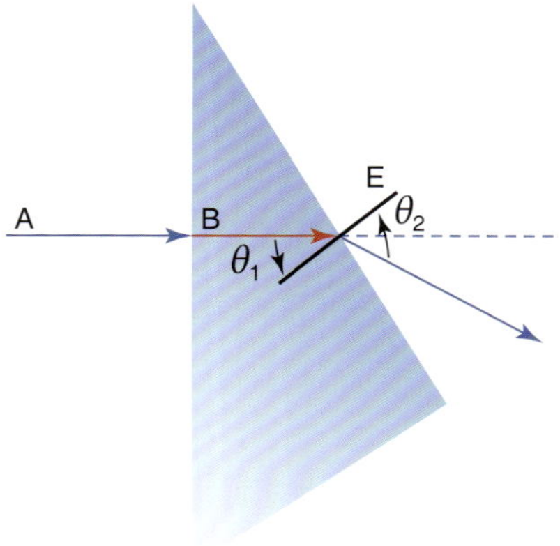

Figure 1-E1 Calculating the power of a prism in Prentice position.

Fresnel Prisms

The power of a prism is related to the angle formed by its sides, not its thickness. Nevertheless, when ground into a spectacle lens, a prism can make one edge of the lens quite thick. An alternative is a Fresnel prism (Figure 1-7), in which the angled surface is broken up into a series of much smaller prismatic surfaces at the same angle.

Fresnel Press-On prisms, fabricated out of flexible plastic, can be applied to a spectacle lens with the base in any orientation. The optical quality of a press-on prism is not as good as a prism ground into a spectacle lens. However, prism ground into a spectacle lens is expensive and increases the weight and thickness of the lens. Moreover, often a prism is required only temporarily, especially in adults (for example, when used on a trial basis in the office), or may need to be changed in strength frequently. Fresnel Press-On prisms can be quite useful in these situations.

例 1–1

应用 Snell 定律计算 Prentice 棱镜位置的棱镜屈光力。

棱镜的取向使入射光线（A）垂直于棱镜的第一表面，并与该表面的法线（N）平行。光线（B）没有偏离该表面并传递到第二表面，它不垂直于该表面或与法线平行（E）（图 1–E1）。因此，光线偏离法线，是因为它从高折射率（n_1 = 1.5）的介质传播到空气（n_2 = 1.0）。偏向量依据 Snell 定律，$n_1\sin\theta_1=n_2\sin\theta_2$。

例如，对于棱镜顶角 θ_1 为 30°，Snell 定律给出（1.5）（0.5）=（1.0）（$\sin\theta_2$），因此 $\sin\theta_2$= 0.75，或 θ_2= 48.6°。因此，入射光线和离开棱镜的偏离光线之间的角度是 $\theta_2-\theta_1$= 18.6°。因为 tan（18.6）= 0.3365，所以棱镜量是 33.65 棱镜度。

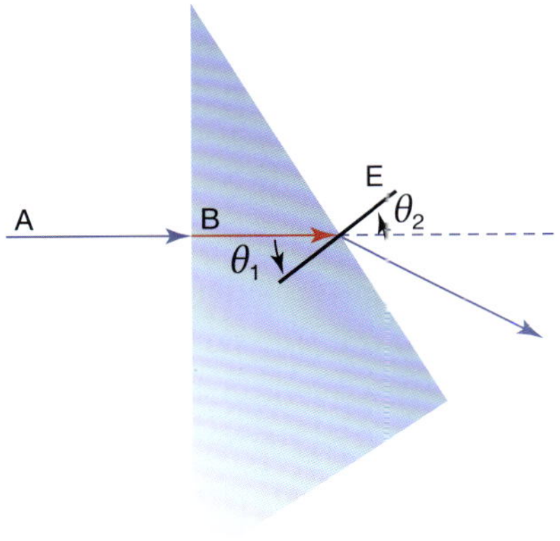

图 1–E1　计算 Frentice 方位的棱镜屈光度。

Fresnel 棱镜

棱镜焦度与其侧边形成的角度有关，而与其厚度无关。可是，当把棱镜磨成镜片时，会使镜片的边缘变得很厚。也可以采用 Fresnel 棱镜（图 1–7），在这种棱镜中，成角的面是以相同的角度构成一系列小的棱镜面。

由柔性塑料制成的 Fresnel 压贴棱镜能够把基底贴在任何方向上。压贴棱镜的光学质量不如磨成的镜片，但是，棱镜眼镜价格昂贵，并且增加了其重量和厚度。此外，人们通常只是暂时使用棱镜，特别是成年人（例如在办公室工作时使用），或者需要经常更换棱镜度。在这种情况下，Fresnel 压贴棱镜非常有用。

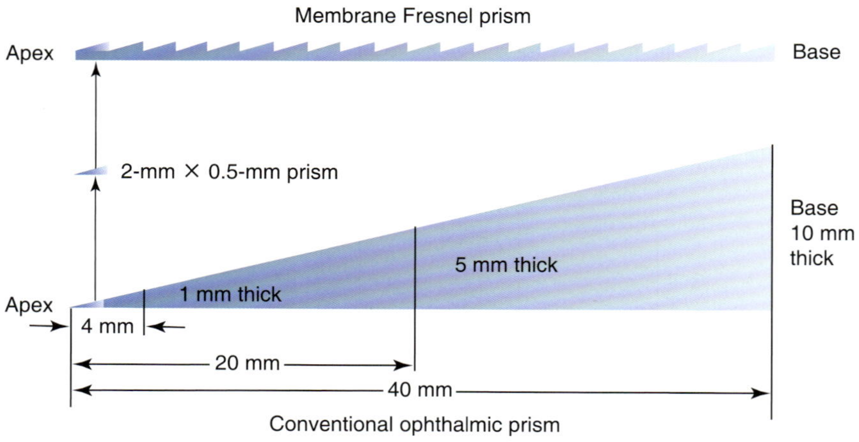

Figure 1-7 Fresnel prism. A Fresnel prism is a collection of small prisms placed parallel to each other. Both prisms have the same power but the Fresnel prism is thinner. *(Redrawn from Duane TD, ed. Clinical Ophthalmology. Hagerstown, MD: Harper & Row; 1976: vol 1, chap 52, fig 52-2.)*

Critical Angle: Total Internal Reflection

Most applications of Snell's law envision light traveling from a less dense (lower n) medium, such as air, into a more dense (higher *n*) medium, such as water or glass. In this situation, as we have seen, the light bends toward the surface normal. If the direction of light transmission is reversed, the light will bend away from the surface normal as it enters the less dense medium. However, if the angle of incidence exceeds the *critical angle* specified by the formula $\sin \theta_{crit} = n_2/n_1$, Snell's law cannot be satisfied, as no angle has a sine greater than 1.0. The result is *total internal reflection* (TIR)—the light is totally reflected at the interface and cannot pass from the denser medium to the less dense medium (Figure 1-8). For an interface between air and an aqueous tissue, the critical angle is about 48°. This prevents a view of the anterior segment angle from the exterior of the eye without optical tricks, such as the use of a goniolens (Figure 1-9).

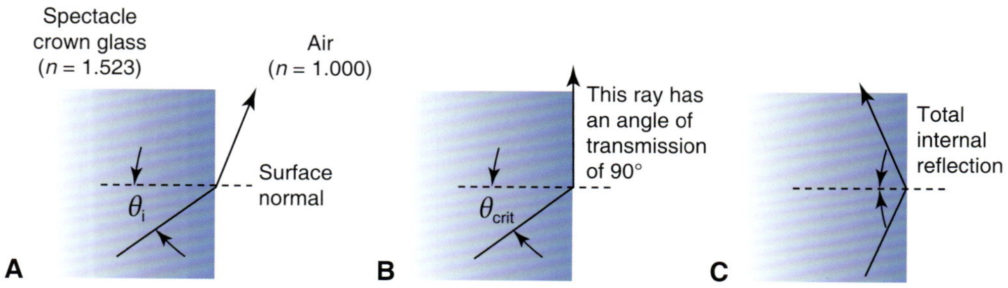

Figure 1-8 Total internal reflection. **A**, When light travels from one medium to a less-dense (lower-n) medium, the rays bend away from the surface normal. **B**, At the critical angle, θ_{crit}, the refracted light travels in the optical interface. **C**, Beyond the critical angle, all light is reflected by the interface. In **A** and **B**, light is also reflected by the interface (not shown). *(Illustration developed by Kevin M. Miller, MD, and rendered by C. H. Wooley.)*

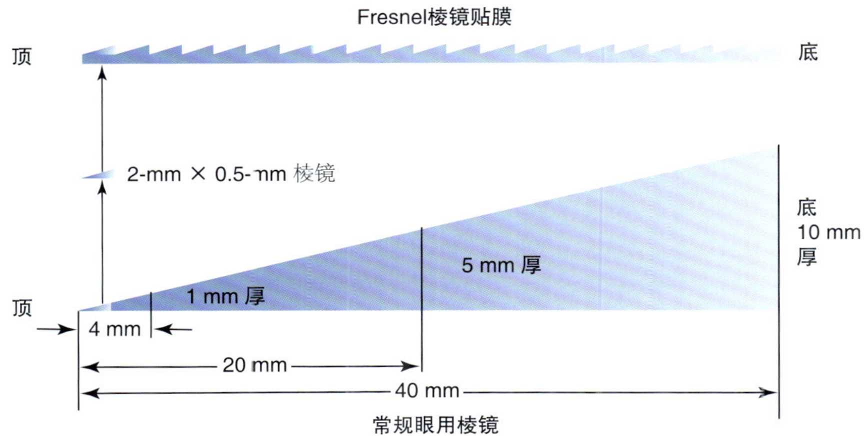

图 1-7 Fresnel 棱镜。Fresnel 棱镜是一组相互平行的小棱镜的集合体。图中 2 种棱镜屈光力相同，但 Fresnel 棱镜会更薄。*（译者注：资料来源见前页原文。）*

临界角：全内反射

在应用 Snell 定律时，大部分情况下会设想光从光疏（低 n）的介质如空气，传播到光密（高 n）的介质如水或玻璃中。如我们所见，在这种情况下，光线向法线方向偏折。如果光的传播方向相反，当它进入低密度介质时就会向远离法线的方向偏折。但是，如果由公式 $\sin\theta_{crit} = n_2/n_1$ 得出入射角超过*临界角*，则无法满足 Snell 定律，因为角的正弦值不会大于 1.0。结果就是*全内反射*（TIR）——光在界面上发生完全内反射，而不能从光密的介质传播到光疏的介质（图 1-8）。对于空气和房水之间的界面，临界角应为 48°，所以如果不借助光学手段（如前房角镜），就不能从眼睛外部看到眼房角（图 1-9）。

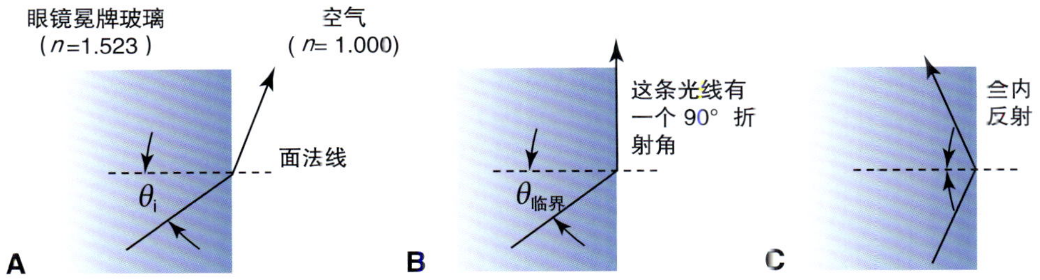

图 1-8 全内反射。**A.** 当光从一种介质传播到一种密度更低（低折射率）的介质时，光线就会向远离法线的方向偏折。**B.** 在临界角（$\theta_{临界}$）上，折射光线在光学界面中传播。**C.** 超过临界角时，所有光线都由界面反射。在 A 和 B 中，光也可以由界面反射（未示出）。*（译者注：资料来源见前页原文。）*

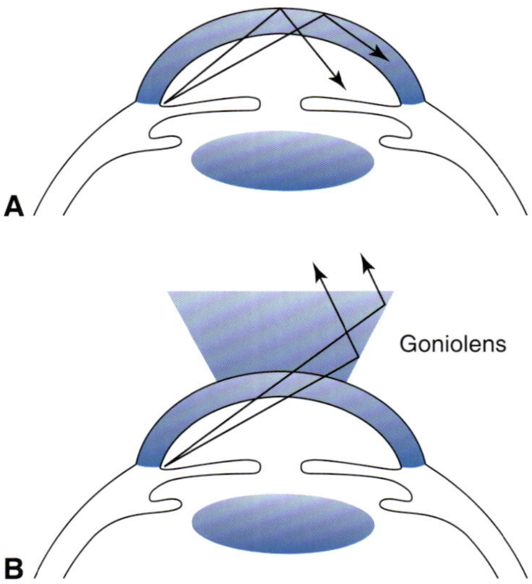

Figure 1-9 Total internal reflection at the cornea–air interface. **A**, Light from the anterior chamber angle undergoes total internal reflection (TIR) at the air–tear-film interface. **B**, A goniolens (contact lens) prevents TIR and allows visualization of the angle structures. *(Illustration developed by Kevin M. Miller, MD, and rendered by C. H. Wooley.)*

Section Exercises 1-1

1.1 Compute the critical angle for the cornea-air interface. The formula for the critical angle is sin $\theta_{crit} = n_2/n_1$. For the cornea–air interface,

$$\sin\,\theta_{crit} = \frac{n_2}{n_1} = \frac{1.00}{1.33} = 0.75$$

so $\theta_{crit} = 48.75°$.

Refraction by a Single Curved Surface

The next simplest refracting system is a single curved surface separating regions of different refractive indices. Several simplifying assumptions are appropriate: we assume that the surface is circularly symmetric about a central axis (in this context referred to as the "optic axis"), and that an incident ray of light is coplanar with the optic axis (that is, we ignore "skew" rays). If we assume that the rays of light travel in close proximity to the optic axis and make only small angles with the optic axis (the "paraxial regime"), we may deduce the following 2 equations from Snell's law, simple geometry, and the "small-angle" trigonometric approximations (Appendix1.1):

$$\frac{n_1}{u} + P = \frac{n_2}{v} \qquad \text{(vergence equation)}$$

$$P = \frac{(n_2 - n_1)}{r} \qquad \text{(lensmaker's equation)}$$

Here n_1 and n_2 are the refractive indices of the regions to the left and to the right of the refracting interface, u is the (signed) distance from the source object point to the refracting interface, v is the (signed) distance from the refracting interface to the image of the source object point, and r is the (signed) radius of curvature of the refracting interface. The sign convention for u, v, and r is that distances to the left of the interface are taken as negative numbers; distances to the right of the interface are taken as positive numbers. Light is assumed to travel from left to right. The quantity P is referred to as the *power* of the refracting interface.

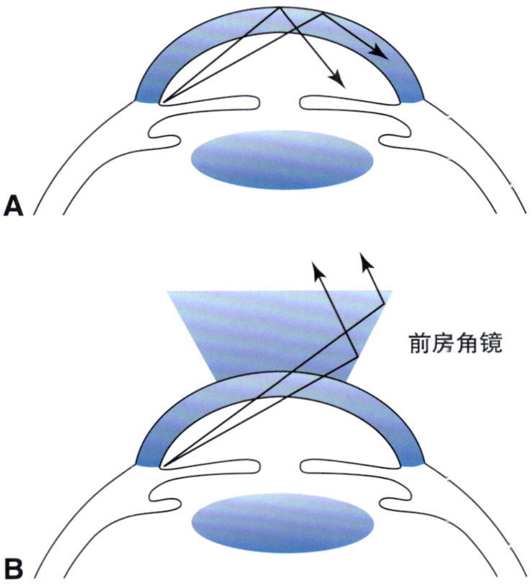

图 1–9　角膜 – 空气界面的全内反射。**A**. 从前房角射入的光线在空气 – 泪膜界面处发生全内反射（TIR）。**B**. 前房角镜（接触式）阻止了全内反射，可以观察到房角结构。（译者注：资料来源见前页原文。）

阶段练习 1–1

1–1　计算角膜 – 空气界面的临界角。临界角的计算公式是 $\sin\theta_{临界} = n_2/n_1$。对于角膜 – 空气界面：

$$\sin\theta_{临界}=\frac{n_2}{n_1}=\frac{1.00}{1.33}=0.75$$

所以 $\theta_{临界}=48.75°$。

单曲面的折射

最简单的折射系统是一个将不同折射率区域分开的曲面。有几个简化假设：假设曲面是关于中心轴（这里称为“光轴”）圆形对称的。假设光线在靠近光轴处传播，且与光轴间的角度很小（近轴区），由 Snell 定律、简单几何学和近似“小角度”三角函数（附录 1.1）导出 2 个公式：

$$\frac{n_1}{u}+P=\frac{n_2}{v}\quad（聚散方程）$$

$$P=\frac{(n_2-n_1)}{r}\quad（透镜制作商方程）$$

这里 n_1 和 n_2 分别指折射界面左侧和右侧的折射率，u（带符号）指发光物点到折射界面的距离，v（带符号）指折射界面到像的距离，r（带符号）指折射界面的曲率半径。u、v 和 r 的符号规则如下：界面左侧的距离用负号表示，界面右侧的距离用正号表示。假设光从左到右传播。P 指折射面的*屈光力*。

If either medium is air, the term n_1/u or n_2/v reduces to a simple reciprocal—$1/u$ or $1/v$, respectively—and is referred to as the *object vergence* or *image vergence*. If the refractive index of either medium is greater than 1.0, the quantity n_1/u or n_2/v is referred to as the *reduced vergence* (even though these quantities are larger than the simple reciprocals). In either case, the vergences (or reduced vergences) are frequently abbreviated as $n_1/u = U$ or $n_2/v = V$, and the vergence equation takes the simple form:

$U + P = V$

Both the vergences U and V and the refractive power P have the units of reciprocal meters, which in this context is called the *diopter*, abbreviated D. In many cases, especially regarding the human eye, measurements must *always* be converted to units of meters for purposes of the vergence equation, although typical distances are more conveniently measured in centimeters or millimeters. The distance equivalents of some common dioptric values are listed in Table1-2.

Table 1-2 Some Common Dioptric Values and Their Distance Equivalents

Diopters	Distance	Approximate Distance
0.25	4 m	
0.50	2 m	
1.00	1 m	
1.25	80 cm	
1.50	$\frac{2}{3}$	66–67 cm
2.00	50 cm	
2.50	40 cm	
3.00	$\frac{1}{3}$	33–34 cm
4.00	25 cm	
5.00	20 cm	
6.00	$\frac{1}{6}$	16–17 cm
7.00	$\frac{1}{7}$	14–14.5 cm
8.00	12.5 cm	
9.00	$\frac{1}{9}$	11–11.5 cm
10.00	10 cm	

This simple geometry, with a single curved refracting surface separating 2 regions of different refractive index, seldom arises in practice. An important exception involves the aphakic eye. Because such an eye has no lens, as a first approximation, we may ignore the interface between the cornea and the aqueous humor, which decreases the refractive power of the air–cornea interface byabout10%. (See Example I-6 in the Quick-Start Guide.)

如果两者中任一介质是空气，则 n_1 / u 或 n_2 /v 可分别简化为倒数 $1 / u$ 或 $1 /v$，称为*物的聚散度*或*像的聚散度*。如果两者中任意一种介质的折射率大于 1.0，则 n_1/u 或 n_2/ v 被称为*简化聚散度*（尽管这些数值比它们的倒数大）。在这 2 种情况下，聚散度（或简化聚散度）通常缩写为 $n_1/u=U$ 或 $n_2/ v=V$。聚散度公式的简化形式如下：

$$U + P = V$$

聚散度 U 和 V 以及屈光力 P 的单位都是 m^{-1}，称为*屈光度*，符号为 D。在许多情况下，特别是对于人眼，为使用聚散度方程，测量值必须*总要*转换成以 m 为单位。尽管典型的距离测量是更方便地用 cm 或 mm 来作单位的。表 1–2 列出了一些常见屈光度值的距离等价物。

表1–2　常见的屈光度和等量距离A

屈光度	距离	近似距离
0.25	4 m	
0.50	2 m	
1.00	1 m	
1.25	80 cm	
1.50	2/3	66~67cm
2.00	50 cm	
2.50	40 cm	
3.00	1/3	33~34cm
4.00	25 cm	
5.00	20 cm	
6.00	1/6	16~17cm
7.00	1/7	14~14.5cm
8.00	12.5 cm	
9.00	1/9	11~11.5cm
10.00	10 cm	

这是由 2 个具有不同折射率的区域组成的单球面的简单几何，临床很少见。其中非常重要的特殊情况是无晶状体眼。对于无晶状体眼，为了取近似值，需要忽略角膜和房水之间的界面，从而降低约 10% 的空气 – 角膜界面的折射率。（参见《快速入门指南》中的例 I–6。）

EXAMPLE 1-2

Apply the lensmaker's equation to compare the power of an intraocular lens (IOL) in air and in an aqueous medium (n = 1.33).

$$P = \frac{n_2 - n_1}{r} \quad \text{(lensmaker's equation)}$$

Consider a lens implant that is planoconvex, with the convex side facing the cornea, and has a radius of curvature of the curved surface of 8.0 mm. The index of refraction of the lens implant is 1.5.
The power of the anterior surface in air is

$$P_{air} = \frac{1.5 - 1.0}{0.008\ \text{m}} = +62.5\ \text{D}$$

The power of the posterior surface of the same lens in air is 0, so the net power of the lens is+62.5 D.

If the same lens is placed in aqueous humor, with n_2 = 1.333, the power of the anterior surface is

$$P_{aqueous} = \frac{1.5 - 1.333}{0.008\ \text{m}} = +20.90\text{D}$$

and the power of the flat posterior surface is again 0. Therefore, an intraocular lens implant in air has approximately 3x the nominal labeled power of the lens.

Section Exercises 1-2~1-6

Vergence equation problems. Thin lenses in air: in each case, given values of u (the distance from source to lens) and P (lens power), find v (the distance from lens to image).

$$\frac{n_1}{u} + P = \frac{n_2}{v} \quad \text{(vergence equation)}$$

$$U + P = V \quad \text{(vergence equation, simple form)}$$

1–2 $U = -\infty, P = +4$ D
In air, $U = 1/u$ *and* $V = 1/v$, so
$(1/-\infty) + (+4\ \text{D}) = 1/v$
$+4 = 1/v$
$v = 1\ /\ 4\ \text{D} = +0.25\ \text{m}$

1–3 $u = -4$ m, $P = +2$ D
Again, in air, $U = 1/u$ *and* $V = 1/v$, so
$(1/-4\ \text{m}) + (+2\ \text{D}) = 1/v$
$+1.75\ \text{D} = 1/v$
$v = 1/1.75\ \text{D} = +0.57\ \text{m}$

1–4 $u = -1$ m, $P = +2$ D
$(1/-1\ \text{m}) + (+2\ \text{D}) = 1/v$
$+1\ \text{D} = 1/v$
$v = +1\ \text{m}$

1–5 $u = -0.5$ m, $P = +2$ D

例 1–2

应用透镜制作商方程比较人工晶状在空气和房水介质中屈光力的不同（n = 1.33）。

$$P=\frac{n_2-n_1}{r} \quad \text{（镜片制作商方程）}$$

考虑到人工晶体是平凸的，凸面朝向角膜，且其曲面的曲率半径为 8.0mm，人工晶体的折射率为 1.5。

则在空气中，其前表面的屈光力为：

$$P_{空气}=\frac{1.5-1.0}{0.008\ \text{m}}=+62.5\ \text{D}$$

在空气中，同一透镜的后表面屈光力为 0，透镜的净屈光力为 +62.50 D。

如果把同样的透镜置于 n_2 = 1.333 房水中，则透镜前表面的屈光力为：

$$P_{房水}=\frac{1.5-1.333}{0.008\ \text{m}}=+20.90\text{D}$$

且透镜后表面平坦部的屈光力仍为 0。因此，在空气中，人工晶体的屈光力约比在正常房水中的大 3 倍。

阶段练习 1–2~1–6

聚散度公式的问题。空气中的薄透镜：在每种情况下，给定的 u 值（从发光物点到透镜的距离）和 P（棱镜焦度），求出 v（透镜到像的距离）。

$$\frac{n_1}{u}+P=\frac{n_2}{v} \quad \text{（聚散度方程）}$$

$$U+P=V \quad \text{（简单聚散度方程）}$$

1–2　$U=-\infty, P=+4$ D

空气中, $U=1/u$ ，$V=1/v$, 所以

$(1/-\infty)+(+4\ \text{D})=1/v$

$+4=1/v$

$v=1/4\ \text{D}=+0.25$ m

1–3　$u=-4$ m, $P=+2$ D

空气中，$U=1/u$ ，$V=1/v$，所以

$(1/-4\ \text{m})+(+2\ \text{D})=1/v$

$+1.75\ \text{D}=1/v$

$v=1/1.75\ \text{D}=+0.57$ m

1–4　$u=-1$ m, $P=+2$ D

$(1/-1\ \text{m})+(+2\ \text{D})=1/v$

$+1\ \text{D}=1/v$

$v=+1$ m

1–5　$u=-0.5$ m, $P=+2$ D

$(1/-0.5\text{ m}) + (+2\text{ D}) = 1/v$
$-2\text{ D} + (+2\text{ D}) = 0 = 1/v$
$v = \text{infinity}$

1-6 $u = -0.4\text{ m}, P = +2\text{ D}$
$(1/-0.4\text{ m}) + (+2\text{ D}) = 1/v$
$(-2.5\text{ D}) + (+2\text{ D}) = -0.5\text{ D} = 1/v$
$v = 1/-0.5\text{ D} = -2\text{ m}$

. Thin lenses in water: rework Section Exercises 1-3~1-6 but with the image space filled with an aqueous medium.

Section Exercises 1-7~1-10

1-7 $u = -4\text{ m}, P = +2\text{ D}$
Because the image space is filled with an aqueous medium, $V = 1.33/v$, so
$(1/-4\text{ m}) + (+2\text{ D}) = 1.33/v$
$-0.25\text{ D} + (+2\text{ D}) = +1.75\text{ D} = 1.33/v$
$v = 1.33/+1.75\text{ D} = 0.76\text{ m}$

1-8 $u = -1\text{ m}, P = +2\text{ D}$
$(1/-1\text{ m}) + (+2\text{ D}) = 1.33/v$
$-1\text{ D} + (+2\text{ D}) = +1\text{ D} = 1.33/v$
$v = 1.33/1\text{ D} = 1.33\text{ m}$

1-9 $u = -0.5\text{ m}, P = +2\text{ D}$
$(1/-0.5\text{ m}) + (+2\text{ D}) = 1.33/v$
$(-2\text{ D}) + (+2\text{ D}) = 0 = 1.33/v$
$v = 1.33/0 = \text{Infinity}$

1-10 $u = -0.4\text{ m}, P = +2\text{ D}$
$(1/-0.4\text{ m}) + (+2\text{ D}) = 1/v$
$(-2.5\text{ D}) + (+2\text{ D}) = -0.5\text{ D} = 1.33/v$
$v = 1.33/-0.5\text{ D} = -2.66\text{ m}$

Two-Sided Lenses

More typical than the 1-sided lenses we have discussed are 2-sided lenses, with front and back refractive surfaces. These surfaces separate the denser medium of the lens from the surrounding medium, usually air or a watery tissue such as aqueous or vitreous humor. In many cases, if the distance between the front and back surfaces is small, we may treat the lens as a single refracting object with power $P = P_1 + P_2$, where P_1 and P_2 are the (signed!) powers of the front and back lens surfaces. (Notice that, for example, for a typical biconvex lens in air, both the front surface and the back surface have positive power, as the both the numerator and the denominator in the lensmaker's equation for the back surface are negative numbers.) This is referred to as the *thin-lens approximation.*

(1/−0.5 m) + (+2 D) = 1/v
−2 D + (+2 D) = 0 = 1/v
v = 无穷远

1–6　$u = -0.4$ m, $P = +2$ D
(1/−0.4 m) + (+2 D) = 1/v
(−2.5 D) + (+2 D) = −0.5 D = 1/v
v = 1/−0.5 D = −2 m

水中的薄透镜：复习部分练习 1–3~1–6，但图像处于水介质中。

阶段练习 1–7~1–10

1–7　$u = -4$ m, $P = +2$ D
因为像处于水介质中，V=1.33/v，所以
(1/−4 m) + (+2 D) = 1.33/v
−0.25 D + (+2 D) = +1.75 D = 1.33/v
v = 1.33/+1.75 D = 0.76 m

1–8　$u = -1$ m, $P = +2$ D
(1/−1 m) + (+2 D) = 1.33/v
−1 D + (+2 D) = +1 D = 1.33/v
v = 1.33/1 D = 1.33 m

1–9　$u = -0.5$ m, $P = +2$ D
(1/−0.5 m) + (+2 D) = 1.33/v
(−2 D) + (+2 D) = 0 = 1.33/v
v = 1.33/0 = 无限远

1–10　$u = -0.4$ m, $P = +2$ D
(1/−0.4 m) + (+2 D) = 1/v
(−2.5 D) + (+2 D) = −0.5 D = 1.33/v
v = 1.33/−0.5 D = −2.66 m

双面透镜

双面透镜比单面透镜更为常见，它有前后 2 个折射面。这 2 个面将密度较高的透镜与周围的介质，通常是空气或水样组织（如房水或玻璃体）分离开来。如果前后表面之间的距离很小，可以视为一个透镜，其屈光力为 $P=P_1+P_2$，其中 P_1 和 P_2（带符号）分别是前表面和后表面的屈光力。（请注意，空气中的双凸透镜，前后表面的屈光力值均为正值，因为在透镜制作商方程中，后表面的分子和分母都是负数。）我们称之为*薄透镜近似*。

In some cases, such as the crystalline lens of the normal human eye or intraocular lens implants, we cannot ignore the separation between the front and back surfaces of a lens. The power of such a "thick lens" for paraxial rays is given, to a first approximation, by the formula

$$P = P_1 + P_2 - \left(\frac{t}{n}\right) P_1 P_2$$

where P_1 and P_2 are the powers of the front and back surfaces of the lens, respectively, t is the distance between them (ie, the thickness of the lens) in meters, and n is the refractive index of the lens material. This formula reduces to the thin-lens approximation as the lens thickness approaches 0.

Principal Planes

The thin-lens approximation treats the front and back lens surfaces as if they coincide, and we use their common location as the position of the lens to calculate the object and image vergences, as we did in the Quick-Start Guide. Unlike the thin-lens case, we do not immediately know how to measure the distance from a source object to a thick lens (or from the lens to the image location) in order to apply the vergence equation. It is helpful to consider a diagram (Figure 1-10). Recall from the Quick-Start Guide that the focal point F of a lens is the location of the image of light from a very distant object (at a distance $f = 1/P$).

Here, rays from a distant object at left are brought to a focal point F_2 on the right side of the lens. But careful inspection shows that the refraction takes place in 2 steps: (1)as the rays cross the front surface of the lens,(2) and as they cross the back surface. If we extend the incident rays and the exiting rays (shown by the dotted lines in Figure 1-10), they cross at an apparent single refracting surface—the second, or "back," *principal plane*— located within the lens substance. That plane, indicated by the vertical line, passes through the optic axis at H_2. Similarly, rays that originate from the front focal point, F, and emerge from the lens as parallel rays appear to have been refracted at a different internal plane—the first, or "front," principal plane)—which passes through the optic axis at H_1 (Figure 1-11).

These apparent refracting planes provide the appropriate locations for the calculation of object and image vergence, respectively. The intersections H_1 and H_2 of the principal planes with the optic axis are known as the first and second (or "front" and "back") *principal points.*

The location of the principal planes depends on the lens design and on the refractive indices of the material in the object space, lens, and image space. For "meniscus lenses," such as those used for spectacles, with 1 convex surface and 1 concave surface, the principal planes may lie outside the lens itself (Figure 1-12).

在某些情况下，如对于正常人眼的晶状体或人工晶状体，我们不能忽略晶状体前后表面的距离。以下公式可计算出这种近轴光线通过厚透镜的近似屈光力

$$P=P_1+P_2-\left(\frac{t}{n}\right)P_1P_2$$

其中 P_1 和 P_2 分别是透镜的前后表面的屈光力，t 是它们之间的距离（即透镜的厚度），单位是米，n 是折射率。当透镜厚度接近 0 时，这个公式可简化为薄透镜公式。

主平面

如《快速入门指南》所述，把透镜的前后表面重合视为薄透镜近似值，并且将它们的共同位置作为“透镜的位置”，来计算物和像的聚散度。与薄透镜不同，其不能应用聚散度公式，可以即刻知道如何测量从物到厚透镜的距离（或从透镜到像的距离）。下图可以帮助我们理解（图 1–10）。《快速入门指南》中指出：透镜的焦点 F 是无限远物体的像的位置（距离 f=1/P）。

此处，光线从左侧一个无限远物体会聚到透镜右侧的焦点 F_2。但是仔细观察发现，折射是分 2 个步骤进行的：①光线穿过透镜的前表面；②光线穿过透镜的后表面。如果延长入射光线和出射光线（如图 1–10 中的虚线所示），它们相交于一个折射面——第二或“后”*主平面*位于透镜内。用 H_2 处通过光轴的垂直线表示。同样的，来自前焦点 F 的光线，以平行光线从透镜中出来，在透镜内，光线在另一个位置的平面发生了折射，这个平面即第一或“前”主平面，它在 H_1 处通过光轴 (图 1–11)

这 2 个折射面可以分别计算出精准的物和像的位置。主平面与光轴的 H_1 和 H_2 交点被称为第一和第二（或“前”和“后”）*主点*。

主平面的位置取决于透镜的设计以及物体空间、透镜和像的空间材料的折射率。如用于眼镜的新月透镜，有一个凸面和一个凹面，其主平面位于透镜外（图 1–12）。

EXAMPLE 1-3

Derive the "thick-lens formula" for a 2-sided lens in air:

$$P = P_1 + P_2 - \left(\frac{t}{n}\right) P_1 P_2$$

Suppose the front surface has power P_1, the lens has refractive index n and thickness t, and the back surface has power P_2 (Figure 1-E3). at the front surface, a paraxial ray with zero vergence is refracted and intersects the optic axis at v, where $0 + P_1 = n/v$, or $v = n/P_1$. the reduced vergence of the refracted ray as it reaches the back surface is $n/(v - t) = n/[(n/P_1) - t]$. After the ray is refracted at the back surface, it meets the optic axis at distance v_2 from the back surface of the lens, and the exiting vergence is

$$\frac{1}{v_2} = \frac{n}{\left(\frac{n}{P_1}\right) - t} + P_2 = \frac{nP_1}{n - tP_1} + P_2$$

$$= \frac{P_1}{(1 - \left(\frac{t}{n}\right) P_1)} + P_2$$

$$= \frac{1}{(1 - \left(\frac{t}{n}\right) P_1)} [P_1 + P_2 \, (1 - \left(\frac{t}{n}\right) \, P_1)]$$

$$= \frac{1}{(1 - \left(\frac{t}{n}\right) P_1)} [P_1 + P_2 \, \left(\frac{t}{n}\right) \, P_1 P_2]$$

For small values of t, this approaches $P = P_1 + P_2 - (t/n)P_1P_2$.

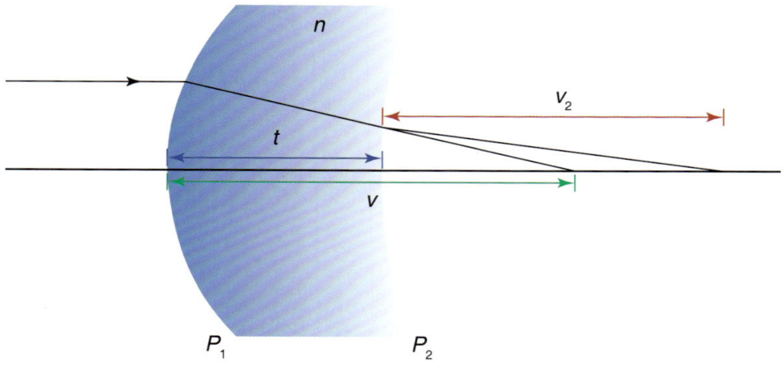

Figure 1-E3 Calculating the power of a "thick lens." Here v is the distance from the front lens surface to the point where the ray refracted by the front lens surface intersects the optic axis. The powers of the front and back surfaces are P_1 and P_2, respectively. *(Courtesy of Scott E. Brodie, MD, PhD.)*

例 1–3

推导出空气中双面透镜的“厚透镜公式”：

$$P = P_1 + P_2 - \left(\frac{t}{n}\right) P_1 P_2$$

假设前表面的屈光力为 P_1，透镜的折射率为 n，厚度为 t，而后表面的屈光力为 P_2（图 1–E3）。在前表面的近轴光线经折射后在 v 处与光轴相交，聚散度为 0，即 $0 + P_1 = n/v$，或 $v = n/P_1$ 到达折射光线后表面的简化聚散度约为 $n/(v - t) = n/[(n/P_1) - t]$。光线经后表面折射，在 v_2 处与光轴相交，其出射光聚散度：

$$\frac{1}{v_2} = \frac{n}{\left(\frac{n}{P_1}\right) - t} + P_2 = \frac{nP_1}{n - tP_1} + P_2$$

$$= \frac{P_1}{\left(1 - \left(\frac{t}{n}\right) P_1\right)} + P_2$$

$$= \frac{1}{\left(1 - \left(\frac{t}{n}\right) P_1\right)}\left[P_1 + P_2 \left(1 - \left(\frac{t}{n}\right) P_1\right)\right]$$

$$= \frac{1}{\left(1 - \left(\frac{t}{n}\right) P_1\right)}\left[P_1 + P_2 \left(\frac{t}{n}\right) P_1 P_2\right]$$

当 t 值越小时，越接近 $P = P_1 + P_2 - (t/n) P_1 P_2$。

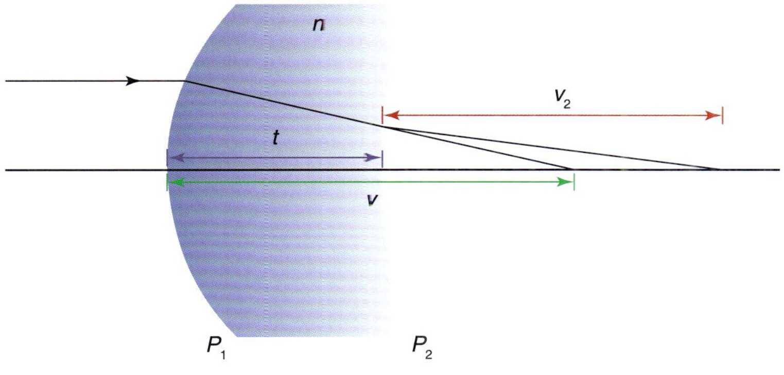

图 1–E3　计算“厚透镜”的屈光力。v 是从透镜前表面到由透镜前表面折射的光线与光轴相交的距离。前表面和后表面的屈光力分别为 P_1 和 P_2。*（译者注：资料来源见前页原文。）*

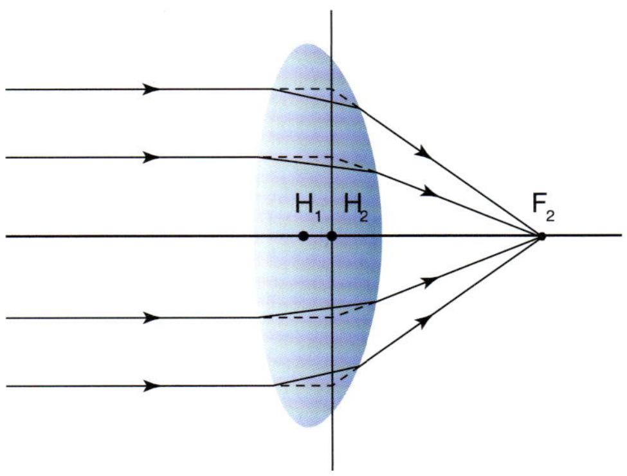

Figure 1-10 Ray tracing for parallel incident light rays striking a thick convex lens. Notice that the rays appear to bend at an internal plane at H_2. *(Redrawn from Creative Commons illustration by Bob Mellish.)*

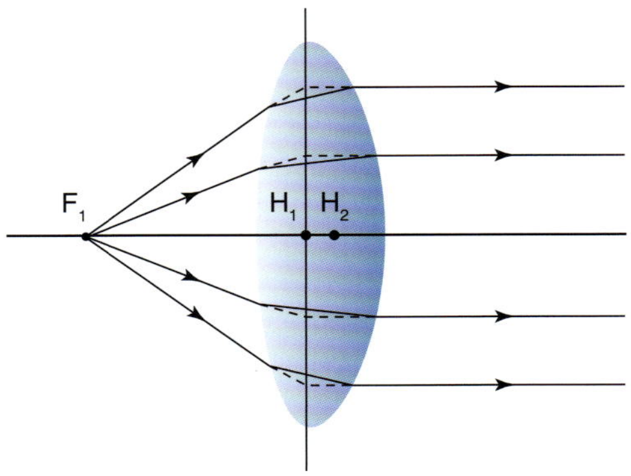

Figure 1-11 Ray tracing for rays emerging from the first focal point, F_1, striking a thick convex lens. Notice that the rays appear to be refracted at a different plane than the incident parallel rays shown in Figure 1-1. *(Redrawn from Creative Commons illustration by Bob Mellish.)*

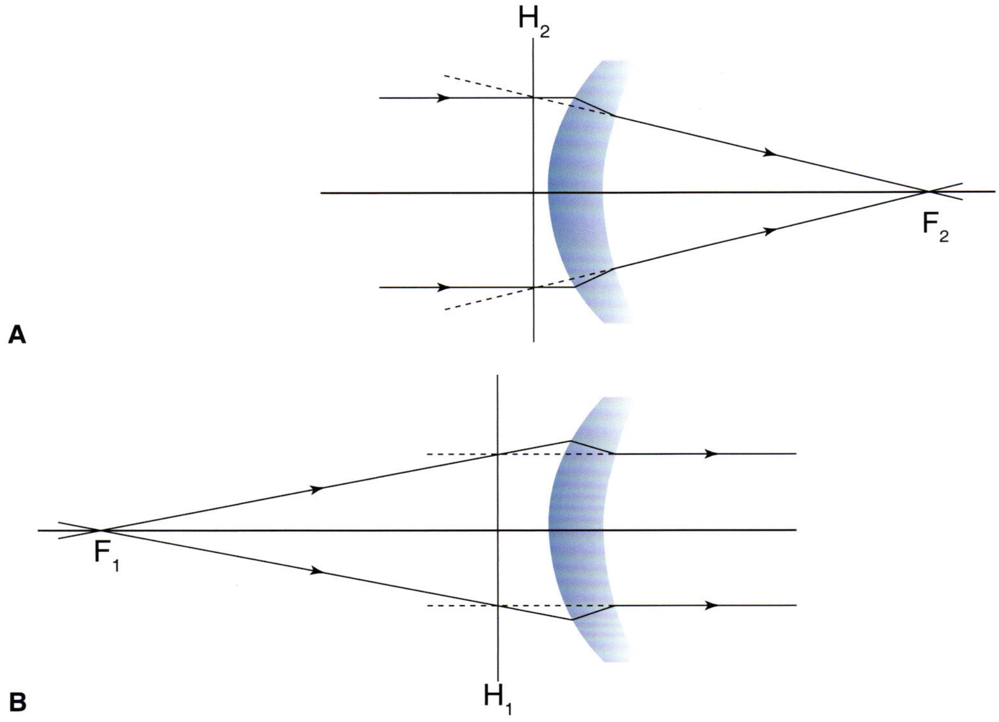

Figure 1-12 Ray tracing for a meniscus lens in air. Notice that the principal planes H_1 and H_2 lie outside the lens.

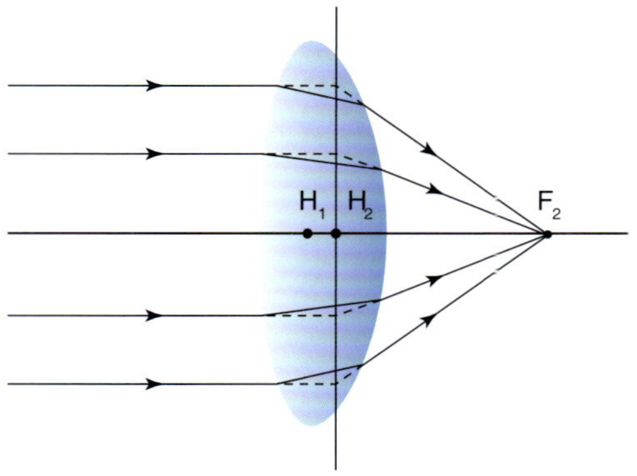

图 1–10　平行入射光线穿过厚凸透镜的光路图。请注意，光线在 H_2 处平面偏折。*（译者注：资料来源见前页原文。）*

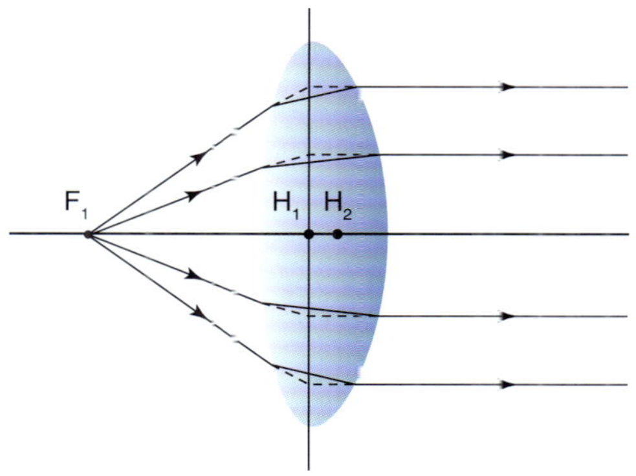

图 1–11　来自第一焦点 F_1 的光线穿过厚凸透镜的光路图。请注意，如图 1–1 所示，光线在另一个位置的平面发生了折射，而不是入射到平行光线处。*（译者注：资料来源见前页原文。）*

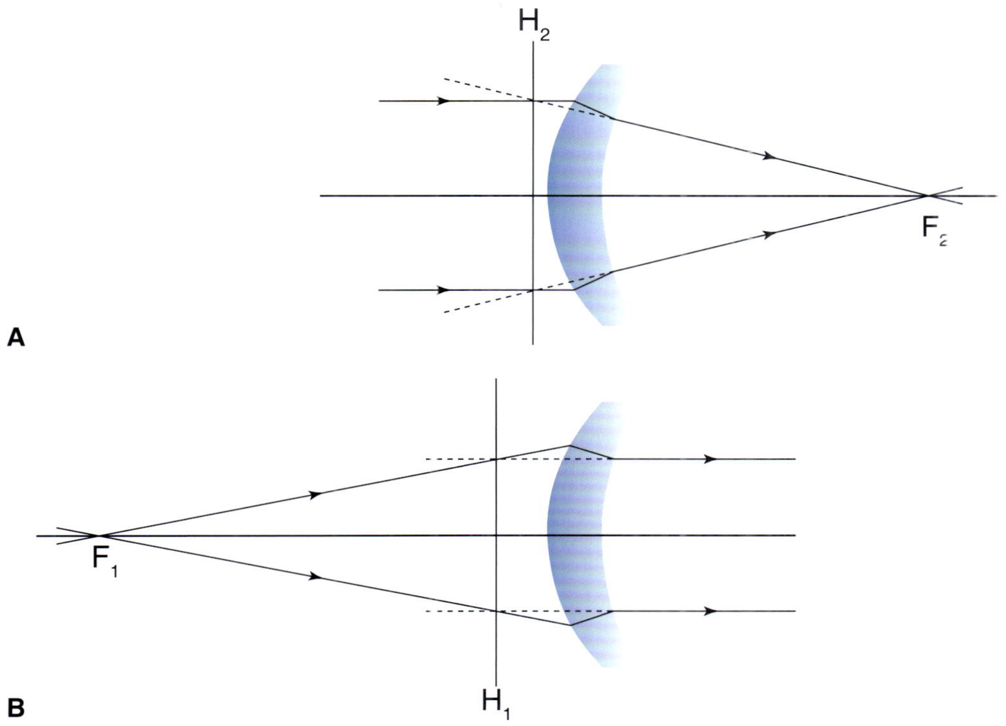

图 1–12　空气中半月板透镜的光路图。请注意，主平面 H_1 和 H_2 位于透镜外。

Calculations of the location of the principal planes are beyond the scope of this book. Fortunately, for most purposes involving ophthalmic lenses in air, such as spectacle corrections and contact lenses, the thin-lens approximation is adequate. However, most calculations of refraction within the eye, where the thickness of the lens is a large fraction of the axial length, may require more detailed treatment.

Depth of Focus and Depth of Field

The preceding discussion has tacitly implied that there is one exact image location. Anyone who has focused an optical instrument has noticed that the best focus is small region, rather than a point, where the image neither improves nor blurs. This typically small but definite region is the *depth of focus* (Figure 1-13). We can conveniently describe it in terms of the range of effective correcting lens powers (in diopters) that permit adequate image clarity.

Depth of focus is a property of the imaging system, not of the image, and it varies from lens to lens. As discussed in the Quick-Start Guide, a pinhole has an infinite depth of focus; lenses have a far more restricted depth of focus.

Whereas depth of focus is the range of *image* locations over which an object remains sharply focused, *depth of field* is the range of *object* locations that will be sharply focused at a single image location (Figure 1-14). Clinically, depth of field is important for prescribing bifocals and trifocals for presbyopia. Even when the depth of focus is small, the depth of field can be large, depending on various factors.

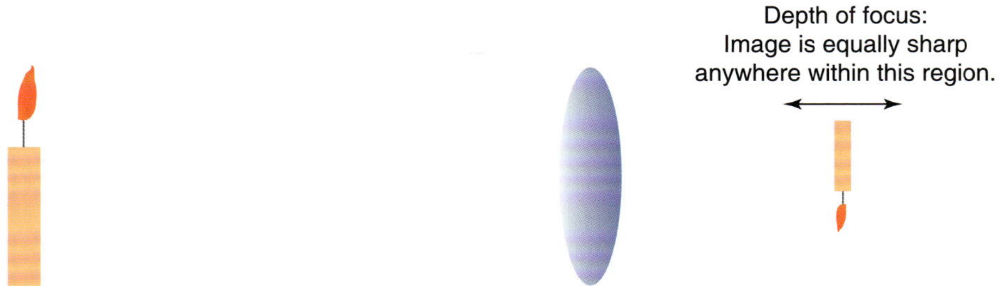

Figure 1-13 Depth of focus. An image is equally sharp anywhere within the indicated region. *(Courtesy of Edmond H. Thall, MD.)*

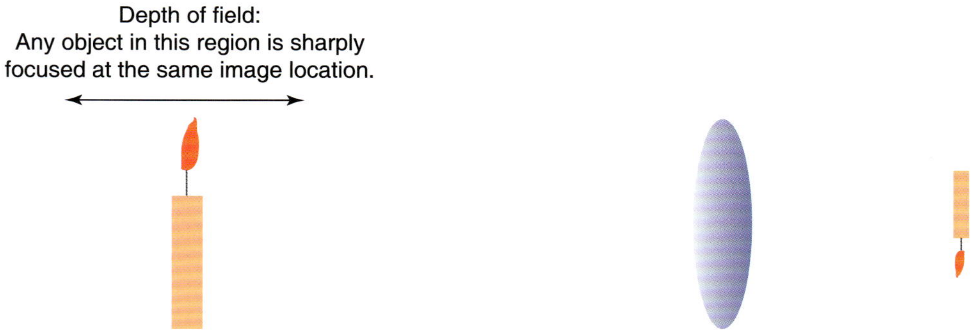

Figure 1–14 Depth of field. Any object within the depth of field will appear sharply focused in the image. *(Courtesy of Edmond H. Thall, MD.)*

主平面位置的计算超出了本书的范围。在空气中应用的多数眼用透镜，如眼镜和接触镜，都可视为薄透镜近似。而大多数的眼内折射，其透镜厚度占眼轴轴长的很大一部分，则需要谨慎对待。

焦深和景深

前面详细讨论了一个精准的成像位置。任何关注光学仪器的人都知道，最好的焦点不是一个点，而是一个很小的区域，这个区域的像清晰度不变。这个小而确定的区域就是*焦深*（图 1–13）。依据允许范围内形成足够清晰度的像的有效矫正镜头屈光力（单位为 D），我们可以方便地描述焦深。

焦深是成像系统的一种特性，而不是像的特性，而且会因透镜不同而有不同。如《快速入门指南》中所描述的那样，针孔具有无限焦深，透镜则是有限焦深。

焦深是一个物体保持清晰聚焦的*像*位置范围，而*景深*是*物*的位置范围。在该范围内的物可在单一位置清晰成像（图 1–14）。临床上，老视的双焦和三焦镜的景深是非常重要的。即使焦深很小，景深也可能很大，这取决于各种因素。

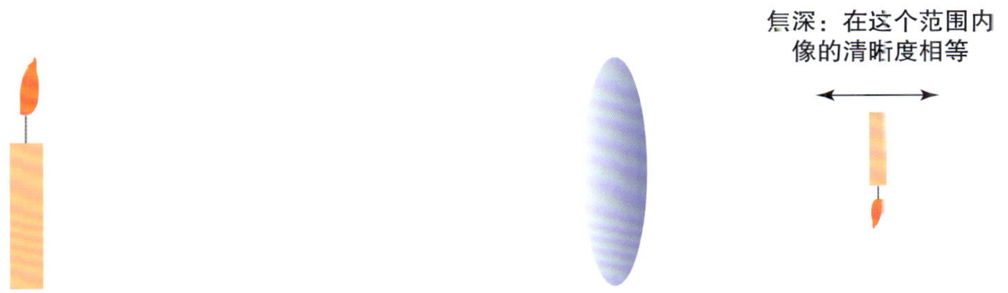

图 1–13　焦深。像在一定范围内的清晰度相同（*译者注：资料来源见前页原文。*）

图 1–14　景深。该范围内的任何物体的像都是清晰的。（*译者注：资料来源见前页原文。*）

General Refracting Systems

Refracting systems can be built up from multiple combinations of lenses of arbitrary thickness and various compositions of optical media, such as types of glass with different refractive indices. Regardless of the complexity, for paraxial rays, such systems can be characterized by a single pair of principal planes and a single refractive power, *P*.

This is a remarkable simplification. We can ignore everything that takes place at the numerous optical interfaces within such an optical system, and proceed by simply determining the object vergence at the first principal plane, adding the power *P*, and then locating the image by referencing the exiting vergence to the second principal plane (Figure 1-15).

EXAMPLE 1-4

Principal planes. Redo Section exercises 1-3–1-6 for a complex lens system with principal planes separated by 1.0 cm = 0.01 m and net power P = +2.0D.

Assume the object distances are referenced to the front principal plane. Then the image distances are the same as before, when referenced to the second principal plane, and are thus 1.0 cm greater than the answers to Section exercises 1-3–1-6.

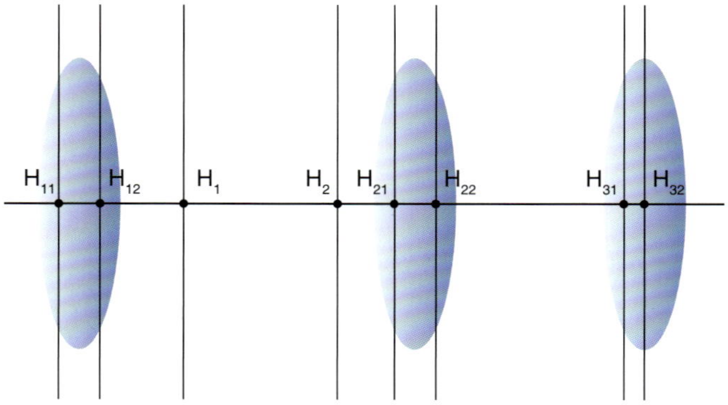

图 **1-15** References for a compound optical system. Each lens has its own power and pair of principal planes, as indicated by subscripts 11 and 12, 21 and 22, and 31 and 32. The combined system has an equivalent or "net" power and a single pair of principal planes representing the entire system, indicated by H_1 and H_2. *(Courtesy of Edmond H. Thall, MD.)*

Section exercise 1-11~1-14

Redo Section Exercises 1-3~1-6 for a lens system with net power P = +10D.

1–11 $u = -4.0$ m, $P = +10$ D
$v = 1/9.75$ D $= 0.10256$ m from the second principal plane

1–12 $u = -1.0$ m, $P = +10$ D
$v = 1/9.00$ D $= 0.111$ m from the second principal plane

1–13 $u = -0.5$ m, $P = +10$ D
$v = 1/8.0$ D $= 0.125$ m from the second principal plane

1–14 $u = -0.4$ m, $P = +10$ D
$v = 1/7.50$ D $= 0.1333$ m from the second principal plane

普通折射系统

折射系统可以是由多种任意厚度的透镜和各种光学介质组合，例如不同折射率的镜片。无论多复杂，对于近轴光线，这类系统可以由 1 对主平面和 1 个屈光力 P 组成。

我们做一个简化。在这样的光学系统中，忽略所有不同光学界面，只需简单地确定物体在第一主平面上的聚散度，再加屈光力 P；然后参考相对于第二个主平面出射的聚散度，来确定像的位置（图 1–15）。

例 1-4

主平面，复习阶段练习 1–3~1–6 复合透镜系统，其主平面间距 1.0cm=0.01m，总屈光力 P=+2.00D。

假设物距是相对于前主平面，像距和以前一样相对于第二主平面，那么就比阶段练习 1–3~1–6 的结果要远 1.0cm。

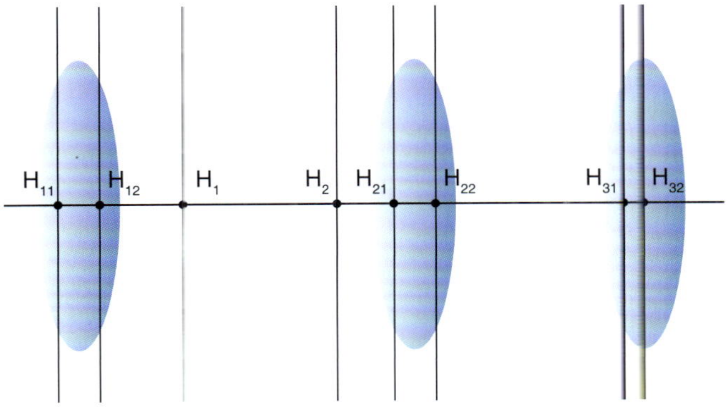

图 1–15　复合光学系统的示意图。每个镜片都有自己的折射率和一对主平面，如图中的下标显示的 11 和 12，21 和 22，31 和 32。复合光学系统有一个等效或“净”屈光力，以及一对用来表示整个光学系统的主平面，由 H_1 和 H_2 表示。*（由 Edmond H. Thall 医学博士提供。）*

阶段练习 1–11~1–14

用净屈光力 P=+10.00D 的透镜系统重新计算 1–3~1–6 题。

1–11　$u = -4.0$ m，$P = +10$ D

$v = 1/9.75$　D=0.10256m　距第二个主平面

1–12　$u = -1.0$ m，$P = +10$ D

$v = 1/9.00$　D=0.111m　距第二个主平面

1–13　$u = -0.5$ m，$P = +10$ D

$v = 1/8.0$　D=0.125m　距第二个主平面

1–14　$u = -0.4$ m，$P = +10$ D

$v = 1/7.50$　D=0.1333m　距第二个主平面

EXAMPLE 1-5

Principal planes and distant objects. the Gullstrand mathematical model closely approximates the human eye. (the Gullstrand model eye is discussed in Chapter 3.) the net power of the entire refracting system of the model eye is P= +58.64 D; the refractive index of the vitreous humor is 1.336, and the second (posterior) principal plane is located 1.602 mm behind the anterior corneal surface. Locate an image of a distant object as formed by the Gullstrand model eye with relaxed accommodation.

The image is located according to the vergence equation: 0 + 58.64 D = 1.336/ν, so ν = 0.02278 m, or 1.602 + 22.78 = 24.382 mm from the anterior corneal surface. For comparison, the axial length is 24.40 mm.

EXAMPLE 1-6

Effectivity of lenses. Suppose a lens of power P in air places the image of a distant object at a distance u to the right of the lens. To move the lens t meters to the right while preserving the image location, how must you adjust the power of the lens?

In its new position, the lens will form the image at a distance $u_2 = u - t$ to the right of the lens (as $v = 0$). Thus, the power P_2 of the moved lens should be $P_2 = 1/(u - t) = 1/(1/P - t) = P/(1 - tP)$. Indeed, the same formula applies for divergent lenses, with the initial image location to the left of the lens, so long as the proper sign conventions are observed. This adjustment is referred to as the correction for the *effectivity of lenses.*

The effectivity of lenses comes into play, for example, when we convert a spectacle correction to the corresponding contact lens correction. For example, a hyperopic correction will place the image of a distant object at the far point of the eye (the location conjugate to the fovea with relaxed accommodation—see the Quick-Start Guide). In this case, the far point is behind the retina, and the effectivity calculation requires that the power of the correcting contact lens be greater than the power of the equivalent spectacles. For example, for a spectacle correction of+4.00D worn at the standard vertex distance of 13.75 mm from the corneal apex, the power of the equivalent contact lens is+4.00D/[1-(0.01375 m)(4.00D)]= +4.232 D, which suggests that the contact lens power should be increased by ¼ D. this correction is negligible for lenses weaker than about 3 D.

Gaussian Optics

To calculate the location of the principal planes, we must know the details of the refractive events within the lens system. In practice, this is usually done by means of an elegant formalism known as *Gaussian optics* (or Gaussian reduction). The details are beyond the scope of this book, but the basic idea is as follows: the paraxial approximation is effectively a linearization of Snell's law. We can therefore express the approximation in terms of 2 types of "linear operators." (1) The "translation operator" describes the propagation of a light ray through a medium of refractive index n over a distance t. This is, in essence, equivalent to the step of recalculating the vergence of light from a source object (or image created by a previous refracting surface) as referenced to the next refracting surface in an optical system. (2) The "refraction operator" describes the change in vergence at a curved optical interface of radius r between media of refractive indices n_1 and n_2. It is the equivalent of adding P to find the vergence of light exiting from a refractive interface. We can represent each of these operators in an appropriate coordinate system by a suitable 2 × 2 matrix. We can then use matrix multiplication to calculate the net action of a sequence of refractive events at the various refractive surfaces in a complex optical system.

例 1–5

主平面和远距离物。Gullstrand 数学模型非常接近人眼。（Gullstrand 模型眼在第 3 章中有讨论）。模型眼的整个折射系统的净屈光力为 $P= +58.64$ D；玻璃体房水的折射率为 1.336，第二（后）主平面位于角膜前表面后 1.602 mm。用 Gullstrand 眼模型，在调节放松状态下，对远处物体的成像进行定位。

根据聚散度方程，成像位置在：0 + 58.64 D = 1.336 /v，所以 v= 0.02278m，或距前角膜表面 1.602 + 22.78 = 24.382mm 处。相比之下，眼轴的长度是 24.40mm。

例 1–6

透镜的有效性。假设空气中有一个屈光力为 P 的透镜，将一个远物体成像于透镜右侧的距离 u 处。要在保持像位置的同时将透镜向右移动 t m，须如何调整透镜的屈光力？

透镜将在右侧其新的位置 $u_2= u-t$ 距离处成像（因为 $v = 0$），因此，移动透镜的屈光力 P_2，应该为 $P_2 = 1/(u - t) = 1/(1/P - t) = P/(1 - tP)$。事实上，只要遵循适当的符号约定，同样的公式也适用于发散透镜，此时像的位置在透镜的左侧。这种调整过程称为*透镜的有效性*矫正。

当我们将框架眼镜转换成接触镜时，透镜的有效性就发挥了作用。例如，远视矫正将会使远处物体成像于眼的远点位置（在调节放松的时候，这个点与黄斑中心共轭。参照《快速入门指南》）。在这种情况下，远点位于视网膜后面，根据有效性计算公式，矫正的接触镜度数大于框架镜。例如，一个 +4.00D 框架镜，标准顶点距 13.75mm，等效接触镜是：+4.00D/[1–（0.01375 m）(4.00D)]= +4.232 D，即接触镜度数增加 1/4D。当度数小于 3.00D 时，这种矫正可忽略不计。

Gauss 光学

为了计算主平面的位置，我们必须了解透镜系统中折射的细节。实际上，这通常是通过一个精确的 *Gauss 光学*（或 *Gauss* 消去法），这些超出了本书的范围，但基本思想是：近轴近似法是 Snell 定律的线性化。因此，可以用 2 种“线性算符”来表示近似。①“转换算符”描述了光线通过折射率 n 的介质传播距离 t。其实，这相对于以光学系统的另一个折射面为参考，重新计算来自发光物体（或由前一折射面成的像）的光束聚散度。②“折射算符”描述了在 n_1 和 n_2 介质之间、半径为 r 的弯曲光学界面处聚散度的变化。相当于加入 P，求出从折射界面发出的光束聚散度。我们可以用匹配的 2 × 2 的矩阵在适当的坐标系表示每一个算符，然后用矩阵乘法来计算复杂光学系统中，各折射面折射结果的净作用。

Real and Virtual Objects and Images

In analyzing the action of a (perhaps complex) sequence of refracting surfaces, we have seen that we can treat each surface in turn by considering the image formed by each surface in the sequence as the source object for the next. From the point of view of the next refracting surface in the sequence, it makes no difference whether the source is an actual source of emitted (or reflected) light or the image of such a source formed by the previous refracting surfaces in the system. We cannot tell by looking at such a beam of light whether it comes from a physical object or the image formed by the previous optics. Nevertheless, it is often helpful to keep track of whether the rays that form an image actually converge at the image location (*real images*), such as the image of a distant object formed by a converging lens, or only appear to diverge from the image location (*virtual images*), such as the image of a distant object formed by a diverging lens (see the Quick-Start Guide).

We can make a similar distinction between the apparent objects that are imaged by successive refractive surfaces. Such an apparent object from which light appears to diverge as it approaches a lens surface is considered a *real object* for that surface; an apparent object toward which light appears to converge as it approaches a refracting surface is a *virtual object* for that surface (Figure 1-16). Evidently, the distinction between "real" and "virtual" objects depends on the context—that is, the location of the lens surface which will form the next image of the object in turn.

In practice, the distinction is straight forward. An *image* is real if it is located on the same side of the lens as the image rays (that is, with the light traveling from left to right, to the right of the lens that forms it; strictly, to the right of the second principal plane), and virtual if it is located on the other side of the lens where the image rays do not exist. An *object* is real if it is located on the same side of the lens as the object rays (that is, with the light traveling from left to right, to the left of the lens that is about to form an image of it; strictly, to the left of the first principal plane), and virtual if it is on the other side of the lens where the image rays do not exist.

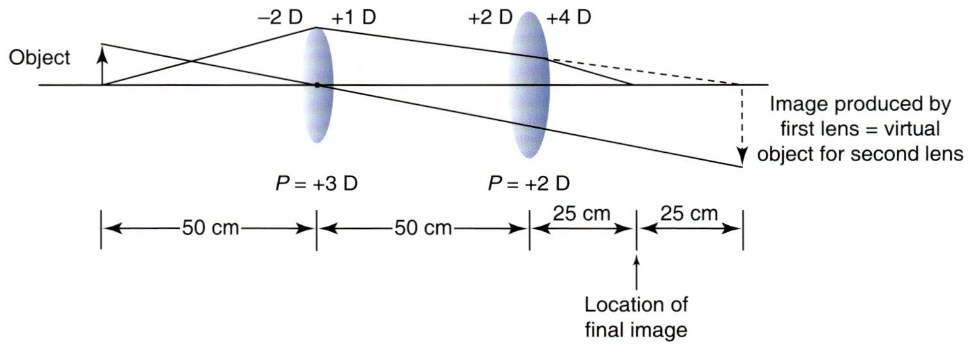

Figure 1-16 Ray tracing for a system of 2 convex lenses in air. The real image formed far to the right by the first lens becomes a virtual object for the second lens. *(Courtesy of Edmond H. Thall, MD.)*

EXAMPLE 1-7

For Section exercises 1-3~1-6, determine which images are real and which are virtual. Images in 1-31 and 1-4 are real, and image 1-6 is virtual.The "imaging" in 1-5 is afocal—that is, the optical system does not form an image at a finite location.

实的和虚的物和像

在分析一个（或复杂的）系列折射面的光学行为时，可以依次将每个折射面形成的像作为下一个折射面的发光物体。对于各折射面中的下一个折射面来讲，发光物体发射（或反射）的是实际光，还是来自系统中前一个折射面形成的像，这都没有区别。因为无法判断这样一束光，它究竟是来自一个真实物体还是之前的光学系统形成的像。然而，却有助于跟踪形成像的光线是否会聚在像的位置（*实像*），例如远处物体通过凸透镜成的像；或者只出现从像的位置发散（*虚像*），如远处物体通过一个凹透镜所成的像（参见《快速入门指南》）。

我们可以对连续折射面成像的表观物作出类似的区分。当光线接近透镜表面时，好像是从该物发出的发散光，这样的物体是该折射面的*实物*；当光线接近折射面时，好像光束会聚到该物体，这样的物体是该折射面的*虚物*（图 1–16）。显然，“真实”和“虚拟”物体之间的区别取决于具体情况，即透镜表面的位置将依次形成物的下一个像。

实际上，这种区别是显而易见的。如果*像*与像方光线位于透镜的同一侧（即当光线从左向右传播，到达形成像的透镜的右侧，严格地说，在第二个主平面的右边），那么该像就是真实的；如果像位于像方光线的透镜的另一边，像就是虚像。如果一个*物*与物方光线位于透镜的同一侧，那么这个物就是实物（即当光线从左向右传播，位于形成像的透镜的左边，严格地说，在第一个主平面的左边），如果它是在像方光线不存在的透镜那边，就是虚物。

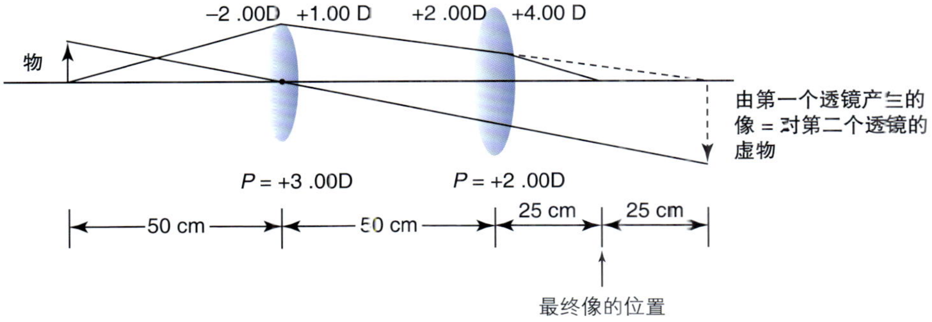

图 1–16 在空气中 2 个凸透镜组成的光学系统的光线追踪图。由第一个凸透镜在其右侧很远的地方成的真实像成为第 2 个透镜的虚物。*（译者注：资料来源见前页原文。）*

例 1–7

针对性阶段练习 1–3~1–6 中，确定哪些像是实像，哪些像是虚像。图 1–3 和图 1–4 中的像是实像，图 1–6 中的是虚像。图 1–5 中的“像”是无焦点的，即光学系统不会在有限的位置形成像。

Transverse Magnification

Optical systems are frequently employed to obtain images of a more convenient size for study than the original objects. Magnifiers and microscopes provide enlarged images of inconveniently small objects; telescopes and binoculars provide smaller, more conveniently located images of immense objects that are very far away. The relocation of images is described by the vergence equation. Magnification is also readily determined in this context. For objects of finite size and distance, *transverse magnification*—the ratio of the height (or distance from the optic axis) of an image to the height of the original source object—is the most appropriate description. Transverse magnification (sometimes referred to as "lateral magnification" or "linear magnification") is denoted by M_T. For lenses in air, a simple calculation with similar triangles (Figure 1-17) gives $M_T = h_2/h_1 = v/u$. Here, u and v carry the same sign conventions as used in the vergence equation. (If the lens separates media of refractive indices n1 and n_2, the corresponding formula is $M_T = n_1v/n_2u$. The refractive index for the object medium multiplies the image distance and vice versa!) Negative values of M_T indicate images that are upside-down (inverted), not images that are reduced in size ("minified"), which correspond to values of M_T less than 1 in absolute value.

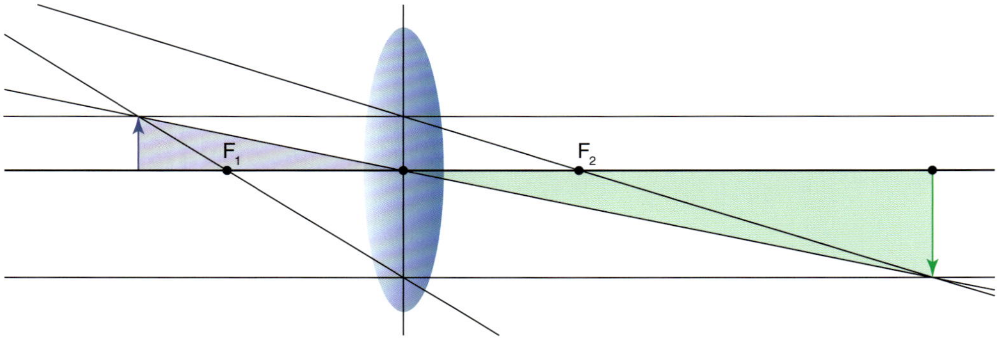

Figure 1-17 Ray tracing for a convex lens used as a magnifier in air. Notice how the principal ray through the central point of the lens creates similar triangles, indicating that the transverse magnification is proportional to the ratio of image distance to object distance. *(Illustration developed by Scott E. Brodie, MD, PhD.)*

Section Exercises 1-15~1-18

Compute the transverse magnification for the setups in Exercises 1-3–1-6.

1–15 $u = -4$ m, $P = +2$ D, $v = +0.57$ m
$M_T = v/u = +0.57$ M/-4 m $= 0.14$

1–16 6$u = -1$ m, $P = +2$ D, $v = 1$ m
$M_T = v/u = -1$ m/1 m $= -1$

1–17 $u = -0.5$ m, $P = +2$ D, $v =$ infinity
$M_T = v/u =$ infinity/-0.5 m $=$ null

1–18 $u = -0.4$, $P = +2$ m, $v = -2$ m
$M_T = v/u = -2$ m/-0.4 m $= +5$

横向放大率

光学系统通常用于获得比原物体更便于研究的像。放大镜和显微镜用于放大较小的物体，望远镜和双筒望远镜用于给距离很远的体积巨大的物体提供更小更便捷的定位像。像的再定位可通过聚散度方程计算，同时可以得出放大倍数。对于有限大小和距离的物体，*横向放大率*[像的高度（或距光轴的距离）与发光物体高度的比值]是最合适的描述。横向放大率（或称为“横向放大”、“线性放大”）用 M_T 表示。空气中的透镜，用一个“相似三角形”的简单计算（图 1–17）：$M_T = h_2/h_1 = v/u$。这里，u 和 v 遵守与聚散度方程相同的符号规定。（如果透镜两边是不同的 2 个折射率为 n_1 和 n_2 的介质，则相应的公式是 $M_T = n_1v/n_2u$。物所在介质的折射率乘以像的距离。反之亦然！）M_T 的负值表示图像是倒置的（颠倒的），而不是像的变小（“缩小”）。像缩小时，M_T 的绝对值应小于 1。

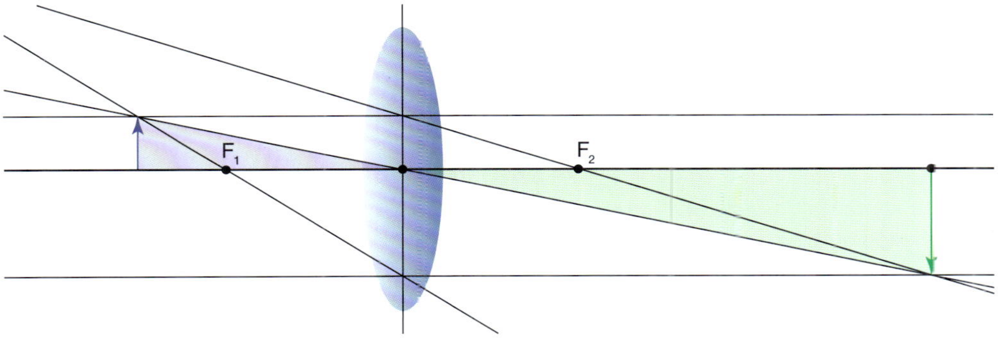

图 1–17　空气中凸透镜系统作为放大镜的光线追踪图。通过透镜中心点，主光学形成相似三角形，提示横向放大率与像距和物距之比成比例。*（由 Scott E. Brodie 医学博士提供。）*

阶段练习 1–15~1–18

计算练习 1–3~1–6 里的横向放大率。

1–15　$u = -4$ m, $P = +2$ D，$v = +0.57$ m

$M_T = v/u = +0.57$ M/-4 m $= 0.14$

1–16　$6u = -1$ m，$P = +2$ D，$v = 1$ m

$M_T = v/u = -1$ m/1 m $= -1$

1–17　$u = -0.5$ m，$P = +2$ D，v=无限远

$M_T = v/u$ =无限远 /-0.5 m = 空值

1–18　$u = -0.4$, $P = +2$ m, $v = -2$ m

$M_T = v/u = -2$ m/-0.4 m $= +5$

Axial (Longitudinal) Magnification

As we have seen, a thin lens in air produces a transverse magnification described by the simple equation $M_T = v/u$. If the source "object" is in fact an assemblage of objects, or an extended object with a palpable axial dimension (measured along the optic axis), the image will also exhibit an axial extent, or apparent thickness. We can show (for example, by differentiating the vergence equation) that the apparent thickness of the image—the *axial*, or longitudinal, *magnification* for a refracting system in air—is given by

$$M_L = (M_T)^2$$

Figure 1-18 illustrates this relationship.

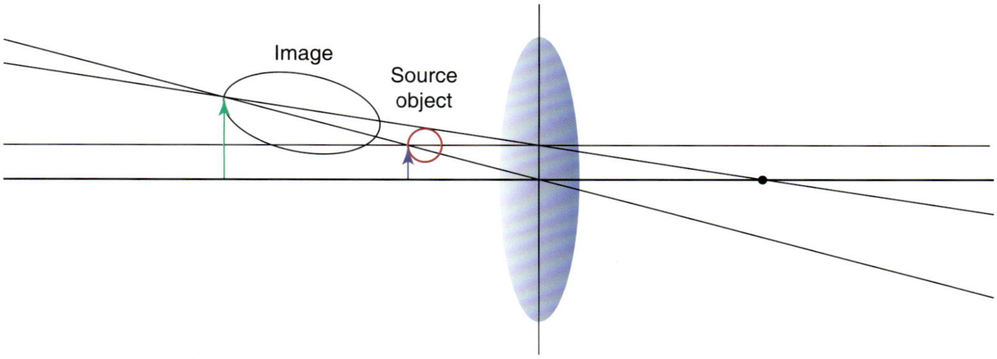

Figure 1-18 Ray tracing for a convex lens in air. The source object is the red circle; its image is the ellipse. Notice the considerable distortion caused by the disparity between transverse and axial magnifications. *(Illustration developed by Scott E. Brodie, MD, PhD.)*

This effect leads to a substantial distortion of the images seen by direct or indirect ophthalmoscopy. Although it is difficult to appreciate image depth with the monocular view through the direct ophthalmoscope, the aerial image seen with the indirect ophthalmoscope is generally seen stereoscopically. Depending on the power of the condensing lens used, the distortion factor may vary as much as fourfold in changing from a 14-D lens to a 30-D lens. The overall stereoscopic effect is reduced by the small inter pupillary distance of the periscopic viewing system but, nevertheless, the perceived shape of fundus features, such as tumors or optic disc excavation, is typically somewhat exaggerated.

轴向（纵向）放大率

正如我们所见，一个在空气中的薄透镜会产生一个横向的放大率，用简单方程描述为 $M_T = v/u$。如果源“物体”实际上是一堆物的集合，或轴向延长的物（沿光轴测量），则像也显示出轴向的延长，或者厚度。我们可以表示（如通过对聚散度方程的微分）这个像的视厚度——空气中的折射系统的*轴向*（或纵向）*放大率*，由如下公式算得：

$$M_L = (M_T)^2$$

图 1-18 描述了这种关系。

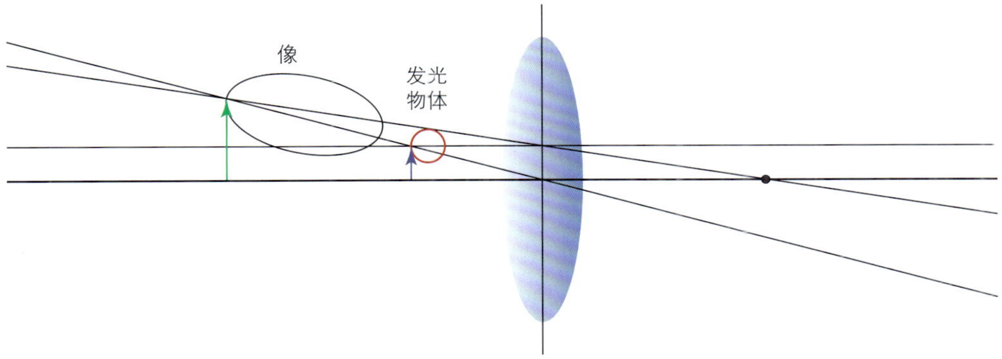

图 1-18 凸透镜在空气中的光线追踪图。发光物体是红圈，像呈椭圆。注意由于横向放大率和纵向放大率所导致的相当大的变形。*（译者注：资料来源见前页原文。）*

这种效应会导致通过直接或间接检眼镜时看到的像明显失真。虽然直接检眼镜的单目注视很难判断图像深度，但间接检眼镜看到的虚像一般是立体的。根据所使用的透镜的屈光力不同，从 14-D 透镜到 30-D 透镜的失真度可能相差 4 倍。潜望镜观察系统的小瞳距使整体的立体效果下降，但观察到的眼底改变，如肿瘤或视盘凹陷往往都会被放大。

EXAMPLE 1-8

Compute the relative apparent thickness of the retinal features as seen by indirect ophthalmoscopy with a 15-D, 20-D, and 30-D condensing lens. (Assume a total power for the eye of 60D.)

The transverse magnification of an indirect ophthalmoscope is equal to the ratio of the power of the eye (about 60D) to the power of the condensing lens (similar to the formula for the power of a Keplerian telescope). The axial magnification is given by $M_L = (M_T)^2$. Although the apparent thickness (or depth) of retinal features is reduced by the periscopes built into the indirect ophthalmoscope (which reduce the effective interocular distance of the examiner) compared with normal viewing, the *relative* depth of fundus features is unaffected. The ratio of the transverse magnification provided by 15D, 20D, and 30D condensing lenses is then 4×, 3×, and 2×, respectively, so the relative axial magnifications are in the ratios of 16 : 9 : 4, respectively. Thus, the apparent retinal thickness as seen with a 15 D condensing lens is nearly double that seen with the 20D lens, and 4 times that seen with the 30D lens.

Conjugate Points

Points that form an object–image pair are said to be *conjugate* to one another, or to form a conjugate pair. Because the paths of light rays are reversible, each point in a conjugate pair is the image of the other. In the case of a source object infinitely far to the left of an optical system, this "point at infinity" is considered conjugate to the back (second) focal point, F_2, to the right of the lens. Similarly, the front (first) focal point, F_1, is conjugate to the point infinitely far to the right of the lens. Notice that the front and back focal points are *not* conjugate to each other. In air, the front and back focal points are located at a distance $f = 1/P$ from the front and back principal planes, respectively.

Ray Tracing

In practice, it is often instructive to trace the paths of light rays as they traverse a lens system. Ray tracing can provide a helpful check on computations based on the vergence equation. For a thin convex lens in air, it is convenient to depict the source object as a vertical arrow, with its tail on the optic axis and its head at a distance—say, h—from the optic axis. We take a central vertical line to be the common location of the front and back principal planes. The ray from the tail of the arrow through the center of the lens on the optic axis passes undeviated. To locate the image of the arrow, we can trace 2 rays that originate at the tip of the arrow. The ray that propagates parallel to the optic axis is bent at the common principal plane and passes through the back focal point, F_2. The ray from the tip of the arrow through the front focal point, F_1, is bent at the common principal plane and redirected to continue parallel to the optic axis, where it eventually crosses the (refracted) path of the previous ray, locating the image of the tip of the arrow. In general, we can also use a third ray, from the tip of the arrow through the (common) principal point on the optic axis (the "center" of the lens) to confirm the construction. By symmetry, this ray will emerge from the lens as if undeviated (though in fact it makes a slight zigzag as it enters and exits the lens) and should also intersect the point of intersection of the previous 2 rays (see Fig 1-17).

The various cases of interest with the source object arrow located at different distances from a thin convex lens, at the front focal point, and between the front focal point and the lens are illustrated in Figure 1-19. The ray tracing for a thin concave lens in air is shown in Figure 1-20.

例 1-8

计算通过带 15-D、20-D 和 30-D 聚光透镜的间接检眼镜所观察到的视网膜特征的相对表观厚度（假设眼的总屈光力为 60.00D）。

间接检眼镜的横向放大率等于眼屈光力（约 60D）与聚光透镜的屈光力之比（类似于开普勒望远镜的屈光力公式）。轴向放大率由 $M_L = (M_T)^2$ 给出。虽然与正常观察相比，间接检眼镜内置的观测镜减少了视网膜特征的相对表观（或深度）（减少了检查者的有效眼间距离），但是眼底特征相对深度并不受影响。15D、20D 和 30D 聚光透镜的横向放大率分别为 4×、3×、2×，因此相对轴向放大率之比为 16∶9∶4。因此，15D 聚光透镜的表观视网膜厚度几乎是用 20D 透镜看到的 2 倍，是用 30D 透镜看到的 4 倍。

共轭点

形成物与像的点为一一对应的点，彼此*共轭*，或称为共轭对。因为光路的可逆性，所以共轭对中的每个点都是另一个点的像。如果点光源在光学系统的左边无限远处，这个“无限远处的点”是与透镜右边的后焦点 F_2（或第二焦点）共轭的。同样地，前焦点 F_1（或第一焦点）与透镜右侧无限远的点共轭。注意前焦点和后焦点相互不是共轭的。在空气中，前、后焦点分别位于与前、后主平面的距离 $f = 1/P$ 处。

光线追踪

在实践中，跟踪光线穿过透镜系统时的路径是有用的。光线追踪可以对聚散度方程的计算进行检验。对于空气中的薄凸透镜，将发光物体描绘成垂直的箭头，其尾端在光轴上，头部是与光轴间的距离 h。取中心垂直线作为前、后主平面的共同位置。箭尾发出的光线通过光轴上透镜的中心而不发生偏移。要定位箭头的像，我们可以追踪箭头尖端发出的 2 条射线。平行于光轴传播的光线在共同主平面上弯曲，并通过后焦点 F_2。从箭头尖端穿过前焦点 F_1 的光线，在公共主平面上弯曲，然后再重新定向，继续平行于光轴，最终穿过前一条线的（折射）路径，定位箭头尖端的像。一般情况下，我们也可以用第三条线，从箭头的尖端穿过光轴上（共同）的主点（透镜的“中心”）来确认。根据对称性，该光线从透镜发出，未偏移（虽然它在进入和离开透镜时实际上会有一个轻微的曲折），并且与前 2 条线的交点相交（见图 1-17）。

图 1-19 显示发光物体箭头位于薄凸透镜的不同距离时，前焦点上和前焦点与透镜之间的不同情况。空气中薄凹透镜的光线追踪如图 1-20 所示。

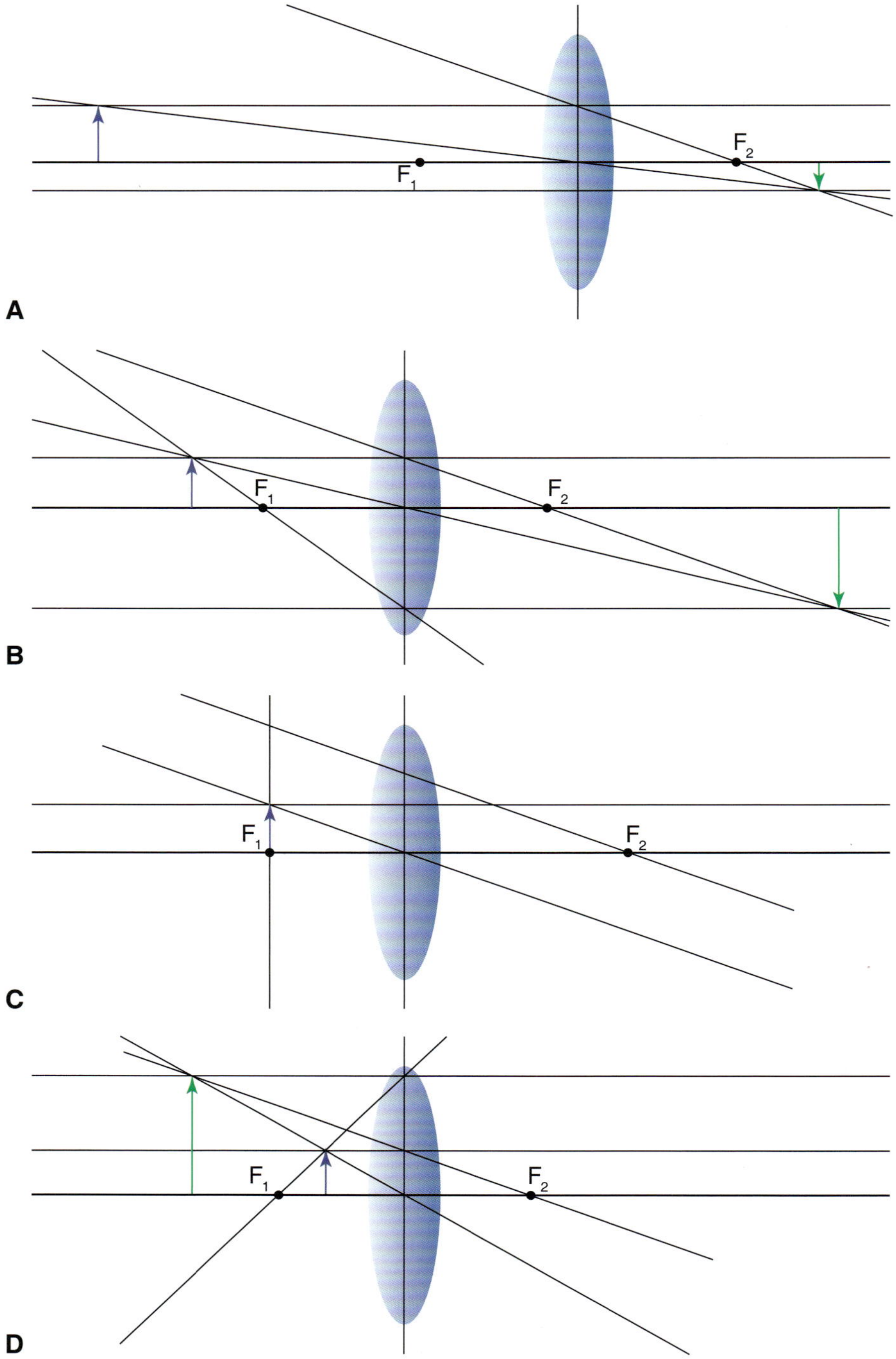

Figure 1-19 Ray tracing for a simple convex lens in air. The blue arrow represents a movable object; the green arrow shows the corresponding image location and size. Points F_1 and F_2 are the front and back focal points of the lens, respectively. **A**, Source object far to left; real image (inverted and minified) is on opposite side of lens. **B**, Source object at left, near first focal point; real image (inverted and enlarged) is on opposite side of lens. **C**, Source object coincides with first focal point; "image" is at infinity. **D**, Source object between first focal point and lens; virtual image (upright and enlarged) is seen to left of source object. *(Illustration developed by Scott E. Brodie, MD, PhD.)*

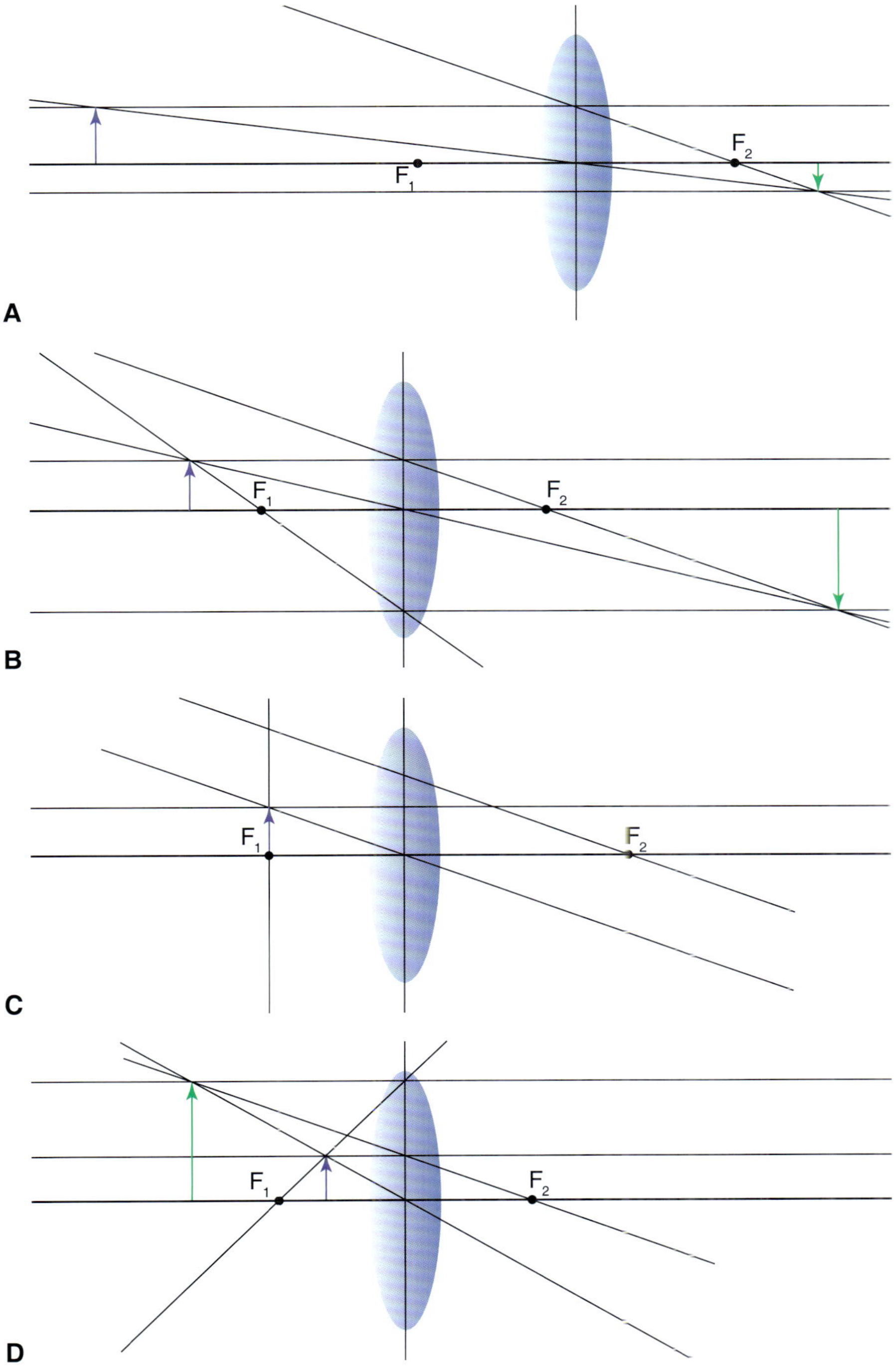

图 1-19　一个简单的凸透镜在空气中的光线追踪图。蓝色箭头表示一个可移动的物体，绿色箭头表示相应的像位置和大小。点 F_1 和点 F_2 分别是透镜的前焦点和后焦点。**A**. 发光物体远离左侧，形成实像（是倒立和缩小的）在透镜的另一侧。**B**. 发光物体在左边、第一焦点的附近，形成实像（是倒立和放大的）在透镜的另一侧。**C**. 发光物体与第一焦点重合，“像”在无穷远处。**D**. 发光物体位于第一焦点与透镜之间，虚像（是直立和放大的）位于发光物体左侧。*（译者注：资料来源见前页原文。）*

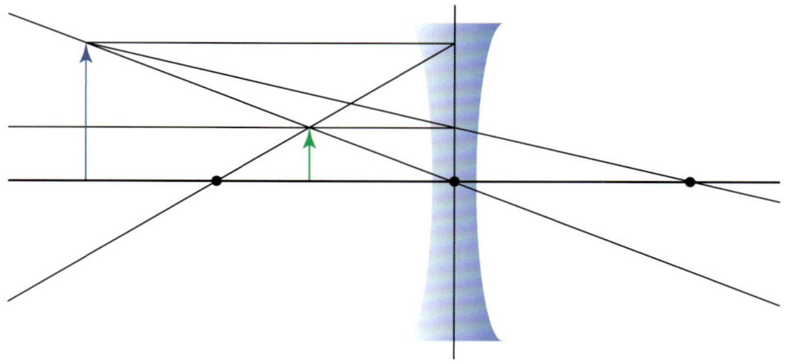
A

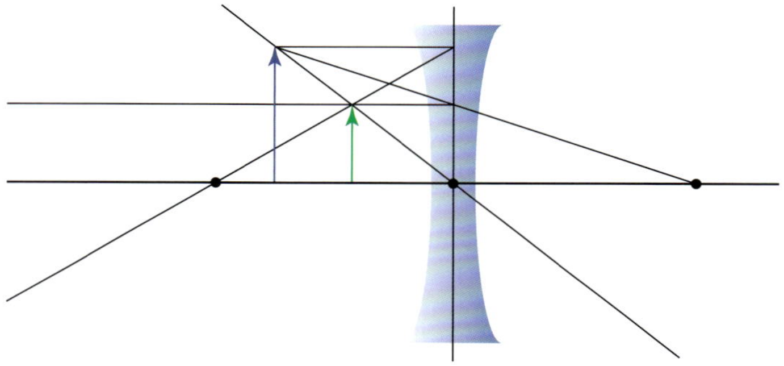
B

Figure 1-20 Ray tracing for a concave lens in air. The blue line represents a movable object; the green line shows the corresponding image location and size. **A**, Source object at left. Virtual image, minified, lies between focal point and the lens. **B**, Moving the object between focal point and lens produces similar virtual image, though with less image minification. *(Illustration developed by Scott E. Brodie, MD, PhD.)*

Section Exercises 1-19~1-22

Draw the ray-tracing diagrams for Exercises 2–5:

1-19 See Figure 1-19A.

1-20 See Figure 1-19B.

1-21 See Figure 1-19C.

1-22 See Figure 1-19D.

Nodal Points

Consider a thick lens (Figure 1-21). Gaussian reduction can be used to show that there is a pair of conjugate points on the optic axis for which an object ray directed at one of these points, N_1, making an arbitrary small angle, θ, with the optic axis will, on exiting the lens, appear to emerge from the other point, N_2, at the same angle θ with the optic axis.

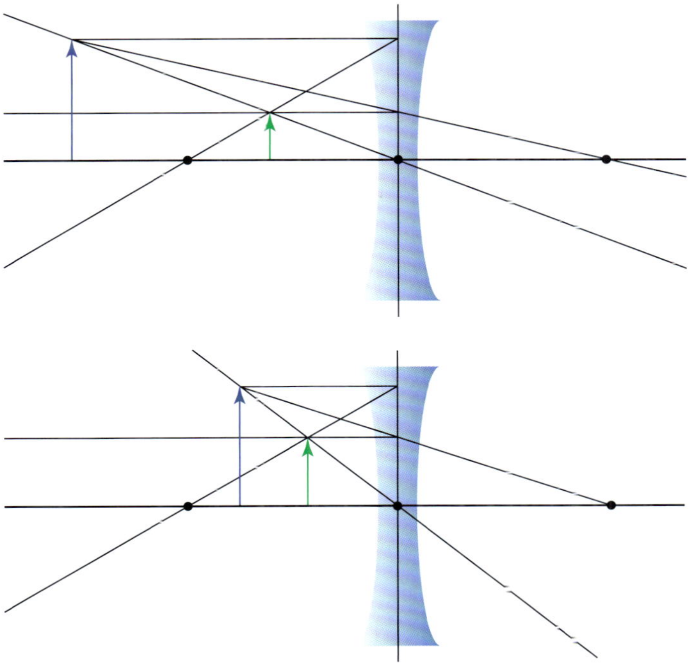

A

B

图 1–20　一个凹透镜在空气中的光线追踪图。蓝线表示一个可移动的物体，绿线表示相应的像位置和大小。**A**. 发光物体位于凹透镜左边，虚像（是缩小的）位于焦点和透镜之间。**B**. 将物体移动到焦点和透镜之间，产生相同的正立虚像，但像是缩小的。*（译者注：资料来源见前页原文。）*

阶段练习 1–19~1–22

画出练习 2–5 的光线追踪图：

1–19　见图 1–19A。

1–20　见图 1–19B。

1–21　见图 1–19C。

1–22　见图 1–19D。

节点

考虑一个厚透镜（图 1–21）。高斯简化可用于表示光轴上的一对共轭点，物体的光线与光轴成任意小角 θ 入射至其中的一个点 N_1，离开透镜时，似乎从另一点 N_2 发出，且与光轴成角 θ。

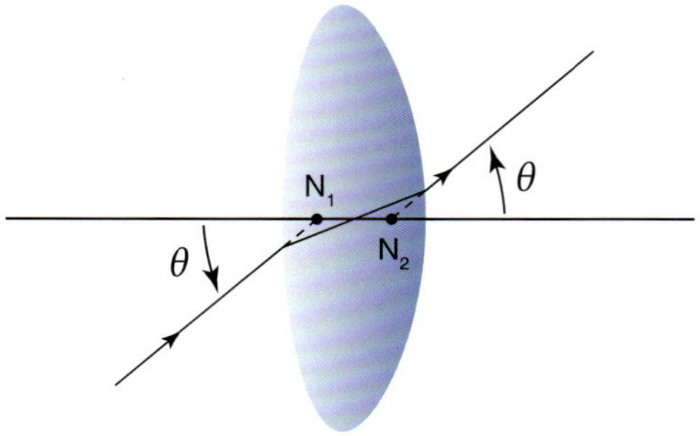

Figure 1-21 Nodal points of a thick convex lens in air. The inclination of an incident ray through the first nodal point equals the inclination of the exiting ray as it apparently emerges from the second nodal point. *(Redrawn from Creative Commons illustration by Bob Mellish.)*

The points N_1 and N_2 are referred to as the front (or first) and back (or second) *nodal points*, respectively. They serve, for ray tracing in a general optical system, as an analogue for the central point in a thin lens, and have a role similar to that of the front and back principal planes for determining object and image vergence. When the refractive indices n_1 and n_2 are equal, the nodal points coincide with the principal points. Nodal points are particularly useful for determining image size (Example 9-1).

It is tempting to draw an analogy between the role of the nodal points in ray tracing and the "fulcrum-like" action of a pinhole aperture, as described in Part 1 of the Quick-Start Guide. In both cases, the angles between the incident and emergent rays and the optic axis for rays passing through the pinhole or nodal points are equal. But this analogy is potentially misleading for optical systems with finite apertures. For these systems (unlike simple pinholes), it is *not* true that all the light passes through the nodal points, only that the unique rays that do pass through the nodal points preserve the same simple geometry as the rays passing through a pinhole aperture. In particular, a small posterior subcapsular lens opacity does not cause a disproportionate reduction in visual acuity by virtue of its proximity to the posterior nodal point of the eye. (Such an opacity may, however, be an effective scatterer of light, greatly reducing a patient's contrast sensitivity.)

EXAMPLE 1-9

In the reduced model eye, the eye's refracting surfaces are replaced by idealized air–water interfaces. The nodal point of the reduced model eye is 17 mm in front of the retina. Using this nodal point, calculate the retinal image size of a target of light 1.0 cm in diameter on a bowl-shaped background (as in the Goldmann perimeter) viewed at 33 cm. (the reduced model eye is discussed in Chapter 3.)

A nodal point 17 mm in front of the retina is about 7 mm behind the anterior corneal surface. By similar triangles, image height/1.0 cm = 17 mm/ 337 mm = 0.050 cm = 0.50 mm.

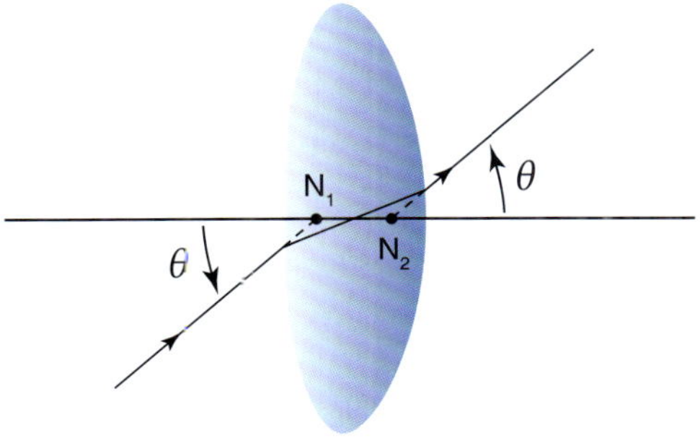

图 1–21　空气中厚凸透镜的节点。通过第一节点的入射光线倾斜等于第二节点出射光线的倾斜。*（译者注：资料来源见前页原文。）*

N_1 和 N_2 分别称为前（或第一个）节点和后（或第二个）节点。在普通光学系统中进行光线追踪时，它们类似于薄透镜的中心点，在确定物和像的聚散上作用类似于前、后主平面。当折射率 n_1 和 n_2 相等时，节点与主点重合。节点用于确定像的大小（例 1–9）。

在光线追踪中，就像在《快速入门指南》的第一部分中描述的那样，将节点的作用和针孔孔径的“支点”作用之间做一个类比。在这 2 种情况下，入射光线和出射光线与光轴之间的角度和与通过针孔或节点光线的角度是相等的。但是这种类比对于有限孔径的光学系统可能具有误导性。对于这些系统（不像简单的针孔），并不是所有的光都通过节点。只有通过节点的光线与通过针孔的光线才具有相同的简单几何学特征。尤其是，一个小的后囊下晶状体混浊并不会由于它靠近眼睛的后节点而导致视力的不成比例的下降。（然而这种混浊产生光的散射，大大降低了患者的对比敏感度。）

例 1–9

在简化模型眼中，眼的屈光面取代理想的空气 – 水界面。简化模型眼的节点位于视网膜前 17mm。利用这个节点，计算观察眼前 33cm 处球形背景中如 Goldmann 视野计直径 1.0cm 光标的视网膜像大小（简化模型眼在第 3 章讨论。）

视网膜前 17mm 的节点约在角膜前表面后 7mm 处。通过相似三角形，像高 /1.0 cm = 17 mm/ 337 mm = 0.050 cm = 0.50 mm。

The Reduced, or Equivalent, Optical System

A complex multiple lens system can always be analyzed sequentially, but the process is tedious and must be repeated from the beginning for each source object location. However, we can calculate an equivalent optical system consisting of just 1 pair of principal planes, 1 pair of focal points, 1 pair of nodal points, and 1 power. The paraxial properties of this equivalent system, called the *reduced optical system*, are identical in every respect to the original system consisting of multiple lenses. Thus, once the equivalent system is determined, we need only a single vergence equation calculation to locate the image of any object. A simplified reduced model for the human eye (Figure 1-22) is discussed in Chapter 3.

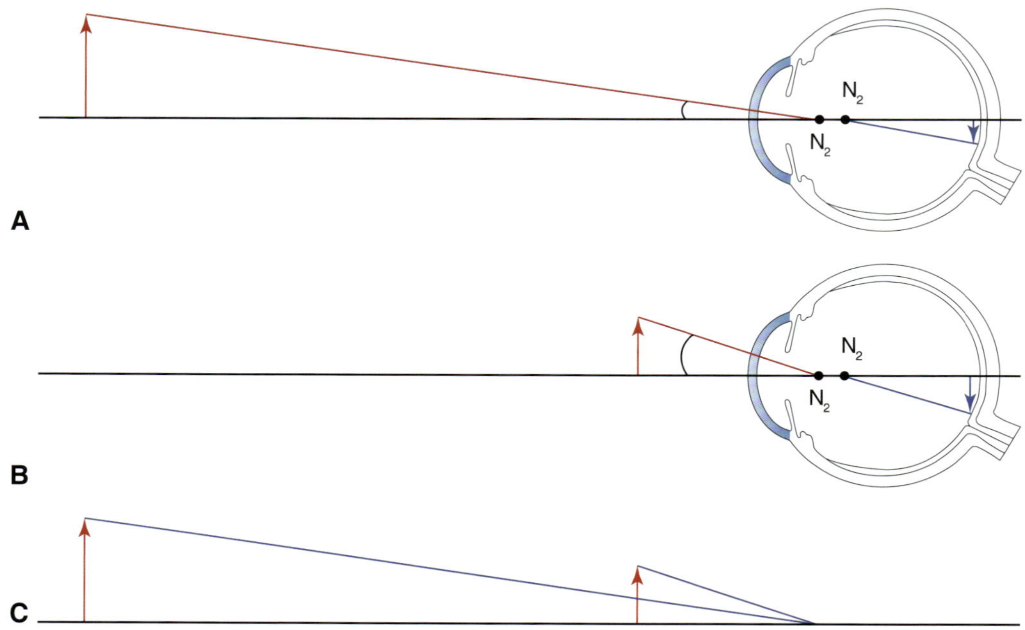

Figure 1-22 Reduced optical system for the human eye. The retinal image size (apparent size) of an object depends in part on the angle subtended at the object nodal point N_1. **A** small object close to the eye can subtend a larger angle than a large but distant object. This is the basis of the magnification produced by a telescope. The object in **A** is twice the size of the object in **B**. However, the object in B is 4 times closer to N_1 than the object in **A**. Therefore, the angle the object in **B** subtends is twice as large as the angle the object in A subtends. **C**, The 2 angles are directly compared. *(Courtesy of Edmond H. Thall, MD.)*

EXAMPLE 1-10

Draw the ray tracing for the general case of a thick lens with positive power and distinct principal planes and nodal points.

Suppose the source object is more distant from the front of the lens than the anterior focal point, and the lens sits with air to the left and water (an optically "denser" medium) to the right. The nodal points are displaced toward the denser medium.The ray tracing is as shown in Figure 1-E10. (The lens surfaces are omitted for clarity.)

简化光学系统或等效光学系统

一个复杂的多透镜系统总是可以按顺序进行分析，但是这个过程很繁琐，每次都要从发光物体的位置开始。然而，我们可以计算出一个由一对主平面、一对焦点、一对节点和一个屈光力组成的等效光学系统。这一等效系统称为*简化光学系统*，其旁轴特性在各个方面都与由多个透镜组成的原系统相同。因此，一旦确定了等效系统，我们只需要一个聚散度方程来计算任何物体的成像位置。人眼的简化模型（图 1–22）将于第 3 章讨论。

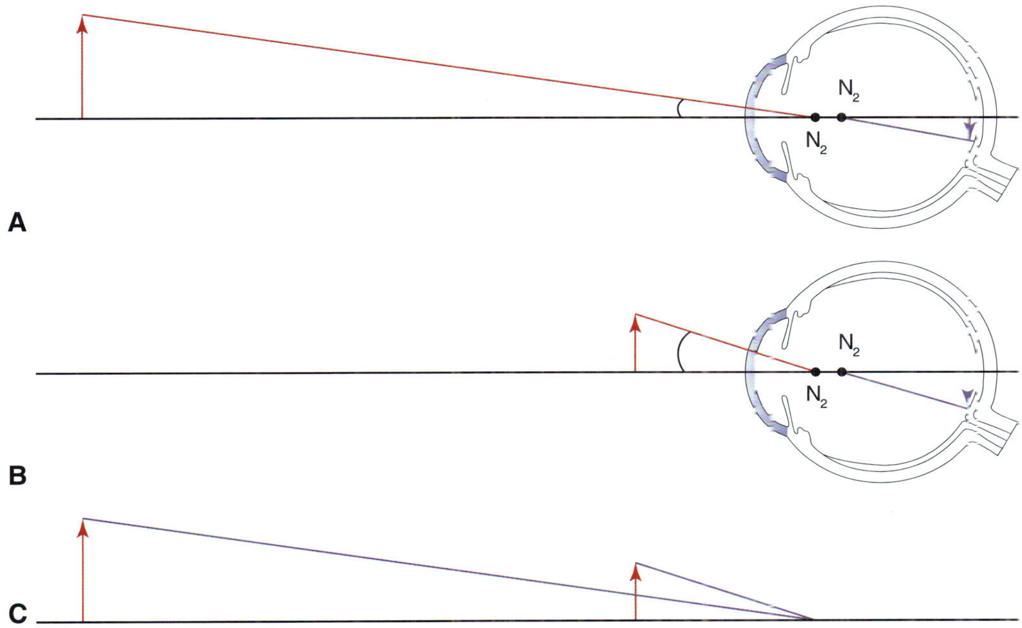

图 1–22　人眼的简化光学系统。物体的视网膜像大小（视尺寸）部分取决于物体节点 N_1 处的夹角。一个靠近眼睛的小物体可以比一个大而远的物体形成更大的夹角。这就是望远镜放大的基础。**A** 中的物体是 B 中的物体大小的 2 倍，但是 B 中的物体距离 N_1 的距离是 A 中的物体距离 N_1 的 4 倍。因此，**B** 中的物体与光轴的夹角是 A 中物体夹角的 2 倍。**C**.2 个角度的直接比较。*（译者注：资料来源见前页原文。）*

例 1–10

画出具有正屈光力、2 个主平面和节点的厚透镜在一般情况下的光线追踪图。

假设发光物体比前焦点离透镜前部更远，且透镜左侧是空气，右侧是水（一种光学上“光密”的介质）。节点向光密的介质移动。其光路追踪如图 1–E10 所示。（为了清晰起见，镜头表面省略了。）

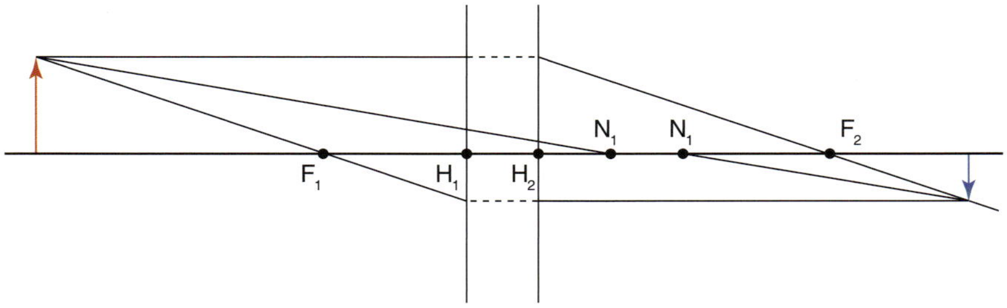

Figure 1-E10 Ray tracing for a general optical system with distinct principal planes and nodal points

Aberrations

The paraxial theory of image formation discussed above is necessarily an idealization of the behavior of real optical systems. The goal of *stigmatic imaging*—recombining the light passing through a finite aperture from an extended object to project all the energy from each object point to a single image point simultaneously—is never perfectly achieved in practice. Even at the best possible focus, light from a single object point is distributed over a small area of the image. Each image point receives light predominantly from one object point but also receives some light from neighboring object points. The image point resembles but does not duplicate the object point. Because rays do not focus perfectly stigmatically, the image does not contain as much detail as the original object. This discrepancy is referred to in general as the *aberration* of an optical system.

Point Spread Function

The region over which light from a single object point is spread in a pinhole camera is a "blur circle" (see the Quick-Start Guide). Strictly, the word *circle* is somewhat misleading. Even with simple ray tracing through a small circular aperture, the image region is typically an ellipse, not a circle. Light from any single object point tends to focus to an irregularly shaped smudge. Moreover, within the smudge light is usually not evenly distributed; some areas are brighter than others. The distribution of light (from a single object point) in the image is aptly named the *point spread function* (PSF), because it describes how light from a single object point spreads out in the image.

An image is therefore composed of multiple partially overlapping smudges, one smudge for each object point. The point spread function is a quantitative description of the smudge and is quite useful because we can deduce all the imaging characteristics of an optical system from the PSF. (The process for extracting image information from the PSF requires advanced mathematics beyond the scope of clinical practice.)

As we have seen, imaging for incident rays near the optic axis is, to an excellent approximation, stigmatic, but rays outside the paraxial region do not focus stigmatically. The size of the paraxial region depends on several factors and varies from lens to lens. The paraxial region can be quite large but typically is small—a few millimeters or less. Nevertheless, the paraxial region is very important because paraxial rays focus stigmatically. Rays outside the paraxial region account for most aberrations.

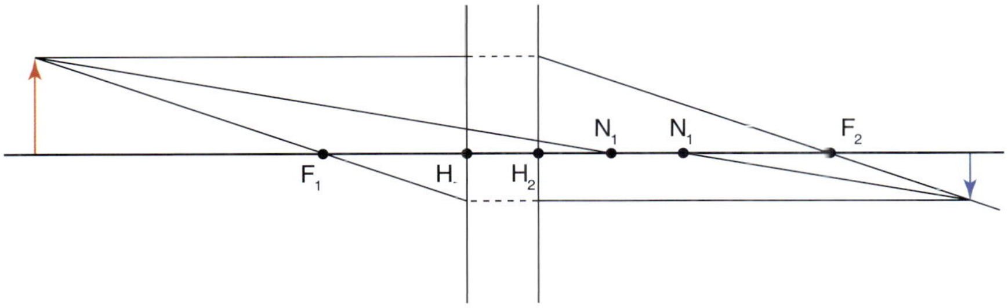

图 1–E10 有 2 个主平面和节点的一般光学系统的光路追踪图。

像差

以上成像的近轴理论是理想化的光学系统。*共点成像*是将来自扩展物体的通过有限孔径的光线重新组合，使每个物体点的所有能量同时投射到单个像点上，而这个目的在现实中从未完美实现。即使在最好的聚焦下，来自单个物体点的光也会分布在像的一个小区域上。每个像点主要从一个物点接收光线，但也会从邻近的物点接收一些光线。像点跟物点类似但不是单纯的复制。因为光线不能完全聚焦，所以像并不包含发光物体的很多细节，这种差异统称为光学系统的*像差*。

点扩散函数

从单个物点发出的光通过针孔相机成像的区域是一个“模糊的圆”（参见《快速入门指南》）。严格来说，“圆”这个词有误导性。即便通过一个小的圆形孔径进行简单的光线追踪，图像区域也通常是一个椭圆，而不是圆。任何一个物点发出的光都会聚焦成不规则形状的光斑。而且，这个光斑也不是均匀分布的，有些区域会更明亮。光（来自单一物点）在图像中的分布被形象地称为*点扩散函数*（PSF），因为它描述了来自单一物点的光如何在像中扩散。

因此，一个像由多个部分重叠的光斑组成，每个光斑对应一个像点。点扩散函数是对光斑的定量描述，它非常有用，因为可以从点扩散函数推导出光学系统的所有成像特性。（从点扩散函数中推导图像信息的过程需要用到超出临床范畴的高等数学。）

正如我们看到的，近轴区域入射光的像是近似于完美的共点成像，但在近轴区域以外的光线，就不能共点聚焦（或消像散聚焦）。近轴区域的大小取决于各种因素，这要根据透镜而不同。近轴区域可以相当大，但通常只有几毫米甚至更小。尽管如此，近轴区域非常重要，因为近轴光线可以共点聚焦。而在近轴区域以外的光线会产生大部分像差。

The vergence equation and transverse magnification equation are based entirely on paraxial rays, completely ignoring rays outside the paraxial region. Paraxial rays alone are enough to calculate image location, size, and orientation to sufficient accuracy. However, to understand image quality, brightness, and depth of focus, we must consider nonparaxial rays. For instance, image quality is diminished because rays do not focus stigmatically. Because paraxial rays do focus stigmatically, it is the nonparaxial rays that determine image quality. We can say nothing about image quality based on paraxial rays alone.

Moreover, the notion of optical power applies to the paraxial region only. There is no such thing as refractive power outside the paraxial region. This is in stark contrast to corneal topographic power maps that assign a "power" to every point on the cornea, even the periphery. However, corneal power maps define power in 2 ways (axial and tangential), and neither is consistent with the correct definition of refractive power as we have used it in this chapter. In the early 1950s, lens designers developed *wavefront theory*, the appropriate way to analyze the optical properties of imaging systems beyond the paraxial regime, especially aberrations.

Wavefront Theory

In geometric optics, the movement of light obeys *Fermat's principle*, which states that light travels between 2 points *only* along the fastest path (Appendix 1.2). Thus, a stigmatic focus can be achieved only when each of the paths from object to image point requires precisely the same amount of time.

We can construct a spherical surface centered on the image point such that all light moving along image rays must cross the arc of that surface simultaneously to achieve a stigmatic focus. This surface is called the *reference sphere* (Figure 1-23).

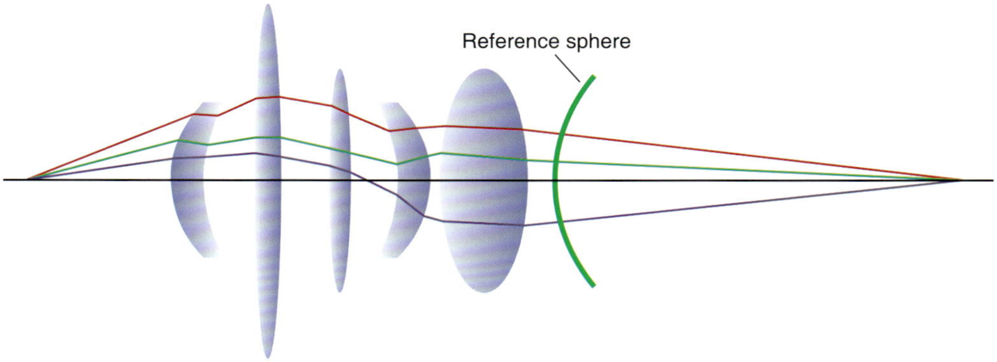

Figure 1-23 The reference sphere, a spherical arc centered on the image point. *(Courtesy of Edmond H. Thall, MD.)*

A geometric *wavefront* is an isochronic (equal-time) surface. We can construct a wavefront anywhere along a group of rays originating from a single object point. All light from a given object point crosses the wavefront simultaneously. If the wavefront that intersects the vertex of the reference sphere is also spherical, then the focus is stigmatic. However, a wavefront is in general irregularly shaped. The difference between the wavefront and the reference sphere is the wave aberration (Figure 1-24).

聚散度方程和横向放大率方程是完全基于近轴光线基础上计算的，完全忽略了近轴区域以外的光线。近轴光线可以精确计算像的位置、大小和方向。然而，为了理解像的质量、亮度和焦深，还必须考虑非近轴光线。例如，非共点聚焦的光线会造成像质下降。因为近轴光线是共点聚焦，而非近轴光线决定了像的质量。仅有近轴光线是无法评价成像质量的。

此外，屈光力的概念只适用于近轴区域，在近轴区域之外不存在屈光力。这与角膜地形图的屈光力形成了鲜明的对比，地形图给角膜的每个点，甚至包括周边的点都赋予了一个“屈光力”。然而，角膜屈光力图对屈光力的定义有 2 种方式（轴向和切线向），这 2 种方式都不是本章所使用的准确的屈光力定义。在 20 世纪 50 年代初期，透镜设计师形成了*波前理论*，这是一种分析非近轴区域成像系统的光学特性，特别是像差的最佳方法。

波前理论

在几何光学中，光的运动遵循 *Fermat 原理*，即光在 2 点之间*只沿*最快的路径传播（附录 1.2）。因此，只有当从物点到像点的每条路径需要完全相同的时间时，才能形成一个共点焦点。

我们可以构建一个以像点为中心的球面，这样沿着成像点光束的所有光线都会同时通过这个球弧，聚焦形成共点焦点。这个表面被称为*参考球面*（图 1–23）。

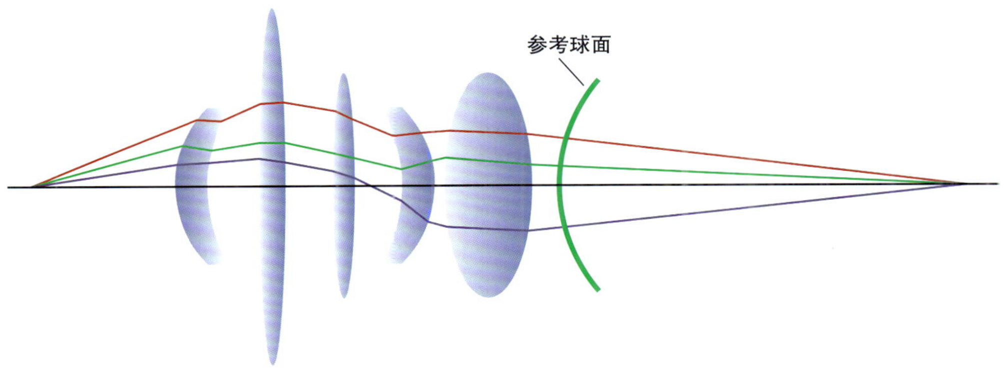

图 1–23　参考球面。以像点为中心的球面弧。*（译者注：资料来源见前页原文。）*

几何*波前*是个等时面（等时间）。我们可以沿着一组来自单一物点发出的光线的任何地方构造波前。所有来自给定物点的光线将同时穿过波前。如果与参考球顶点相交的波前也是球形的，则焦点是共点的。然而，波前通常是不规则的。波前和参考球面的差异就是波前像差（图 1–24）。

It is a common misconception that *wavefront* refers in some way to the wave nature of light. Geometric optics ignores the wave nature of light. (See Appendix 2.1 for a brief discussion of the wave nature of light, an aspect of physical optics.) A geometric wavefront is a surface of equal time, regardless of whether light is a wave or a particle. The term *isochrone* might be more descriptive, but for historical reasons the term *wavefront is* entrenched.

The wavefront aberration is a smooth but irregularly shaped surface, typically something like the shape of a potato chip or corn flake. The mathematical description of the wavefront aberration may at first seem daunting, but conceptually it is straightforward.

Consider first a toric surface (see the Quick-Start Guide). A *toric surface* is the combination of 2 "more fundamental" surfaces: a sphere and a cylinder. We can represent any toric surface as the sum of a certain amount of sphere and a certain amount of cylinder. The fundamental shapes sphere and cylinder never change from one toric surface to another; only the amount of sphere and cylinder (and the cylinder orientation) changes. Sphere and cylinder are the only fundamental shapes required to define any toric surface or for that matter to express any amount of regular astigmatism. The same idea applies to wavefront aberration, except more than 2 fundamental shapes are required. Every wavefront aberration is the sum of the same fundamental shapes. The amount of each shape varies from patient to patient, but the fundamental shapes themselves never change.

The most common set of fundamental reference shapes used for this purpose is known as the *Zernike polynomials*, which are mathematical functions defined on a disc-shaped region. The first several Zernike polynomials closely resemble simple combinations of the wavefront aberrations that we commonly encounter with simple optical systems. A detailed discussion of this material is far beyond the scope of this text; a brief qualitative discussion follows.

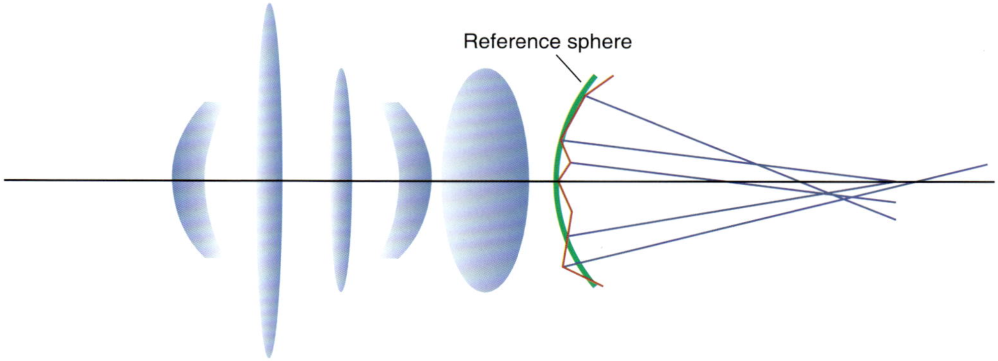

Figure 1-24 The wavefront and wavefront aberration. The actual wavefront is irregularly shaped, and the image is not stigmatic. The difference between the actual wavefront and the reference sphere is the wave aberration[Wave ? wavefront]. *(Courtesy of Edmond H. Thall, MD.)*

The most fundamental aberrations were initially described in the nineteenth century by Philipp Ludwig von Seidel. They are known as *Seidel aberrations*—spherical aberration, coma, astigmatism, curvature of field, and distortion (Figure 1-25):

- *Spherical aberration* is a disparity in focal length for rays from a single axial object point that are refracted at different distances from the center of the lens.
- *Coma* is a disparity in focal length for rays from a single *off-axis* object point that are refracted at different distances from the center of the lens.

常常将*波前*误解为是光的波动性。几何光学不考虑光的波动性。（关于光的波动性，即物理光学特性，请参阅附录 2.1）几何波前是一个等时间面，不考虑光是波还是粒子。“*等时*”一词可能更具有描述性，但由于历史原因，*波前*一词根深蒂固。

波前像差是一种光滑但形状不规则的面，类似于土豆片或玉米片的形状。对波前像差的数学描述乍一看似乎令人生畏，但从概念上讲却是直截了当的。

我们先来看看复曲面（参见《快速入门指南》）。*复曲面*是 2 个“最基本的”表面的组合：一个球面和一个柱面。我们可以把任意一个复曲面表示成一定数量的球面和一定数量的柱面的总和。基本球面和柱面不会从一个曲面变化到另一个曲面，只有球面和柱面波的数量（和柱面的方向）会发生变化。球面和柱面波是定义复曲面或以表达任何数量的规则散光的唯一基本形状。同样的，这个概念也适用于波前像差，只是波前像差需要 2 个以上的基本波形叠加。每个波前像差都是相同的基本波形叠加起来的。每个波形的数量因个体而异，但是基本波形不变。

最常见的用以描述最基本参考波形的常见集合被称为 *Zernike 多项式*，它是定义在一个圆盘样区域上的数学函数。Zernike 多项式的前几项，与在简单光学系统中遇到的波前像差的简单组合非常相似。对该多项式的详细讨论远远超出了本文的范围，因此，我们将进行下面的简单讨论：

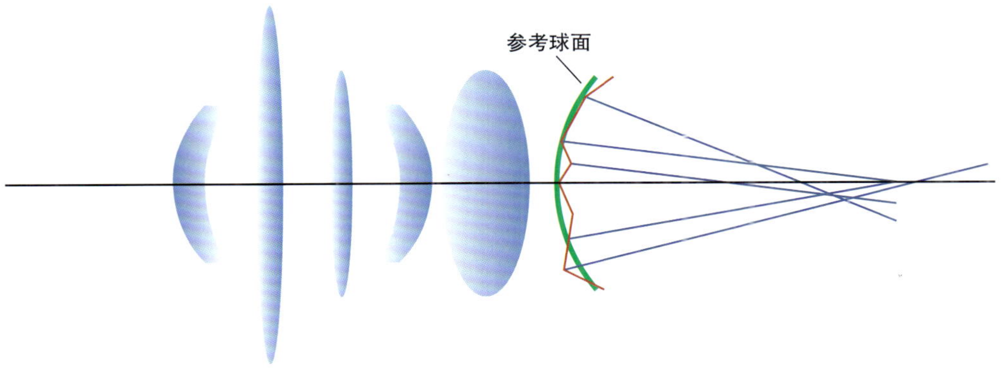

图 1–24　波前和波前像差。实际波面形状是不规则的，像不是对称的。实际波前与参考球面之间的差就是波前像差。*（译者注：资料来源见前页原文。）*

最基本的像差是在 19 世纪由 Philipp Ludwig von Seidel 首先提出的，被称为 *Seidel 像差*——球差、彗差、像散、场曲和畸变（图 1–25）：

- *球差*是从单一轴物点发出的光线，在距透镜中心不同距离处折射后，焦距的差异。
- *彗差*是从单一离轴物点发出的光线，在距透镜中心不同距离的折射后，焦距的差异。

- *Curvature of field* is a disparity in focal length for objects at different distances from the optic axis.
- *Astigmatism* is the disparity in focal length for rays from a single object point that are incident at different meridians of the lens (see the Quick-Start Guide).
- *Distortion* is a disparity intransverse magnification for objects at different distances from the optic axis.

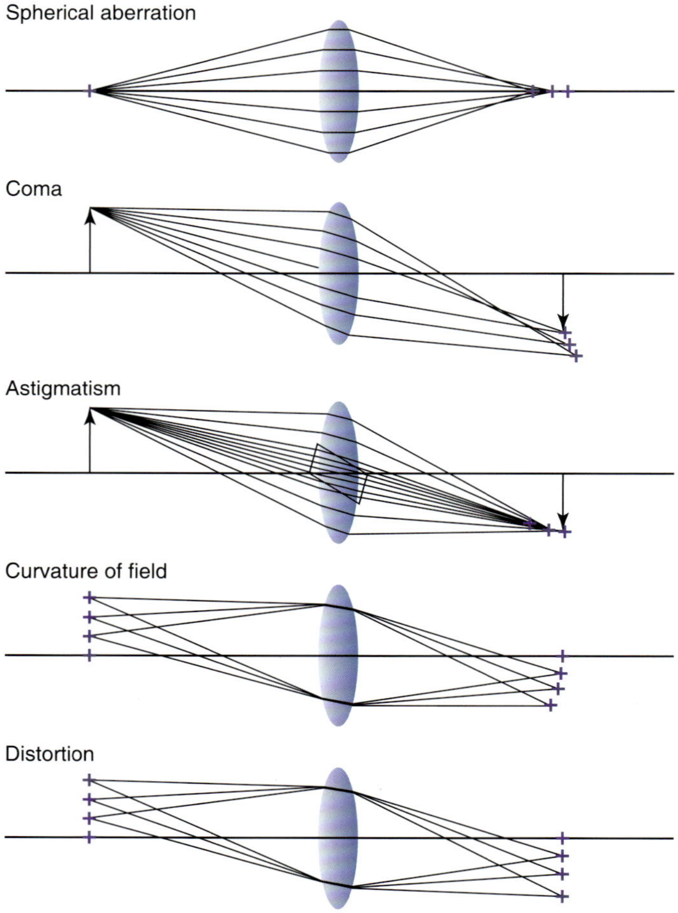

Figure 1-25 Schematic depiction of the classic Seidel aberrations. *(Courtesy of Edmond H. Thall, MD.)*

The low-order Zernike polynomials closely mirror basic optical image manipulations and the classic Seidel aberrations. (Figure 1-26 depicts the lowest-order Zernike polynomials.) For example, the first-order Zernike polynomial aberration named *tilt* is, in essence, equivalent to a prismatic deviation.

The second-order Zernike polynomial aberrations are referred to as *defocus*, corresponding to myopia and hyperopia, and astigmatism, which corresponds to the potato chip–like waveform surface created by a spherocylindrical lens.

The Seidel aberrations are third-order Zernike polynomial aberrations. These include coma, which corresponds to a lobular asymmetry in the waveform surface.

In myopia, the wavefronts are displaced relative to the reference sphere (Figure 1-27). The wavefront is spherical but has a smaller radius than the reference sphere, and the wave aberration is parabolic.

- *像散*是从单一物点的光线，在透镜的不同子午线入射后，焦距的差异。（见《快速入门指南》）。
- *场曲*是物体在距视轴不同距离时，焦距的差异。
- *畸变*是距视轴不同距离的物体在横向放大上的差异。

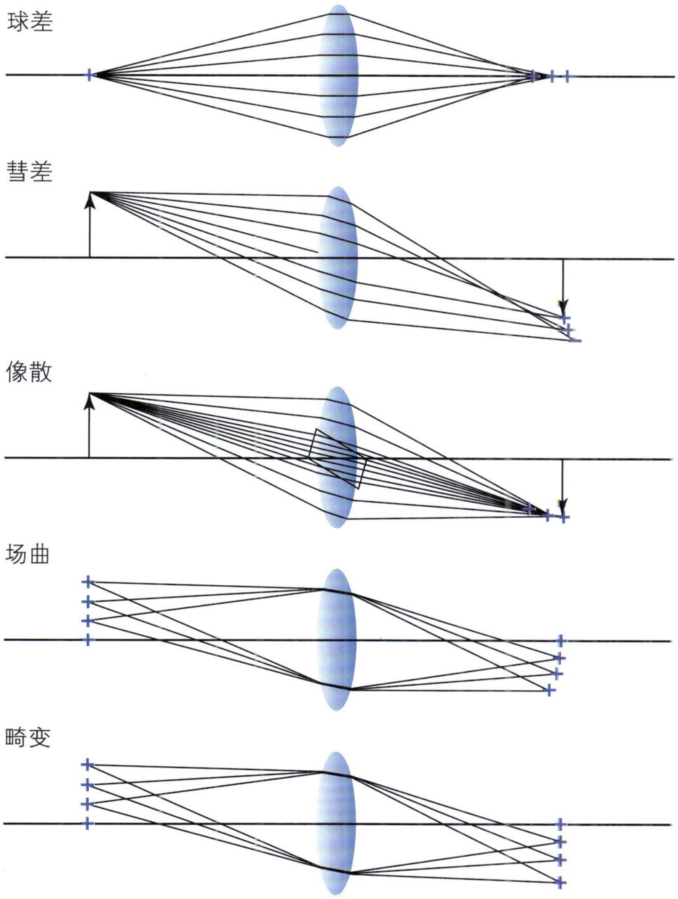

图 1–25　经典的 Seidel 像差的示意图。*（译者注：资料来源见前页原文。）*

低阶 Zernike 多项式反映了基本光学图像处理和经典 Seidel 像差。（图 1–26 描述了最低阶 Zernike 多项式。）例如，一阶 Zernike 多项式的像差叫*倾斜*，在本质上等同于棱镜偏移。

二阶 Zernike 多项式像差称为*离焦*，对应于近视、远视和散光，对应于球柱镜产生的薯片状波面。

Seidel 像差是三阶 Zernike 多项式像差。这些包括彗差，对应于不对称小叶状的波面。

对于近视而言，波前相对于参考球面有位移（图 1–27）。其波前为球形，但半径小于参考球面，波像差为抛物线。

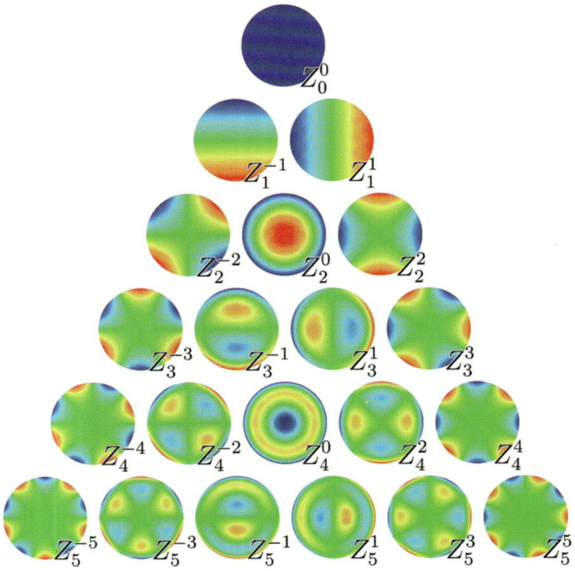

Figure 1-26 Low-order depictions of the first several Zernike polynomials, labeled according to standard notation. Top row: "piston" aberration affects only the phase of light waves and is not ordinarily detectable. Second row: "tilt" corresponds to misdirection of wave propagation, akin to prismatic deviations, shown as vertical or horizontal. Third row: the outer functions show astigmatic aberrations; the middle function shows variations in focal point with circular symmetry, akin to defocus and/or spherical aberration. Bottom row: the middle 2 functions are lobular wavefront errors, akin to classical coma; the outer functions ("trefoil") show a threefold symmetry sometimes seen as a complication following refractive surgery procedures, such as LASIK. *(Illustration by Wikipedia user Zom-B via Creative Commons.)*

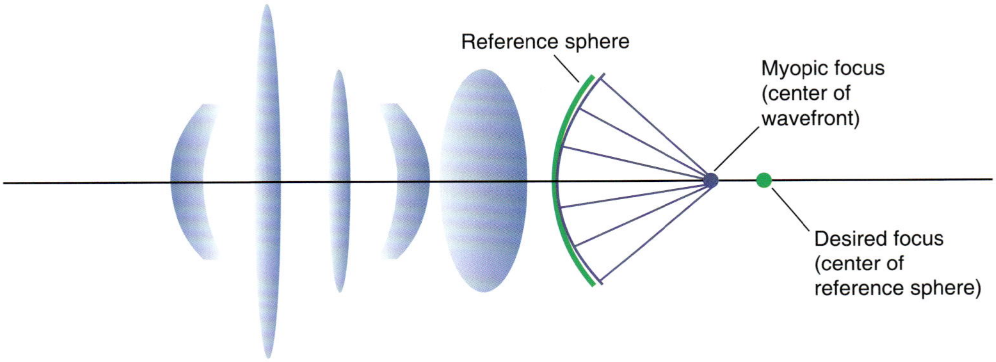

Figure 1-27 Myopia. In pure myopia, the focus is still stigmatic. Therefore, the actual wavefront is also a sphere but with a smaller radius than the reference sphere. The wave aberration has a parabolic shape. *(Courtesy of Edmond H. Thall, MD.)*

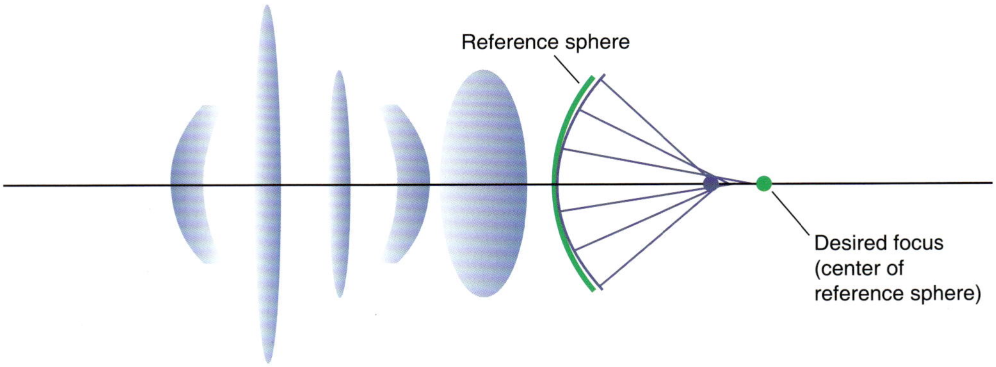

Figure 1-28 Positive spherical aberration. The peripheral rays focus anterior to the paraxial rays. The wave aberration has a bowl shape—flat centrally, then strongly curved toward the edge. *(Courtesy of Edmond H. Thall, MD.)*

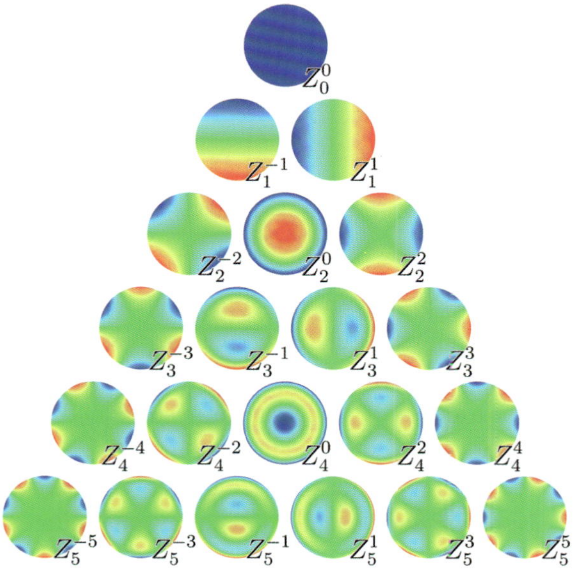

图 1–26　根据标准注释表示的前几个 Zerrike 多项式中描述的低阶像差。第一行："活塞"像差只影响光波的相位，通常不易觉察。第二行："倾斜"对应于波的传播方向错误，类似于棱镜偏移，分为垂直偏移或水平偏移。第三行：外函数表示像散像差；中间的函数表示具有圆形对称的焦点的改变，类似于离焦和 / 或球差。最下面一行：中间的 2 个函数是小叶波前误差，类似于经典的彗星；外部的函数（"三叶草"）显示出三频对称性，有时视为屈光手术后的并发症，例如 LASIK。*（译者注：资料来源见前页原文。）*

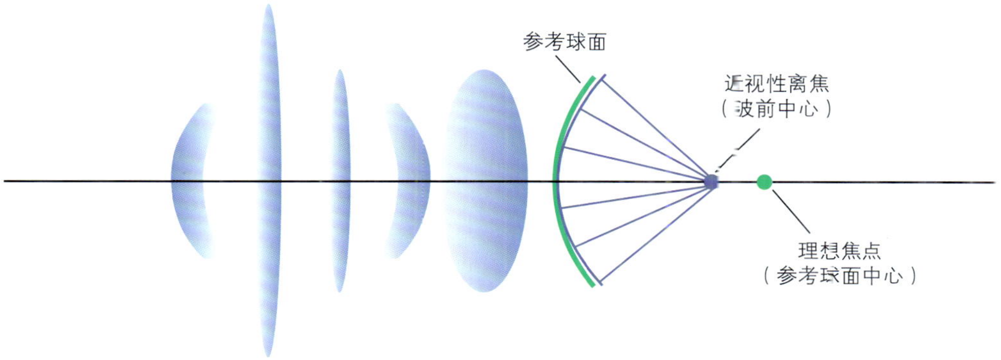

图 1–27　近视。对单纯近视而言，焦点仍然是像散矫正的。因此，实际的波前也是一个球体，但半径小于参考球体。波像差呈抛物线形。*（译者注：资料来源见前页原文。）*

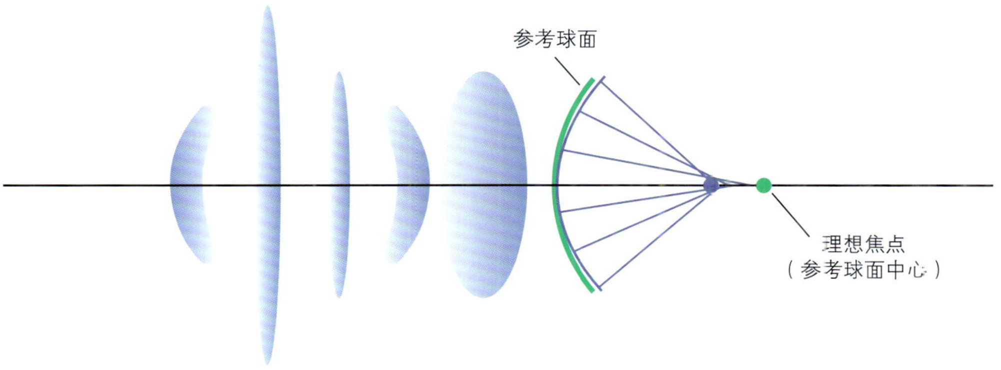

图 1–28　正球差。周边光线聚焦于近轴光线之前。波像差像碗一样，中心平坦，周边明显弯曲。*（译者注：资料来源见前页原文。）*

In positive spherical aberration, rays at the edge of the wavefront focus anteriorly to central (paraxial) rays (Figure 1-28). The wave aberration is bowl shaped. Spherical aberration shifts the position of best focus anteriorly. This aberration is strongly pupil dependent: as the pupil of a patient with positive spherical aberration dilates, the shift in best focus renders the patient more myopic. The condition is known as *night myopia* and can be treated by prescribing spectacles with an extra -0.50D in the distance correction for use at night or in low light.

Chromatic Aberration

In addition to these "monochromatic" aberrations, images produced by white light may also be degraded by *chromatic aberration*, the spreading apart of colors of white light by a lens system. This effect is caused by dispersion, by which the index of refraction of a material medium may vary with the wavelength of the light passing through it. Just as a prism bends blue light more strongly than it bends red light, in practice, a convex lens will create a focal point for blue light anterior to the one for red light, so the eye is typically about 0.5 D more myopic for images formed in blue light than in red light. This disparity is the basis for the Lancaster red-green ("duochrome") test for accommodative control (see the Quick-Start Guide).

Astigmatism

The basic properties of toric (spherocylindrical) lenses were introduced in the Quick- Start Guide. Unlike a rotationally symmetric lens (eg, sphere), which produces a point image of a point object, a toric lens always produces 2 linear "images" of a single point. As we have seen, the 2 focal lines are perpendicular to each other—one parallel to the cylinder axis, the other perpendicular to the cylinder axis. The focal lines are found at different distances from the lens, according to the vergence equation for the maximal and minimal powers of the principal meridians of the lens.

The Conoid of Sturm

The geometric figure that is formed by the rays of light leaving an astigmatic lens is called the *conoid of Sturm* (Figure 1-29). The *circle of least confusion* is the circular cross section of the conoid of Sturm that is halfway between the 2 focal lines—in terms of diopters, not linearly. (Notice that the circle of least confusion in Figure 1-30 is closer to the vertical focal line than to the horizontal one.)

Consider again the spherocylinder of Example 1-9. There are 2 focal lines separated by 75 cm. The region between these 2 linear foci is the conoid of Sturm. Starting at the linear focus in the 30° meridian 25 cm from the lens and proceeding farther to the right, the focus changes from a line to an ellipse with the long axis in the 30° meridian. Farther to the right, the ellipse becomes a circle; then another ellipse with the long axis in the 120° meridian, and eventually a line in the 120° meridian.

The Spherical Equivalent

The *spherical equivalent* (*SE*) is the "average" power of a toric lens. For instance, a +2.00 +3.00 × 010 cylinder has a power of +2.00D in the 10° meridian and +5.00D in the 100° meridian. The average is +3.50D, which is the SE power. If the lens is described in spherocylindrical notation, we calculate the SE as the sum of the sphere and half the cylinder power. For instance, a +2.00 - 5.00 × 020 spherocylinder has the SE of -0.50D.

We can use the SE to calculate the location of the circle of least confusion. For example, when the SE is +3.50D and the object vergence is -1.00D, the circle of least confusion is +2.50D, or 40 cm to the right of the lens.

在正球差中，波前边缘的光线聚焦于中心（近轴）光线前（图 1–28）。波像差呈碗状。球差将最佳聚焦位置前移。这种像差的瞳孔依赖性很强：当正球差患者的瞳孔扩大时，最佳聚焦的移动会使患者更加近视。这种状况称为“*夜间近视*”，它可以通过在夜晚或者暗光下配带 −0.50D 眼镜来治疗。

色差

除了“单色”像差之外，白光产生的像也可能由于*色差*而使成像质量下降，通过透镜系统使白色光分散成多种颜色。这种效应是由色散引起的。通过色散，介质的折射率可能随穿过介质的光的波长而变化。如同棱镜使蓝光的弯曲比红光更明显。实际上，凸透镜的蓝光焦点在红光前。所以，蓝光在眼内形成的像比红光形成的像偏 0.50D “近视”。这种差异是 Lancaster 红绿测试（双色试验）进行调节控制的基础（见《快速入门指南》）。

散光

复曲面透镜的基本性能见《快速入门指南》。旋转对称的透镜（如球面）能产生点物体的点像，与其不同的是，复曲面透镜总是能产生单一点的 2 个线状“像”。正如我们所见，这 2 条焦线互相垂直——一条平行于柱镜轴，另一条垂直于柱镜轴。根据透镜主子午线的最大和最小屈光力的聚散度方程，可以在距透镜不同距离处找到焦线。

Sturm 光锥

离发散光透镜的光线形成的几何图形称为 *Sturm 光锥*（图 1–29）。*最小弥散圆*是 Sturm 光锥形成的。它位于 2 个焦线的 1/2 处的圆形截面，用屈光度表示，不是线性的。（请注意，图 1–30 中最小弥散圆更接近垂直焦线，而不是水平焦线。）

思考一下案例 1–9 中的球柱镜。有 2 条焦距为 75cm 的焦线，这 2 个焦线之间的区域就是 Sturm 光锥。30° 子午线的焦线，距离透镜 25cm，行进到右侧更远处，焦点从一个线变成了一个长轴在 30° 子午线的椭圆。再往右一点，椭圆就成了一个圆；然后成为一个长轴在 120° 子午线的椭圆，并最终成像在 120° 子午线。

等效球镜

等效球镜（*SE*）是一个复曲面透镜的“平均”屈光力。例如，+2.00 / +3.00 × 010 的柱镜在 10° 子午线上的屈光力是 + 2.00D，100° 子午线的屈光力是 + 5.00D，平均屈光力是 +3.50D，这就是等效球镜。如果透镜是用球柱镜方法描述的，我们用球镜和 1/2 柱镜之和来计算等效球镜。例如，一个 + 2.00 / −5.00 × 020 的球柱镜，等效球镜是 −0.50D。

我们可以通过等效球镜计算最小弥散圆的位置。例如，当等效球镜为 +3.50D，物像聚散度为 −1.00D，那么最小弥散圆是 +2.50D，即位于透镜右侧 40cm 处。

EXAMPLE 1-11

A point source is 1 m to the left of a +2.00 +3.00 × 030 toric lens. Where are the images? The object vergence is -1.00D. the lens has a power of+5.00D in the 120° meridian and therefore produces a linear image oriented in the 30° meridian corresponding to an exiting vergence of +4.00D, or 25 cm to the right of the lens. The lens also has a power of +2.00D in the 30° meridian and therefore produces a linear image oriented in the 120° meridian with an exiting vergence of+1.00D, or 1 meter to the right of the lens. The object point and both linear images are real.

Suppose the object point is 25 cm to the left of the same lens. Where are the linear images? Using the same methods, we get a linear image oriented in the 30° meridian+1.00D, or 1 meter to the right of the lens. Also, there is a linear image in the 120° meridian with a vergence of -2.00D, or -50 cm to the left of the lens. In this case, the object point and the linear image in the 30° meridian are real, but the linear image in the 120° meridian is virtual.

Next, consider a pure cylinder such as+2.00×180 and an object 1 m to the left of the lens. The object vergence is again -1.00D, and one linear image is -1.00D+(+2.00D)= +1.00D to the right of the lens, real, and oriented along the 180° meridian. the second linear image is -1.00D + (+0.00D) = -1.00D, or 1 meter to the leftof the lens, virtual, and oriented in the 90° meridian. So, the vertical image is virtual and in the same location as the object.

The notion of a virtual linear image at the object can be confusing, but consider the Maddox rod, which is an array of parallel cylinders of high power. The virtual images these cylinders produce are used to test ocular alignment (Figure 1-E11).

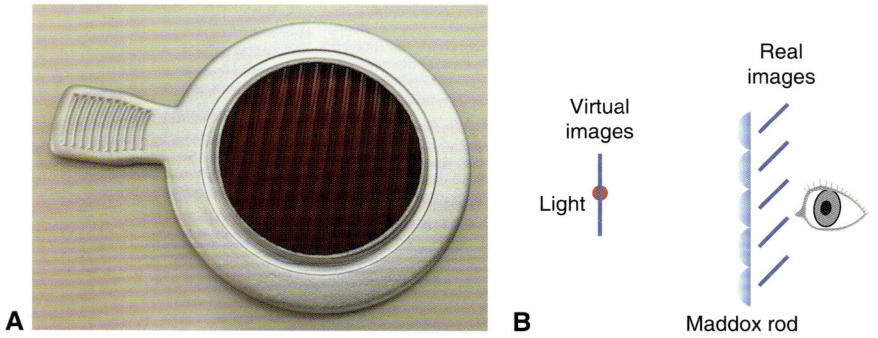

Figure 1-E11 Maddox rod. **A**, Maddox rod, an array of high-power parallel cylinders. **B**, The cylinders produce real images parallel to, and a few millimeters behind, the cylinders and virtual images perpendicular to the axis through the object. The real images are too close to the eye for the patient to see them. Only the virtual images are visible. *(Part A courtesy of Scott Brodie, MD, PhD; part B courtesy of Edmond H. Thall, MD.)*

例 1-11

点光源位于 +2.00 +3.00 × 030 的复曲面镜左侧 1m 处 此时像在哪里? 物的聚散度为 -1.00D，透镜在 120° 子午线的屈光力为 +5.00D，因此在 30° 子午线上产生一个线状像，该像的聚散度为 +4.00D，或这个像位于镜片右侧 25cm 处。这个透镜同时在 30° 子午线上有 +2.00D 的屈光力，因此在 120° 子午线上产生一个线性像，该像的聚散度为 +1.00D，或这个像位于镜片右侧 1m 处。物点和 2 条线状像都是实像。

假设物点位于同一个透镜的左侧 25cm 处。线状像又在哪里? 用同一种方法，得知 30° 子午线上的线状像聚散度为 +1.00D，或该像位于镜片右侧 1m 处。同样的 120° 子午线上的线状像聚散度为 -2.00D，相当于位于透镜左侧 -50cm 处。在这种情况下，物点和 30° 子午线上的线状像是实像，但是 120° 子午线上的线状像是虚像。

接下来，考虑一个单纯的柱镜，例如 +2.00 × 180 和一个位于镜片左侧 1m 位置的物体。物的聚散度依然是 -1.00D，一个线状像是 -1.00D +(+2.00D)=+1.00D，位于透镜右侧，实像，位于 180° 子午线。另一个线状像是 -1.00D + (+0.00D) = -1.00D，位于透镜左侧 1m 处，虚像，位于 90° 子午线。所以，垂直像是虚像，同物体位置一样。

物体的虚线状像概念令人混淆，可以参考 Maddox 杆，它是由许多高屈光力的平行柱镜组成，就是通过柱镜产生的虚像来检测眼位。(图 1-E11).

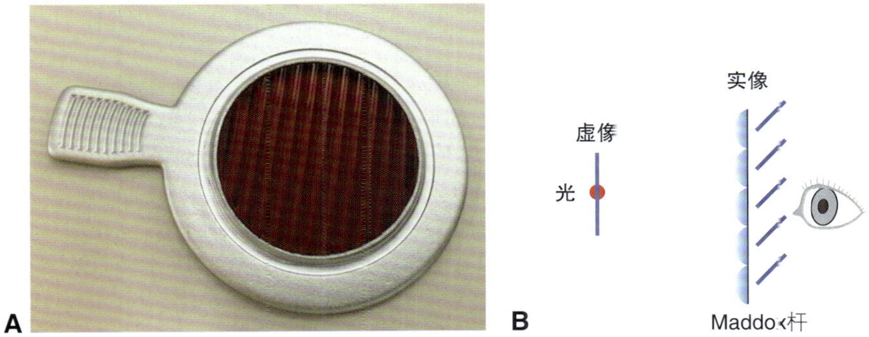

图 1-E11 Maddox 杆。**A**. Maddox 杆，一组由高屈光力组成的平行圆柱。**B**. 柱镜产生的实像平行于柱镜，且在其后几毫米处，虚像垂直于柱镜轴。实像距离眼睛太近，不能看到。只有虚像可以看到。*(译者注: 资料来源见前页原文。)*

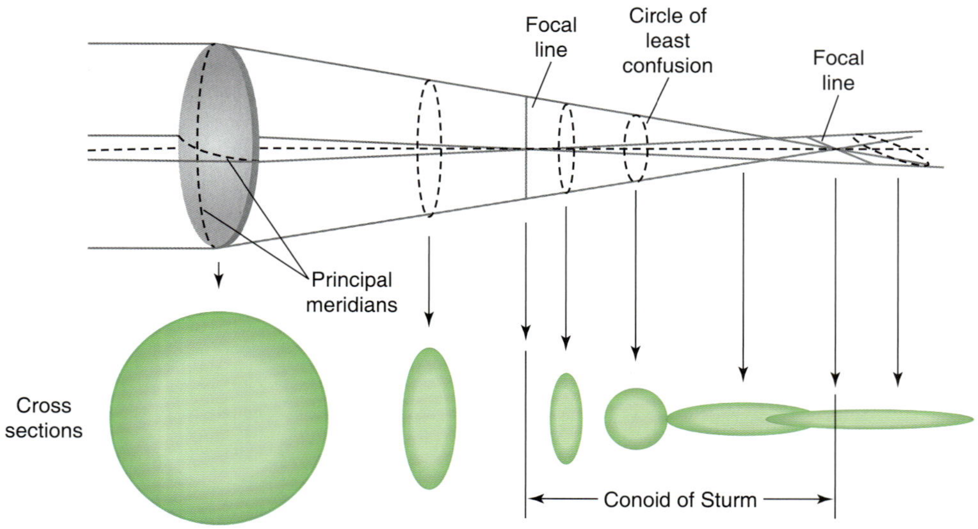

Figure 1-29 Conoid of Sturm, the geometric figure formed by the rays of light leaving an astigmatic lens. The circle of least confusion is the circular cross section of the conoid of Sturm that is halfway (in diopters, not linearly) between the 2 focal lines. *(Reproduced from Guyton DL et al., Ophthalmic Optics and Clinical Refraction. Baltimore: Prism Press; 1999.)*

The Power Cross

Any spherical, toric (spherocylindrical), or purely cylindrical lens can be represented graphically by a *power cross.* A spherical lens has the same power at every meridian. A toric lens has a different power at every meridian that varies between a maximum and a minimum value. The maximum and minimum powers are always in meridians that are 90° apart. The power cross shows the maximum and minimum powers and their meridians.

A pure cylinder has zero power along its axis and either highest positive or lowest negative power perpendicular to its axis. The rule is "the power of a cylinder is perpendicular to its axis." For instance, a +2.00 × 015 cylinder has zero power in the 15° meridian and +2.00D power in the 105° meridian (Figure 1-30).

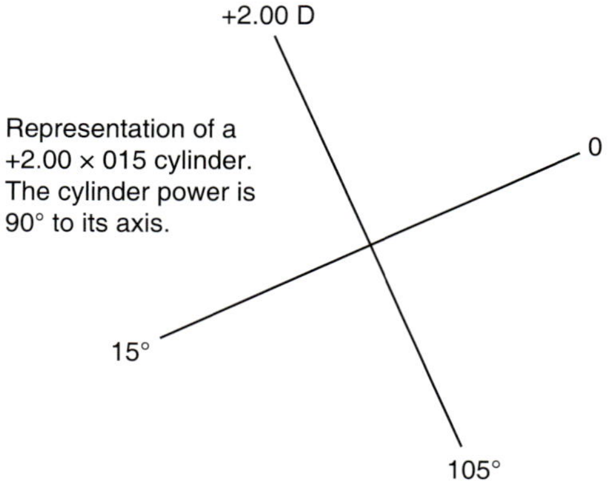

Figure 1-30 Power-cross representation of a +2.00 × 015 cylinder. The power of a cylinder is 90o to its axis. *(Courtesy of Edmond H. Thall, MD.)*

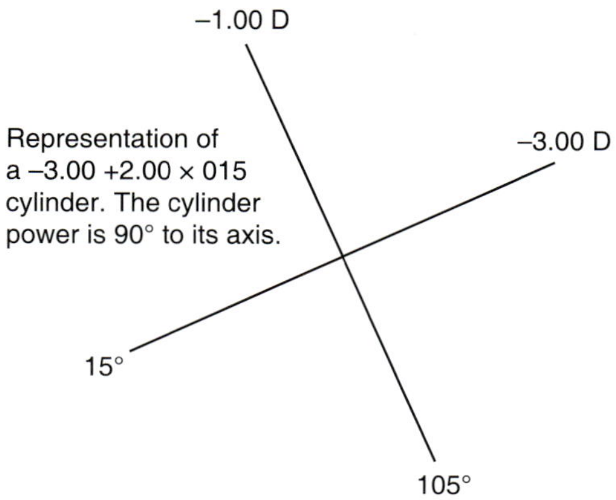

Figure 1-31 Power-cross representation of a –3.00 +2.00 × 015 cylinder. Again, the power of a cylinder is 90o to its axis. *(Courtesy of Edmond H. Thall, MD.)*

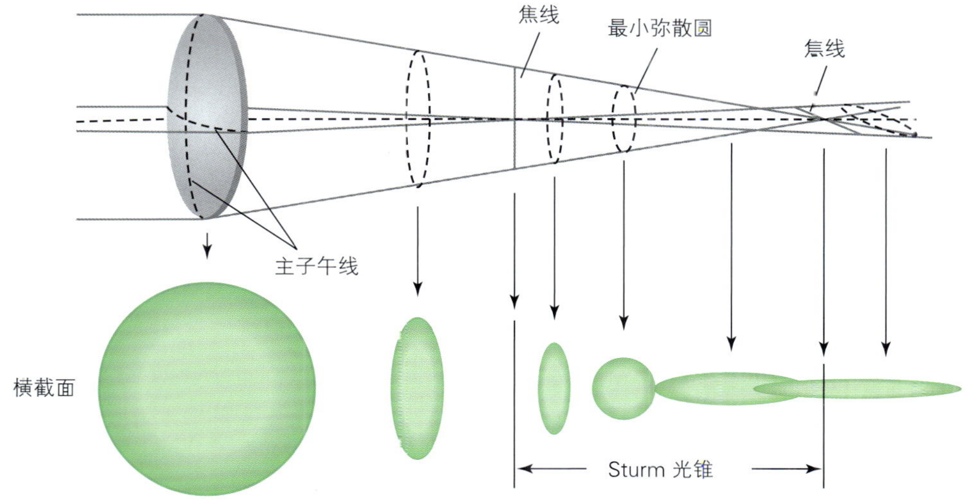

图 1–29　Strum 光锥，离发散光镜后的光线形成的一种几何图形。最小弥散圆是 Sturm 光锥在 2 个焦线的 1/2 处（度数上的，不是距离上的）的圆形截面。*（译者注：资料来源见前页原文。）*

屈光力十字

任何球面、复曲面（球柱面）或者单纯的柱面透镜都可以用*屈光力十字*来表示。球面透镜在每个子午线上都有同样的屈光力。复曲面镜片在每一个子午线上，屈光力不同，并且屈光力是在最小到最大之间变化的。最大和最小的屈光力轴向总是呈 90°。所以，屈光力十字用来表示最大和最小屈光力，以及它们的子午线。

一个单纯的柱镜，在其轴向上没有屈光力，却存在垂直于其轴的屈光力最高或最低。这个规则就是“柱镜的屈光力总是垂直于它的轴”。例如，+2.00×015 的柱镜，在 15° 子午线上屈光力为零，105° 子午线上屈光力是 +2.00D（图 1–30）。

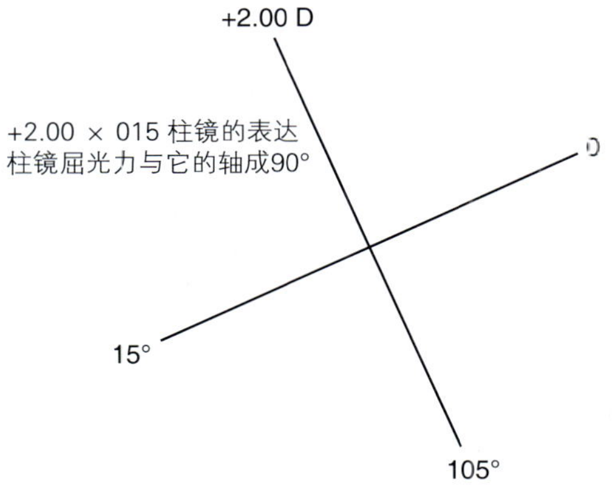

图 1–30　+2.00×015 柱镜的屈光力十字表示。柱镜的屈光力垂直于其轴向。*（译者注：资料来源见前页原文。）*

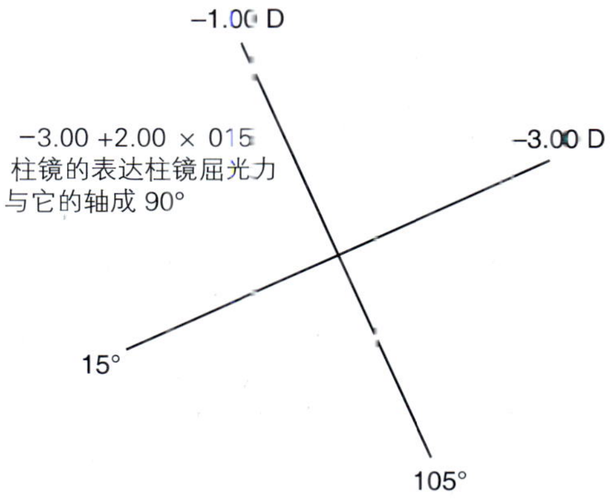

图 1–31　–3.00 / +2.00×015 柱镜的十字表示。柱镜的屈光力垂直于其轴向。*（译者注：资料来源见前页原文。）*

As discussed in the Quick-Start Guide, a -3.00 +2.00 × 015 toric lens has a -1.00D power in the 105° meridian and -3.00D in the 15° meridian (Figure 1-31). Using spherocylinder notation, we can always represent the same toric lens in 2 ways—a plus cylinder form and a minus cylinder form—which can lead to confusion. To convert from one form to the other ("transposition" of the spherocylindrical specification):

- The new sphere is the algebraic sum of the old sphere and cylinder.
- The new cylinder has the same value as the old cylinder but with opposite sign.
- The axis needs to be changed by 90°.

One advantage of the power cross is that any toric lens has only 1 power-cross representation.

However, we can use a power cross to combine spherocylinders only when their power-cross meridians are identical. For instance, what is the result of combining a +2.00 +1.00 × 080 lens with a +3.00 -2.00 × 080 lens? Using a power cross to represent each lens, we can simply add the powers in the corresponding meridians (Figure 1-32).

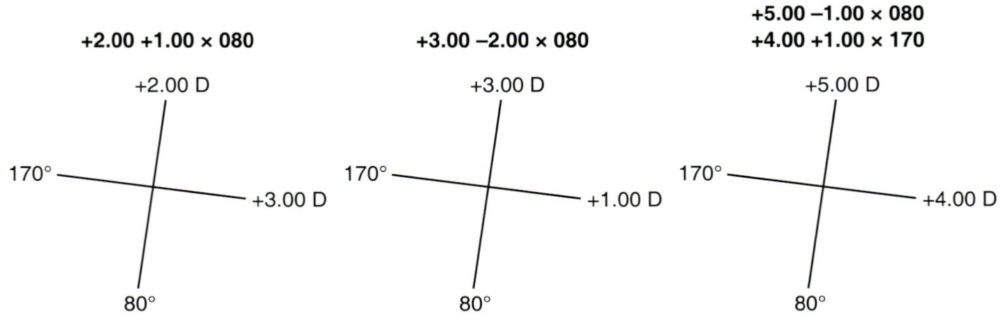

Figure 1-32 Combination of spherocylinders with identical meridians. *(Courtesy of Edmond H. Thall, MD.)*

EXAMPLE 1-12

Use the power-cross representation of astigmatic lenses to show how an astigmatic refractive error can be corrected with a cylinder lens of the same power as the astigmatic error, placed 90° away from the lens representing the astigmatic error, and combined with a spherical lens of the opposite sign.

Suppose the "excess" power in the eye is equivalent to a cylindrical +1.00 × 180 lens. the power-cross representation of this lens is 0.0 @ 180°, +1.00 @ 90°. placing a lens with power-cross representation of +1.00 @ 180°, 0.0 @ 90° in front of this eye yields a net excess power of +1.00 @ 180°, +1.00 @ 90°, equivalent to a spherical lens of power +1.00D. We can correct this net spherical error by using an additional spherical lens of power -1.00D, for a net correcting lens of -1.00 + 1.00 × 90, because the power of a correcting cylinder is 90° away from the axis of that correcting cylinder.

正如在《快速入门指南》中讨论的，–3.00 + 2.00 × 015 的复曲面透镜，在 105° 子午线上的屈光力是 –1.00D，在 15° 子午线上的屈光力是 –3.00D（图 1 – 31）。使用球柱镜表示法，可以用 2 种方式表示相同的复曲面透镜——一种是正柱镜形式，另一种是负柱镜形式，这可能会导致混淆。从一种形式转换为另一种形式的方法如下（球柱镜转换规则）：

- 新的球镜度是旧的球镜度和柱镜度的代数和。
- 新的柱镜度和旧的柱镜的值相同，符号相反。
- 轴向改变 90° 。

屈光力十字的优点在于，任何复曲面镜都只有一种屈光力十字的表示方法。

然而，只有当球柱镜的屈光力十字的子午线相同时，我们才能使用屈光力十字联合球柱镜。例如，1 个 +2.00 +1.00 × 080 和 1 个 +3.00 –2.00 × 080 的镜片组合后的屈光力结果是多少？我们可以用光学十字法分别表示出每一个镜片度数，然后简单地将每个镜片相对应轴向上的屈光力值相加即可（图 1–32）。

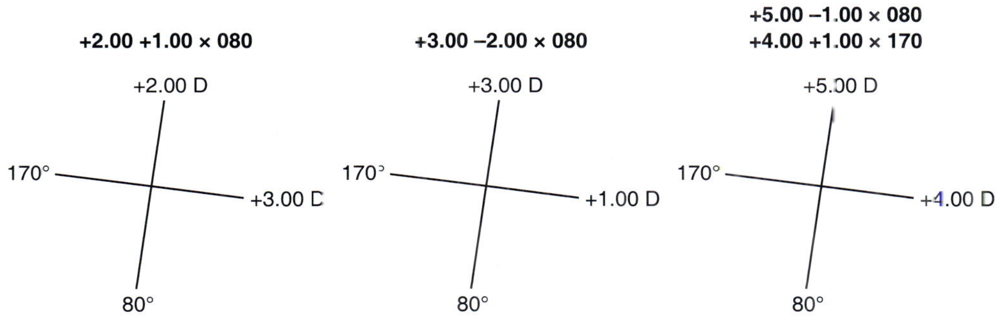

图 1–32　相同子午线的球柱镜的联合。*（译者注：资料来源于前页原文。）*

例 1–12

为了说明如何用柱镜矫正一个相同度数的散光，我们使用屈光力十字表示一个散光镜片，并在距镜片 90° 放置一个镜片来代表散光度，然后叠加一个相反度数的球镜。

假设眼睛附加的屈光力相当于一个 +1.00× 180 的柱镜，这个柱镜的屈光力十字是 0.0 @ 180° ，+1.00 @ 90° 。在眼前面放置一个屈光力十字为 +1.00D@180° ，0.0 @ 90° 的镜片，产生额外的 +1.00 @ 180° ，+1.00 @ 90° 的净屈光力，就相当于 +1.00D 的球镜度。我们可以用一个附加的 –1.00D 的球镜来净矫正 –1.00 + 1.00 × 90，因为矫正的柱镜和矫正的轴向呈 90° 。

Section Exercises 1-23~1-26

Practice transposition of astigmatic lenses—ie, convert between the plus cylinder and minus cylinder. For example:

+1.00 +2.00 × 80 = +3.00 -2.00 × 170

1-23 +1.00 -2.00 × 80
-1.00 +2.00 × 170

1-24 -2.00 -3.00 × 10
-5.00 +3.00 × 100

1-25 -2.00 +1.00 × 10
-1.00 -1.00 × 100

1-26 -1.00 -0.75 × 180
-1.75 +0.75 × 90

Power-Versus-Meridian Graph

The (paraxial) power of a spherocylinder varies in every meridian according to the equation

$$P_\theta = P_S + P_C \sin^2(\theta - \phi)$$

Here P_θ is the power in the meridian at angle θ from the horizontal (measured counterclockwise, as seen facing the patient), P_S is the power of the spherical component of the spherocylinder, P_C is the power of the cylindrical component, and ϕ is the cylinder axis.

For instance, a +3.00 D cylinder with an axis at 020 has a power in the 050 meridian given by

$$P_{050} = +3.00\text{ D}\,[\sin^2(50 - 20)] = +0.75\text{ D}$$

A power-versus-meridian graph (PVMG) represents the power in every meridian (Figure 1-33). Like a power cross, a toric lens has only 1 PVMG. Whether specified in plus cylinder or minus cylinder form, the PVMG is the same. However, the PVMG is a more complete representation of a spherocylinder—unlike a power cross, which shows power in only 2 meridians, a PVMG shows power in all meridians. We can use the PVMG to represent the combination of spherocylinders at any axes in a single representation without the need for a separate calculation for cylinders and spheres. We can algebraically add the $\sin^2$ formulas for meridional power of 2 thin spherocylindrical lenses in contact and simplify according to the usual rules for trigonometric functions, regardless of whether the cylinder axes coincide.

阶段练习 1–23~1–26

练习散光透镜的转换——例如正柱镜和负柱镜的转换。例如：

+1.00 +2.00 × 80 = +3.00–2.00 × 170

1–23　+1.00–2.00 × 80
　　　–1.00 +2.00 × 170
1–24　–2.00 –3.00 × 10
　　　–5.00 +3.00 × 100
1–25　–2.00 +1.00 × 10
　　　–1.00 –1.00 × 100
1–26　–1.00 –0.75 × 180
　　　–1.75 +0.75 × 90

屈光力 – 子午线图

根据方程，球柱镜（近轴）屈光力在每个子午线都会发生改变：

$$P_\theta = P_S + P_C \sin^2(\theta - \phi)$$

这里 P_θ 是从水平线到 θ 角的子午线屈光力（面对患者，逆时针方向测量），P_S 是球柱镜中的球镜成分，P_C 是柱镜成分，ϕ 是柱镜轴。

例如，+3.00D 柱镜轴向 20° 在 50° 子午线的屈光力为

$$P_{050} = +3.00\text{D} [\sin^2(50 - 20)] = +0.75\ \text{D}$$

屈光力 – 子午线图（PVMG）表示了每个子午线方向的屈光力（图 1–33）。与屈光力十字一样，复曲面镜只有 1 个屈光力 – 子午线图。不论正柱镜或负柱镜，屈光力 – 子午线图是相同的。然而，屈光力 – 子午线图是球柱镜更完整的表述，但与只显示 2 个屈光力子午线的屈光力十字不同，屈光力 – 子午线图显示所有方向的屈光力子午线。我们可用 PVMG 代表任意轴向的球柱镜和，不需要单独计算球镜和柱镜。无论柱镜轴重合与否，根据三角函数的一般规则化简，我们都可以用代数方法加入 2 个薄球柱镜子午屈光力的 $\sin^2$ 公式。

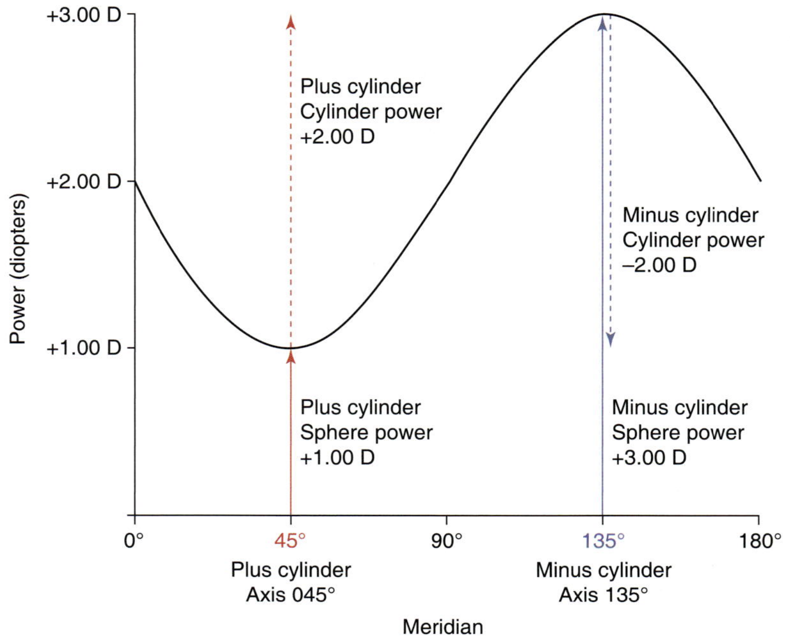

Figure 1-33 Power-versus-meridian graph (PVMG) of a toric lens. There is only 1 PVMG for any toric lens. To read the spherocylinder power in plus cylinder form (red arrows), look at the trough (lowest point on the graph). The (vertical) distance between the trough and the horizontal axis is the sphere power P_S; the cylinder axis is the meridian of the trough. The (positive) cylinder power is the distance from the trough to the peak (highest point on the graph). For minus cylinder form, the distance of the peak from the horizontal is the sphere power P_S; the cylinder axis is the meridian of the peak. The (negative) cylinder power is the distance from the peak to the trough. *(Courtesy of Edmond H. Thall, MD.)*

Jackson Cross Cylinder

A *Jackson cross cylinder (JCC)* is a spherocylindrical lens with equal but opposite powers in the perpendicular principal meridians. The JCC is conveniently mounted with a handle oriented between the principal meridians in such a way that twirling the handle quickly exchanges the 2 meridians. (See the Quick-Start Guide.) Exercise 1-27 is an example of a JCC. A JCC may be of any power and always has the SE of zero. Thus, a JCC is any spherocylindrical lens with the SE of zero. We can fabricate such a lens by grinding a cylinder on 1 surface, paired with a sphere of half the power and opposite sign of the cylinder on the opposite surface.

Section Exercises 1-27–1-30

Calculate some spherical equivalents.

1-27 Refraction: –1.00 +2.00 × 180
SE: (–1.00D) + (2.00D/2) = 0
This example has the SE of zero and thus is equivalent to a cross cylinder lens.

1-28 Refraction: –1.00 +4.00 × 180
SE: (–1.00D) + (4.00D/2) = +1.00D

1-29 Refraction: –1.00 +2.00 × 90

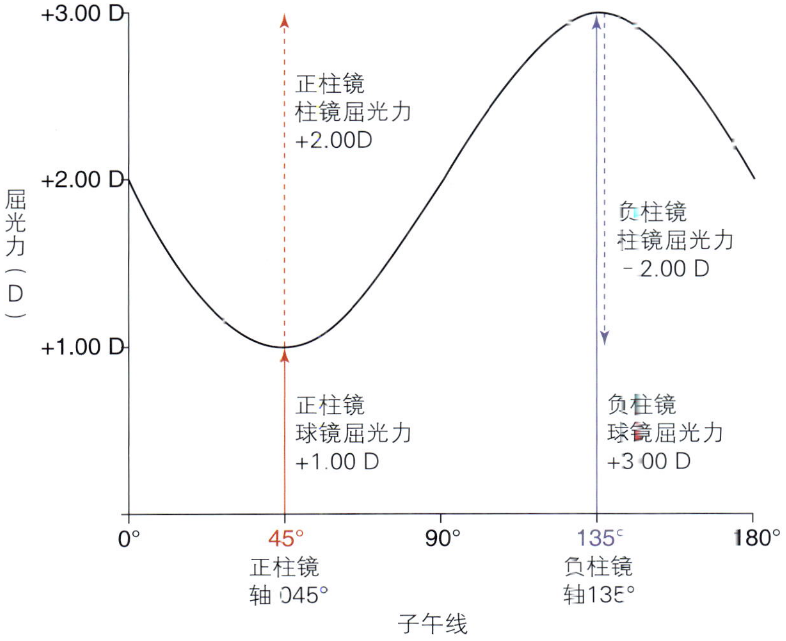

图 1-33 复曲面镜的屈光力 - 子午线图（PVMG）。只需一幅图可表示任意复曲面镜。图示以正柱镜形式的球柱镜屈光力（红色箭头），在波谷处（图的最低点）。波谷与横轴（垂直）距离为球镜度 P_S，柱镜轴是波谷子午线，（正的）柱镜是波谷到波峰（图的最高点）的距离。对于负柱镜形式，波峰到横轴的距离为球镜 P_S，柱镜是波峰子午线，（负的）柱镜是波峰到波谷的距离。*（译者注：资料来源见前页原文。）*

Jackson 交叉柱镜

Jackson 交叉柱镜（*JCC*）是一种有 2 条互相垂直且度数相等但符号相反的主子午线的球柱透镜。JCC 手柄置于主子午线之间，便于迅速翻转、交换两主子午线的相互位置（参见《快速入门指南》）。练习 1-27 举例说明 JCC。因此，JCC 可以是任意等效球为 0 的球柱镜。我们可以在一个平面上磨制柱镜，在另一个平面上磨制 1/2 球镜度数但符号相反的柱镜。

阶段练习 1-27~1-30

计算等效球镜：

1-27 验光：-1.00 +2.00 × 180
　　等效球镜：（-1.00D）+（2.00D/2）= 0
　　本例等效球镜为 0，因此是一个交叉柱镜。

1-28 验光：-1.00 +4.00 × 180
　　等效球镜：（-1.00D）+（4.00D/2）= +1.00D

1-29 验光：-1.00 +2.00 × 90

SE: (–1.00D) + (–2.00D/2) = –2.00D
1-30 Refraction: –5.00 –6.00 × 90
SE: (–5.00D) + –6.00D/2) = –8.00D

Mirrors

The effect of smooth mirrors on the paths of light rays is governed by the *law of reflection*. Sometimes referred to as the law of specular reflection, this law states that the *angle of reflection*, between the reflected ray and the surface normal (line perpendicular to the reflecting surface) at the point of reflection, equals the *angle of incidence*, between the incident ray and the surface normal.

Plane mirrors simply reverse the direction of propagation of light, without altering vergence. This effect is often described as a "reversal of the image space." Curved mirrors, in addition to reversing the image space, also add or subtract vergence. For paraxial rays, we can draw a simple geometric construction, akin to the derivation of the vergence equation and the lensmaker's equation, to demonstrate a similar vergence equation for mirrors (Appendix 1.3). We use the following conventions:

$$P = \frac{-2}{r}$$

$$\frac{1}{u} + P = \frac{1}{\text{“v”}}$$

Here

- we assume the incident light travels from left to right in the usual way;
- r is the (signed!) radius of curvature of the mirror, with the usual sign conventions(a mirror concave to the left has a *negative* number as its radius, so the power P of such a mirror is a *positive* number; a mirror convex to the left has a positive number as its radius, so the power P is a negative number);
- "v" is the distance from the mirror to the image in the reversed image space—rays converging from right to left are considered to have *positive* vergence; rays diverging from right to left are considered to have *negative* vergence. We use quotation marks around the letter "v" to remind you of the change in sign convention necessary when you use the vergence equation for mirrors rather than for lenses.

Notice that the refractive index does *not* appear in these equations—the law of reflection does not include a correction for refractive index.

So, for example, parallel rays moving from left to right, striking a mirror concave to the left, emerge traveling right to left with positive vergence. They converge on the focal point of the mirror at half the radius of the mirror, to the left of the mirror. Conversely, parallel rays moving from left to right that strike a mirror convex to the left emerge diverging from right to left, with an apparent focus (a virtual image) at distance $r/2$ to the right of the mirror.

It is often useful to clarify these unusual sign conventions by ray tracing. For mirrors, we recognize 3 special rays: (1) the ray through the center of curvature of the mirror (not the vertex on the optic axis, as for lenses) is the undeviated ray; (2) the ray that strikes the vertex is reflected at an angle equal to the angle of incidence; and (3) the ray that propagates parallel to the optic axis passes through the focal point of the mirror, which is halfway between the mirror surface and the center of curvature.

等效球镜：（$-1.00D$）+（$-2.00D/2$）$=-2.00D$
1-30　验光：$-5.00\ -6.00\times 90$
等效球镜：（$-5.00D$）$+-6.00D/2$）$=-8.00D$

面镜

光滑的镜面对光线路径的影响是由反射定律决定的。有时称为镜面*反射定律*，它指出反射点处的反射光线与法线（垂直于反射面）的*反射角*等于入射光线与法线之间的*入射角*。

平面镜仅简单地逆转光的传播方向，不改变聚散度。这种结果通常被描述为“像空间的反转”。曲面镜除了反转图像空间外，还会增加或减少聚散度。对于近轴光线，我们可以画简单的几何图，类似于聚散度方程和透镜制作商方程的推导，来阐释一个相似的镜面聚散度方程（附录 1.3）。我们使用以下约定：

$$P=\frac{-2}{r}$$

$$\frac{1}{u}+P=\frac{1}{\text{“}v\text{”}}$$

这里，

- 我们假定入射光线从左向右传播；
- r（有正负号！）是镜面的曲率半径，遵守符号规则（左边凹面镜的半径为*负*，所以镜面屈光力 P 为*正*；左边凸面镜的半径为*正*，所以镜面屈光力 P 为*负*）；
- “v”是倒像空间的镜像距离——光线从右向左会聚为*正*聚散，光线从右向左发散为*负*聚散。我们用引号括起字母“v”是提醒注意，当使用镜面而非透镜聚散度方程时需要遵守符号规则。

注意，屈光介质没有出现在方程中——反射定律不包括屈光介质矫正。

例如平行光线从左向右传播，与左边是凹面的镜面相交，光线传播从右向左发生会聚。光线的会聚焦点在镜面左侧 1/2 半径处。相反，平行光线从左向右传播，与左侧是凸面的镜面相交，使光线传播从右向左发生发散，虚焦点（虚像）在镜面右侧 1/2 r 处。

用光线传播来阐明这些特殊的符号规则是很有用的。对于镜面，我们需要认识 3 种特殊光线：①通过镜面曲率中心的光线（不同于透镜光轴的顶点）是不偏向光线；②光线在顶点处反射角与入射角相等；③光线沿光轴平行传播通过镜面的焦点，焦点位于镜面和曲率中心的 1/2 处。

Only a couple of examples occur commonly in practice: a large-radius concave mirror, such as those used as cosmetic or shaving mirrors, with source object closer than the focal point, and a small-radius convex mirror, such as those used in rear-view mirrors on automobiles (Figure 1-34). The cornea is used as a small-radius reflecting surface to measure the corneal curvature (keratometry).

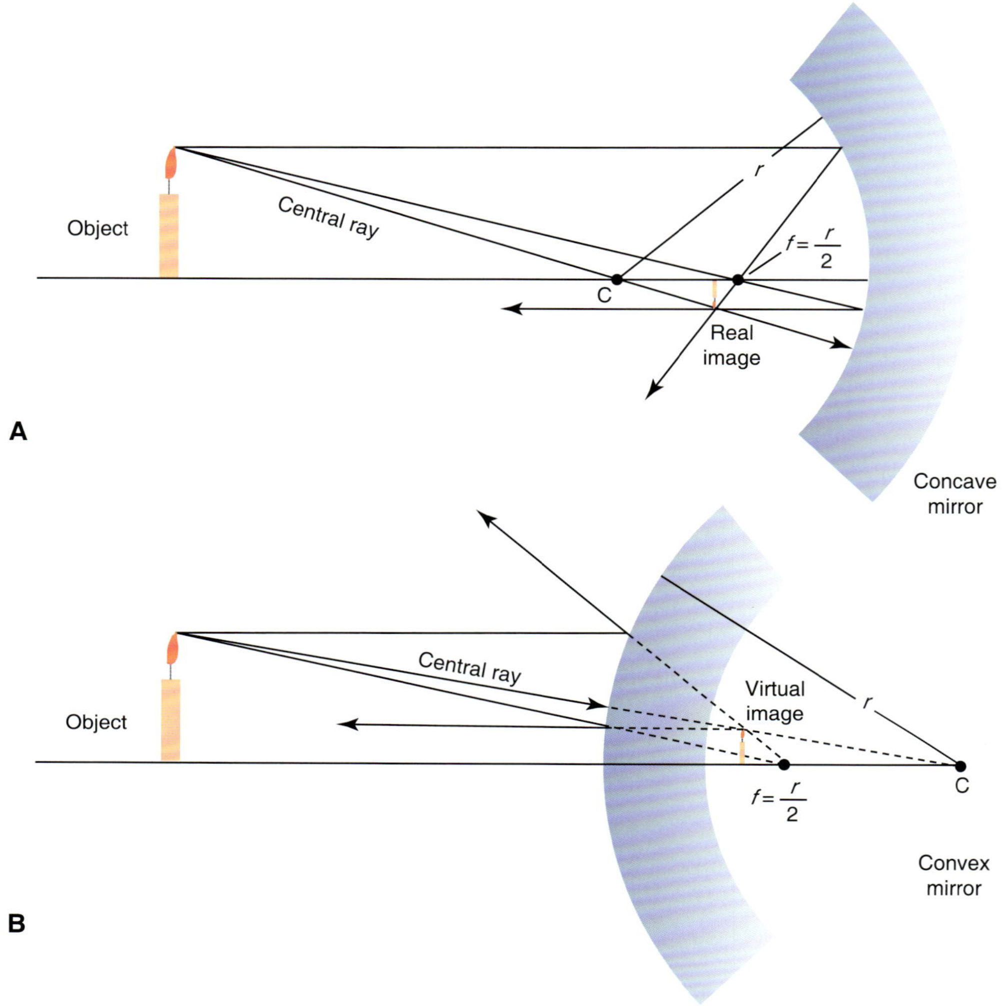

Figure 1-34 Ray tracing for concave (**A**) and convex (**B**) mirrors. The central ray for mirrors is different from the central ray for lenses in that it passes through the center of curvature ("C") of the mirror, not through the center of the mirror. *(Illustration developed by Kevin M. Miller, MD, and rendered by C. H. Wooley.)*

实际应用：大曲率半径的凹面镜，如化妆镜或剃须镜，发光物体比焦点近；小曲率半径的凸面镜，如汽车后视镜（图 1-34）。角膜是一种小曲率半径的反射面，可用来测量曲率半径（角膜曲率计）。

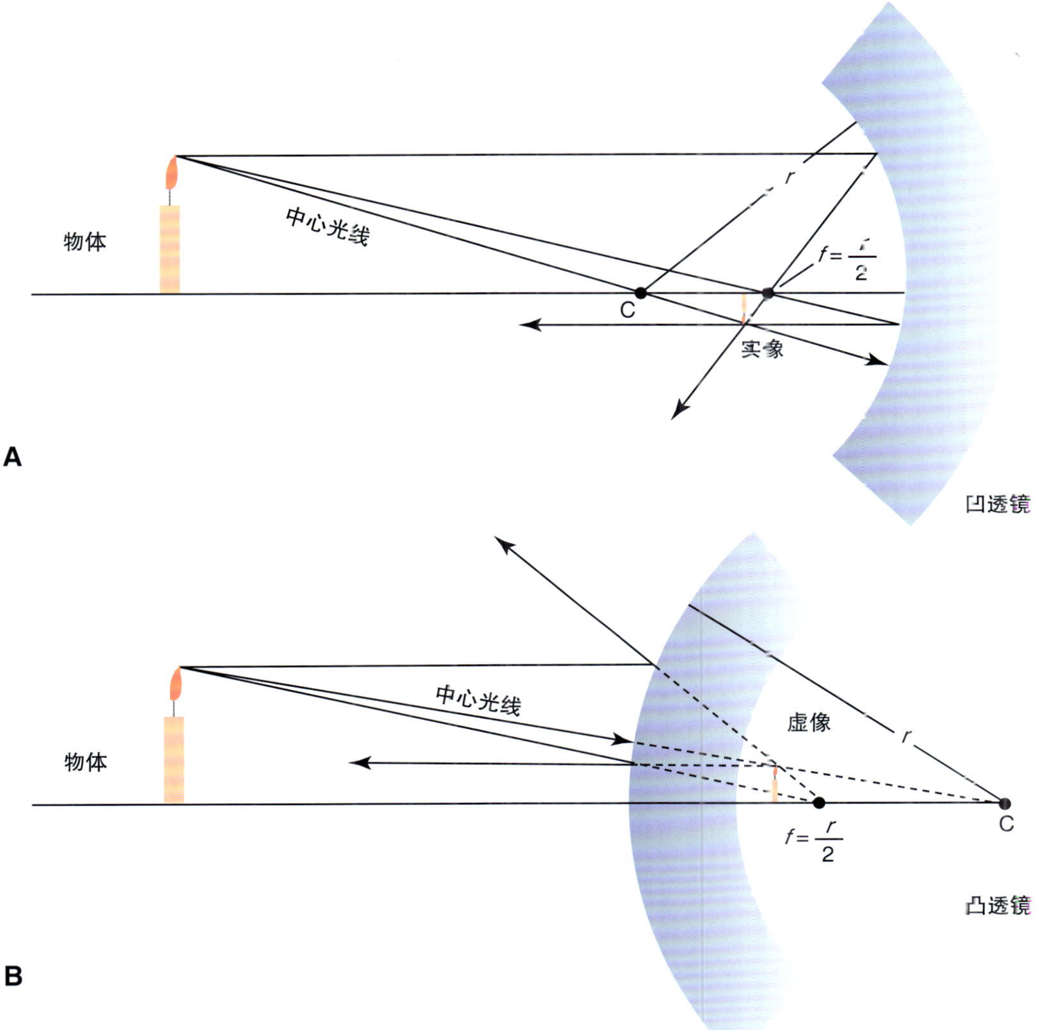

图 1-34 光线在凹面镜（**A**）和凸面镜（**B**）的追踪。镜面的中央光线不同于透镜的中央光线，它通过镜面曲率半径中央（“C”），而不通过镜面中央。*（译者注：资料来源见前页原文。）*

EXAMPLE 1-13

Show the ray tracing for a shaving mirror, and compute the image location and magnification.

For a concave mirror to work as a magnifier, suitable as a shaving or cosmetic mirror, the source object (such as your face) must be closer to the mirror than the focal point. Suppose the radius of the mirror is, say, -2.0 m; then the focal point is 1.0 m to the left of the mirror. The power of the mirror is -2/-2.0 m = +1.0D. If the source object is at u = -0.5 m, the vergence equation gives 1/"v " = 1/-0.5 D + 1.0D and "v" = -1.00 m, so the image is located 1 m away from the mirror. The minus sign implies that the image is 1 m to the right of the mirror, as the image space is "reversed" (Figure 1-E13). Thus, the image is twice as far "behind" the mirror as the source was in front of the mirror, and similar triangles yield a magnification factor of +2.0.

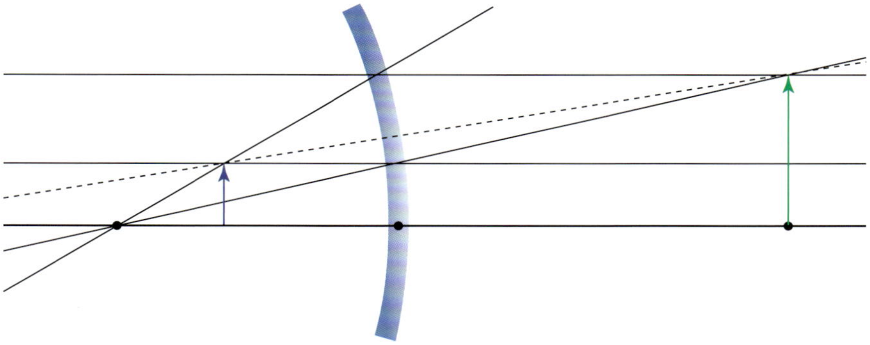

Figure 1-E13 Ray tracing for a concave shaving mirror.

Section Exercises 1-31

Show the ray tracing for the image of a "muscle light" as reflected in the human cornea, as in the Hirschberg test for the measurement of strabismus (see BCSC Section 6, *Pediatric Ophthalmology and Strabismus*). This diagram is depicted in Figure 1-34B.

Telescopes

Galilean, or terrestrial, *telescopes* consist of a lower-power positive lens (the objective) and a higher-power minus lens (the ocular, or eyepiece) separated by the difference in their focal lengths. *Keplerian*, or astronomical, *telescopes* consist of a lower-power positive objective lens and a higher-power positive eyepiece separated by the sum of their focal lengths (Figure 1-35). (Technically, the separation of the lenses is $f_1 - f_2$ for both types of telescopes because f_2 is negative for the Keplerian telescope.) We can easily construct both types by using trial lenses. The Galilean telescope produces an upright image; the Keplerian, an inverted image. However, by placing prisms inside the Keplerian telescope, we can achieve an upright image. Most binoculars are Keplerian telescopes with inverting prisms.

In both types of telescope, an object ray parallel to the optic axis is conjugate to an image ray parallel to the axis. Consequently, the system considered as a whole has no focal points, and hence it is termed an afocal system. Also, considered as a whole, telescopes have no principal planes and no nodal points.

例 1–13

说明剃须镜的光线追踪，并且计算像的位置和放大率。

凹面镜作为放大镜使用，如剃须镜或化妆镜，点光源（例如你的脸）必须比焦点更靠近镜子。假设镜子的半径为 −2.0m，焦点在镜子左侧 1.0m 处。镜子的屈光力为 −2/−2.0m=+1.00D。如果发光物体在 u=−0.5m 处，根据聚散度方程 1/“v”=1/−0.50D+1.00D 和“v”=−1.00m，因此，像位于镜子 1m 处。负号提示，像在镜子右侧 1m 处，因为像空间“反转”了（图 1–E13）。相对于镜子前面的物体，像在镜子“后面”2 倍距离远的地方，相似三角形导出放大倍数为 +2.00D。

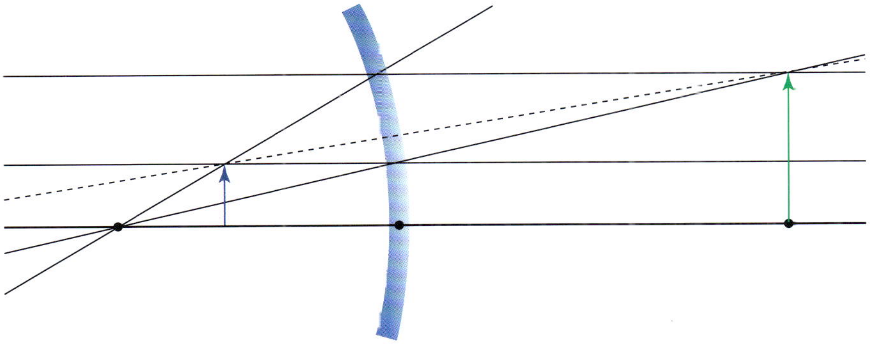

图 1–E13　凹面镜的剃须镜光线追踪图。

阶段练习 1–31

1–31　显示反射在人类角膜上的“肌光”像的光线踪迹，就像在测量斜视的 Hirschberg 检查（参看 BCSC 第 6 册《*小儿眼科与斜视*》）。图解描述参看图 1–34B。

望远镜

Galileo 望远镜，又称陆地*望远镜*是由一个低焦度正透镜（物镜）和一个高焦度负透镜（目镜）组成，并通过不同焦距分隔。kepler 望远镜，又称天文*望远镜*，是由一个低焦度正透物镜和一个高焦度正透目镜组成，并通过它们的焦距之和分隔（图 1–35）。（严格来讲，2 种望远镜的透镜分隔都是 f_1-f_2，因为 kepler 望远镜的 f_2 是负的。）我们可以用试验透镜制作这 2 种望远镜。Galileo 望远镜是正立的像，kepler 望远镜是倒立的像。然而，在 kepler 望远镜内放置棱镜可以将像正立。多数双目镜为放置反向棱镜的 kepler 望远镜。

2 种望远镜中，物体光线平行进入光轴形成与光轴平行的共轭的像。整体上，系统没有焦点，为无焦点系统，也没有主平面和主节点。

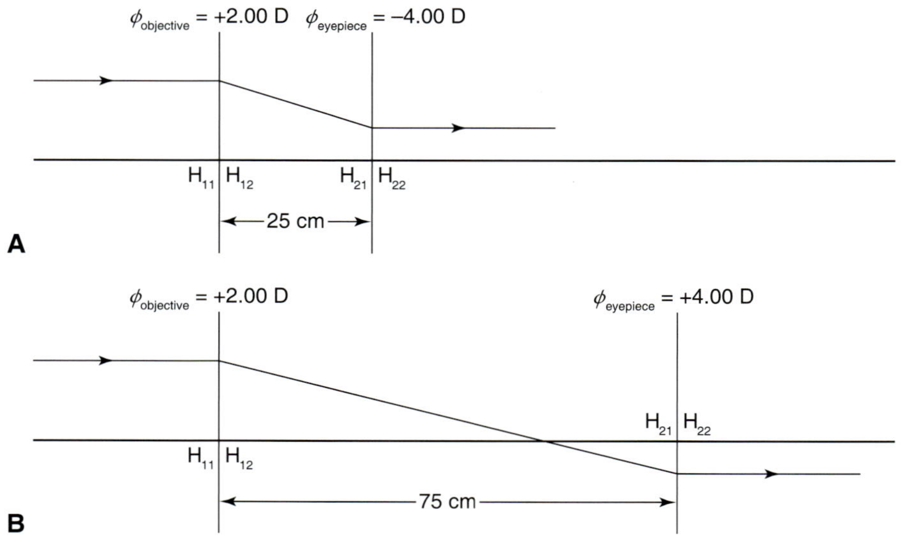

Figure 1-35 Ray tracing for 2 types of telescopes. **A**, A Galilean telescope consists of the objective (a lower-power plus lens) and the eyepiece, or ocular (a higher-power minus lens), separated by the difference of their focal lengths. **B**, A Keplerian telescope consists of a lowpower plus lens (objective) and a higher-power plus lens (eyepiece). In both cases, an object ray parallel to the axis is conjugate to an image ray parallel to the axis. Consequently, although the individual lenses have focal points, the system as a whole does not. *(Courtesy of Edmond H. Thall, MD.)*

Both types of telescope produce images smaller than the original object: $M_T = -P_1/P_2$. In the examples shown in Figure 1-36, the image is half the size of the object (note the distance between the horizontal entering ray and the horizontal exiting ray). However, the image appears larger because it is much closer to the eye. In those examples, the image appears 4 times closer than the original object. Because the image is half the size of the original object but 4 times closer, the angle the image subtends and the appearance of the image are twice as large as the original object.

In general, we use telescopes to view objects at very great ("astronomical") distances, for which transverse magnification is of little interest. It is more useful to describe the magnification in such a system in terms of the ratio of the angular separation between source objects as seen without the telescope and the angular separation between their images as seen through the telescope. We can show with careful ray tracing that this ratio, the *angular magnification*, is given by

$$M_a = \frac{-P_{eyepiece}}{P_{objective}}$$

Telescopes are often prescribed as visual aids for visually impaired patients (see Chapter 9). The Galilean telescope is generally preferred for visual aids because it is shorter than the Keplerian and produces an upright image. The Keplerian telescope can produce an upright image only by incorporating inverting prisms, which increase the weight of the visual aid. However, Keplerian telescopes gather more light than Galilean telescopes do—a quality that is advantageous in some situations.

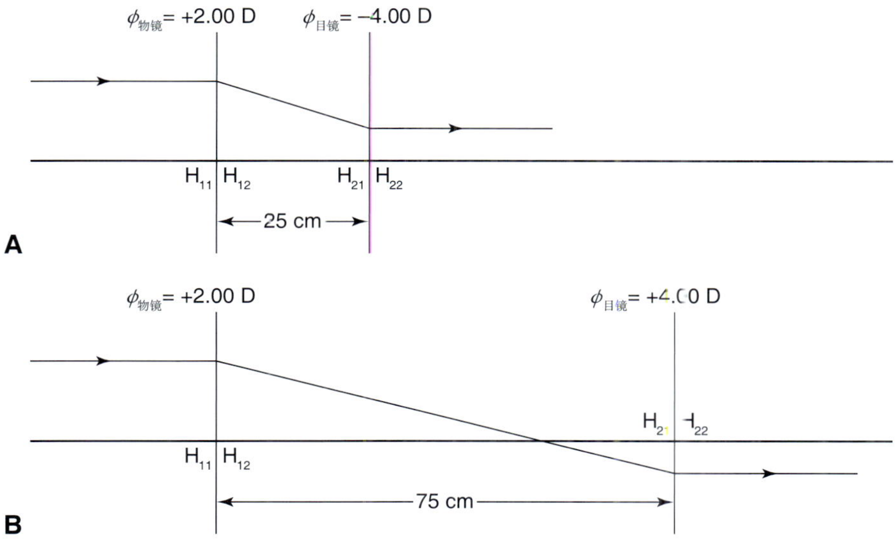

图 1–35　2 种望远镜的光线追踪。**A** Galileo 望远镜由物镜（低焦度正透镜）和目镜（高焦度负透镜）组成，由不同焦距分隔。**B**. kepler 望远镜由目镜（低焦度正透镜）和目镜（高焦度负透镜）组成。2 种透镜中，物体光线平行进入光轴形成与光轴平行的共轭的像。因此，尽管每个透镜有焦点，整体系统是无焦点的。*（译者注：资料来源见前页原文。）*

2 种望远镜成像都小于原物体：$M_T = -P_1/P_2$。在图 1–36 示例中，像是物体的 1/2（注意水平入射光线和水平出射光线之间的距离）。然而，由于像非常靠近眼部，因此被放大了。在这些例子中，像比物近 4 倍。由于像的大小是物的 1/2，但距离近 4 倍，所以，像的夹角和像的大小是原物体的 2 倍。

总之，我们使用望远镜观察非常远的物体（天文上的），这样的横向放大率可以忽略。用角间距描述系统放大率，即不用望远镜看到的发光物体的角间距和用望远镜看到的像的角间距的比率。我们可以采用光线追踪推出这个比率，*角放大率*即

$$M_a = \frac{-P_{目镜}}{P_{物镜}}$$

望远镜经常作为视觉损害患者的助视器（参见第九章）。Galileo 望远镜更常作为助视器，因为它较 kepler 望远镜短且成正像。kepler 望远镜只有联合反转棱镜才成正像，这会增加助视器的重量。但是，kepler 望远镜聚光优于 Galileo 望远镜——这在某些情况下具有优势。

Appendix 1.1

Derivation of the Vergence Equation and the Lensmaker's Equation from Snell's Law

Consider Figure 1-A1. A light ray traveling from left to right (shown in dark green) is incident on a curved refracting surface with radius of curvature r and center of curvature C on the optic axis OC. Suppose the index of refraction to the left of the surface is n_1, to the right of the surface, n_2, (shown with $n_2 > n_1$). The incident ray strikes the axis at distance u from the vertex, O, of the refracting surface and meets the surface at a height h from the axis, making an angle, α, with the optic axis. The incident ray makes an angle θ with the surface normal and is then refracted such that it makes, say, a smaller angle, σ, with the surface normal to the right of the refracting surface. The refracted ray (shown in light green) meets the axis at a distance v from the vertex, forming an angle β with the axis. The angle subtended by the height h at the center of the circle is denoted by γ.

In the paraxial regime, angles θ, σ, α, β, and γ are small (that is, h is substantially smaller than r). We use the "small-angle approximation" from trigonometry: for small angles ϕ,

$$\phi = \sin \phi = \tan \phi$$

With this approximation, Snell's law, $n_1 \sin \theta = n_2 \sin \sigma$, simplifies to

$$n_1\theta = n_2 \sigma \qquad (1)$$

Similarly, using the tangent approximation for angles α, β, and, γ, and in the same spirit ignoring the discrepancy between the foot of the perpendicular from the point of incidence and O, we have

$$\alpha = \frac{h}{u};\ \beta = \frac{h}{v};\ \gamma = \frac{h}{r} \qquad (2)$$

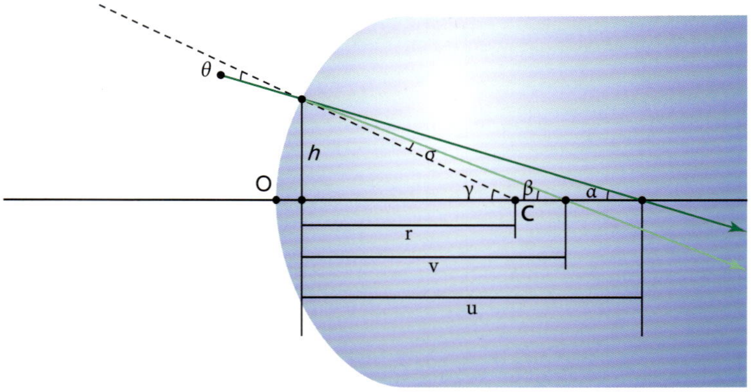

Figure 1-A1 Geometry for deriving the vergence equation and the lensmaker's equation from Snell's law.

Finally, from geometry (the "exterior-angle theorem" and the fact that "opposite" angles are equal), we observe that

$$\gamma = \theta + \alpha \text{ and } \gamma = \beta + \sigma$$

附录 1.1

聚散度方程和透镜制作商方程的推导

思考图 1–A1。从左到右的光线（深绿色示）入射在弯曲的折射面上，曲率半径为 r，由率半径中心为 C，位于光轴 OC 上。假设屈光介质在折射面左侧为 n_1，右侧为 n_2（$n_2 > n_1$）。入射光线在距折射面顶点 O 的 u 处与轴相交，与折射面相交点距离轴高为 h，与轴形成夹角 α。入射光线与曲面法线形成夹角 θ，在右边介质与曲面面法线折射成较小的夹角 σ。折射光线（浅绿色示）在距折射面顶点 v 处与轴相交，形成夹角 β。在 h 处延长至圆心，形成夹角 γ。

在近轴区，θ，σ，α，β 和 γ 是非常小的（即 h 远比 r 小）。我们用三角函数里的“小角度近似值”：对于角 ϕ，

$$\phi = \sin \phi = \tan \phi$$

用这个近似值，Snell 定律有，$n_1 \sin \theta = n_2 \sin \sigma$，近似于

$$n_1 \theta = n_2 \sigma \quad (1)$$

类似的，用角 α、β 和 γ 切线近似值，并且用同样的原理忽略入射点垂直角和 O 的差异，我们有

$$\alpha = \frac{h}{u}; \beta = \frac{h}{v}; \gamma = \frac{h}{r} \quad (2)$$

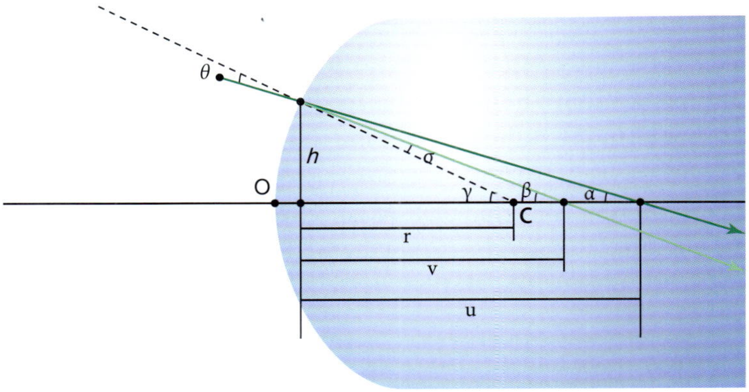

图 1–A1　通过 Snell 定律推导聚散度方程和 Lensmaker 方程的几何图

最终，通过几何（“外角定理”和对角相等），我们发现

$$\gamma = \theta + \alpha \text{ and } \gamma = \beta + \sigma$$

so

$$\theta = \gamma - \alpha \text{ and } \sigma = \gamma - \beta \qquad (3)$$

From here, it is only algebra: substituting Eq. (3) into Eq. (1) gives

$$n_1(\gamma - \alpha) = n_2(\gamma - \beta)$$

so

$$\gamma(n_2 - n_1) = n_2\beta - n_1\alpha \qquad (4)$$

Substituting Eq. (2) into Eq. (4) gives

$$\left(\frac{h}{r}\right)(n_2 - n_1) = n_2\left(\frac{h}{v}\right) - n_1\left(\frac{h}{u}\right)$$

Clearing the common factor h and rearranging yields

$$\frac{n_1}{u} + \frac{(n_2 - n_1)}{r} = \frac{n_2}{v}$$

Equating $(n_2 - n_1)/r$ with P yields both the vergence equation and the lensmaker's equation at once!

Appendix 1.2

Fermat's Principle

The basic rules of geometric optics (straight-line propagation of light in homogeneous media, the law of refraction, and Snell's law) are readily interpreted as a manifestation of Fermat's principle. This interpretation is frequently stated as the observation that the path of a light ray between 2 fixed points is the path that takes the least time. Thus, in a homogeneous medium, where the shortest path between the 2 points obviously corresponds to the path that takes the least time, it follows that light travels in straight lines.

Similarly, a simple geometric construction confirms that, of all reflecting paths connecting 2 points on the same side of a smooth reflecting surface, the path with the angle of incidence equal to the angle of reflection is the shortest. In this sense, the law of refraction is likewise a manifestation of Fermat's principle (Figure 1-A2A).

The proof of Snell's law is only slightly more difficult. Consider Figure 1-A2B. Among the paths shown between points A and B, the shortest (straight-line) path is not the path of least travel time, as we can save time by changing from, say, Path 3 to Path 2 to reduce the portion of the travel time in glass, where the speed of light is slower than that in air.Eventually, the trade-off works the other way, as in Path 1.We can determine the optimal path by calculating the distance in air and in glass for each possible inflection point and dividing by the speed of light in each medium.

所以

$$\theta = \gamma - \alpha \text{ 和 } \sigma = \gamma - \beta \qquad (3)$$

由此，只有一个代数式，替换公式（3）到公式（1），有

$$n_1(\gamma - \alpha) = n_2(\gamma - \beta)$$

所以

$$\gamma(n_2 - n_1) = n_2\beta - n_1\alpha \qquad (4)$$

将公式（2）代入公式（4）有

$$\left(\frac{h}{r}\right)(n_2 - n_1) = n_2\left(\frac{h}{v}\right) - n_1\left(\frac{h}{u}\right)$$

提取公因数 h，整理得

$$\frac{n_1}{u} + \frac{(n_2 - n_1)}{r} = \frac{n_2}{v}$$

将（$n_2 - n_1$）/r 用 P 表示，最终得出聚散度方程和 Lensmaker 方程！

附录 1.2

Fermat 原理

几何光学的基本原理（光在均匀介质中的直线传播、折射定律和 Snell 定律）很容易被解释为 Fermat 原理。这种解释经常被描述为：光线路径在 2 个定点之间时间最短。因此，在均匀介质中，2 点之间的最短路径显然对应于耗时最短的路径，它遵循光沿直线传播。

同样的，一个简单的几何结构证明，在连接光滑反射面的同侧 2 点的所有反射路径中，入射角等于反射角的路径最短。从这个意义上说，折射定律同样是 Fermat 原理的一种表现（图 1–A2A）。

Snell 定律的证明稍有难度。分析图 1–A2B。在点 A 和点 B 之间，最短（直线）的路径不是最短时间路径，我们可通过改变例如从路径 3 变到路径 2，来减少在玻璃中传播的时间，由于光线在玻璃中传播的速度比在空气中慢。最终，这是另一种方式，同路径 1。我们可以通过计算空气到玻璃的距离确定光线路径的折射点，并通过每种介质中的光速将其分开，从而得到最佳路径。

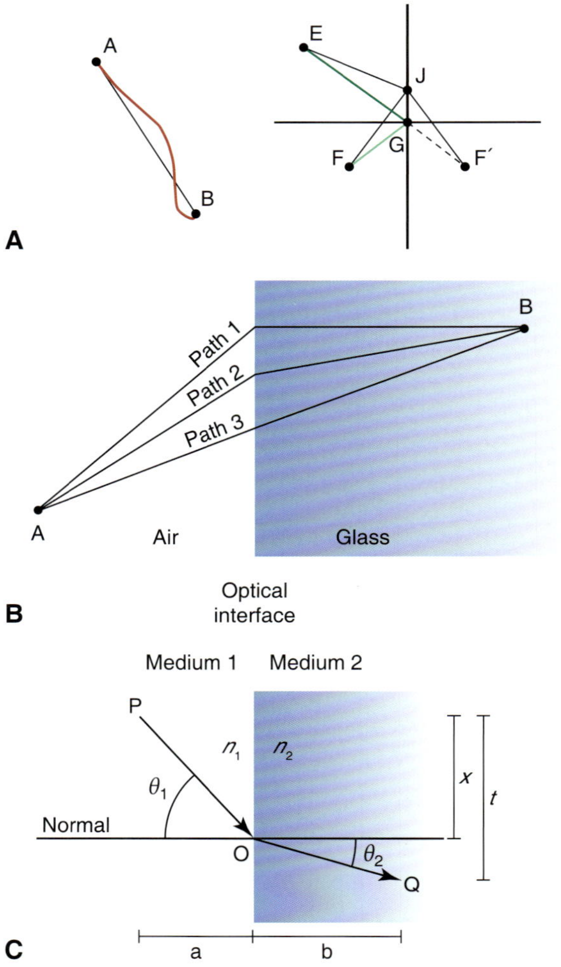

Figure 1-A2 **A**, Left: The straight path between points A and B is the shortest and thus takes the least time among all possible paths from A to B. Right: Light reflecting from point E to point F takes the shortest possible path when the extension of the straight path from E to the mirror reaches the mirror-image point F′ along a straight line. That extension locates the point of reflection at G, such that the angle of incidence equals the angle of refraction. Other possible paths, such as that through point J, are longer and take more time. **B**, Because light travels faster through air than through glass, Path 3 is not the path of shortest travel time. Path 2 saves time overall by spending less time in glass. **C**, Geometry for demonstration of Snell's law from Fermat's principle.

Using the geometry shown in Figure 1-A2C, we denote the distance traveled through a medium 1 and a medium 2 as d_1 and d_2, respectively. Then

$$d_1 = \sqrt{a^2 + x^2} \quad 和 \quad d_2 = \sqrt{b^2 + (l - x)^2}$$

where x is the vertical distance traversed through medium 1 and l is the total vertical distance traversed through both media. We divide by the speed of light in each medium (which is c/n_1 *or* c/n_2, respectively, where c is the speed of light in a vacuum) and add the 2 values to get the total travel time T:

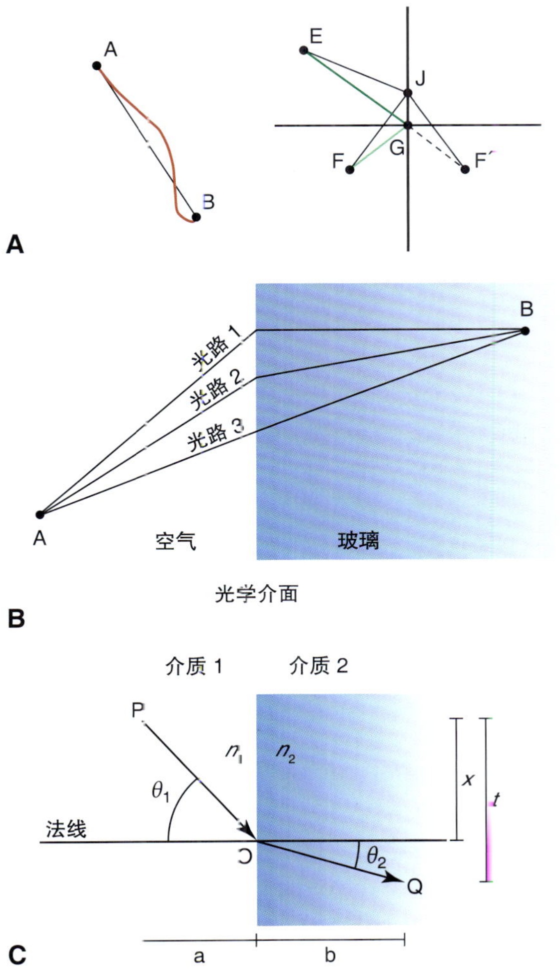

图 1–A2　A. 左图：通过点 A 和 B 的直线最短，因此耗时最短。右图：光线从点 E 折射到点 F 路径最短，从点 E 延长直线通过镜面到像点 F'，延长线交点为 G，入射角等于折射角。其他可能的路径，例如通过点 J，距离和耗时均较长。**B**. 由于光线在空气中传播较在玻璃中传播快，因此路径 3 不是耗时最短的。路径 2 在玻璃中总体耗时较短。**C**. 通过 Fermat 原理得出的 Snell 原理的几何图。

应用图 1–A2C 中的几何图，我们分别用 d_1 和 d_2 表示介质 1 的传播距离和介质 2 的传播距离，然后得出，

$$d_1=\sqrt{a^2+x^2} \text{ 和 } d_2=\sqrt{b^2+(l-x)^2}$$

这里 x 是通过介质 1 的垂直距离，l 是通过 2 种介质的总垂直距离。我们用每种介质的光速区分（分别为 c/n_1 或 c/n_2，是真空中的光速），然后加入 2 个值得到总传播时间 T：

$$T=\sqrt{a^2+x^2}\left(\frac{n_1}{c}\right)+\sqrt{b^2+(l-x)^2}\left(\frac{n_2}{c}\right)$$

To minimize the total transit time, we seek the value of x for which the *derivative* of the transit time, $\mathrm{d}T/\mathrm{d}x$, is equal to 0. Dredging up our knowledge of freshman calculus (and canceling the common factor of c), we obtain

$$\frac{n_1 x}{\sqrt{a^2+x^2}}-\frac{n_2(1-x)}{\sqrt{b^2+(l-x)^2}}=0$$

But careful inspection of Figure 1-A2C indicates that the fractions in this equation are in fact the sines of the angles of incidence and refraction, respectively—that is,

$$n_1 \sin\theta_1 = n_2 \sin\theta_2$$

which is Snell's law.

Appendix 1.3

Derivation of the Vergence Equation for Mirrors

Consider Figure 1-A3. The incident ray (shown in dark green) moves from left to right and would intersect the optic axis at u if the ray did not first intersect the mirror (here drawn convex to the left, with radius of curvature r) at height h above the optic axis. The direction of the reflected ray (shown in light green) is determined by the law of reflection, so the angle $\gamma/2$ between the incident ray and the mirror's surface normal (drawn as a dashed line) equals the angle $\gamma/2$ between the surface normal and the reflected ray. The reflected ray travels from right to left, but if extended, it would intersect the optic axis at v. The angles between the optic axis and the reflected ray, radius of curvature to the point of reflection, and incident ray are denoted α, θ, and β, respectively.

In this case, the direction of the reflected ray is determined by the law of reflection instead of Snell's law. We have:

$$\alpha = \gamma + \beta \qquad (1)$$

$$\alpha = \theta + \gamma/2$$

$$\gamma = 2\alpha - 2\theta \qquad (2)$$

Inserting Eq. (2) into Eq. (1) gives

$$\alpha = 2\alpha - 2\theta + \beta$$

$$T=\sqrt{a^2+x^2}\left(\frac{n_1}{c}\right)+\sqrt{b^2+(l-x)^2}\left(\frac{n_2}{c}\right)$$

为了减少总传播时间，我们要求出传播时间的导数 dT/dx 等于 0 的 x 值。这里会用到我们大学入学时的微积分知识（取消公因数 c），我们得到

$$\frac{n_1 x}{\sqrt{a^2+x^2}}-\frac{n_2(1-x)}{\sqrt{b^2+(l-x)^2}}=0$$

注意观察图 1–A2 中的 C，方程中的分数实际上分别是入射角和折射角的正弦值，即

$$n_1 \sin\theta_1 = n_2 \sin\theta_2$$

这就是 Snell 定律。

附录 1.3

镜面聚散度方程的推导

思考图 1–A3。入射光线（深绿色所示）从左向右传播，如果光线没有先相交于视轴上方 h 点的镜面（此处为凸面向左，曲率半径为 r），则入射光线将与视轴在 u 点相交。反射光线的方向（亮绿色所示）是由反射定律决定，所以入射光和镜面法线（画虚线）之间的 $\gamma/2$ 角等于镜面法线和反射光线之间的 $\gamma/2$ 角。反射光线从右到左传播，但如果延长反射光线，会与光轴相交于 ν。光轴和反射光线的夹角、到反射点的曲率半径和入射光线分别用 α、θ 和 β 表示。

在这种情况下，反射光线的方向由反射定律决定，而不是由 Snell 定律决定。我们有

$$\alpha = \gamma + \beta \quad (1)$$

$$\alpha = \theta + \gamma/2$$

$$\gamma = 2\alpha - 2\theta \quad (2)$$

将（2）代入（1）得出

$$\alpha = 2\alpha - 2\theta + \beta$$

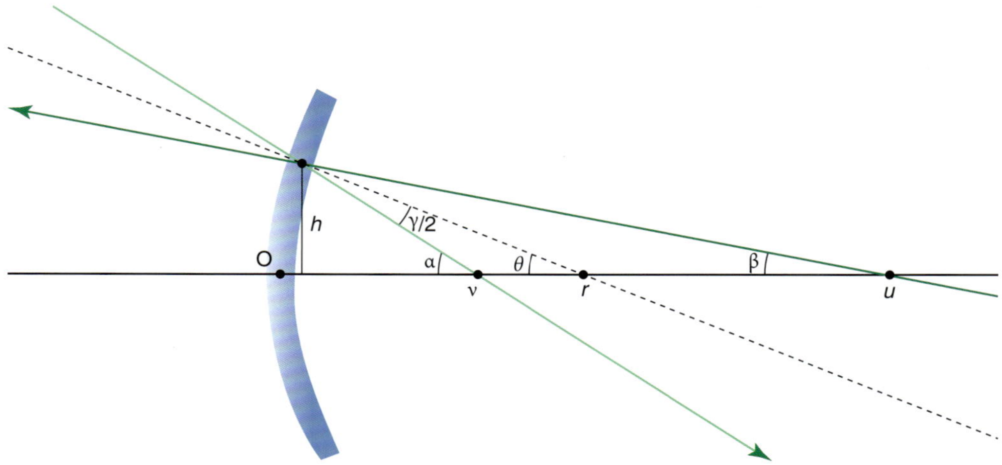

Figure 1-A3 Geometry for deriving the vergence equation for mirrors from the law of reflection. *(Illustration developed by Scott E. Brodie, MD, PhD.)*

so

$$\alpha = 2\theta - \beta$$

Using the small- angle approximations for α, β, and θ (as in Appendix 1.1), we have

$$\frac{h}{v} = 2\frac{h}{r} - \frac{h}{u}$$

Canceling the common factor h and rearranging gives

$$\frac{1}{u} - \frac{2}{r} = -\frac{1}{v}$$

Identifying $P = -2/r$ as the power of the mirror, and interpreting the minus sign on the right side of the equation as indicating a vergence of "1/v" in the "reversed" image space, yields the vergence equation for mirrors.

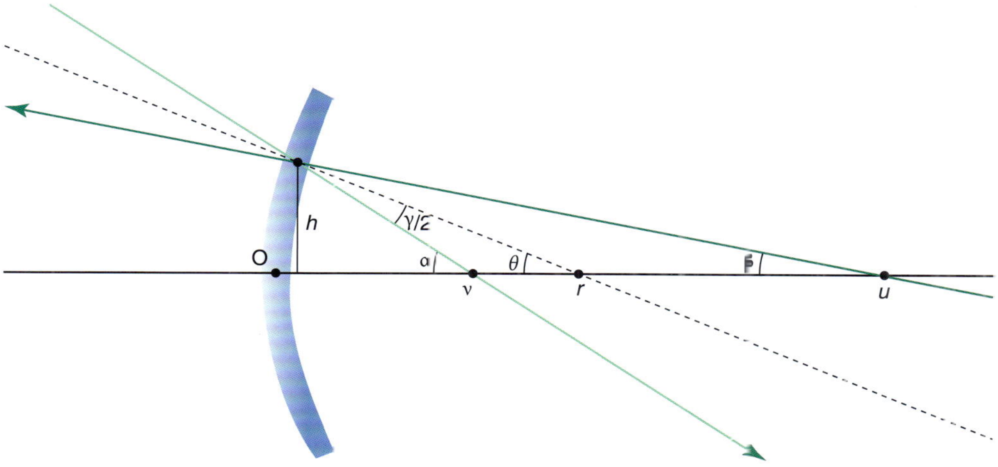

图 1–A3　从反射定律推导出镜面聚散度方程的几何形式。*（译者注：资料来源见前页原文。）*

因此

$$\alpha = 2\theta - \beta$$

用 α 、β 、θ 小角度近似（参见附录 1.1），我们有

$$\frac{h}{v} = 2\frac{h}{r} - \frac{h}{u}$$

提取公因数 h 并删除，重新整理，得

$$\frac{1}{u} - \frac{2}{r} = -\frac{1}{v}$$

将 $P = -2/r$ 作为镜面屈光力，将方程右边的负号理解为“$1/v$”在“反转”的像空间的聚散度，推出镜面的聚散度方程。

（翻译　杨亚军 朱丹 张宁 孙西宇 // 审校 石一宁 // 章节审校 魏瑞华）

CHAPTER 2

Physical Optics

This chapter includes related videos, which can be accessed by scanning the QR codes provided in the text or going to www .aao .org /bcscvideo section03.

Highlights

- quantum electrodynamics: unifying theory of light
- phenomena of light: polarization, coherence and interference, and diffraction
- measures of light: radiometry, photometry, and conversion between radiometric and photometric outputs
- lasers and therapeutic laser–tissue interactions
- light hazards

Glossary

Coherence The ability of light to produce interference phenomena.

Diffraction Refers to light "spreading out beyond the edges" of a small aperture or "bending around the corners" of an obstruction, into a region where—using strictly geometric optics reasoning—we would not expect to see it, and sets a limit on the resolution that can be achieved in any optical instrument. With a circular aperture such as the pupil, for example, the image of a point source of light formed on the retina—the point spread function (PSF)—in the absence of aberrations, takes the form of alternating bright and dark rings surrounding a bright central spot, the Airy disc, rather than a point.

Geometric scattering Scattering of light by particles that occurs if the particle size is much larger compared to the wavelength of incident light. The interaction of light with the particle is usually sufficiently described by the laws of geometric optics (refraction and reflection). The formation of a rainbow, for example, is sufficiently described by refraction and reflection by raindrops.

Interference Interference reveals the correlation between light waves and occurs when 2 light waves are brought together (superposition of waves), reinforcing each other and resulting in a wave of greater amplitude (ie, *constructive* or *additive interference*), or subtracting from each other and resulting in a wave of lower amplitude (ie, *destructive* or subtractive *interference*), depending on their relative phase.

第 2 章

物理光学

本章包括相关视频，可通过扫描文本提供的二维码或访问 www .aao.org /bcscvideo section03。

重点

- 量子电动力学：光的统一理论。
- 光的现象：偏振，相干、干涉和衍射。
- 光的度量：辐射测量、光度测量，以及辐射测量和光度输出之间的转换。
- 激光和治疗性激光组织作用。
- 光危害。

术语

相干 是光产生干涉现象的能力。

衍射 是指光经过小孔或障碍物时，会漫出小孔边缘或绕过障碍物 进入一个严格遵循几何光学但无法看到的区域，继续传播的现象。在没有像差的情况下点光源通过圆孔，如瞳孔，在视网膜上成像——点扩散函数（PSF），在明亮中心点周围形成明暗交替环，即 Airy 斑，而并非一个点。

几何散射 如果粒子的大小比入射光的波长大很多，就会发生光的散射。光与粒子的相互作用可以用几何光学定律（折射和反射）来描述。如彩虹的形成可以用雨滴的折射和反射来描述。

干涉 干涉揭示了光波之间的相互关系，当 2 个光波聚集在一起（波的叠加），相互增强，产生更大振幅的波（即*构造干涉*或*相长干涉*），或相互削弱，产生振幅较低的波（即*相消性干涉*或相减干涉），这些都取决于它们的相对相位。

Laser Initially the acronym for Light Amplification by Stimulated Emission of Radiation.

Mie scattering Scattering of light produced by particles whose size is the same order of magnitude as the wavelength of incident light. Mie scattering caused by water droplets contributes to the white appearance of clouds. Similarly, Mie scattering caused by a cataract accounts for the whitish appearance of the lens under slit-lamp examination.

Photometry A measurement of the human visual system's psychophysical response to light. Basically, photometry can be considered a subtype of radiometry that considers the varying sensitivity of the eye to different wavelengths in the visible spectrum.

Polarization Light is said to be polarized when the orientation of the electric field, as it oscillates perpendicularly to the direction of propagation, is not random. The polarization state can be pictorially represented by the path that the tip of the electric field vector traces with time as viewed along the propagation axis looking toward the source, and can be linear, circular, or elliptical.

Quantum electrodynamics The quantum theory of the interaction of light and matter that resolves the wave–particle confusion. The theory describes most of the phenomena of the physical world—including all observed phenomena of light—except for gravitational and nuclear phenomena

Radiometry Refers to the direct measurement of light in any portion of the electromagnetic spectrum. In contrast to the photometric measurements, radiometric measurements weight equally the energy transmitted at every wavelength of the electromagnetic spectrum..

Rayleigh scattering Wavelength-dependent scattering that occurs when light interacts with particles much smaller than the wavelength of the light. The blue appearance of the sky during daytime and its reddish appearance during sunrise or sunset is due to Rayleigh scattering by atmospheric gas molecules. The bluish appearance of the cornea and lens (particularly noticeable in young eyes) under slit-lamp examination is also due to Rayleigh scattering by stromal collagen and lenticular fiber cells.

Introduction

The previous discussions of *geometric optics* in this book disregard the wavelength and photon character of light. These discussions work with the artificial construct of light rays and show how light behaves on a large scale compared with the dimensions of interest.

Physical optics goes beyond ray tracings and vergence calculations and deals with the properties of light on smaller scales, providing explanations for many of the phenomena of the physical world, such as *polarization*, *coherence*, *interference*, and *diffraction*, for which the ray approximation of geometric optics is insufficient.

激光　是英文受激发射的辐射光放大的第一个字母的缩写。

Mie 散射　指与入射光波长相同数量级的粒子所产生的光散射。水滴产生的 Mie 散射使云彩呈现白色外观。同样的，白内障引起的 Mie 散射致使裂隙灯下晶状体呈现白色外观。

光度测量　是人类视觉系统对光的心理–物理反应的测量。基本上，光度测量是辐射测量的亚型，它考虑的是眼睛对可见光谱中不同波长的敏感度的变化。

偏振　当电场的方向与传播方向垂直振荡时，光就会被极化。极化状态可以用沿传播轴向光源方向的电场矢量尖端随时间的轨迹表示，可以是线性的、圆形的或椭圆形的。

量子电动力学　是光与物质相互作用的量子理论，它解决了波–粒混淆。这个理论描述了大多数物理世界的现象，包括除了万有引力和核现象之外的所有可观察到的光的现象。

辐射测量　指对电磁光谱的任何部分光的直接测量。与光度测量不同的是，辐射测量等量测量了电磁波谱各波长传播的能量。

Rayleigh 散射　波长依赖性散射，当光与比光波长小得多的粒子相互作用时发生。白天天空呈蓝色，日出或日落时天空呈红色，这都是由于大气气体分子 Rayleigh 散射形成的。在裂隙灯检查下角膜和晶状体呈蓝色（在年轻人眼睛中尤为明显），这也是由于基质胶原蛋白和晶状体纤维细胞的 Rayleigh 散射造成的。

引言

前一节讨论的*几何光学*，忽略了光的波长和光子特性。这些讨论与光线的人工构造有关，并揭示了宏观上光的行为。

*物理光学*超出了光线追踪和聚散度计算，是在微观上研究光的性质，并解释了许多物理现象，如*偏振*、*相干*、*干涉*和*衍射*，而几何光学的光线近似是不能解释这些现象的。

What Is Light?

Visible Light

In ophthalmic optics, the term *light* generally refers to visible light, which is just a very narrow portion of a long scale, analogous to a musical scale, in which there are "notes" both higher and lower than we can perceive (Fig 2-1). The visual perception of these notes—specified by *frequency* (ν) and *wavelength* (λ) along the "scale" of light (*the electromagnetic spectrum*) and related to each other via the "speed of light" ($c = \nu \lambda \approx 3 \times 10^8$ m/s in a vacuum)—is what we call (spectral) *color*.

Although the visible spectrum is normally considered to run from 400 nm to 700 nm (Table 2-1), the boundaries are not precise. Under certain conditions, such as with sufficiently intense light, the eye's sensitivity extends into the infrared and ultraviolet (UV) regions. As another example, in aphakia, without the UV absorption of the natural lens, the retina can detect wavelengths well below 400 nm.

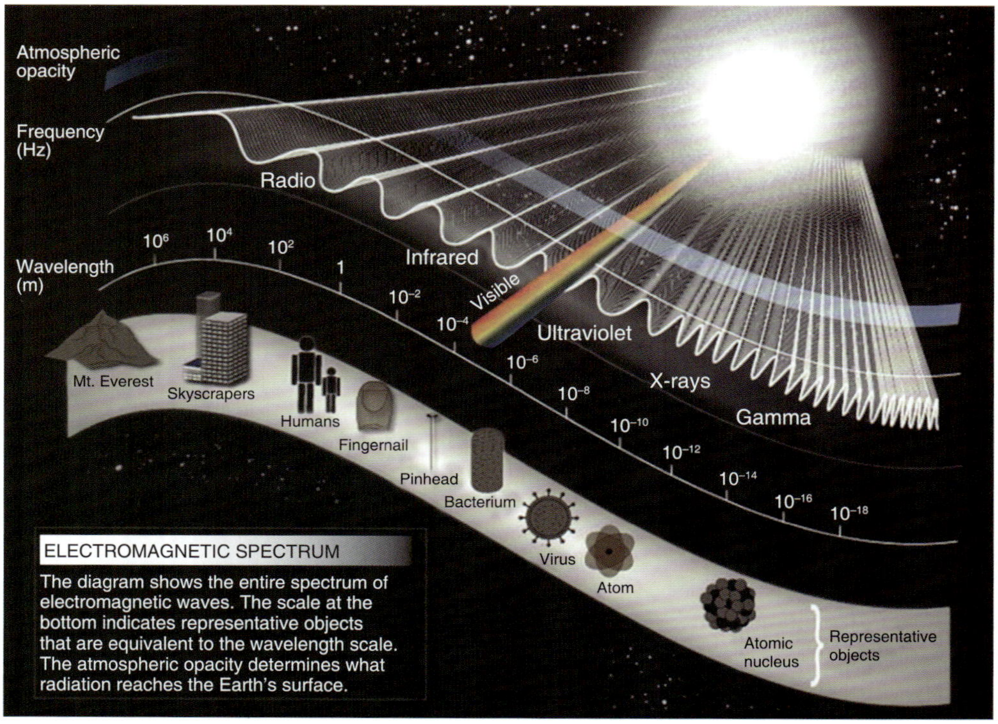

Figure 2-1 The electromagnetic (EM) spectrum. The spectrum is divided into several regions according to the wavelength or frequency of light. Note that visible light is just a very narrow portion of the entire EM spectrum. *(Courtesy of NASA.)*

光是什么?

可见光

在视光学中，*光*这个术语通常指的是可见光，只是光谱中很窄的一部分，类似于音乐音阶，其中有比我们所能感知到的更高或更低的“音符”（图 2–1）。这些光波的视觉感知的*频率*（ν）和*波长*（λ）沿着光谱（*电磁频谱*）排列，通过光速（$c = \nu\lambda \approx 3 \times 10^8$ m / s，在真空中）形成相互关系，即我们所说的（光谱）的*颜色*。

可见光谱通常是从 400~700nm（表 2–1），但边界并不精确。在某些条件下，如在足够强烈的光线下，眼睛的敏感度会延伸到红外线和紫外线（UV）区域。另一个例子是，在无晶状体眼中，没有自然晶状体的紫外线吸收，视网膜可以感受到远低于 400 nm 的波长。

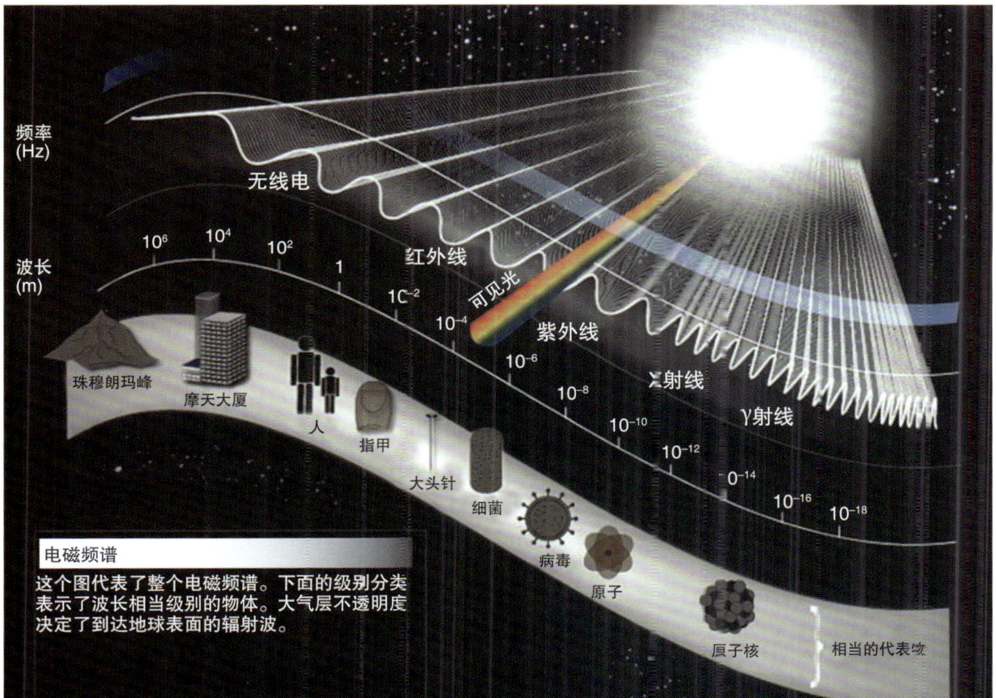

图 2–1　电磁波（EM）光谱。光谱根据光的波长或频率分为几个区域。请注意，可见光只是整个 EM 光谱中非常狭窄的一部分。*（译者注：资料来源见前页原文。）*

Table 2-1 Visible Spectrum and Approximate Color Associations

Color	Wavelength, nm (In Vacuum)
(Infrared)	>700
Red	620
Orange	610
Yellow	580
Green	540
Blue	480
Violet	450
(Ultraviolet)	<400

Wave or Particle?

The earliest comprehensive theories on the nature of light were advanced around the turn of the 17th century. In 1690, Christiaan Huygens put forward a *wave theory* of light, demonstrating how light waves might superimpose (interfere) to form a wavefront, similar to water waves (Fig 2-2), and travel in a straight line (in accordance with the ray approximation of geometric optics). As such, Huygens's wave theory covered little of what we would call physical optics today and was soon overshadowed by Isaac Newton's particle viewpoint. Newton suggested that light was made of particles—he called them "corpuscules." The *particle theory* of light took precedence and was accepted essentially unchallenged for over a century.

In the early 19th century, Thomas Young's double-slit experiment appeared to prove the wave-like behavior of light, via the observation of bright and dark bands (fringes) upon illumination of a barrier with 2 narrow openings, very similar to the interference pattern that results from the superposition of water waves. Later that century, James Clerk Maxwell formulated light entirely as a wave; that is, as the propagation of electromagnetic waves (Fig 2-3A) according to his Maxwell equations. Thus, for many years after Newton, as interference, diffraction, and other phenomena were readily explained by waves, the wave model became the dominant theory of the nature of light.

However, it is now clear that light also exhibits properties of particles, as seen in experiments with instruments that are sensitive enough to detect very weak light. An example of such an instrument is a photomultiplier, which produces "clicks" when light is shone on it. According to the wave theory, these clicks should become less loud as the intensity of the impinging light is decreased. In reality, these clicks remain equally loud, but decrease in frequency. Thus, light can be thought of as something like raindrops, with each little "drop" being called a photon.

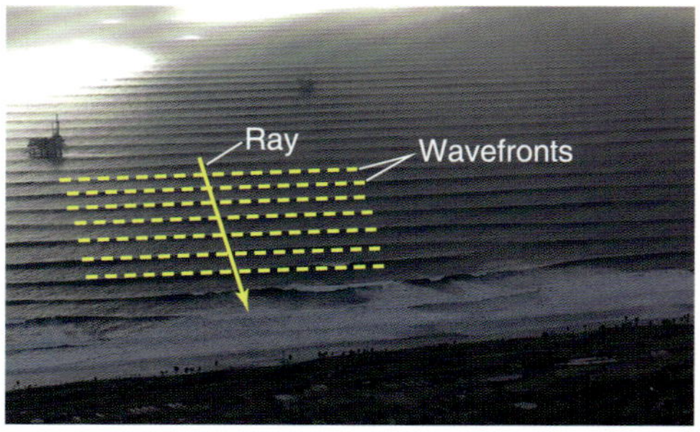

Figure 2-2 A wavefront is an imaginary construct that can best be understood in the example of water waves. Note that wavefronts are perpendicular to the ray direction. *(Photo- graph by Sang Pak, modified by Kristina Irsch, PhD.)*

表2-1　可见光谱和近似色彩相关

颜色	波长（真空中）/nm
（红外线）	>700
红色	620
橙色	610
黄色	580
绿色	540
蓝色	480
紫色	450
（紫外线）	<400

波还是粒子？

最早的关于光本质的理论是 17 世纪初提出的。1690 年，Christiaan Huygens 提出了*光波理论*，论证了光波如何叠加（干扰）形成类似于水波波前（图 2-2），并沿直线传播（符合几何光学的光线近似）。因此，Christiaan Huygens 波理论几乎没有涉及我们今天所说的物理光学，很快就被 Newton 的粒子观点所掩盖。Newton 认为光是由称之为“微粒”的粒子构成的。光的*粒子理论*在 1 个多世纪的时间里一直处于领先地位，基本上没有受到任何挑战。

在 19 世纪早期，Thomas Young 的双缝实验证明了光的波动行为。通过在一个有 2 个狭窄开口的挡板上观察明暗条纹（条纹），与水波叠加产生的干涉图样非常相似。随后，James Clerk Maxwell 把光完全视为一种波，即电磁波遵循 Maxwell 方程传播（图 2-3A）。因此，在 Newton 之后，由于干涉、衍射和其他现象很容易用波来解释，光波模型成为光本质的主导理论。

现在已经很清楚的是光也表现出粒子的特性，就像在实验中所看到的那样，这些仪器非常灵敏，可以探测到非常微弱的光。如光电倍增管，当光线照射到它时，光电倍增管就会发出“咔嗒”声。根据波动理论，当照射光的强度降低时，“咔嗒”声就会变得不那么响亮。实际上这些“咔嗒”声依然响亮，但是频率降低了。因此，光可以被认为是类似雨滴的东西，每个小“雨滴”被称为光子。

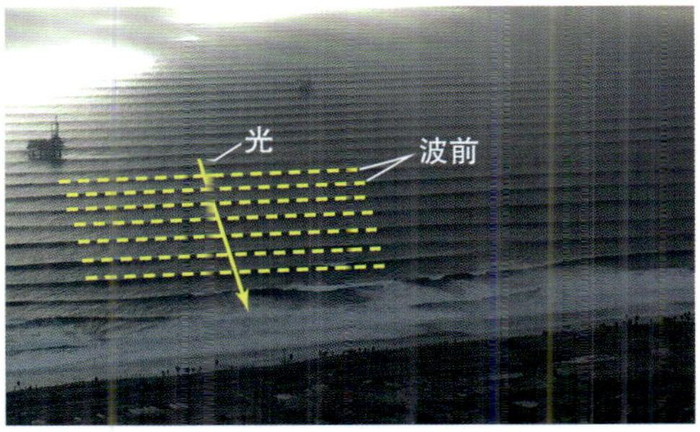

图 2-2　波前是一种假想的结构，参考水波最容易理解。注意波前垂直于光线方向。*（译者注：资料来源见旬页原文。）*

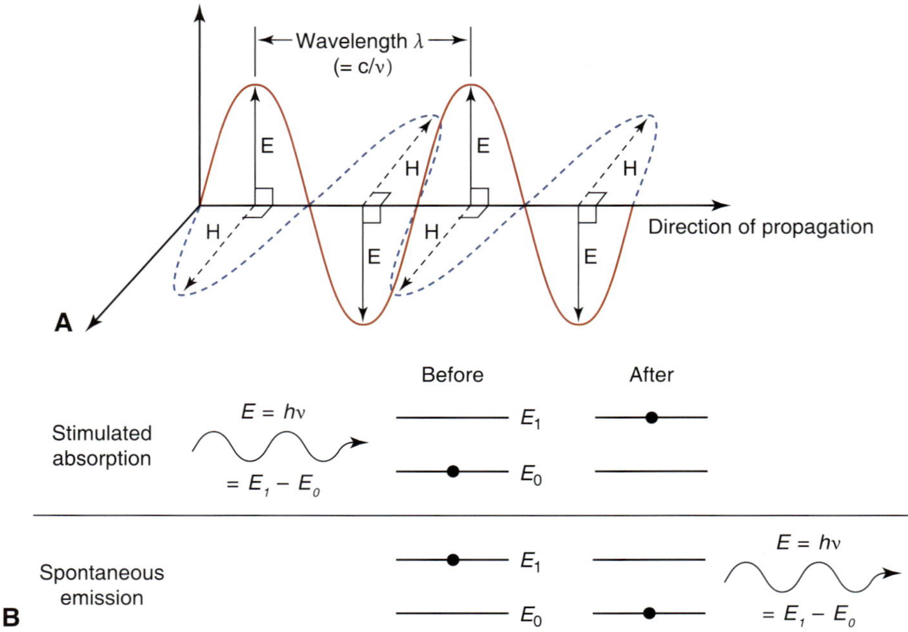

Figure 2-3 Electromagnetic wave theory and quantum theory. **A**, According to electromagnetic wave theory, light may be described as a transverse electromagnetic wave, whose oscillating electric (E) and magnetic (H) fields are both perpendicular to each other as well as to the direction that the light travels. The wavelength (λ) and frequency (ν) of light are related to each other via the "speed of light" ($c = \nu \lambda \approx 3\times10^8$ m/s in vacuum). **B**, According to quantum theory, electrons in atoms (or molecules) exist in nonradiating states, with each state being associated with a specific energy level. In a process called stimulated absorption, an electron moves between its lowest energy (ground) state (E_0) and an excited state (E_1) after picking up (absorbing) a photon or quantum of energy ($E = E_1 - E_0 = h_\nu$). Similarly, a photon is given off (emitted) when an electron moves from a higher energy state to a lower one (spontaneous emission). *h* is the Planck constant. *(Illustration part A by Kristina Irsch, PhD. Part B Reproduced with permission from Steinert RF, Puliafito CA. The Nd:YAG Laser in Ophthalmology: Principles and Clinical Applications of Photodisruption. Philadelphia: Saunders; 1985. Redrawn by C. H. Wooley and modified by Kristina Irsch, PhD.)*

In the early 20th century, Albert Einstein postulated light as the sum of individual packets (quanta) of energy, and thus was born the word *photon* and the quantum theory of light (Fig 2-3B). This influenced the formation of the concept of *a wave–particle duality* of light, which was not a very satisfactory theory, but rather represented a state of confusion, as to exactly which model to use in each circumstance. Maxwell's theory of electromagnetism (which fails to explain the observations with very dim light falling on photomultipliers) had to be modified to conform with the concepts of *quantum mechanics* (essentially a description of the motion of electrons in matter).

A new theory—*quantum electrodynamics* (*QED*)—the quantum theory of the interaction of light and matter, developed by a number of physicists in 1929 and clarified by Richard Feynman and 2 other physicists, Julian Schwinger and Sin-Itiro Tomonaga, in 1948, unites Maxwell's equations of electricity and magnetism with quantum mechanics. It thereby resolves the wave–particle confusion by stating that light is made of particles, not in the ordinary sense to be able to predict exactly what will happen in any given experiment, but rather it leaves us with being able to calculate only probabilities of an event.

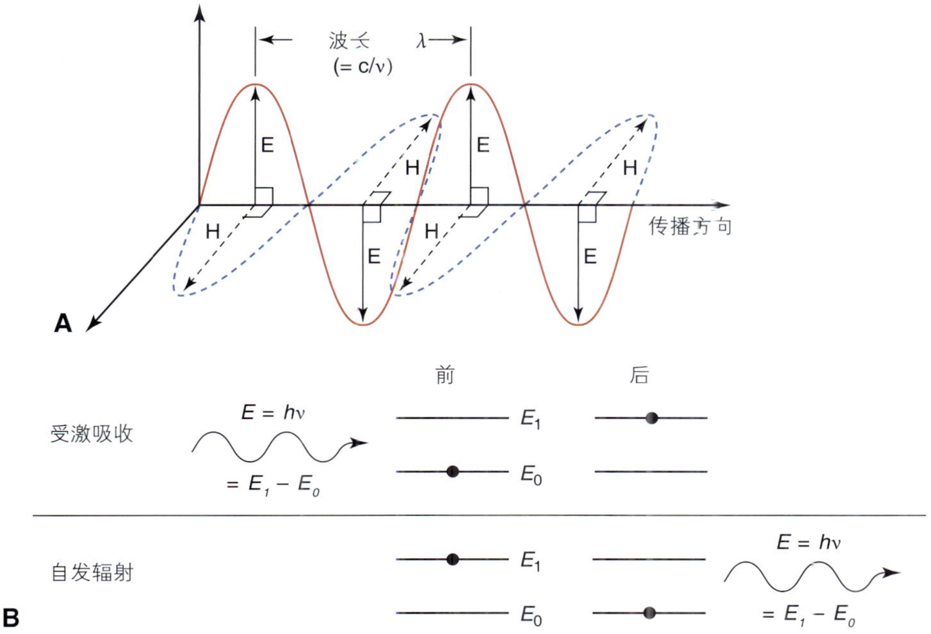

图 2–3　电磁波理论和量子理论。**A.** 根据电磁波理论，光可以被描述为横向电磁波，其振荡电场（E）和磁场（H）既相互垂直，并与光的方向传播垂直。光的波长（λ）和频率（ν）通过光的速度相互关联（$c = \nu\lambda \approx 3 \times 10^8$ m/s，真空中）。**B.** 根据量子理论，原子（或分子）中的电子以非辐射状态存在，每个状态都与特定的能量水平相关联。在一个被称为受激吸收的过程中，电子在最低能量（地面）状态（E_0）和接（吸收）光子或量子的能量（$E = E_1 - E_0 = h\nu$）的激发状态（E_1）之间移动。同样地，当电子从高能量状态到低能量状态（自发发射）时，就会发出（发射）光子。h 是普朗克常数。*（译者注：资料来源见前页原文。）*

在 20 世纪早期，Albert Einstein 假设光是单个能量包（量子）的总和，因此诞生了*光子*和光的量子理论（图 2–3B）。这影响了光的*波粒二象性*的概念的形成，这不是一个很令人满意的理论，而是代表了一种混乱的状态，即在某种情况下究竟该如何使用哪种模型。Maxwell 的电磁学理论（它不能解释非常微弱的光落在光电倍增管上的观测现象）必须修正，以符合*量子力学*的概念（本质上是对物质中电子运动的描述）。

一种新的理论——*量子电动力学（QED）*——光和物质相互作用的量子理论，在 1929 年由多位物理学家提出，并且在 1948 年由 Richard Feynman 和另外 2 名物理学家 Julian Schwinger 和 Sin-Itiro Tomonaga 将 Maxwell 电磁方程与量子力学相结合，阐明了光是由粒子构成的，用以解决波 – 粒混淆。但不是通常意义上能够准确预测在任何给定的实验中会发生什么，而是只能够计算事件的概率。

Thus, contrary to what is taught in many ophthalmology and ophthalmic optics text books, there is one theory that explains all the properties of light we know: QED. Note that for most purposes, in practice it suffices to consider the wave-like behavior of light (see Fig 2-3A) for phenomena at the macroscopic level, and the simple quantum-view of the light (see Fig 2-3B) at the microscopic level, as will be illustrated.

Feynman RP. *QED: The Strange Theory of Light and Matter*. 2nd ed. Princeton: Princeton University Press; 2006.

Quantum Electrodynamics: Unifying Theory of Light

Quantum electrodynamics describes most of the phenomena of the physical world, except for gravitational and nuclear phenomena. All these phenomena can be essentially deduced from 3 basic actions, each of which occurs with a certain probability that can be calculated using the tools of the theory: (1) a photon goes from point to point, (2) an electron goes from point to point, and (3) an electron emits (or absorbs) a photon. Qualitatively, the theory boils down to photons, which make up the light, going from one electron to another, and electrons, which make up the matter, picking up and giving off photons while moving about.

Refraction and Reflection

Both refraction (transmission) and reflection are the result of the interaction of light and matter, that is, of photons with electrons in the atoms and molecules inside the refractive and/or reflective medium.

We learned in Chapter 1 that light changes speed and direction when moving from one medium to another. However, the individual photons do not go slower inside the material. Slowing of the light is caused by the electrons throughout the material scattering the photons, and the degree to which there is scattering is called the refractive index for that particular medium. Similarly, light is not reflected off a surface. In reality, the photons are scattered by the electrons in the material, the net result of which is the same as if the photon hit and was reflected by only the surface.

Here's what essentially happens during refraction and reflection: a photon arrives from the outside, hits an electron, and is picked up (*absorption*) by the electron; the electron continues a bit, and then a new photon is emitted. This dance of photons and electrons is called *scattering* of light. Thus, in refracted and reflected light, the photon that emerges from the process is not the same photon as the one that went in. Thus, the behavior of light in classical optics reflects the net result rather than the actual path of the photon, providing a convenient approximation to describe the phenomena we are familiar with.

因此，与许多眼科和眼科光学教科书所教的相反，有一种理论可以解释我们所知道的光的所有性质：量子电动力学 QED。注意，在大多数情况下，只需要在宏观上考虑光的波动行为（见图 2–3A）和在微观上考虑光的简单量子观（见图 2–3B）。

Feynman RP. *QED: The Strange Theory of Light and Matter*. 2nd ed. Princeton: Princeton University Press; 2006.

量子电动力学：光的统一理论

除了引力和核现象以外，量子电动力学描述了大部分物理现象。基本上所有的这些现象都可以推导出 3 个作用，每个都以一定的概率出现，使用该理论的工具可以计算：①光子的点对点运动；②电子的点对点运动；③ 1 个电子发射（或吸收）1 个光子。从定性角度上说，这个理论可以归结为光子，它构成了光，从一个电子到另一个电子，而电子构成了物质，在移动的过程中接收并释放光子。

折射与反射

折射（透射）和反射都是光和物质相互作用的结果。也就是说，光子的产生是电子在折射和（或）反射介质里的原子和分子相互作用的结果。

我们在第 1 章学习过，当光从一种介质移动到另一种介质时，会改变其速度和方向。然而，单个光子在材料内部的运动并不慢。光的减慢是由整个材料中的电子散射光子引起的，散射的程度被称为特定介质的折射率。同样，光不会从表面反射。实际上，光子是由材料中的电子散射的，其结果与光子撞击的结果相同，只是在表面上反射。

这是折射和反射过程：一个光子从外面到达，击中一个电子，然后被电子*吸收*；电子继续运动，然后一个新的光子发射出来。这种光子和电子的跳跃叫作光的*散射*。在折射和反射的光中，从这个过程中产生的光子与进入的光子是不同的。因此，在经典光学中的光行为是光子作用的结果，而不是实际路径，这为我们提供了一个用于描述熟悉现象的近似值。

Scattering

The scattering of light by an electron in an atom is the phenomenon that accounts for reflection and transmission (refraction) in a medium. Light scattering is also responsible for the visible appearance or perception of color and may be divided into 3 regimes— *Rayleigh scattering, Mie scattering,* and *geometric scattering*—according to the dimensions of the scattering medium with respect to the wavelength of the incident light. Note that the Tyndall effect, a term commonly used in ophthalmology and chemistry for scattering of light by colloidal suspensions, does not describe a separate scattering regime, but rather the effect of the light beam becoming visible. For example, normally you cannot see a beam of light in water or the aqueous humor. Shining a flashlight beam in a glass of water after adding a few drops of milk is an excellent demonstration of the Tyndall effect. The milk proteins will stay suspended in the water (a colloid suspension), making the beam visible. Similarly, if we can see the beam of light in the aqueous humor during slit-lamp examination, this is an indication of inflammation, in other words an indication resulting from the presence of suspended protein in the aqueous.

Rayleigh scattering

Rayleigh scattering occurs when light interacts with particles much smaller than the wavelength of the light. The degree of this form of scattering varies strongly with wavelength, more precisely, inversely to its fourth power. Therefore, the probability that light will scatter is much higher for shorter wavelengths (higher frequencies), such as blue light, than for longer wavelengths (lower frequencies), such as red light.

The effect of Rayleigh scattering of sunlight on gas molecules that make up the Earth's atmosphere is what produces the blue appearance of the sky during daytime and its reddish appearance during sunrise or sunset. This is because during daytime, when the sun is overhead, the highly scattered blue end of the spectrum that is emitted by the sun reaches your eye from all directions, whereas the weakly scattered redder wavelengths miss your line of sight. At sunrise and sunset, with the sun at the horizon, it is the weakly scattered red end of the spectrum that can still be seen, passing the atmosphere towards your eyes almost undeviated, while the blue light that is scattered off misses your line of sight.

The bluish appearance of the cornea and lens (particularly noticeable in young eyes) under slit-lamp examination is also due to Rayleigh scattering by stromal collagen and lenticular fiber cells.

Mie scattering

Mie scattering is produced by particles whose size is the same order of magnitude as the wavelength of incident light. Unlike Rayleigh scattering, this form of scattering, on average, does not vary strongly with wavelength and tends to be stronger in the forward direction than in any other direction.

Mie scattering contributes to the white appearance of clouds. This is because the water droplets that make up the cloud are of comparable size to the visible wavelengths, so that the probability of being scattered is about identical for the different wavelengths (or frequencies) in the white sunlight, and the clouds therefore appear to be white.

In the eye, age-related increase in scattering is mostly associated with an increase in Mie scattering by cataract formation, which adds a strong forward, but less wavelength- dependent, component to the Rayleigh scattering (the predominant scattering component in healthy young eyes). Mie scattering caused by a cataract accounts for the whitish appearance of the lens under slit-lamp examination. The increase in forward scattering is what results in decreased contrast of the patient's retinal image, and hence increased glare sensitivity.

散射

原子中电子对光的散射会引起介质中的反射和透射（折射）现象。光散射也形成了可见的外观或颜色的感知，并可根据散射介质的量度和入射光的波长分为 *Rayleigh 散射*、*Mie 散射*和*几何散射* 3 种状态。请注意，Tyndall 效应是眼科和化学领域常用于描述胶体悬浮液对光的散射的术语，它并不描述一个单独的散射区，而是描述了光束变得可见的效应。例如，一般看不到水中或房水中的光束，加了几滴牛奶后，打开手电筒，就可以观察到水中的光束，这也证实了 Tyndall 效应。牛奶蛋白悬浮在水中（胶体悬浮），使光束可见，同样地，裂隙灯检查时看到房水中的光束，这是炎症的迹象。换句话说，这是由于在房水中存在悬浮的蛋白。

Rayleigh 散射

光线和比光线波长小得多的粒子相互作用时会产生 Rayleigh 散射。这种散射的程度随波长有很大变化，更准确地说，与波长的四次方成反比。因此，与波长较长的（频率较低）红光相比，波长较短的（频率较高）蓝光的光散射概率要大得多。

阳光的 Rayleigh 散射对地球大气的气体分子的影响是：在白天天空呈蓝色，在日出或日落时天空呈淡红色。这是因为在白天，当太阳在头顶的时候，太阳发出的光谱的高度分散的蓝端从各个方向到达你的眼睛，而微弱分散的更红的波长会错过你的视线。日出日落时，太阳在地平线上，我们仍然可以看到光谱中微弱散射的红端，它几乎没有偏离方向地将大气中的红光传递到你的眼睛，而散射出去的蓝光却偏离了你的视线。

裂隙灯检查下角膜和晶状体呈蓝色（在年轻的眼睛中尤为明显），这也是由于基质胶原蛋白和透镜纤维细胞的 Rayleigh 散射造成的。

Mie 散射

Mie 散射是由与入射光波长相同数量级的粒子产生的。与 Rayleigh 散射不同的是，这种散射形式一般不会随波长而剧烈变化，而是在正前方比在其他方向上更强。

Mie 散射有助于云的白色外观。这是因为组成云团的水滴的大小与可见光波长相当，因此在白色阳光下散射的概率与不同波长（或频率）是相同的，所以云团看起来是白色的。

在眼睛中，与年龄相关的散射增加主要与白内障形成导致的 Mie 散射增加有关，而白内障增强了前向的、与波长无关的 Rayleigh 散射（这是健康年轻眼睛中的主要散射成分）。Mie 散射导致了在裂隙灯下检查晶状体的白色外观。前向散射的增加导致患者视网膜像对比度降低，从而增加了眩光敏感性。

Geometric scattering

If the particle size is much larger compared to the wavelength of incident light, the interaction of light with the particle is usually sufficiently described by the laws of geometric optics (refraction and reflection). For example, refraction and reflection are sufficient to explain the formation of a rainbow. This is because raindrops are larger than water droplets in clouds and can be considered as merely refracting and reflecting the white sunlight from their surfaces. This nicely illustrates how at the macroscopic level, the quantum behavior of light can be conveniently disregarded.

Phenomena of Light

Although QED can account for all observed phenomena of light, several macroscopic phenomena of light, such as polarization, coherence, and interference, can completely, and more easily, be explained by Maxwell's classical theory of electromagnetic waves. In this context, light may therefore be described as a transverse electromagnetic wave, whose oscillating electric and magnetic fields are both perpendicular to each other as well as to the direction that the light travels (see Fig 2-3A).

Polarization

Fundamentals

As the magnetic field is always perpendicular to and proportional to the electric field, it may be conventionally ignored when considering polarization, so only the electric field need be described for simplicity. The orientation of the electric field, as it oscillates perpendicularly to the direction of propagation, defines the state of polarization. Note that the electric-field vector, which is shown oriented in a single plane in Figure 2-3A, typically changes rapidly and randomly, resulting in randomly polarized light that is said to be *unpolarized*. When the movement of the electric field vector is not random, the light is said to be polarized. Pictorially, the polarization state can be represented by the path that the tip of the electric field vector traces with time as viewed along the propagation axis looking toward the source (Lissajous figures). Figure 2-3A depicts *linearly polarized light*, with the electric field vector being constrained to a single plane; when viewed head-on it traces a single line. In *circularly polarized light*, the electric field vector rotates, tracing a corkscrew pattern as the light propagates. Viewed head-on, the pattern mapped out by the tip of the electric-field vector is a circle. In *elliptically polarized light*, which represents a more general case of circular polarization, the electric-field vector rotates and at the same time changes its amplitude as the light propagates, tracing an ellipse instead of a circle when viewed head-on.

Polarized light can be produced in a number of ways. One way to produce complete or *partially polarized light* is by reflection. Partial polarization, as the name implies, is a mixture of unpolarized and polarized light (linear, circular, or elliptical). Fresnel showed that the polarized component of reflected light tends to be linear, parallel to the interface. Reflected light is completely polarized if the angle of incidence equals the *Brewster angle*:

$$\text{Brewster Angle} = \tan^{-1}\frac{n_{\mathrm{t}}}{n_{\mathrm{i}}}$$

几何散射
如果粒子的大小比入射光的波长大得多，那么光与粒子的相互作用可以用几何光学定律（折射和反射）描述。如折射和反射解释了彩虹的形成。这是因为雨滴比云里的水滴大，仅仅折射和反射了表面的白色阳光。这很好地说明了在宏观上，可以忽略光的量子行为。

光的现象

虽然量子电动力学（QED）可以解释所有观察到的光的现象，但是一些光的宏观现象，如偏振、相干和干涉，完全可以更容易地用 Maxwell 经典电磁波理论来解释。因此，在这种情况下，光可以被描述为横向电磁波，其振荡的电场和磁场既相互垂直，又垂直于光的传播方向（看图 2–3A）

偏振

基本原理
由于磁场总是垂直于电场，并且与电场成正比，所以在考虑极化时，通常可以忽略它，只简单描述电场。电场的方向，当它垂直于传播方向振荡时，就定义了极化的状态。请注意，图 2–3A 所示的电场矢量在一个平面上定向、迅速而随机地变化导致偏振光的*去偏振*。当电场矢量的运动不是随机的时，光就被称为偏振光。从图上看，极化状态可以用沿着传播轴向光源方向的电场矢量尖端随时间的轨迹来表示（Lissajous 图形）。图 2–3A 描述了*线偏振光*，电场矢量限定在一个平面上，当正面观察时，它会追踪一条直线。在*圆偏振光*中，电场矢量旋转，会随着光的传播沿着螺旋形轨迹运动，从正面看，由电场矢量的尖端绘出的图形是一个圆。在*椭圆偏振光*中，这是一种更普遍的圆偏振，电场矢量在旋转的同时也随着光的传播而改变其振幅，当正面观察时绘出的是一个椭圆而不是圆形。

偏振光可以以多种方式产生。产生完全或部分偏振光的一种方法是反射。*部分偏振*，顾名思义，是非偏振和偏振光（线、圆形或椭圆形）的混合。Fresnel 实验表明，反射光的偏振分量趋于线性，与界面平行。如果入射角等于 *Brewster 角*，反射光就是完全偏振：

$$\text{Brewster 角} = \tan^{-1}\frac{n_t}{n_i}$$

where n_t and n_i are the refractive indices of the transmitted and incident media, respectively. At the Brewster angle, all the *reflected* light is linearly polarized, but not all the linearly polarized light is reflected. Consequently, the *transmitted* light is a mixture of linearly and randomly polarized (commonly referred to as unpolarized) light—that is, it is partially polarized.

Applications and clinical relevance

Ophthalmic applications of polarization are numerous, some of which are discussed briefly here. Polarizing sunglasses are sometimes useful for reducing glare from reflected sunlight. Reflected light is somewhat polarized parallel to the reflecting surface, and in most environments, reflecting objects tend to be horizontal. In boating, for example, sunlight reflected from the water surface is partially polarized, usually horizontally, as is light reflected from a road surface or from the hood of a car. Even the sky acts as a partial polarizer by means of the scattering properties of air molecules. Accordingly, sunglasses incorporate vertically oriented linear polarizers (polarizing filters) to block the horizontally polarized component of reflected light.

Several stereopsis tests incorporate the use of linear polarizers. The well-known Stereo Fly test, for example, displays 2 slightly displaced images that linearly polarize light in perpendicular meridians. The person wears glasses containing linear polarizers, also at right angles to each other; each eye sees just 1 of the images, thus a single 3-dimensional (3D) image is perceived by someone with normal 3D or stereoscopic vision.

Polarized light is used in some ophthalmic instruments, such as the scanning laser polarimeter (discussed in Chapter 8). The retinal nerve fiber layer is birefringent, which means that polarized light travels through it at different speeds depending on whether the polarization is along or across the fibers. This retardation is linearly related to the thickness of a birefringent medium. Scanning laser polarimetry employs this effect to determine the thickness of the nerve fiber layer, for glaucoma diagnostic purposes.

Coherence and Interference

Fundamentals

Coherence describes the ability of light to produce interference phenomena. Interference reveals the correlation between light waves and occurs when 2 light waves are brought together (superposition of waves), reinforcing each other and resulting in a wave of greater amplitude (ie, *constructive* or additive *interference*), or subtracting from each other and resulting in a wave of lower amplitude (ie, *destructive* or subtractive *interference*), depending on their relative phase (Fig 2-4). Figures 2-5 and 2-6 illustrate the concepts of coherence and interference of light.

其中 n_t 和 n_i 分别为透射介质和入射介质的折射率。在 Brewster 角，所有的*反射*光都是线偏振的，但不是所有的线偏振光都是光线反射的。因此，*透射*光是线偏振和无偏振（通常称为非偏振）光的混合物，即部分偏振。

应用与临床的相关性

偏振光在眼科的应用很多，其中一些在这里简要讨论。偏振光太阳镜有时有助于减少反射日光的眩光。反射光是与反射面平行偏振光，在大多数情况下，反射物是水平的，如在划船时，从水面反射的阳光是部分偏振的，通常是水平的，就像从路面或汽车引擎盖反射的光一样。通过空气分子的散射特性，天空也作为部分偏振器。因此，太阳镜加入了垂直方向的线偏振器（偏振滤光片），可以阻断反射光的水平偏振成分。

立体视觉测试采用了线偏振器。如立体苍蝇测试呈现了两个轻微位置差异、且相互垂直的线偏振图像。戴着相互成直角的线偏振镜的人，每只眼睛只能看到其中的一幅图像，因此具有正常 3D 或立体视觉的人可以感知到一个三维（3D）图像。

偏振光常用于一些眼科仪器，如扫描激光偏振计（在第 8 章中讨论）。视网膜神经纤维层是双折射的，这意味着偏振光通过它的速度是不同的，这取决于偏振是沿着纤维还是穿过纤维。这种延迟与双折射介质的厚度呈线性关系。扫描激光偏振测量仪就是利用这种效应来确定神经纤维层的厚度，可以用于青光眼的诊断。

相干和干涉

基本原理

相干性描述了光产生干涉现象的能力。干涉揭示了光波之间的相互关系，当 2 个光波聚集在一起（波的叠加）时，或相互加强，产生更大振幅的波（即*相长*或相加*干涉*），或相互相减而产生在振幅较低的波（如*相消*或相减*干涉*），这都取决于相对像位（图 2–4）。图 2–5 和图 2–6 说明了光的相干和干涉的概念。

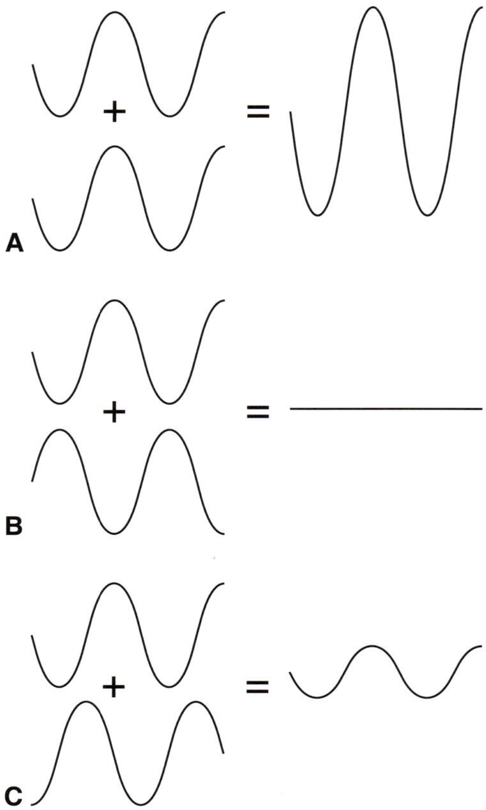

Figure 2-4 Superposition of waves of identical frequency and amplitude produces stable interference patterns. **A**, Waves overlap in phase—peaks coincide with peaks and troughs with troughs—producing a resultant wave of twice the amplitude. **B**, Waves overlap out of phase—the peak of one wave coincides with the trough of the other—and the waves cancel. **C**, Waves partially overlap— neither completely in nor out of phase— producing a wave of intermediate amplitude (between zero and twice the amplitude). *(Illustration developed by Edmond H. Thall, MD, and redrawn by C. H. Wooley.)*

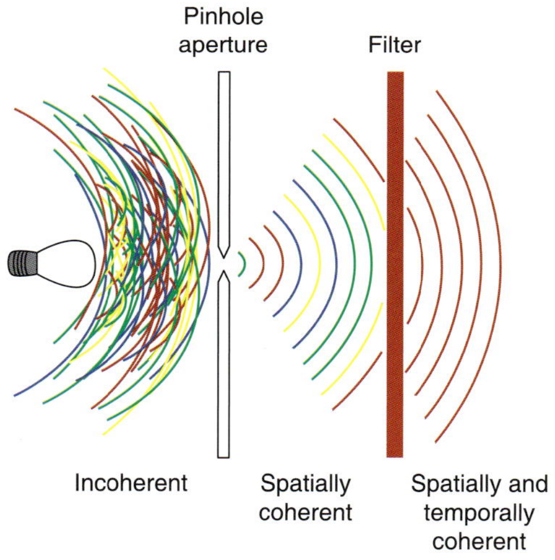

Figure 2-5 Pictorial explanation of coherence. A white light source produces incoherent light, emitting wavefronts of diverse wavelengths and arrangements. If incoherent light is passed through a pinhole aperture, spatial coherence is improved; that is, the resulting wavefronts are more regularly arranged. If spatially coherent light is passed through a narrow-band filter, selecting a narrow band of wavelengths, temporal coherence is improved; that is, the resulting wavefronts also have the same wavelength. *(Illustration developed by Kristina Irsch, PhD.)*

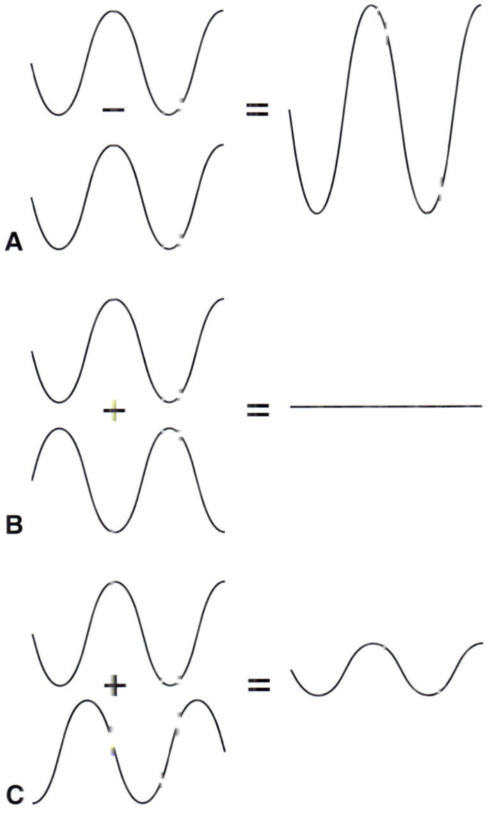

图 2–4　相同频率和振幅的波叠加产生稳定的干涉图。**A**. 相位重叠的波（波峰与波峰、波谷与波谷重合）产生 2 倍振幅的波幅。**B**. 相位交错的波（波峰值与另一波的波谷重合）相互抵消。**C**. 波部分重叠（既不完全在相位内，也不完全在相位外）产生中等振幅的波（振幅在 0~2 倍之间）。*（译者注：资料来源见前页原文。）*

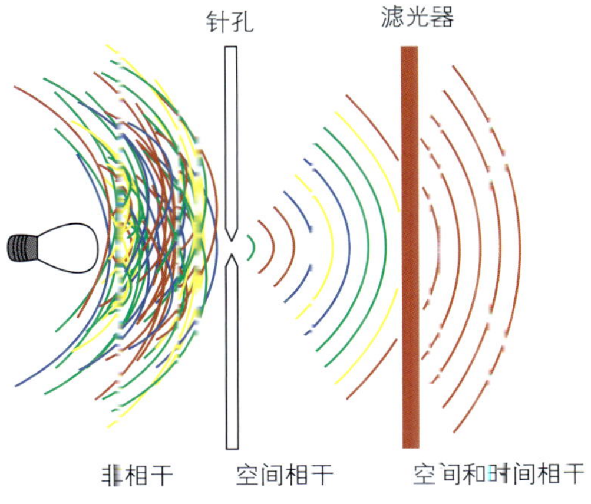

图 2–5　相干图示说明。白光产生非相干光，发出不同波长和排列的波前。非相干光通过针孔时，空间相干性提高，即产生的波前排列更有规律。如果空间相干光通过窄带滤波器，会选择窄波段波长，时间相干性提高，即产生的波前也具有相同的波长。*（译者注：资料来源见前页原文。）*

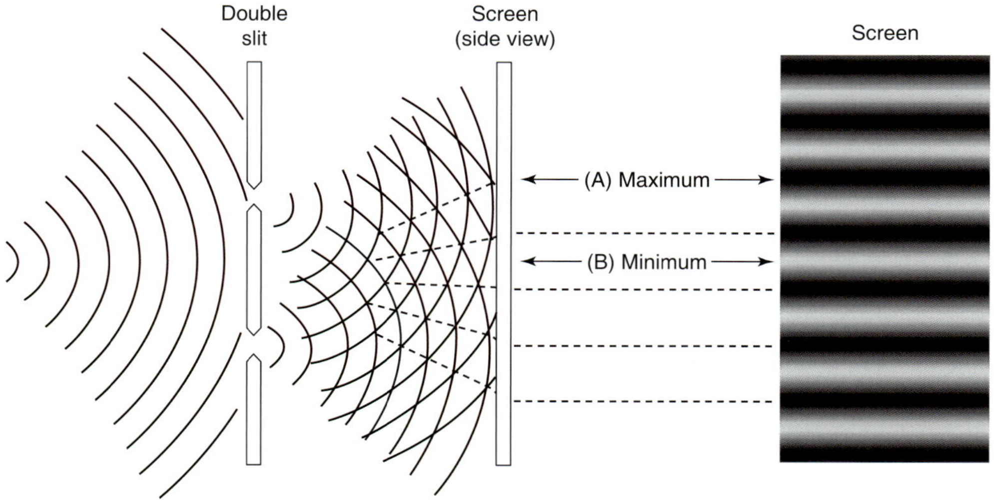

Figure 2-6 Pictorial explanation of interference. Coherent light strikes a double slit or 2 pinhole apertures from which new wavefronts emanate, which are then superimposed on a screen, creating an interference pattern of a series of bright and dark fringes. (A) represents constructive interference. (B) indicates destructive interference. *(Illustration by Jonathan Clark, modified by Kristina Irsch, PhD.)*

In Figure 2-5, a white light source produces incoherent light, emitting wavefronts of diverse wavelengths and arrangements. However, if incoherent light is passed through a pinhole aperture, *spatial coherence* of the light is improved, that is, the resulting wavefronts are more regularly arranged. If spatially coherent light is passed through a narrow- band filter, selecting a narrow band of wavelengths (we will discuss later how these filters work), *temporal coherence* of the light is improved, that is, the resulting wavefronts have the same wavelength, thereby making the light monochromatic. Laser light is highly coherent. However, as shown here, coherent light can be produced even without a laser, but at the expense of discarding a large amount of the light.

Figure 2-6 illustrates the basic concept of Young's double-slit experiment, discussed earlier. If coherent light strikes a double slit or 2 pinhole apertures, new wavefronts emanate, which then are superimposed on a screen. Note that the curved lines represent the crests of the waves at a particular instant. Where the crests coincide (eg, at A), a maximum of intensity is produced (constructive interference); where the crest of one wave coincides with the trough of the other wave (B) intensity is minimized (destructive interference). An interference pattern of a series of bright and dark fringes is observed on the screen, representing areas of constructive and destructive interference respectively.

The concepts of coherence length and coherence time, which are essential in the understanding of the basic principle of optical coherence tomography (OCT; see Chapter 8), can be best understood in the example of interferometry. In interferometry, as illustrated in Figure 2-7, light is split into 2 beams, and the beam backscattered from a sample is then compared (superimposed) with the beam that has traveled a known time from a reference mirror. Interference between the 2 light beams occurs only when the optical distances traveled by the light in both the sample and reference paths (arms) match to within the coherence length of the light. In other words, *coherence length* is the maximum path difference for good visibility of interference fringes. Likewise, *coherence time* is the maximum transit time difference for which interference fringes are still observable.

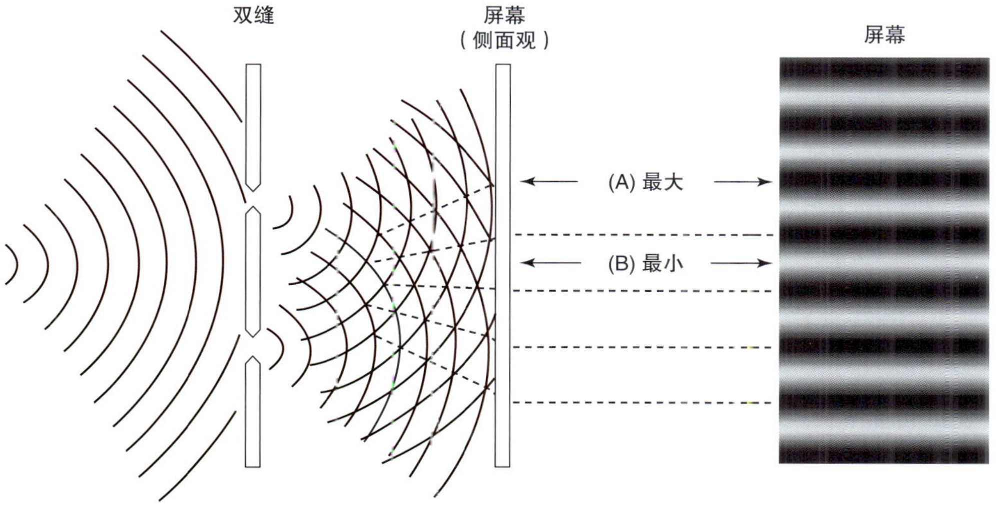

图 2–6 干涉的图示说明。相干光从一个双缝或双针孔中发出新的波前，然后叠加在屏幕上，形成一系列明暗条纹的干涉图样。（A）表示相长干涉。（B）表示相消干涉。*（译者注：资料来源见前页原文。）*

在图 2–5 中，白色光源产生非相干光，发出不同波长和排列的波前。但是，如果非相干光通过针孔，光的*空间相干性*就会得到改善，即产生的波前排列更有规律。如果空间相干光通过窄带滤光器，选择窄波段的波长（将在后面讨论滤光器如何工作），光的*时间相干性*就会得到改善，即与产生的波前具有相同的波长，从而产生单色光。激光是高度相干的。然而，正如这里所示，即使没有激光也能产生相干光，但却会丢失大量的光。

图 2–6 展示了前面讨论的 Young 双缝实验的基本概念。如果相干光照射到双缝或双针孔，会产生新的波前，叠加在屏幕上。注意，曲线代表了某一特定时刻的波峰。波峰重合（如 A 点）处的强度最大（相长干涉）；一个波的波峰与另一个波的波谷重合处（B）的强度最小（相消干涉）。屏幕上可以观察到一系列明和暗条纹的干涉图案，分别表示相长干涉和相消干涉的区域。

相干长度和相干时间的概念对于理解光学相干断层成像基本原理至关重要（OCT，见第 8 章），这可以在干涉测量仪中得到最好的理解。在干涉测量仪中，如图 2–7 所示，光被分成 2 束，然后将从样品中散射出来的光束与从参考镜中经过已知时间的光束进行比较（叠加）。2 束光之间的干扰只发生在光在样品和参考路径（臂）上的传播距离都在光的相干长度内的情况下。换句话说，*相干长度*是干涉条纹可见的最大路径差。同样地，*相干时间*是干涉条纹可见的最大时间差。

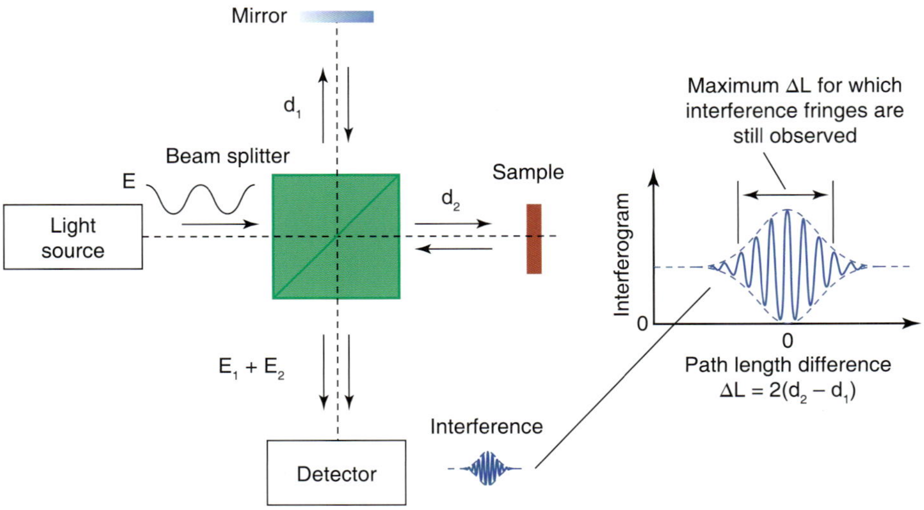

Figure 2-7 Basic concept of interferometry. Light is split into 2 beams, and the beam that has traveled an unknown time and distance (d_2) from a sample is compared (interfered) with the beam that has traveled a known time and distance (d_1) from a reference mirror. An interference pattern is detected only when the optical distances traveled by the light in both the sample and reference paths match to within the coherence length of the light (ΔL). *(Illustration developed by Kristina Irsch, PhD.)*

Both coherence time and length are inversely proportional to the *spectral bandwidth* of the light source (ie, the frequency or wavelength range over which sources emit light). Note that a source with a narrow spectral bandwidth (light of nearly a single wavelength or wholly monochromatic; eg, laser light) has a high temporal coherence, whereas a source with a broad bandwidth (light of multiple wavelengths; eg, white light) has a low temporal coherence (Fig 2-8).

Hence, when a narrow-bandwidth source is used to perform interferometry (eg, conventional laser interferometry), interference fringes will occur over a long range of path length differences between the 2 beams (Video 2-1). In low-coherence interferometry— using a broadband light source—on the other hand, interference occurs only when the time traveled by the light in the reference and sample arms is nearly equal, within the coherence length of the source. Low-coherence interferometry therefore enables greater sensitivity in separating out reflections, especially when from a sample with multiple, closely spaced reflecting surfaces (Video 2-2).

VIDEO 2-1 Concept of conventional (laser) interferometry.
Animation developed by Kristina Irsch, PhD.
Access all Section 3 videos at www.aao.org/bcscvideo_section03.

VIDEO 2-2 Concept of low-coherence interferometry.
Animation developed by Kristina Irsch, PhD.

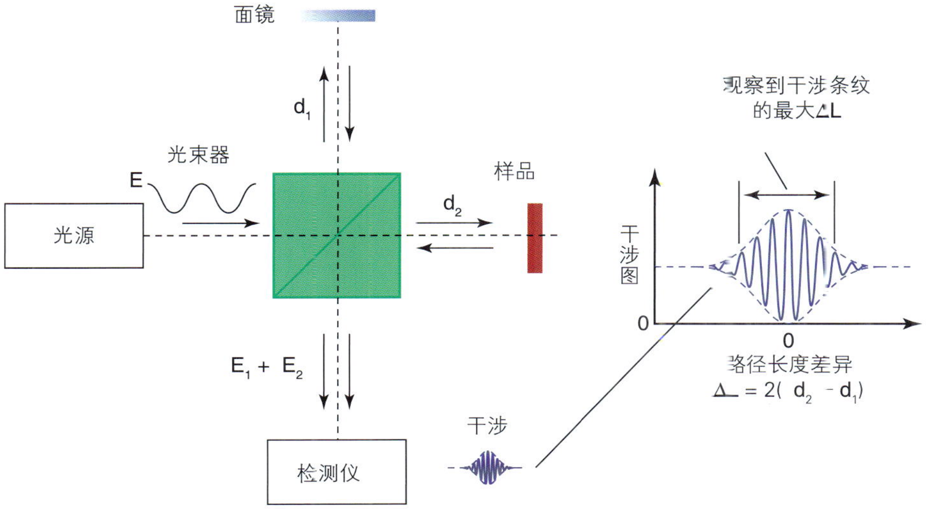

图 2–7　干涉测量仪的基本概念。光被分成 2 束，将从未知的时间和距离（d_2）的样本光束，与从已知时间和距离（d_1）参考镜的光束进行比较（干涉）。只有当样本和参考路径的光程在光相干长度（ΔL）内相匹配，可以检测到一个干涉图。*（译者注：资料来源见前页原文。）*

相干时间和长度都与光源的*光谱带宽*成反比（即光源发出光的频率或波长范围）。注意，具有窄光谱带宽的光源（近单一波长或完全单色的光，如激光）具有高时间相干性，而具有宽频带（多波长光，如白光）具有较低的时间相干性（图 2–8）。

因此，当使用窄带宽光源进行干涉测量（如传统的激光干涉测量仪）时，干涉条纹会出现在 2 个光束之间的路径长度差较长的范围内（视频 2–1）。而在宽带宽光源的低相干干涉测量仪中，只有在光源的相干长度内，光在参考光和光臂中经过的时间几乎相等时，才会发生干涉。因此，低相干干涉仪在分离反射时，特别是当从具有多个密集反射表面的样品中分离反射时，会更为灵敏（视频 2–2）。

视频2–1　传统（激光）干涉测量仪的概念。*（译者注：资料来源见前页原文。）*
在www.aao.org /bcscvideo _ Section 03中访问所有的第三册视频。

视频2–2　低相干干涉测量仪的概念。*（译者注：资料来源见前页原文。）*

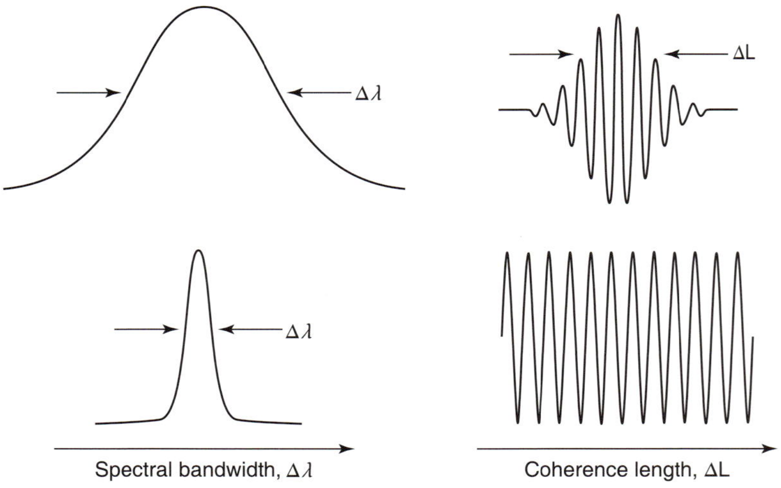

Figure 2-8 Inverse relationship between spectral bandwidth of a light source and its coherence length. A source with a broad bandwidth (light of multiple wavelengths; eg, white light) has a short coherence length (upper panel), whereas a source with a narrow spectral bandwidth (light of nearly a single wavelength or wholly monochromatic; eg, laser light) has a long coherence length (lower panel). *(Illustration developed by Kristina Irsch, PhD.)*

Applications and clinical relevance

One familiar application of interference in ophthalmic optics is the use of *antireflection coatings* on spectacle lenses (Fig 2-9). To decrease unwanted reflections from the surfaces of spectacle lenses, a thin film of a transparent material with a refractive index that is different from the lens is deposited on the lens surface, so that some light will be reflected from the back surface and an equal amount will be reflected at the front surface. These reflected waves—if the thickness of this deposited film is chosen such that it is one-quarter of a specified wavelength of light—will be one-half wavelength out of phase, resulting in complete destructive interference and therefore eliminating the reflections.

The use of *narrow-band interference filters*, such as in fluorescein and indocyanine green angiography, as well as autofluorescence imaging (discussed in Chapter 8), is another application of interference in ophthalmology. To produce very sharp boundaries and separate excitation from fluorescent light, a thin film of a transparent material is deposited on a glass substrate, similar to the previous example but this time with a thickness that is a multiple of the desired wavelength and surfaces that are partially reflecting. Multiple reflections of light with the desired wavelength, from the front and back surfaces of this deposited film, will exit in phase and reinforce each other, whereas light of other wavelengths will exit out of phase and cancel each other (Fig 2-10). Modern narrow-band filters exist that consist of several thin layers of transparent materials allowing only light of wavelengths within a few nanometers to get transmitted while blocking everything else.

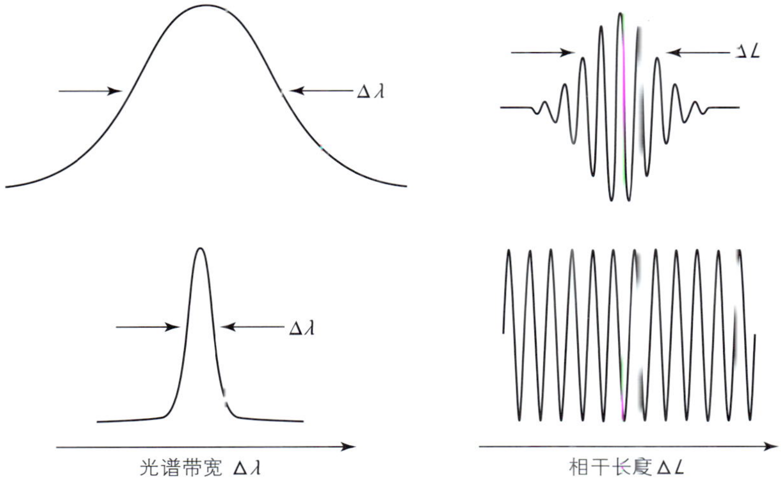

图 2-8　光源光谱带宽与其相干长度的反比关系。宽频带光源（多波长光，如白光）具有较短的相干长度（上图），而光谱带宽较窄的光源（接近单一波长或完全单色的光，如激光）具有较长的相干长度（下图）。*（译者注：资料来源见前页原文。）*

应用与临床相关性

干涉在眼科光学中很常见的应用是眼镜片的减反射涂层（图 2-9）。为了减少不必要的镜片表面的反射，会将折射率不同的透明薄膜涂于镜片表面，这样光从后表面反射，等量光从前表面反射。如果选择的薄膜厚度在指定波长的 1/4 时，就会使这些反射波的 1/2 波长偏离相位，造成完全的相消干涉，从而消除反射。

使用*窄带干涉滤光片*，如荧光素和吲哚菁绿血管造影以及自荧光成像（第 8 章讨论），都是干涉在眼科的另一种应用。为了产生非常尖锐的边界和从荧光光分离的激发现象，而将透明材料的薄膜涂于玻璃基板上，类似于前面的例子，但这次的厚度应该是所需波长和部分反射表面的倍数。从沉积膜的前表面和后表面多次反射到所需波长的光线，会在相位出现，并相互增强，而其他波长的光线会偏离相位出现，并相互抵消（图 2-10）。现代的窄带滤光器是由几层薄薄的透明材料组成的，只允许波长在几纳米范围内的光通过，而阻断其他所有光的通过。

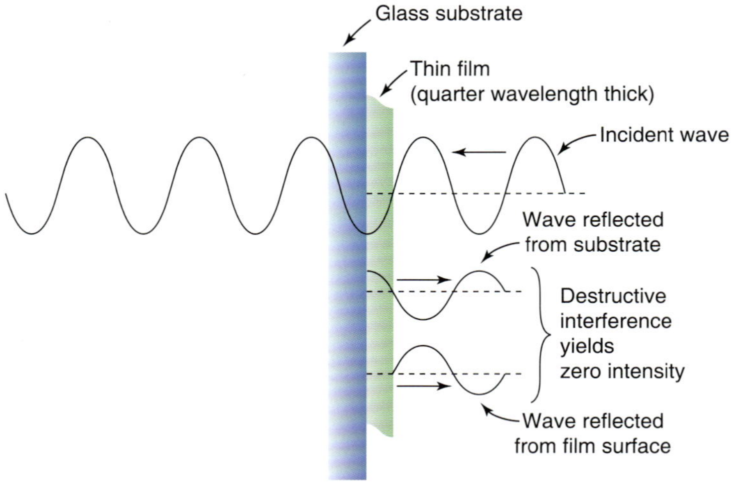

Figure 2-9 Antireflection coating on a spectacle lens. The thickness of the thin film deposition is chosen such that it is one-quarter of a specified wavelength of light, which results in complete destructive interference and therefore eliminates the reflections. *(Redrawn by C. H. Wooley.)*

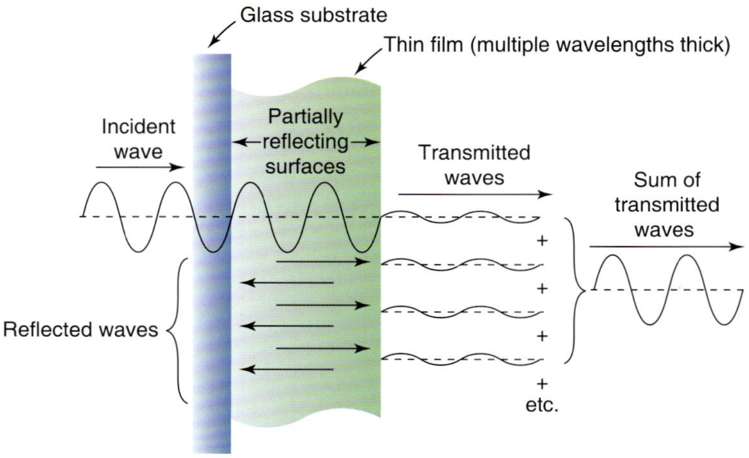

Figure 2-10 Interference filter. Multiple reflections from the front and back surfaces of the deposited film (multiple of a specified light wavelength thick) exit in phase and reinforce each other, whereas light of other wavelengths exits out of phase and cancels each other. *(Redrawn by C. H. Wooley.)*

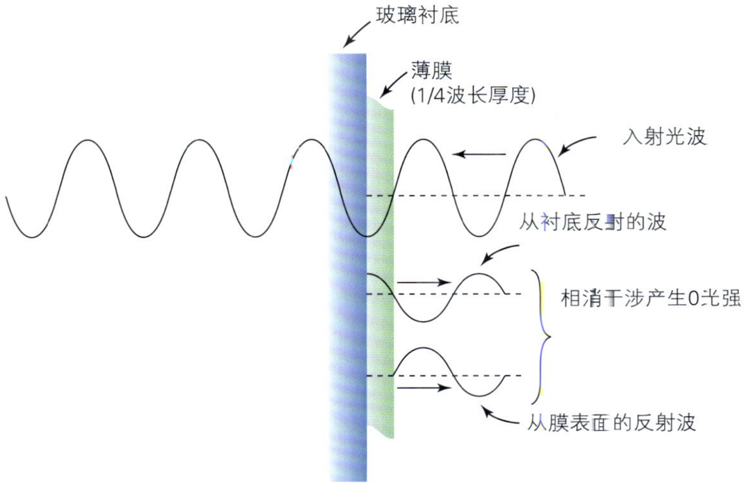

图 2–9　眼镜镜片上的减反射涂层。选择薄膜沉积的厚度为 1/4 指定波长，导致完全的相消干扰，从而消除反射。*（译者注：资料来源见前页原文。）*

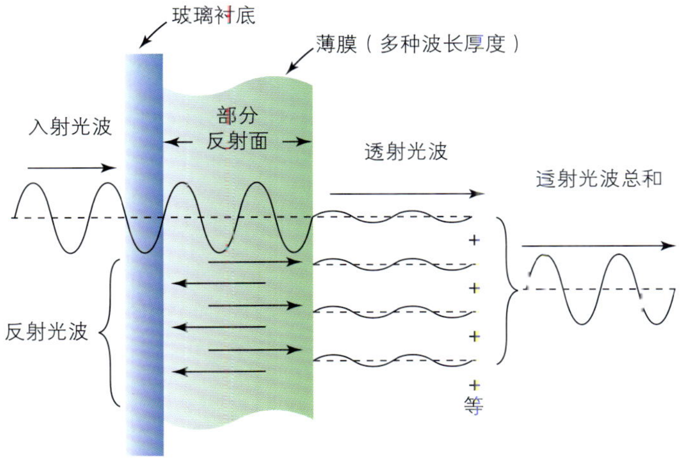

图 2–10　干涉滤波器。沉积膜的前表面和后表面的多次反射（特定波长厚度相乘），相位发出，相互增强，而其他波长的光偏离相位发出，相互抵消。*（译者注：资料来源见前页原文。）*

Diffraction

Fundamentals

If we try to pass light through a very small hole, we will realize that it actually does not go in a straight line, but rather spreads out. This apparent "spreading out beyond the edges" of an aperture or "bending around the corners" of an obstruction, into a region where—using strictly geometric optics reasoning—we would not expect to see it, is referred to as *diffraction*. Diffraction may be thought of as light, when encountering an obstacle, scattering off in different directions at the edges. What really happens, of course, is light interacts with the electrons in the material, most noticeably with the electrons at the edges.

While a more detailed description of diffraction is beyond the scope of this text, we can appreciate that once light scatters off in different directions, it usually interferes with other parts of the diffracted light. Hence, in classical wave theory, the phenomenon of diffraction of light, as it passes beyond an obstacle of comparable size to its wavelength, is generally described as interference effects of the emerging light.

The consequence of these interference effects created by diffraction on apertures is that it sets a limit on the resolution that can be achieved in any optical instrument, which immediately brings us to applications and clinical relevance in ophthalmology.

Applications and clinical relevance

All apertures produce diffraction to some extent, even an opening as large as the pupil of an eye. Thus, we are constantly aware of its effects in ophthalmology.

With a circular aperture, such as the pupil, in the absence of aberrations, the image of a point source of light formed on the retina— the point spread function (PSF)— takes the form of alternating bright and dark rings surrounding a bright central spot, the Airy disc (Fig 2-11), rather than a point. This pattern is the consequence of diffraction and its associated interference effects. The latter are apparent by the concentric bright and dark rings that are analogous to the fringes observed in Young's double- slit experiment (see Fig 2-6). Most of the energy is concentrated in the central disk, so the outer rings are usu-ally ignored. The dia meter of the Airy disc is given by the equation

$$\text{Airy Disc Diameter} \approx 2.44\lambda \frac{f}{D}$$

where D is the diameter of the aperture (pupil) and f is the focal length—the distance from the aperture to the diffracted image. This equation illustrates that longer wavelengths (eg, red light) have a larger Airy disc than shorter wavelengths (eg, blue light) and therefore diffract more. Similarly, diffraction increases as the pupil size decreases.

Under photopic lighting conditions, the pupil of the human eye is around 2–3 mm in diameter. With pupil sizes less than that (for a person with emmetropia), diffraction effects become visually significant, limiting visual acuity. For an eye with a 3-mm-diameter pupil (and f-number, that is f/D, of about 5), for example, and a 555-nm light source, corresponding to the maximum photopic sensitivity of the retina (see the section Measures of Light), the Airy disc diameter is approximately 7.4 µm, encompassing the outer segments of roughly 11 photoreceptors. The smallest resolvable detail is approximately equal to the Airy disc radius. An Airy disc of 3.7 µm radius corresponds roughly to 20/15 visual acuity.

衍射

基本原理

如果让光通过一个很小的孔，就会发现实际上光并不是沿着一条直线，而是向外扩散。这种“超过了孔的边缘”或“在障碍物后弯曲”的扩散，进入一个严格使用几何光学推理不会看到它的区域，被称为*衍射*。衍射是光遇到障碍时，在边缘的不同方向散射。实际上是光与材料中的电子相互作用，而在边缘的电子相互作用最明显。

虽然对于衍射更详细的描述超出了本文的范围，但是我们可以理解，一旦光线分散到不同的方向，它通常会干扰衍射光的其他部分。因此，在经典波理论中，当光通过与波长相当大小的障碍物时的衍射现象称为发射光的干涉效应。

孔的衍射产生的干涉效应的结果是，限制了光学仪器的分辨率　这将应用于眼科和相关临床中。

应用与相关临床

所有的光阑都会在一定程度上产生衍射，即便像眼睛瞳孔一样大的开口也会如此。因此，我们会关注它在眼科的作用。

用一个圆孔，如瞳孔，在没有像差的情况下，让一个点光源在视网膜上的图像——点扩散函数（PSF）——形成了环绕明亮的中央点的明和暗交替环，即 Airy 斑（图 2-11），而不是一个点。这种模式就是衍射及其相关干涉效应的结果。后者呈明暗相间的同心环，与托马斯・杨的双缝实验的条纹相似（见图 2-6）。大部分的能量集中在中央斑，外圈常被忽略。Airy 斑的直径由方程给出

$$\text{Airy 斑的直径} \approx 2.44\lambda\frac{f}{D}$$

其中 D 为孔径（瞳孔），f 为焦距，即孔径到衍射像的距离。这个方程表明，较长的波长（如红光）比较短的波长（如蓝光）的 Airy 斑更大、衍射更多。同样地，衍射随着瞳孔缩小而增大。

在光照条件下，人眼的瞳孔直径约为 2~3mm。瞳孔小于这个值（对于正视眼来说），衍射效应在视觉上非常重要，它限制了视力。一个 3mm 瞳孔直径（f/D 为 5），如 555 nm 光源，对应于最大光敏感度的视网膜（见光的测量一节），Airy 斑直径约 7.4 μm，包括了外段大约 11 个光感受器。最小可分辨值近似等于 Airy 斑的半径。一个 Airy 斑的半径 3.7 μm 对应大约 20/15 视力。

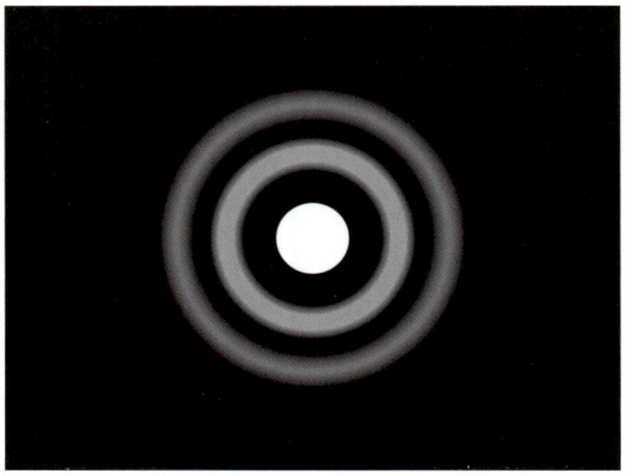

Figure 2-11 Diffraction pattern produced by a small circular aperture. The central bright spot is called an Airy disc. *(From Campbell, CJ. Physiologic Optics. Hagerstown, MD: Harper & Row; 1974:20.)*

Thus, in theory, the larger the pupil size, the smaller the Airy disc and therefore bet- ter visual acuity or higher resolution of the image on the retina. However, in practice (as discussed in Chapter 8), higher-order aberrations occur at larger pupil sizes. While there are ways to correct for wavefront aberrations (adaptive optics, discussed in Chapter 8), we cannot suppress diffraction. It sets an absolute limit on the best resolution obtainable with any optical system, including the eye, and is represented by the Airy disc pattern (see Fig 2-11).

Diffraction can also be used to an advantage in ophthalmic optics, in the creation of bifocal or multifocal lenses. For example, etching a specially designed pattern of closely spaced circular steps on one of the surfaces of a contact or intraocular lens can cause light to diffract, such that the resulting interference effects of the diffracted light create a second near focal point for the lens, with the overall curvature of the lens simultaneously providing distance focus.

Measures of Light

For many clinicians, the measurement of light is one of the most confusing topics in the field of clinical optics. This section will attempt to clarify the subject.

As we learned previously, light is a range of electromagnetic radiant energy, comprising the range of wavelengths to which the eye is ordinarily sensitive—about 400–700 nm. The measurement of light thus naturally derives from more general methods for the measurement of electromagnetic radiant energy—specifically, from general methods to measure the *transfer* of energy by electromagnetic radiation.

Energy is the ability of a system to perform work. Through the insights of physics and thermodynamics, energy is understood to take many forms, including kinetic energy, the energy of objects in motion; potential energy, the energy stored in a system by virtue of its position (such as the height of an object subject to gravity); chemical energy, the potential energy available through chemical reactions; and thermal energy, the energy stored in the temperature of objects. Thus, the units for work and energy are the same—typically joules ($J = kg{\cdot}m^2/s^2$).

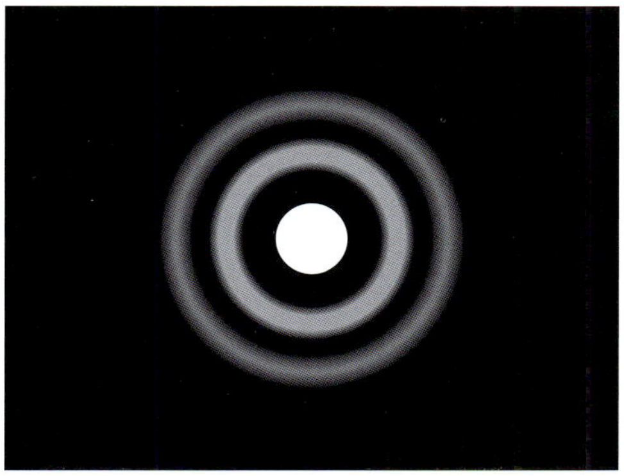

图 2–11　小孔衍射图。中心的亮点被称为 Airy 斑。*（译者注：资料来源见前页原文。）*

因此，从理论上讲，瞳孔越大，Airy 斑衍射越小，视网膜上像的视敏度或分辨率就越高。然而，在实践中（如第 8 章所讨论的），高阶像差发生在直径较大的瞳孔。虽然有纠正波前像差的方法（“自适应光学”，在第 8 章讨论），但我们也不能抑制衍射。它为包括眼睛在内的任何光学系统所能获得的最佳分辨率设置了绝对限制，并以 Airy 斑图案表示（见图 2–11）。

衍射也可以用于眼科光学，如双焦或多焦镜。在接触镜或人工晶体刻蚀一个特别设计的密集环形阶梯时，其衍射光的干涉效应产生透镜的第二个近焦，同时透镜的整体弯曲提供远焦点。

光的测量

对许多临床医生来说，光的测量是临床光学领域中最令人困惑的课题之一。本节将试图阐明这个主题。

正如之前所述，光是一种电磁辐射能量的范围，包括了眼睛敏感的波长范围，为 400~700nm。因此，光的测量就是测量电磁辐射能的方法，具体地说，是从通过电磁辐射测量能量交换的一般方法。

能量是一个系统做功的能力。通过物理学和热力学的学习，能量可以理解为有多种形式，包括动能，运动物体的能量；势能，系统中因其位置（如受重力影响的物体的高度）而储存的能量；化学能，化学反应产生的势能；热能，储存在物体温度中的能量。因此，功和能的单位是相同的，为焦耳（$1\ J = 1\ kg \cdot m^2/s^2$）。

Power is the rate at which energy is transformed or transferred from one form to another. It is measured in units of work (or energy) per unit time, typically joules per second (J/s), or watts (W). Historically, this unit and its multiples have served in most contexts for measuring the rate of energy transfer, from the output of a gasoline engine to the energy required to operate a computer microprocessor chip. The watt is used without difficulty whatever the form of the energy transfer, from mechanical devices, to electrical power lines, to heat generation. Derived quantities are described in simple combinations of units—for example, the productivity of solar panels might be described in units of power per unit area—say, W/m^2.

Radiometry

Measurements of the power transferred by means of electromagnetic radiation are typically described with derived units in accordance with the above scheme (Table2-2). In principle, the fundamental measurement tool for this purpose is the blackbody radiometer. This is an object (frequently realized in the form of a hollow cavity), which absorbs radiant electromagnetic radiation at all wavelengths with equal efficiency. The amount of energy absorbed is determined by measuring the increase in the temperature of the blackbody, and converting heat to energy according to the laws of thermodynamics and knowledge of the heat capacity of the detector, and dividing by the length of time the radiometer was exposed to the radiation. (In practice, radiometers are designed to work only over limited ranges of the electromagnetic spectrum, depending on the physics of the detector employed.)

In practice, care must be taken to account for the geometry of the source of the radiation, and for the geometry of the detector. The simplest case is a point source, radiating equally in all directions—the power output of such a device is appropriately measured simply in watts. But it would be difficult to surround such a point source with a detector, which would simultaneously absorb the output in every direction. Typically, the detector will intercept the radiation over only a small area. In this case (assuming the radiation output to be uniform in every direction), it would be appropriate to normalize the measurement by dividing the energy transfer intercepted by the detector by the solid angle it subtends (in essence, the area of the detector divided by the distance from the point source), thus reporting the energy output of the point source in watts per steradian (W/sr), with the understanding that multiplying by 4π (the total solid angle of the space surrounding a point) would yield the energy output of the point source, in watts. This description of the energy output from a point source is referred to as its *radiant intensity*.

Table 2-2 Comparison of Radiometric and Photometric Units

Radiometric Quantity	SI Unit	Photometric Quantity	SI Unit
Radiant energy, Q_e	joule (J) = watt second (W · s)	Luminous energy, Q_v	lumen second (lm · s)
Fluence, H_e	joules per meter² (J/m²) = (W · s/m²)	Luminous exposure, H_v	lumen second per meter² (lm · s/m²)
Radiant flux, Φ_e	watt (W)	Luminous flux, Φ_v	lumen (lm) = candela steradian (cd · sr)
Radiant intensity, I_e	watts per steradian (W/sr)	Luminous intensity, I_v	candela (cd)
Irradiance, E_e	watts per meter² (W/m²)	Illuminance, E_v	lux (lx) = (cd · sr/m²) = (lm/m²)
Radiance, L_e	watts per meter² per steradian (W/m² · sr)	Luminance, L_v	nit (cd/m²) = (lm/m² · sr)

功率是能量从一种形式转换到另一种形式的速率。测量时以单位时间做的功（或能量）为单位，单位为焦耳每秒（J / s），或瓦特（W）。从历史上看，这个单元及其倍数在大多数情况下测量的是，从汽油发动机的输出到操作电脑微处理器芯片所需要的能量的传递速度。无论能量以何种形式从机械设备、电力线路、热能上产生，它们都能使用瓦特作为单位来表达。派生的量用简单的单位组合来描述，例如，太阳能电池板的生产率可以用单位面积功率作为单位来描述，如 W/m^2。

辐射度学

通过电磁辐射传输的功率的测量，常用导出单元按照上述方案来进行描述（表 2–2）。原则上，用于此目的的基本测量工具是黑体辐射计。这种物体（通常以空腔的形式实现）以相等的效率吸收所有波长辐射的电磁辐射。吸收的能量计算为，黑体增加的温度测量值，以及根据热力学定律和已知热容探测器将热量转化为的能量值，除以辐射计被暴露在辐射中的时间。（实际上，根据所使用的探测器的物理特性，辐射计只能在有限的电磁波谱范围内工作。）

在实践中，必须注意辐射源的几何学，以及探测器的几何学。最简单的例子是点辐射源，它在所有方向上的辐射都是相等的——这种设备的输出功率以瓦特为单位进行测量。但要在这样的点辐射源周围装上探测器是很困难的，因为探测器会同时从各个方向吸收输出。通常，探测器只会在一小块区域内拦截辐射。在这种情况下（假设辐射输出在各个方向均匀），通过将探测器拦截的能量传输除以其所包含的立体角度来进行规范测量（即用探测器的面积除以点辐射源的距离）是合适的。因此，以瓦特每球面度（W/sr）为单位的点辐射源的能量输出乘以 4π（围绕点空间的总立体角），就会得到以瓦特（W）为单位的辐射源的能量输出。对点辐射源输出能量的描述称为*辐射强度*。

表2–2　辐射计量单位与光度计量单位比较

辐射度学量	SI单位	光度学量	SI单位
辐射能量, Q_e	1J=1W·s	发光能量, Q_v	lm·s
积分通量, H_e	$1J/m^2 = 1W·s/m^2$	光照量, H_v	$lm·s/m^2$
辐射流, Φ_e	W	光通量, Φ_v	1lm = 1cd·sr
辐射强度, I_e	W/sr	发光强度, I_v	cd
辐照度, E_e	W/m^2	照度, E_v	$1 x = 1cd·sr/m^2 = 1lm/m^2$
辐射, L_e	$W/m^2·sr$	亮度, L_v	$nit = 1cd/m^2 = 1lm/m^2·sr$

Similarly, if the radiation source is an extended planar object, the appropriate description of its energy output would be in terms of watts per unit area, say W/m^2. This description of the energy output is referred to as the radiant exitance of the extended source. If one prefers to measure the rate at which radiant energy impinges on an extended object, the appropriate units are again, W/m^2, but in this context, the energy transfer is referred to as *irradiance*.

Note that "intensity," depending on the context or the background of the person using the term, can have alternative meanings. In optics and particular laser physics, it generally refers to power density (ie, radiometric irradiance) and most commonly is expressed in watts per square centimeter (W/cm^2).

Photometry

Photometry is the modification of the scheme described above so as to reflect the variable sensitivity of human vision to light of different wavelengths, in contrast to the radiometric measurements, which weight equally the energy transmitted at every wavelength of the electromagnetic spectrum.

This adjustment is based on empirical measurements of the relative sensitivity of human vision to light of the various wavelengths. This weighting curve is referred to as the *spectral luminous efficiency function*, usually denoted by $V(\lambda)$ or V_λ. The photometric measurement of the radiant energy output or input in a system is the summation (or, better, integral) of the energy transfer at each wavelength multiplied by the value of V_λ for that wavelength.

Unfortunately, for historical reasons, unlike the case for radiometric measurements, the derived units for each geometric variant of this process for photometric measurements have been given different names, further complicating these discussions.

The photometric equivalent of the measurement of the total radiant output of a point source is the *lumen* (lm), the V_λ-weighted version of the watt. This quantity is referred to as the *luminous flux*. For example, the output of an ordinary incandescent or light-emitting diode (LED) light bulb (which can be regarded for most purposes as a point source) is now often indicated in lumens. A 60-W incandescent bulb might typically have a light output of 800 lumens. (In contrast, an 800-lumen LED bulb might consume only 12W of power.)

The photometric equivalent of the measurement of the radiant output of a point source per unit of solid angle is the *candela* (cd), or lm/sr. This quantity is referred to as the *luminous intensity* of the point source. For historical reasons, the candela is the primary SI (metric system) unit for the measurement of light, intended to approximate the light output of the standard wax candles which were originally used for this purpose. One cd is defined as the luminous intensity of a source emitting monochromatic radiation at a frequency of 540THz and a radiant intensity of 1/683W/sr. Note that 540THz corresponds to approximately 555nm ($=c \times 10^9 / f = 3 \times 10^8 \times 10^9 / 540 \times 10^{12}$), the wavelength to which the human eye is most sensitive under light-adapted or photopic lighting conditions, and that 1/683 was chosen to make 1cd equal to the old unit, the "candle," which was based on the actual luminous intensity of a wax candle flame.

The photometric equivalent of the measurement of the radiant output of an extended planar source is the $lumen/m^2$. This quantity is referred to as the *luminous exitance*.

Conversely, the photometric equivalent of the measurement of the radiant energy incident on an extended planar surface is also measured in $lumen/m^2$. This quantity is known as the *illuminance*. As a unit for illuminance, the lm/m^2 is known as the *lux*.

同样的，如果辐射源是一个扩展的平面物体，它的能量输出的描述应该是瓦每单位面积，例如 W/m^2。这种对能量输出的描述称为扩展源的辐射出射度。如果测量辐射能量对扩展物体的作用率，则使用单位 W/m^2，但在这种情况下，能量传递被称为*辐照度*。

值得注意的是，根据使用该术语的上下文或背景，“强度”有不同的含义。在光学和特殊的激光物理中，它通常是指功率密度（即辐射辐照度），最常用的单位是瓦特每平方厘米（W/cm^2）。

光度学

*光度学*测定是对上述测量值的修正，以反映人类视觉对不同波长光变化的敏感性，对辐射测量值，在电磁波谱的每个波长辐射能同等加权。

这种调整是基于人类视觉对不同波长光的相对灵敏度的经验测量值。权重曲线被称为*光谱发光效率函数*，常用 $V(\lambda)$ 或 V_λ 表示。对系统的辐射能输出或输入的光度测量，是对每种波长的能量传递之总和（或积分更佳）乘以该波长的 V_λ 值。

与辐射测量不同，由于历史原因，光度测量中每一种几何变量的导出单位都有不同的名称，使这些讨论更加复杂。

点辐射源的总辐射输出的光度学等效测量值单位是*流明*（lm），以 V_λ 的单位瓦特加权，这个量称为*光通量*。如普通白炽灯或发光二极管（LED）灯泡（大多数情况下视为点光源）的输出以流明表示。一个 60W 的白炽灯泡通常有 800lm 的光输出。（相比之下，800lm 的 LED 灯泡可能只消耗 12W 的电能。）

点辐射源，单位立体角辐射输出的光度学等效测量值单位为*坎德拉*(cd)，或 lm/sr。这个量称为点辐射的*发光强度*。由于历史原因，坎德拉是测量光的主要 SI（国际单位制）单位，目的是接近最初用于这一目的的标准蜡烛的光输出。1cd 为源点发出单色辐射的发光强度，其频率为 540 THz、辐射强度为 1/683W/sr。注意，540THz 对应于 555nm（$= c \times 10^9 / f = 3 \times 10^8 \times 10^9 / 540 \times 10^{12}$），是人眼在明适应或适应光的照明条件下最敏感的波长，将 1/683 定义为 1cd，其值约等于以前的单位“烛光”，这也是基于实际蜡烛火焰的发光强度。

扩展平面辐射源辐射输出的光度学等效单位为 lm/m^2。这个量称为*光出射度*。

相反，在扩展平面上入射辐射测量的光度学等效量也以 lm/m^2 为单位。这个量被称为*照度*。作为照度的单位，lm/m^2 被称为勒克斯（lx）。

The spectral luminous efficiency function depends in practice on the state of light adaptation or dark-adaptation of the eye. Most measurements are made under light-adapted conditions, and use the light-adapted (or photopic) efficiency function. Under dark-adapted (scotopic) conditions, the efficiency function shifts toward shorter wavelengths (the Purkinje shift), reflecting the difference between the absorption spectrum of rhodopsin (the visual pigment in retinal rods) and the summed absorption spectra of the 3 visual pigments in the retinal cones. The scotopic spectral luminance efficiency function is often referred to as $V'(\lambda)$ or V'_{λ}. It has a maximum at 507nm, whereas the photopic efficiency function has a maximum at 555nm. In precise work, the choice of luminance efficiency function should be specified.

Further note that the terms *radiance* or *luminance* are not used simply as the counterparts for emitting surfaces of the terms *irradiance* or *illuminance* for absorbing surfaces. Rather, radiance refers to the radiant intensity per unit area, and thus is expressed in units of $W/sr{\cdot}m^2$. The corresponding photometric quantity, luminance, refers to the luminous intensity per unit area, and is thus expressed in units of $cd/m^2 = lm/sr{\cdot}m^2$. This last unit is also referred to as the *nit.* Table2-3 lists other alternative units commonly used to measure illuminance and luminance. To help you develop a "feel" for photometric units, Table2-4 lists photometric values associated with visual functions.

Table 2-3 Various Photometric Units and Their Conversion Factors

Photometric Quantity	SI Unit	Alternative Units and Conversion Factors (Some Are Obsolete)
Illuminance, E_v	lux	1 lux = 1 lm/m^2 = 1 m · cd
		1 phot = 1 lm/cm^2 = 10,000 lux
		1 milliphot = 10 lux
		1 foot-candle = 1 lm/ft^2 = 10.76 lux
Luminance, L_v	nit	nit = 1 cd/m^2
		Stilb = 1 cd/cm^2 = 10,000 nits
		Apostilb = (1/π) cd/m^2 ≈ 0.32 nits
		cd/ft^2 = 10.76 nits
		cd/in^2 = 1550 nits
		1 foot-lambert = 1/π · ft = 3.426/m^2

Table 2-4 Luminance Levels Associated With Various Visual Functions

Visual Function	Luminance (nits)
Best acuity	1000
Cone threshold	10^{-4}
Damage	10^{8}
Limit of rod sensitivity	10^{-7}
Mesopic range	10^{-4}–10
Photopic range	10–10^{8}
Rod saturation	10
Scotopic range	10^{-7}–10^{-4}

光谱光效率函数在实际应用中取决于人眼的明适应或暗适应状态。大多数测量都是在明适应条件下进行的，并使用明适应（明视）效率函数。在暗适应（暗视）条件下，效率函数向较短波长（Purkinje 位移）移动，反映了视紫红质（视杆细胞内视色素）的吸收光谱与视锥细胞内 3 种视色素的总吸收光谱的差异。暗光谱亮度效率函数常称为 $V'(\lambda)$ 或 V'_{λ}。它在 507 nm 处最大，而明适应效率函数在 555 nm 处最大。在精密工作中，应具体选择亮度效率函数。

值得注意的是，*辉度*或*亮度*是用作发射表面的术语，而*辐照度*或*照度*是用作吸收表面的术语，并非是简单的对应项。辐射度是指单位面积的辐射强度，用 $W/(sr \cdot m^2)$ 表示。对应的光度学，亮度是指单位面积的发光强度，用 cd/m^2 或 $lm/(sr \cdot m^2)$ 表示。前一个单位也就是*尼特（nt）*。表 2–3 列出了其他常用的测量照度和亮度的替代单位。为了帮助读者理解光度学单位，表 2–4 列出了与视觉功能相关的光度学值。

表2–3　各种光度单位及其换算系数

光照度	SI 单位	可供选择的单位和换算系数 (有些已经过时)
照度, E_v	lx	1 lx = 1 lm/m^2 = 1 cd·sr/m^2*
		1 ph = 1 lm/cm^2 = 10 000 lx
		1 mph = 10 lx
		1 ft · cd = 1 lm/ft^2 = 10.76 lx
亮度, L_v	nt	1 nt = 1 cd/m^2
		1sb= 1 cd/cm^2 = 10 000 nt
		1asb= (1/π) cd/m^2 ≈ 0.32 nt
		1cd/ft^2 = 10.76 nt
		1cd/in^2 = 1550 nt
		1 ft · L = 1/π · ft = 3.426cd/m^2

** 译者注：此公式原文（见前页）有误，此处予以更正。*

表2–4　与各种视觉功能相关的亮度等级

视功能	亮度 /nt
最佳视力	1000
视锥细胞阈值	10^{-4}
损伤	10^{8}
视杆细胞敏度极限	10^{-7}
中间介适应范围	10^{-4}~10
明适应范围	10~10^{8}
视杆细胞饱和	10
暗适应范围	10^{-7}~10^{-4}

Conversion Between Radiometric and Photometric Outputs

So now that we defined the radiometric and photometric measures of light, how do we convert from one to the other? In other words, if a light source has a known radiometric output, can we determine its corresponding photometric output? Yes, if we know the spectral properties of the lamp, that is, the radiometric output at each wavelength. Then, the output at each wavelength is multiplied by the sensitivity of the eye to that wavelength as well as by the conversion factor that is given by the definition of the candela (according to which there are 683 lumens per watt for 555-nm light), and the results are summed to obtain the total response of the eye to light from that source.

For example, if a light source has a known output in watts, how much is its output in lumens? If we assume a monochromatic light source, such as a 650-nm (red) laser pointer with a photometric power of 5mW, the photoptic weighting factor is 0.096, and therefore the corresponding luminous flux is 0.096 × 0.005W × 683lm/W = 0.33lm. If we had a green (532nm) laser pointer, this value would rise to 0.828 × 0.005W × 683lm/ W = 2.83lm.

Light Sources: Lasers

The classical theory of electromagnetic waves successfully explains "macroscopic" light phenomena, but fails to explain phenomena at the atomic and molecular levels. Quantum theory, as illustrated in Figure2-3B, can explain such phenomena. For the following considerations, it therefore becomes crucial to consider the quantum behavior of light.

According to quantum theory, electrons in atoms (or molecules) exist in *nonradiating* states and each state is associated with a specific energy level. The energy states possible for an atom differ from element to element, and those for a molecule differ from compound to compound. Each element or compound has a unique distribution of energy states. When an electron drops from a higher energy state to a lower one, the difference in energy (E) is radiated as a packet, called a photon, with a characteristic frequency (ν) given by

$$E = h\nu$$

where h is the Planck constant. Similarly, an electron can jump to a higher energy state by absorbing a photon, with the resulting energy absorption equal to the energy difference between states (see Fig 2-3B).

Fundamentals

When an electron absorbs a photon and jumps to a higher energy level (*stimulated absorption*, see Fig 2-3B), usually it quickly drops back to the original level and emits a photon identical in frequency to the one it absorbed (*spontaneous emission*, see Fig 2-3B).

However, atoms of some elements have 2 energy levels that are close together. When a photon is absorbed, the electron jumps to the highest energy level. Instead of dropping back to the original level, the electron first transitions to the slightly lower level without emitting visible energy. Next, it drops to the initial energy level and emits a photon. The emitted photon has less energy than the stimulating, absorbed photon and, therefore, a lower frequency, or longer wavelength (and different perceived color). This phenomenon, called *fluorescence*, occurs only in materials possessing close spacing between energy levels. Its clinical utility derives from the essential feature that the absorbed and emitted photons have a different wavelength and is the basis of fluorescein angiography and macular autofluorescence (discussed in Chapter 8).

辐射和光度输出之间的转换

我们定义了光的辐射测量和光度测量，但如何将两者相互转换？换句话说，如果已知光源的辐射输出，就能够确定它相应的光度输出吗？是可以的，如果我们知道灯的光谱特性，也就知道了每个波长的辐射输出。然后，每个波长的输出乘以眼对该波长的敏感度以及给出的坎德拉转换因子（对于眼睛的 555nm 最敏感波长，需给辐射输出 683lm/W）。对结果进行求和就可以得到眼睛对该辐射源发出光的总反应。

例如，如果已知光源的输出功率，它的输出流明是多少？假设一个单色光源，如光度学功率为 5mW 的 650nm（红色）激光笔，明适应权重因子为 0.096，相应的光通量是 0.096 × 0.005W × 683lm/W =0.33lm。如果有一个绿色激光笔（532 nm），这个值将升至 0.828 × 0.005 W × 683 lm/W =2.83 lm。

光源：激光

经典的电磁波理论成功地解释了“宏观”的光现象，但不能在原子和分子水平上解释光现象。如图 2–3B 所示，量子理论可以解释这种现象。因此，考虑光的量子行为就变得至关重要。

根据量子理论，原子（或分子）中的电子以*非辐射*状态存在，每个状态都与特定的能级有关。原子的能态因元素的不同而不同，分子的能态因化合物的不同而不同。每个元素或化合物都有独特的能态分布。当电子从一个较高的能量状态下降到较低的能量状态时，能量（E）的差异作为一个整体，称为光子被辐射，其频率（ν）为

$$E = h\nu$$

其中 h 是 Planck 常数。同样的，电子通过吸收光子可以跃迁到更高的能级，得到的能量吸收等于能级之间的能量差（见图 2–3B）。

基本原理

当电子吸收光子并跃迁到更高的能级（*受激吸收*，见图 2–3B）时，通常会迅速回落到原来的能级，并发射出与被吸收光子频率相同的光子（*自发发射*，见图 2–3B）。

然而，一些元素的原子有 2 个能级是紧密相连的。当光子被吸收时，电子跃迁到最高能级。电子没有回落到原来的能级，而是先跃迁到稍低的能级，而不发射可见能量。接下来，它下降到初始能级，并发射光子。发射光子与激发、吸收的光子相比，能量较低，因此，频率较低，或波长较长（以及感知颜色不同）。这种现象叫作荧光，只发生在能级间距很近的材料中。其临床应用源于吸收和发射光子具有不同波长这一基本特征，是荧光血管造影和黄斑自发荧光的基础（见第 8 章）。

In most cases, electrons remain in elevated energy states for very short periods. However, the elevated state is sometimes metastable; that is, the electron may remain in the elevated state for several seconds or longer before dropping back down. Such a process describes how light is produced by *phosphorescence*, which is essentially identical to fluorescence except that the transitions take longer. Light resulting from fluorescence stops immediately after removal of the exciting energy, whereas light resulting from phosphorescence persists long after the exciting energy ceases.

A photon of appropriate frequency passing near an electron in a metastable state may stimulate the electron immediately to drop to a lower state and radiate an identical photon (Fig 2-12). Such *stimulated emission* is the basis of the light emission in lasers. In fact, the word *laser* originated as an acronym for Light Amplification by Stimulated Emission of Radiation.

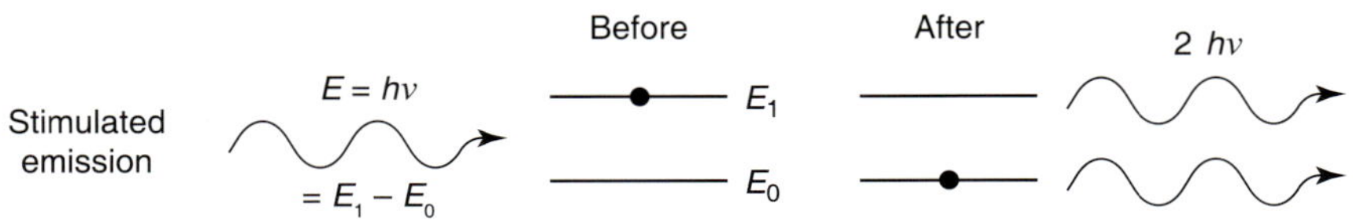

Figure 2-12 In a process called stimulated emission, which is the basis of light emission in lasers, a photon of appropriate frequency passing near an electron in an excited state may stimulate the electron to drop to a lower state and emit an identical photon. *(Reproduced with permission from Steinert RF, Puliafito CA. The Nd:YAG Laser in Ophthalmology: Principles and Clinical Applications of Photodisruption. Philadelphia: Saunders; 1985. Redrawn by C. H. Wooley.)*

Lasers use an *active medium* with an appropriate metastable state. Energy is introduced into the active medium in a variety of ways. For example, *optical pumping* uses a bright incoherent light source to excite a large number of electrons into the metastable state. The active medium is inside a *resonator cavity*, which typically has a fully reflecting mirror on one end and a partially reflecting one on the other; this design causes light to make numerous passes through the active medium, producing more and more photons by stimulated emission with each pass (Fig 2-13).

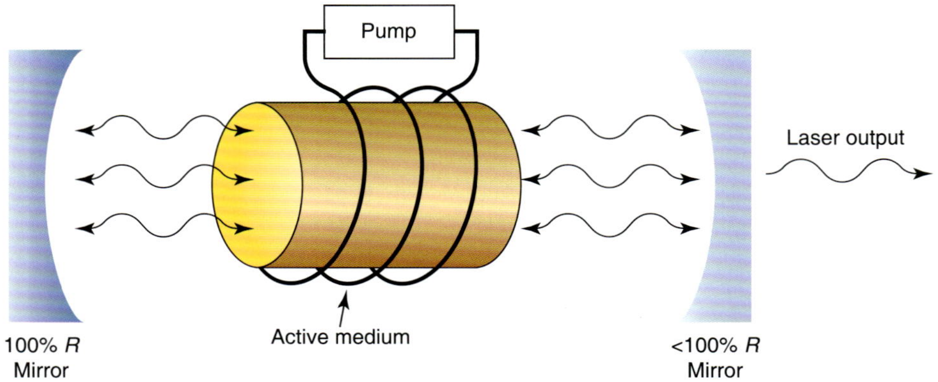

Figure 2-13 Simple schematic of a laser illustrating the active medium within the resonator cavity formed by the mirrors and the pump, which raises a majority of electrons to elevated states (population inversion) in the active medium. One mirror is fully reflective (100% *R*), whereas the other is partially transparent (<100% *R*). As drawn, the mirror is 66% reflective, and the average light wave makes 3 round-trips through the active medium before being emitted. *(Reproduced with permission from Steinert RF, Puliafito CA. The Nd:YAG Laser in Ophthalmology: Principles and Clinical Applications of Photodisruption. Philadelphia: Saunders; 1985. Redrawn by Jonathan Clark.)*

在大多数情况下，电子在很短的时间内处于高能量状态。上升状态有时呈亚稳态，也就是说，电子可能会在上升状态停留几秒钟或更长时间，之后下落。这描述了*磷光*如何产生光。磷光与荧光本质上是相同的，只是转换时间更长。荧光产生的光在激发能被去除后立即停止，而磷光产生的光在激发能停止后仍能长期存在。

适当频率的光子经过亚稳态电子附近时，可立即激发电子降至较低的状态，并辐射出相等的光子（图 2–12）。这种*受激发射*是激光器发射光的基础。事实上，*激光*一词就是通过辐射的受激发射的光放大的缩写。

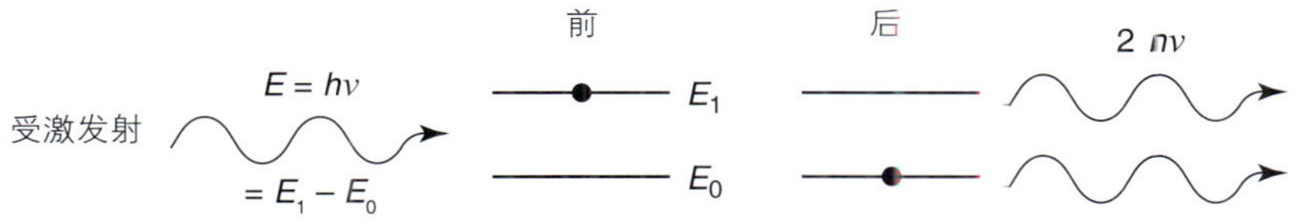

图 2–12　在受激发射的过程中，一个相应频率的光子经过处于激发态的电子附近时，会激发电子降至较低的状态，并发射出相等的光子，这是激光发射光的基础。*（译者注：资料来源见前页原文。）*

激光器使用具有适当亚稳态的*活性介质*。能量以各种方式被引入到活性介质中。例如，*光泵*利用一个明亮的非相干光源激发大量电子进入亚稳态。活性介质位于*谐振腔*内，谐振腔通常是一端为全反射镜，另一端为部分反射镜。这种设计使光在活性介质中可以多次通过，每一次通过就会受激辐射从而产生更多的光子（图 2–13）。

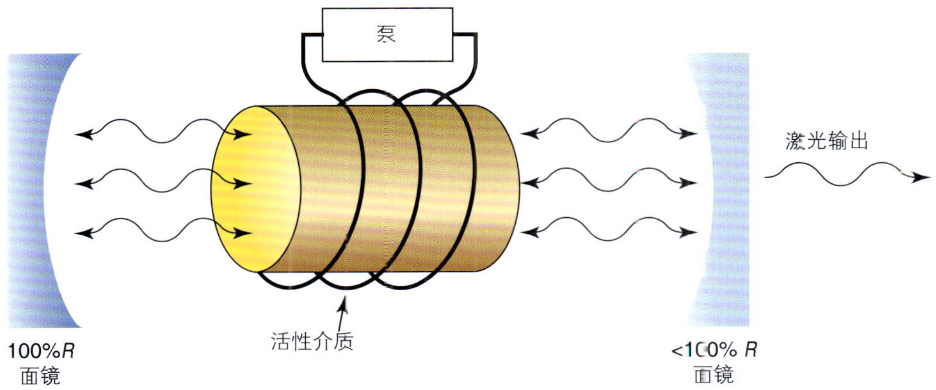

图 2–13　激光器的简单示意图，说明了由反射镜和泵形成的谐振腔内的活性介质，该谐振腔将大多数电子提升到活性介质中的高能态（粒子数反转）。一面镜子是完全反射的（100% *R*），另一面是部分透明的（<100% *R*），如图所示，镜子的反射率为 66%，平均光波在发射前经过活性介质 3 次往返。*（译者注：资料来源见前页原文。）*

Contrary to common belief, lasers are not very efficient light sources. Compared with the amount of energy required to power a laser, the amount of energy produced is modest. The light produced, however, has unique and useful characteristics. Laser light has a very narrow bandwidth (ie, it is nearly a single wavelength or monochromatic) and, consequently, it has high temporal coherence. The coherence length is relatively long—about half the length of the resonator cavity—typically a few centimeters. Lasers are the most intense sources of monochromatic light available.

Although the total energy in laser light may be slight, it can be focused on a very small area to produce a very high energy density (ie, energy that is transferred per square centimeter, or fluence; see Table2-2). Laser light is also highly directional and, depending on the design of the resonator, may also be polarized.

Lasers are usually named after their active medium. The medium can be a gas (argon, krypton, carbon dioxide, argon with fluoride [excimer], or helium with neon), a liquid (dye), a solid (an active element supported by a crystal, such as neodymium: yttrium-aluminumgarnet [Nd:YAG] and titanium: sapphire [Ti:Sapphire]), or a semiconductor (diode).

Lasers may operate continuously (eg, an argon laser for photocoagulation), commonly referred to as *continuous wave*, or in pulses (eg, a Nd:YAG laser for capsulotomy). Modelocking and Q-switching are 2 common methods of producing a *pulsed* output. The details of such methods are beyond the scope of this chapter. Note, however, that while *Q-switching* allows for the production of short pulses (mainly on the order of nanoseconds, ie, 10^{-9} s), it is *mode-locking* that can produce *ultrashort pulses*, with a duration on the order of picoseconds (ie, 10^{-12} s) or less, depending on the properties of the laser. In fact, the pulse duration is mainly dependent on the spectral bandwidth of the laser medium; the larger its spectral bandwidth, the shorter the pulse that can be realized. Thus, ultrashort laser pulses are not monochromatic, and for the generation of femtosecond pulses, a laser with a large spectral bandwidth is required. For a Ti:Sapphire laser with a 128-THz spectral bandwidth, for example, the shortest pulse that can be created would be around 3.4 femtoseconds (ie, 10^{-15} s)

We have learned previously that power is the amount of energy delivered in a given time period. A watt is 1 joule of energy delivered over 1 second. The same joule delivered over a nanosecond has a power of 1 billion watts; over a picosecond, 1 trillion watts; and over a femtosecond, 1 quadrillion watts. Pulsing is a way of increasing the power of a laser's output by delivering a modest amount of energy over a very short period.

Therapeutic Laser–Tissue Interactions

The fundamental process of any therapeutic laser application is the energy transfer to the tissue via absorption of light, which is a function of the nature of the tissue (its distribution of energy states) as well as the wavelength (photon energy) of the light. Therapeutic laser–tissue interactions may be divided into 5 different types (Table2-5), each of which will be discussed in detail: *photochemical interaction*, *thermal interaction*, *photoablation*, *plasma-induced ablation*, and *photodisruption*. These mechanisms are primarily determined by the power density (irradiance) of the laser light and its interaction time (laser pulse duration) with the tissue. All therapeutic laser–tissue interaction mechanisms share a common characteristic, in that all meaningful energy densities (the energy that is transferred to the tissue—fluence) vary typically between 1 and 1000J/cm^2 (Fig 2-14).

Niemz MK. *Laser-Tissue Interactions: Fundamentals and Applications*. 3rd ed. New York: Springer; 2007.

与普遍的看法相反，激光不是很有效的光源。与激光所需的能量相比，激光产生的能量是有限的。然而，激光产生的光具有独特而有用的特性。激光具有非常窄的带宽（即它几乎是一个波长或单色），因此，它具有高度的时间相干性。相干长度相对较长——大约是谐振腔长度的 1/2——通常只有几厘米。激光是最强的可用的单色光源。

虽然激光的总能量可能很小，但它可以聚焦在一个很小的区域，产生很高的能量密度（即每平方厘米传输的能量或通量，见表 2–2）。激光也具有很强的方向性，而且根据谐振腔的设计，它也可以偏振。

激光通常以其活性介质命名。介质可以是气体 [氩、氪、二氧化碳、带氟的氩（excimer）或带氖的氦]、液体（染料）、固体 [由晶体支持的活性元素，如钕 : 钇铝石榴石（Nd:YAG）和钛 : 蓝宝石（Ti:Sapphire）] 或半导体（二极管）。

激光可以连续工作（如用于光凝固的氩激光器），通常被称为*连续波*或脉冲（如用于囊膜切开术的 Nd:YAG 激光器）。模型闭塞和 Q 开关是产生*脉冲*输出的 2 种常用方法。这些方法的细节超出了本章的范围。但是请注意，*Q 开关*允许产生的短脉冲（主要的纳秒，即 10^{-9}s），它是可以产生持续时间的皮秒（即 10^{-12}s）或更低*超短脉冲*的*锁模式*，这取决于激光的性质。事实上，脉冲持续时间主要取决于激光介质的光谱带宽，其频谱带宽越大，可实现的脉冲越短。因此，超短的激光脉冲并不是单色的，要产生飞秒脉冲，需要一个具有较大光谱带宽的激光器。例如，128 THz 光谱带宽，Ti:Sappline 激光可以创建最短的脉冲约 3.4fs（即 10^{-15}s）。

我们以前学过，功率是一定时间内传递的能量。1W 是 1s 传递 1J 的能量。同样的，1J 在 1ns 内传递的能量是 10×10^{8}W；1ps 传递 10^{12}W 的能量；1fs 传递 10^{15}W 能量。脉冲是一种在很短的时间内提供少量的能量来增加激光输出功率的方法。

治疗性激光 – 组织相互作用

任何治疗激光应用的基本过程都是通过吸收光向组织传递能量，这是组织的性质（能量状态的分布）和光的波长（光子能量）的函数。治疗激光与组织的相互作用可分为 5 种不同的类型（表 2–5），每种相互作用将详细讨论：*光化学作用*、*热作用*、*光切除*、*等离子体诱导蚀除*和*光致破裂*。这些机制主要由激光的功率密度（辐照度）及其与组织的相互作用时间（激光脉冲持续时间）决定。所有的治疗性激光 – 组织相互作用机制都有一个共同的特点，即所有有意义的能量密度（转移到组织的能量）通常在 1~1000 J/cm^2（图 2–14）。

Niemz MK. Laser–Tissue Interactions: Fundamentals and Applications. 3rd ed. New York: Springer; 2007

Photochemical interaction

Photochemical interaction, sometimes referred to as *photoactivation*, takes place at long exposure times, ranging from seconds to continuously, and very low power densities or irradiances (typically 1 W/cm^2). This type of interaction is based on the use of a photosensitizing dye (eg, rose bengal, riboflavin, or verteporfin), which serves as a chemical (electron reaction) catalyst. Laser irradiation, at a wavelength coupled to the specific dye used, causes a photochemical reaction only within tissues where the dye is present and when irradiated.

Table 2-5 Laser-Tissue Interaction Types and Associated Mechanisms

Interaction Type	Mechanism
Photochemical interaction	Photocatalysis
Thermal interaction	Increase in temperature
Photoablation	UV dissociation
Plasma-induced ablation	Plasma ionization
Photodisruption	Shock-wave generation

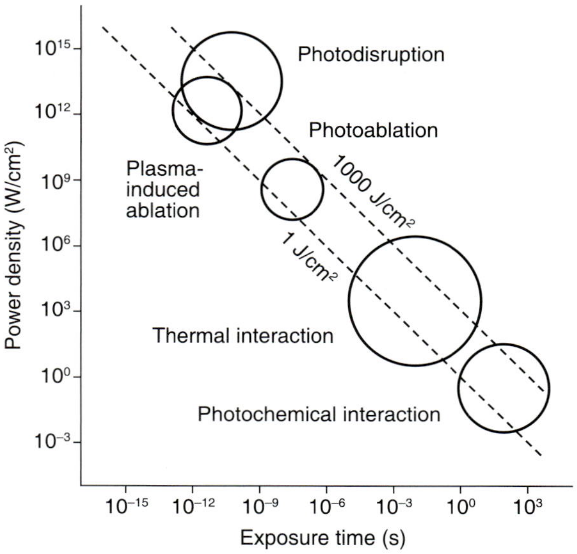

Figure 2-14 Laser-tissue interactions may be divided into 5 different types: photochemical interaction, thermal interaction, photoablation, plasma-induced ablation, and photodisruption. They are primarily determined by the power density (irradiance) and exposure time (pulse duration) of the laser light. All therapeutic laser–tissue interactions share a common characteristic, in that all meaningful energy densities (transferred energy to the tissue) vary typically between 1 and 1000J/cm^2. *(Reproduced with permission from Niemz MK. Laser-Tissue Interactions: Fundamentals and Applications. 3rd enlarged ed. Berlin, Germany: Springer, Berlin, Heidelberg; 2007.)*

光化学作用

光化学作用，有时被称为*光激活*，发生在长时间的曝光，范围从几秒钟到连续性时间，以及非常低的功率密度或辐照度(一般为 1 W/cm²)。这种相互作用是基于光敏染料(如玫瑰孟加拉、核黄素或维替泊芬)作为一种化学(电子反应)催化剂的使用。仅在染料存在的组织内和照射时，激光照射的波长与所使用的特定染料耦合，才会引起光化学反应。

表2-5　激光-组织相互作用类型及机制

相互作用类型	机制
光化学作用	光催化作用
热作用	温度升高
光切除	紫外线分解
等离子体诱导切除	等离子体电离
光致破裂	冲击波的产生

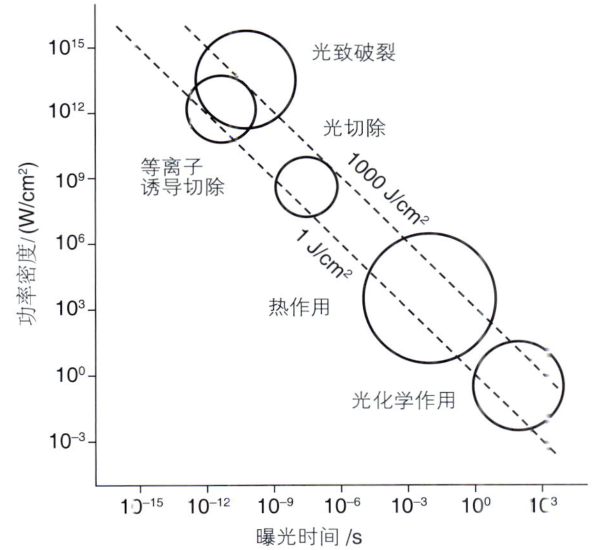

图 2-14　激光与组织的相互作用可分为 5 种不同类型：光化学作用、热作用、光切除、等离子体诱导蚀除和光致破裂。它们主要由激光的功率密度(辐照度)和曝光时间(脉冲持续时间)决定。所有治疗性激光 - 组织的相互作用都有一个共同的特点，即所有有意义的能量密度(转移到组织的能量)通常在 1~1000 J/cm² 之间。
(译者注：资料来源见前页原文。)

This is for example used in photodynamic therapy (PDT), where a photosensitizing agent is injected into the circulation. The blood vessels are then treated with laser irradiation to activate the photosensitizer. A chemical reaction occurs, resulting in thrombosis and closure of the blood vessels. Other than retinal PDT in age-related macular degeneration (AMD), a specific example of this is the treatment of a vascularized cornea with rose bengal and green argon laser irradiation, to thrombose blood vessels and thereby reduce the chance of rejection of a subsequent graft. Another ophthalmic application is the use of ultraviolet-A (UV-A) light after application of riboflavin onto the corneal surface, to promote corneal crosslinking in the treatment of keratoconus.

Thermal interaction

At somewhat shorter exposure times—ranging from microseconds to a minute—and higher power densities—ranging from 10 W/cm^2 to 10^6 W/cm^2—diverse thermal effects at different temperatures may be distinguished (Table2-6 and Fig 2-15). This type of interaction is based on the generation of heat (molecular motion) by the absorption of light.

Photocoagulation, which is associated with protein and collagen denaturation, is the most commonly used thermal laser–tissue interaction in ophthalmic surgery. Natural chromophores or dyes within the tissue absorb light and convert it to heat, which causes denaturation. Their absorption strongly depends on the wavelength of incident light. Thus, laser light of appropriate wavelength must be selected to target specific ocular structures. The main natural chromophores within ocular tissues that are targeted during photocoagulation are hemoglobin (eg, in blood vessels) and melanin (eg, in the iris or deep retinal layers), which strongly absorb wavelengths from about 400 nm to 580 nm. Laser wave lengths longer than 500 nm are generally the preferred choice, in particular when treating near or in the macula, as light between 450 nm and 500 nm is strongly absorbed by the yellow xanthophyll pigments in the macula. Formerly, large argon gas-filled tubes were used to create green laser beams (513 nm), but newer solid-state device scan emit the desired wavelengths, such as frequency-doubled Nd:YAG (ie, one-half of the fundamental 1064-nm wavelength of the Nd:YAG laser, thus 532 nm), or more compact diode lasers.

Table 2-6 Thermal Effects Occurring at Different Temperatures

Temperature	Biological Effect
37°C	—
>42°C	Hyperthermia
>60°C	Coagulation (denaturation of proteins and collagen)
100°C	Vaporization
>100°C	Carbonization
>300°C	Melting

例如在光动力疗法（PDT）中，将光敏剂注入血循环，然后用激光照射血管以激活光敏剂发生化学反应，导致血栓形成和血管闭合。除了视网膜光动力疗法在年龄相关性黄斑变性（AMD）中应用外，一个具体的例子是用玫瑰孟加拉和绿色氩激光辐照血管化的角膜，使其栓塞血管，从而减少随后移植排斥反应的机会。另一种眼科应用是核黄素应用于角膜表面后，利用紫外线 -A （UV-A）光促进角膜交联，治疗圆锥角膜。

热作用

在较短的曝光时间（从微秒到分钟）和较高的功率密度（10~10^6W/cm^2），可以区分不同温度下的不同热效应（表 2-6 和图 2-15）。这种相互作用是建立在吸收光产生热（分子运动）的基础上的。

光凝固是眼科手术中最常用的热激光 - 组织相互作用，它与蛋白质和胶原变性有关。组织内的天然发色团或染料吸收光并将其转化为热，最终导致变性。它们的吸收很大程度上取决于入射光的波长。因此，必须选择适当波长的激光以靶向特定的眼结构。眼内组织中的主要发色团，其光凝固作用靶是血红蛋白（例如，在血管中）和黑色素（例如，在虹膜或深视网膜层中），吸收 400~580nm 的波长。激光波长大于 500nm 通常是优选的选择，尤其是当在黄斑附近或黄斑处理时，因为450~500nm之间的光被黄斑中的黄色叶黄素色素强烈吸收。以前，大型氩气充气管用于制造绿色激光光束（513nm），但更新的固态器件可以发出所需的波长，例如倍频 Nd：AG（即 Nd：YAG 激光的基本 1 064nm 波长的一半，即 532nm）或更致密的二极管激光器。

表2-6　不同温度下的热效应

温　度	生物效应
37°C	—
>42°C	高热
>60°C	凝血(蛋白质和胶原蛋白变性)
100°C	蒸发
>100°C	碳化
>300°C	融化

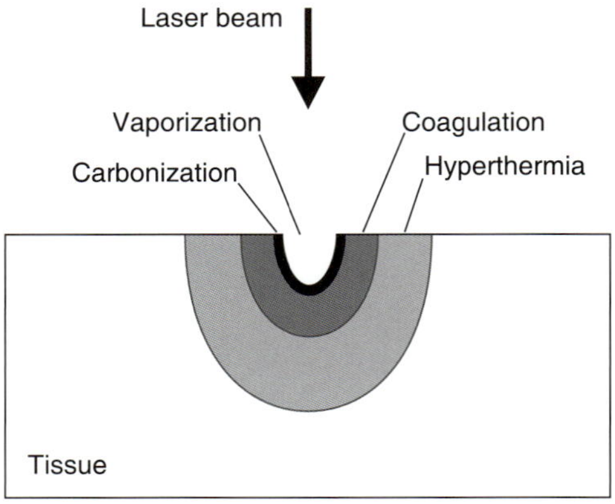

Figure 2-15 Thermal interaction effects inside biological tissue. *(Reproduced with permission from Niemz MK. Laser-Tissue Interactions: Fundamentals and Applications. 3rd enlarged ed. Berlin, Germany: Springer, Berlin, Heidelberg; 2007. Redrawn by Kristina Irsch, PhD.)*

The most common ophthalmic applications of photocoagulation include laser coagulation to prevent retinal detachments, photocoagulation of retinal vessel disease, panretinal photocoagulation in diabetic retinopathy, transpupillary thermotherapy for malignant choroidal melanoma and choroidal neovascularization in AMD, laser trabeculoplasty for open-angle glaucoma, and laser iridotomy for closed-angle glaucoma.

Photocoagulation is also used for photothermal shrinkage of stromal collagen, known as *laser thermo-keratoplasty(LTK)*, in the treatment of hyperopia. The cornea does not absorb enough visible light, even highly concentrated light, to produce a significant temperature increase. However, the cornea is opaque to some infrared wavelengths, thus an infrared laser(eg, holmium: yttrium aluminum garnet [Ho:YAG]) is used in LTK.

Photoablation

If we deliver photons in a short enough time, so that no heat is transferred, and with sufficient energy—typically in the 5 to 7 electron voltage (1 eV ~ 1.602×10^{-19} J) range—then we can directly split molecules, that is, break their covalent chemical bonds. Excimer lasers generating photons with wavelengths in the UV range (eg, a 193-nm argon fluoride excimer laser) are ideally suited for photoablation. This results in ejection of fragments and very clean ablation without necrosis or thermal damage to adjacent tissue. We can think of this type of interaction as "vaporization" without the surrounding thermal effects from Figure 2-15. Typical threshold values for this type of interaction are irradiances of 10^7 to 10^8 W/cm^2 and pulses in the nanosecond range. Photoablation is used in the cornea, which absorbs UV light below around 315 nm, for refractive surgery of the cornea such as photorefractive keratectomy (PRK) and laser in situ keratomileusis(LASIK).

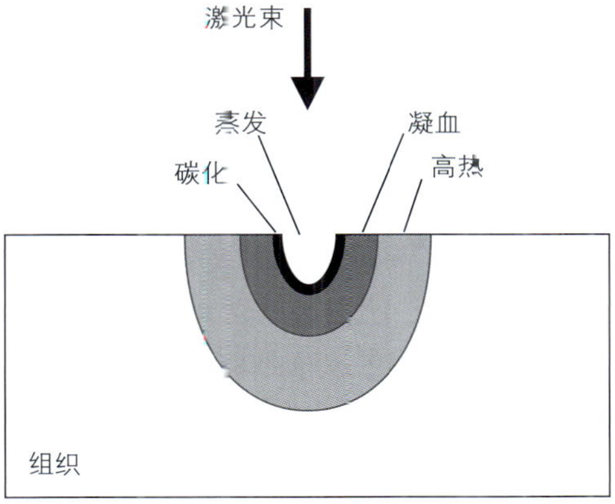

图 2–15　生物组织内部热相互作用效应。*（译者注：资料来源见前页原文。）*

光凝固在眼科应用中最常见的包括激光光凝预防视网膜脱离术、视网膜血管疾病光凝术、糖尿病视网膜病变的全视网膜光凝术、经瞳孔温热疗法治疗脉络膜黑色素瘤和 AMD 的脉络膜新生血管、开角型青光眼的小梁成形术，以及闭角型青光眼的虹膜切开术。

光凝固也用于基质胶原的光热收缩，例如*激光热角膜成形术（LTK）*，多用于治疗远视。角膜不能吸收足够的甚至高度集中的可见光来提升温度。然而，角膜在某些红外波长是不透明的，如红外激光 [例如，钬：钇铝石榴石（Ho：YAG）] 在 LTK 中的使用。

光切除

如果能在足够短的时间内传送光子，那么热量就不会被传递并有足够的能量。通常在 5~7 eV 电子电压（1 eV ≈ 1.602×10^{-19} J）范围内可以直接分裂分子，即打破它们的共价化学键。准分子激光器产生波长在紫外线范围内的光子（例如，193nm 氟化氩准分子激光）非常适合切除。可以做到让碎片切除得非常干净彻底，而且对邻近组织没有坏死或热损伤。可以将这种类型的作用视为没有周围热效应的“汽化”（图 2–15）。这种作用的阈值是辐射率为 10^7~10^8 W/cm^2，脉冲为纳秒范围。吸收 315nm 以下的紫外线的切除应用于角膜屈光手术、光学激光角膜切削术（PRK）和激光原位角膜磨镶术（LASIK）。

Plasma-induced ablation

Under even higher concentrated peak irradiances (but ideally low-pulse energies compared to photo disruption; see Fig 2-14), typically 10^{11} to 10^{13} W/cm^2, and shorter exposure times, in the picosecond and femtosecond range, we can not only break molecules (as during photoablation), but even strip electrons from (ionize) their atoms and accelerate them ("optical breakdown").The accelerated electrons, in turn, can collide with and ionize further atoms, as illustrated in Figure 2-16. This process is called *cascade ionization* and leads to a *plasma formation*, a highly ionized state. It enables a very clean and well-defined removal of tissue without any evidence of thermal or mechanical damage. This type of interaction also makes it possible to transfer energy to transparent media without the use of UV lasers, by creating a plasma that is capable of absorbing non-UV laser photons. Especially in ophthalmology, transparent tissues like the cornea, which is essentially transparent to wavelengths from about 315 nm to 1400 nm, can be treated with non-UV lasers using plasma-induced ablation.

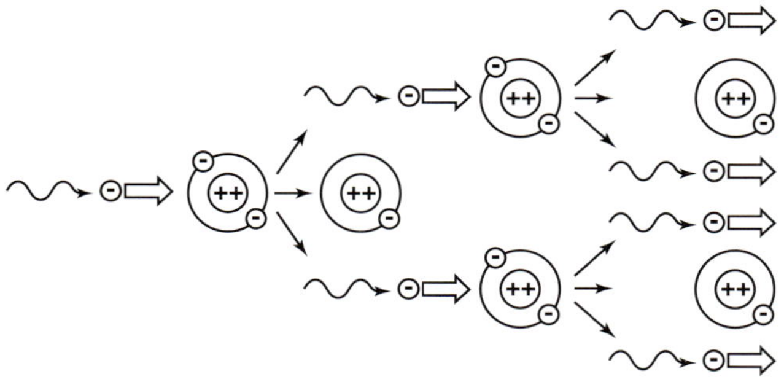

Figure 2-16 Cascade ionization (electrons are stripped from their atoms) leading to plasma formation, a highly ionized state. *(Reproduced with permission from Niemz MK. Laser-Tissue Interactions: Fundamentals and Applications. 3rd enlarged ed. Berlin, Germany: Springer, Berlin, Heidelberg; 2007. Redrawn by Kristina Irsch, PhD.)*

There are secondary mechanical side effects, however, such as the generation of a shock wave (ie, plasma electrons are not confined to the focal volume of the laser beam) and cavitation bubbles. But they do not define the global effect upon the tissue in the plasma-induced ablation process. Note that this kind of ablation is primarily caused by plasma ionization itself (the dissociation of molecules and atoms), which is distinct from the more mechanical interaction process called *photodisruption* and is what is generally attempted with emerging methods of corneal refractive surgery using femtosecond lasers(eg, intrastromal ablation or cutting, and formation of the corneal flap).

Photodisruption

At higher pulse energies (typically 1 to 1000 J/cm^2), and thus higher plasma energies, mechanical side effects become more significant and might even determine the global effect upon the tissue, in which case we refer to the interaction processas photodisruption.

等离子诱导切除

在更高浓度的峰值辐照度下(但在理想状态下,与光爆破能量相比,脉冲能量较低,见图 2–14),通常为 10^{11}~10^{13} W/cm^2，并且曝光时间更短，在皮秒和飞秒的范围内，我们不仅可以破坏分子(如在光消融过程中)，甚至可以从(电离)原子上剥离电子，并加速它们(“光学击穿”)。反过来，加速的电子可以与原子碰撞，并使其电离，如图 2–16 所示，该过程称为*级联电离*，并导致*等离子体形成*，即高度电离状态。它可以非常彻底地将组织清除干净，且不会出现任何热或机械损伤。这种类型的相互作用还可以在不使用紫外线激光的情况下通过产生能够吸收非紫外线激光光子的等离子体将能量转移到透明介质。特别是在眼科学中，可以使用等离子体诱导切除的非紫外线激光处理角膜等透明组织，而角膜对于 315~1400 nm 的波长基本上是透明的。

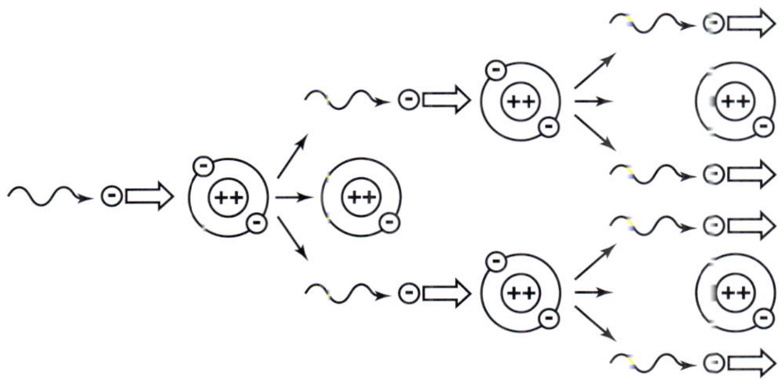

图 2–16　级联电离(电子从其原子中剥离)导致等离子体形成,即高度电离的状态(*译者注：资料来源见前页原文。*)

与此同时，也有一些副反应，例如产生电击波(即等离子体电子不限于激光束聚焦体积)和空化气泡。但它们没有影响等离子诱导的组织消融总体效应。这里需要注意的是，这种消融本身主要是由等离子体电离引起的(分子和原子的解离)，与机械的不同互动过程称为*光致破裂*,通常是作为飞秒激光进行角膜屈光手术的新方法来使用的(例如,基质内消融或切割,以及形成角膜瓣)。

光致破裂

较高的脉冲能量(通常为 1~1000 J / cm^2),越高的等离子体能量,机械副作用也变得更加重要,甚至可能决定总体效应。对于组织结构，我们指的是相互作用的过程，即光致破裂。

The most important ophthalmic application of this photodisruptive interaction is posterior capsulotomy using the Nd:YAG laser. During a photodisruption procedure, it is the mechanical (acoustic) wave and not the laser light itself (as with plasma-induced ablation) that breaks the capsule. Since both interaction mechanisms—plasma-induced ablationas well as photodisruption—rely on plasma generation and graphically overlap(see Fig 2-14), it is not always easy to distinguish between these 2 processes. In fact, most literature sources attribute all tissue effects evoked by ultrashort laser pulses to photodisruption. However, during photodisruption, the tissue primarily is split by mechanical forces, with shock-wave and cavitation effects propagating into adjacent tissue, thus limiting the localizability of the interaction zone. In contrast, plasma-induced ablationis spatially confined to the breakdown region and laser focal spot, with the tissue primarily being removed by plasma ionization itself. The primary distinguishing parameter between the 2 interaction processes is energy density (see Fig 2-14).

Why ultrashort laser pulses?

Per the definition of power (energy per second), the shorter the pulse duration, the higher the power that can be delivered at a given energy. In other words, picosecond or femtosecond (ultrashort) pulses permit the generation of high peak powers with considerably lower pulse energies than nanosecond pulses.

Another consequence of this is that, for ultrashort pulses, especially in the femtosecond range, considerably lower pulse energies are needed to achieve optical breakdown (plasma generation), and therefore purely plasma-induced ablation can be observed. For nanosecond pulses, on the other hand, as illustrated in Figure 2-17, the threshold energy density for optical breakdown is higher, so that purely plasma-induced ablation is not observed, but is always associated with photodisruption. Since disruptive effects can damage adjacent tissue, ultrashort laser pulses are generally preferred (depending on the application).

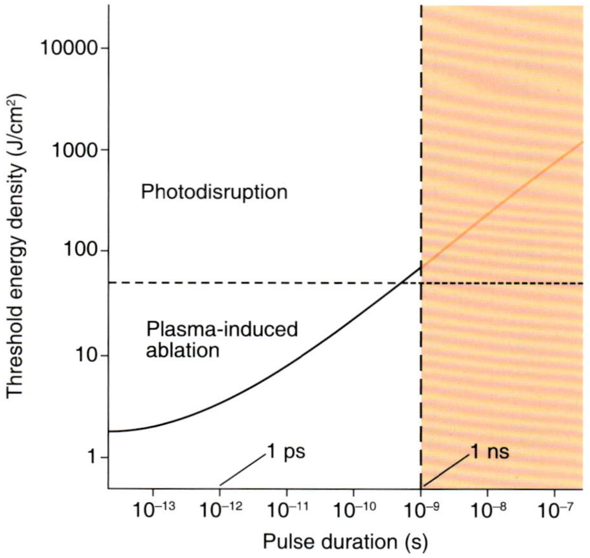

Figure 2-17 Distinction of plasma-induced ablation and photodisruption according to applied energy density. Note that for nanosecond pluses, purely plasma-induced ablation is not observed but always associated with disruptive effects, even at the very threshold for optical breakdown. *(Reproduced with permission from Niemz MK. Laser-Tissue Interactions: Fundamentals and Applications.3rd enlarged ed. Berlin, Germany: Springer, Berlin, Heidelberg; 2007. Redrawn by Kristina Irsch, PhD.)*

这种光致破裂相互作用的最重要的眼科应用是 Nd：YAG 激光进行后囊膜切开术。在光致破裂过程中，它是机械（声）波，而不是激光光本身（如同等离子体诱导消融）打开后囊膜。由于 2 种相互作用的机制（等离子诱导消融以及光致破裂）都依赖于等离子体生成和重叠（见图 2–14）。事实上这两 2 种作用过程并不容易区分。大多数文献将其归因于超短激光脉冲诱发的光致破裂。然而，在光致破裂时，组织主要通过有冲击波力量的机械分裂和空化效应传播到邻近组织，从而限制了相互作用区的局部性。相比之下，等离子体诱导消融在空间上局限于击穿区域和激光焦点，而组织主要通过等离子体电离本身去除。这 2 个反应之间的主要区别参数是能量密度（见图 2–14）。

为什么是超短激光脉冲?
根据功率（每秒能量）的定义，脉冲持续时间越短，给定能量下可以提供的能量越高。换句话说，皮秒或飞秒（超短脉冲）脉冲可产生的高峰值功率脉冲能量要低于纳秒脉冲的。

这样做的另一个结果是，对于超短脉冲，特别是在飞秒中的范围，需要相当低的脉冲能量来实现光学击穿（等离子体产生），因此等离子体诱导切除是可以观察到的。对于纳秒，如图 2–17 所示，为实现光学击穿的脉冲阈值能量密度更高，因此等离子体诱导的消融没有被观察到，但是总是与光致破坏有关。由于破坏性影响会损害邻近组织，超短激光脉冲通常是更好的选择（取决于其应用）。

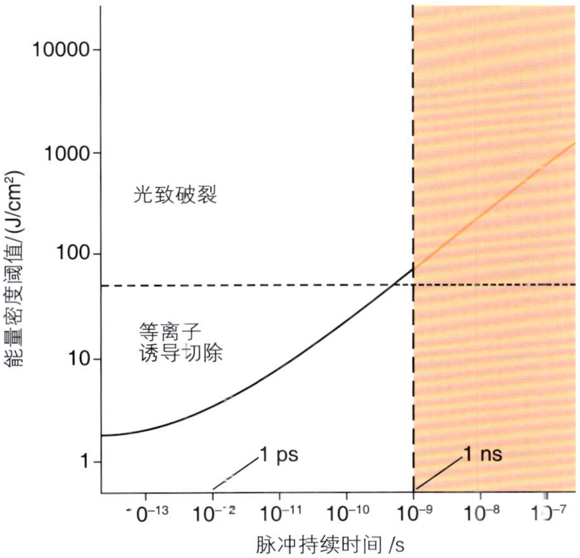

图 2–17　根据应用的等离子体诱导切除和光爆破的区别是能量密度。对于纳秒级脉冲，未观察到纯粹的等离子体诱导的消融总是与破坏性影响有关，即使是在光学的极限分解情况下。（*译者注：资料来源见前页原文。*）

Note that for a laser with high-energy pulses (photodisruption regime), causing disruptive effects that propagate beyond its focal spot, lower repetition rates are needed; incontrast, for a laser with low-energy pulses (plasma-induced ablation regime), higher repetition rates are necessary and produce smoother surface cuts without increasing the time of the procedure (Fig 2-18).

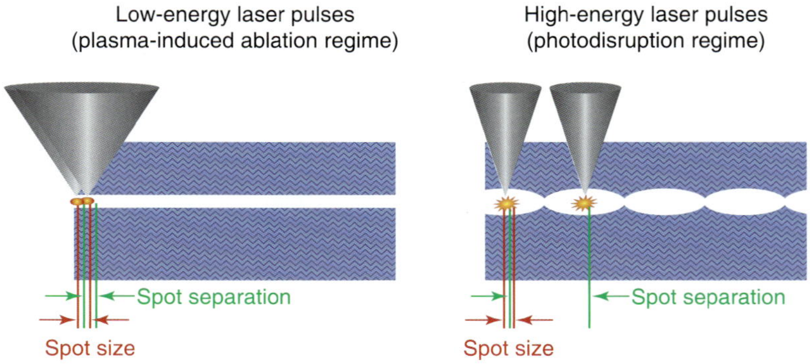

Figure 2-18 Repetition rate versus energy density. For high-energy laser pulses (photodisruption regime), causing disruptive effects that propagate beyond its focal spot, lower repetition rates are needed, whereas for low-energy pulses (plasma-induced ablation regime), higher repetition rates are necessary. Note that the latter will produce smoother surface cuts without increasing the time of the procedure. *(Courtesy of Rowiak GmbH. Modified by Kristina Irsch, PhD.)*

Light Hazards

As with any therapeutic light application, nontherapeutic damage to the eye caused by light is primarily dependent on the wavelength as well as the irradiance and time of light exposure.

For example, the sun itself produces a power density (irradiance) of about 10 W/cm^2,which will rise to 170 W/cm^2 if that sunlight is focused and falls well within the range of thermal interaction (see Fig 2-14); in fact, retinal photocoagulation was first performed by focusing sunlight onto the retina. Similarly, prolonged irradiation or cumulative exposure from the operating microscope or indirect ophthalmoscope through a focusing lens, in particular on the eye with a dilated pupil, may be harmful to the eye. For instance, there is some evidence that cases of post-cataract- extraction cystoid macular edema are related to microscope illumination.

The anterior segment of the eye is essentially transparent to wavelengths from about400 nm to 1400 nm and opaque to light outside that wavelength range, thereby reducing and protecting the subsequent ocular media from direct exposure to UV as well as infrared (IR) light. This is thanks to the crystalline lens essentially blocking UV-A light(315–400 nm) and the cornea essentially blocking UV-B (280–315 nm), UV-C(280 nm and below), as well as IR-Band IR-C (1400 nm to 1 mm) radiation. The filtering properties of anterior-segment components is inherently related to their absorptive capabilities, in case of UV radiation causing breakdown of the absorptive molecules in the cornea and lens, and in case of IR radiation causing a temperature rise and subsequent denaturation of protein in the cornea. Therefore, the anterior segment is not only susceptible to injury from UV irradiation, from which photo keratitis (from short-term exposure to UV-B and UV-C) and cataract (from long-term cumulative exposure) may result, but also to thermal injury from IR radiation. Damage from thermal injury may be caused from any light above 400 nm.

需要注意的是，对于激光高能量脉冲（光致破裂），其造成破坏性传播超出了它的焦点的效果，而且需要的重复率较低。相比之下，对于激光低能量脉冲（等离子体诱导的消融），需要具有更高的重复速率，并且在不增加时间的情况下产生更平滑的表面切割过程(图 2-18)。

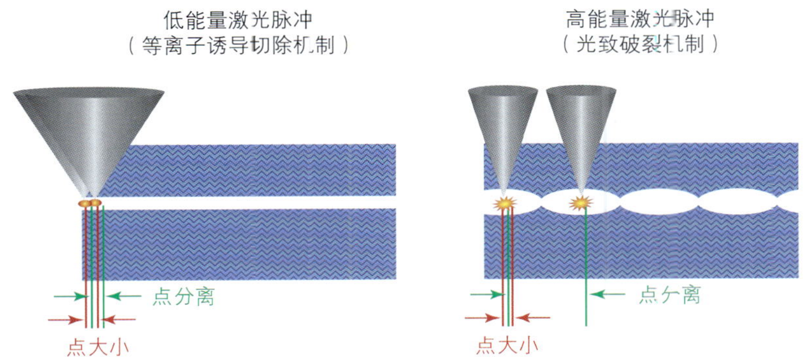

图 2-18　重复率与能量密度。用于高能激光脉冲（光致破裂），造成超出其焦点的破坏性影响，需要较低的重复速率，而对于低能量脉冲（等离子体诱导的消融方式），则需要更高重复率。需要注意的是，后者将产生更平滑的表面切割，但不会增加手术时间。

光的危害

与任何治疗性光应用一样，对眼睛造成非治疗性损伤主要取决于光波长，以及光的辐照度和曝光时间。

例如，太阳本身产生的功率密度（辐照度）约为 10 W / cm^2，如果太阳光在很好的范围内聚焦，则会升至 170 W / cm^2（见图 2-14）。事实上，首次视网膜光凝是将阳光聚焦在视网膜上。同样，在特定的瞳孔散大的情况下，长时间被手术显微镜累积照射或被间接检眼镜照射，可能对眼睛有害。例如，一些证据表明后发性白内障——囊样黄斑水肿与显微镜照射具有相关性。

眼睛的前节对于 400~1400nm 的波长基本上是透明的。并且对该波长范围外的光是不透明的，从而减少并保护后续的眼部介质不直接暴露于紫外线（UV）以及红外（IR）灯。这要归功于晶状体基本上阻挡了 UV-A 光（315~400nm），和角膜基本上阻挡 UV-B（280~315nm）、UV-C（280nm 和以下）以及 IR-B 和 IR-C（1400nm~1mm）辐射。眼前段屈光介质过滤属性与其吸收能力本质上是相关的，在紫外线辐射的情况下，会导致角膜和晶状体可溶解分子破坏，并且在 IR 辐射的情况下，引起温度升高和随后角膜中蛋白质的变性。因此，前节不仅容易受到紫外线照射的伤害，造成角膜炎（从短期来看）和白内障（长期暴露于 UV-B 和 UV-C 可能导致累积暴露），也可能导致热量红外辐射伤害。任何光线都可能导致高于 400nm 的热损伤。

In the retina, natural chromophores, including melanin, hemoglobin, and xanthophyll, as previously discussed, strongly absorb wavelengths from about 400 nm to 580 nm. This makes the retina susceptible to photochemical injury in that region, especially from blue light. Note, that in an aphakic eye, this susceptibility to damage extends to below 400(to about 315 nm) without the UV-A absorption capability of the natural lens, and is the basis for incorporating UV-blocking and blue-blocking chromophores in some intraocular lenses. The retina is also susceptible to thermal injury from optical radiation occurring from the visible to near-infrared wavelengths of 400–1400 nm.

Appendix 2.1

Reconciliation of Geometric Optics and Physical Optics

We have seen how the basic principles of geometric optics are consequences of Fermat's principle. In turn, Fermat's principle can be understood as a consequence of the wave properties of light. Although a rigorous derivation is beyond the scope of this volume, aheuristic description of the concepts can be instructive.

A beam of light propagates as a wave, oscillating perpendicular to the direction oftravel. Two such waves that coincide will interfere with one another. This interference is constructive or destructive, according to whether the peaks and troughs of the waves coincide (see Fig 2-6). If 2 coincident waves of light emanate from a common source, their peaks and troughs coincide whenever the travel time of the 2 waves is identical. In this case, the full strength of the light waves is evident. Conversely, if the travel times of 2 coincident waves differ such that the arrival of their peaks and troughs differ by exactly half a wavelength, the waves cancel each other perfectly, and no light appears to be transmitted.

When small variations in the light path occur, possible paths for which the travel time is essentially unchanged will thus contribute strongly to the resultant image, whereas those paths that vary more strongly in travel time will essentially cancel out. Paths for which small variations (often referred to as "perturbations") of the light path have little effect on travel time are referred to as *extremal* paths. The most familiar of these are the paths of shortest travel time, such as the straight-line paths of light through uniform media. The formal derivation of these observations is the concern of the mathematical subject known as the "calculus of variations," which is beyond the scope of this book.

In rare instances, paths other than those of shortest travel time may also be extremal and are also permitted by the wave properties of light. One important example occurs in fiber-optic light-guides, which are fabricated with a gradient in the refractive index such that the "densest" material is at the center of each fiber. The path down the center of the fiber takes the longest time of all possible nearby light paths, steering the light down the center of each fiber.

在视网膜中，自然发色团，包括黑色素、血红蛋白和叶黄素，都会强烈地吸收 400~580nm 的波长。这使视网膜在该区域容易受光化学伤害，特别是来自蓝光的伤害。值得注意的是，在无晶状体眼中，由于没有了晶状体吸收 UV-A 的能力，以及眼内一些自然发色团结合紫外线和阻挡蓝色的基础，这种对损伤的敏感性可以扩展到 400nm 以下（至约 315nm），视网膜也容易受到从可见的接近红外线波长为 400~1400nm 的光辐射发生的热损伤。

附录 2.1

几何光学与物理光学的一致

我们已经看到了基本的几何光学原理是 Fermat 原理。反过来，Fermat 原理也可以被理解为波的结果，而波又是光的属性。虽然严格的推导超出了本卷的范围，但是概念的描述仍然具有指导意义。

一束光作为波传播，垂直于波的方向振荡前行。2 个这样的波将相互干扰。这种干扰是否具有建设性或破坏性是由波浪的波峰和波谷重合决定（见图 2-5）的。如果 2 个重合的光波来源于一个共同的光源，当 2 个波的传播时间相同时，它们的光的峰和波谷就会重合。在这种情况下，光波的全部强度是显而易见的。相反，如果 2 个波传播时间一致而不同波的峰和谷的到达恰好相差一半波长，波浪就会完全抵消，则不会有光线传播。

当光路发生微小变化时，可能传播时间的路径就基本上没有变化，因此对所得图像有强烈影响，而传播时间变化较大的路径会基本上被抵消了。对传播时间影响非常微小的路径（通常称为“扰动”）称为*极值*路径。其中最常见的是最短的传播时间的路径，如直线通过统一媒体的光路。这就是数学学科中的“变异的微积分”。此理论超出了本书的范围。

在极少数情况下，最短的传播时间也可能是极端的，并且符合光的波动特性。一个重要的例子就是光纤光导，它们用折射率梯度制成“最密集”的材料位于每根纤维的中心。沿着中心的路径光纤占用所有可能的最长时间附近的光路，从而引导着光线每根纤维的中心。

Chapter Exercises

Questions

2.1. Which theory provides the most comprehensive description of light?
- a. wave theory
- b. particle theory
- c. ray theory
- d. quantum electrodynamics

2.2. The Airy disc image on the retina is larger in which circumstance?
- a. The wavelength of light is shortened.
- b. The focal length of the eye is shorter.
- c. The pupil size decreases.
- d. Macular degeneration is present.

2.3. Corneal haze secondary to corneal edema is primarily caused by which light phenomena?
- a. reflection
- b. light scattering
- c. refraction
- d. diffraction

2.4. Which light phenomenon is the underlying basis of optical coherence tomography?
- a. diffraction
- b. interference
- c. fluorescence
- d. polarization

2.5. Which laser–tissue interaction is the basis of laser in situ keratomileusis (LASIK)?
- a. photodisruption
- b. photochemical interaction
- c. plasma-induced ablation
- d. photoablation

2.6. In aphakia, the susceptibility to photochemical injury to the retina is which of the following?
- a. is decreased without the focusing capability of the natural lens
- b. is unchanged
- c. is increased without the ultraviolet absorption of the natural lens
- d. is not an issue

Answers

2.1. **d**. In general, it suffices to consider the wave-like behavior of light for phenomena at the macroscopic level and the simple quantum-view of light at the microscopic level. However, the quantum theory of the interaction of light and matter—quantum electrodynamics—explains all the properties of light we know, resolving the wave-particle confusion.

2.2. **c**. The Airy disc is the central portion of a pattern of light and dark rings formed when light from a point source passes through a circular aperture and is diffracted. The size of the Airy disc increases with smaller pupil size (especially pupil diameter <2.5 mm), longer wavelengths of light, and longer focal lengths. Retinal conditions such as macular degeneration have no effect on the size of the Airy disc.

章节练习

问题

2.1 哪种理论提供了最全面的光线描述？
a. 波动理论
b. 粒子理论
c. 射线理论
d. 量子电动力学

2.2 视网膜上的 Airy 斑光盘图像在哪种情况下更大？
a. 光的波长缩短了
b. 眼的焦距更短
c. 瞳孔大小减小
d. 存在黄斑变性

2.3 继发于角膜水肿的角膜浑浊主要是由哪种光引起的现象？
a. 反射
b. 光散射
c. 折射
d. 衍射

2.4 哪种光现象是潜在的光学相干断层扫描的基础？
a. 衍射
b. 干涉
c. 荧光
d. 偏振

2.5 哪种激光原位角膜磨镶术（LASIK）是激光与组织相互作用的基础？
a. 光致破裂
b. 光化学作用
c. 等离子体诱导
d. 切除

2.6 在无晶状体中，视网膜光化学损伤的易感性是下列哪一个？
a. 减少，由于没有晶体的聚焦
b. 没有改变
c. 增加，由于没有吸收紫外线的晶体
d. 没有答案

答案

2.1 **d**。一般来说，从宏观上，光具有波动性；从微观上，光具有粒子性。然而，量子理论的光与物质的相互作用——量子电动力学，可以解释我们所有的光属性，解决了波粒子混乱。

2.2 **c**。当来自点光源的光通过圆孔并被衍射时，为 Airy 斑形成光明和暗环图案的中心部分。Airy 斑的尺寸随着瞳孔尺寸的减小（特别是瞳孔直径 <2.5 mm），光波和焦距的增长而增加。视网膜黄斑变性等病症对 Airy 斑大小无影响。

2.3. **b**. Light scattering occurs when small particles suspended in a transparent medium interfere with the transmittance of light and cause photons to deviate from a straight path. Short wavelengths of light are scattered more strongly than are longer wavelengths. Larger particles scatter light more intensely than do smaller particles. In a healthy cornea, the tightly arranged and regularly spaced collagen molecules minimize the effects of scattering. When a cornea becomes edematous, excess fluid in the stroma disrupts the regular collagen structure, causing light scattering.

2.4. **b**. Optical coherence tomography (OCT) is an optical analogue to ultrasound imaging, using infrared light instead of sound. The much higher speed of light compared with sound allows for finer resolution, but direct electronic measurement of the shorter "echo" times it takes light to travel from different structures at axial distances within the eye is not feasible. Interferometry enables us to overcome this difficulty. More precisely, OCT uses interference of broadband or tunable coherent light to generate optical sections of the retina and cornea.

2.5. **d**. Laser in situ keratomileusis (LASIK) and photorefractive keratectomy (PRK), common refractive surgeries of the cornea, are based on photoablation using excimer lasers generating photons with wavelengths in the ultraviolet (UV) range that are absorbed within the corneal tissue.

2.6. **c**. In the retina, natural chromophores strongly absorb wavelengths from about 400 nm to 580 nm, which makes the retina susceptible to photochemical injury in that region, especially from blue light. This susceptibility to damage is increased in an aphakic eye, extending to below 400 (to about 315 nm), without the UV-A absorption capability of the natural lens, and is the basis for incorporating UV-blocking and blue-blocking chromophores in some intraocular lenses.

2.3　**b**。当小颗粒悬浮在透明介质中发生光散射时，干扰光的透射率会导致光子偏离。短波长的光会比更长波长的光更强烈地散射。较大的粒子比小粒子光具有更强烈的散射光。在健康的角膜中，紧密排列和定期间隔的胶原分子使散射的影响最小化。当一个角膜变得水肿，基质中多余的液体破坏了常规的胶原蛋白结构，导致光散射。

2.4　**b**。光学相干断层扫描（OCT）是超声波的光学模拟成像，使用红外光代替声音，比起声音来说，红外光的速度要快得多，允许的分辨率也更精细，但直接电子测量较短的“回声”时间需要光从不同的路径传播，而沿眼内轴向距离的结构传播是不可行的。我们要克服这个困难来实现干涉测量。更确切地说，OCT 使用干扰宽带或可调谐相干光来产生视网膜的光学部分和角膜。

2.5　**d**。激光原位角膜磨镶术（LASIK）和屈光性角膜切削术（PRK）是常见的角膜屈光手术，是基于光消融术使用的准分子激光器产生波长在角膜组织吸收范围内的紫外线（UV）的光子。

2.6　**c**。在视网膜中，自然发色团强烈吸收 400~580nm 的波长，这使视网膜易受光化学伤害，特别是蓝光的伤害。在无晶状体眼中，这种对损害的敏感性增加至 400nm 以下（至约 315nm），这是由于没有了晶体对 UV-A 的吸收能力以及一些眼内发色团阻挡紫外线和蓝光的基础。

（翻译　叶璐　王景慧　王顿　魏瑞华 // 审校　石一宁 // 章节审校　魏瑞华）

CHAPTER 3

Optics of the Human Eye

Highlights

- model eyes: Gullstrand model eye, reduced schematic (model) eye
- important axes: principal line of vision, pupillary axis, visual axis, optical axis
- important angles: angle alpha (α), angle kappa (κ)
- measuring vision: visual acuity, contrast sensitivity
- refractive errors: monocular, binocular
- accommodation and presbyopia

Glossary

Accommodation The faculty of the eye to increase the optical power of the lens—may be used to focus on near objects, or to self-correct hyperopic refractive errors.

Against-the-rule astigmatism Astigmatism with the greatest refractive power in the horizontal meridian.

Ametropia Any refractive error—any deviation from emmetropia.

Angle alpha (α) The angle between the pupillary axis and the optical axis.

Angle kappa (κ) The angle between the pupillary axis and the visual axis.

Aniseikonia Disparity in the size of the retinal images formed in the 2 eyes of a patient.

Anisometropia Different refractive errors in the 2 eyes of a patient.

Astigmatism A refractive error in which the power of the eye varies in different meridians.

Contrast sensitivity The ability to detect small spatial variations in the luminance of a visual stimulus; quantitatively, the reciprocal of the contrast threshold.

Contrast sensitivity function The relationship of the contrast sensitivity of an eye as measured using grating test targets to the spatial frequency (spacing) of the gratings.

Contrast threshold The minimum contrast at which a target is detectable.

第 3 章

人眼光学

重点

- 模型眼：Gullstrand 模型眼，简化模型眼。
- 重要的轴线：视觉主线，瞳孔轴，视轴，光轴。
- 重要的角：α 角，κ 角。
- 视觉测量：视力，对比敏感度。
- 屈光不正：单眼，双眼。
- 调节和老视。

术语

调节 眼睛增加晶状体屈光力的功能——可用于聚焦近处物体，也可自行代偿远视屈光不正。

逆规散光 在水平子午线上具有最大屈光力的散光。

屈光不正 任何偏离正视的屈光状态异常。

α 角 瞳孔轴与光轴之间的夹角。

κ 角 瞳孔轴与视轴之间的夹角。

物像不等 双眼视网膜成像不等大。

屈光参差 双眼屈光不正不同。

散光 在不同子午线上屈光力不同的屈光不正。

对比敏感度 在一定视觉刺激亮度的条件下，识别微小空间变化的能力，定量上是对比度阈值的倒数。

对比敏感度函数 使用光栅视标测量的眼睛的对比敏感度与光栅视标的空间频率（间距）之间的关系。

对比度阈值 可看到视标的最小对比度。

Emmetropia The refractive state of an eye which focuses objects at optical infinity on the fovea with relaxed accommodation.

Entrance pupil The image of the anatomical pupil as seen through the cornea.

Gullstrand model eye A detailed schematic eye model developed by Allvar Gullstrand.

Hyperopia A refractive error in which objects at infinity are focused behind the retina, with relaxed accommodation.

Irregular astigmatism A refractive error where the astigmatism varies significantly across the optical aperture of the eye.

Modulation transfer function A function that describes the relationship between the contrast of a visual stimulus and the contrast of the image of the stimulus on the retina, as a function of spatial frequency.

Myopia A refractive error in which objects at infinity are focused in front of the retina, with relaxed accommodation.

Optical axis The line connecting the optical center of the cornea and optical center of the crystalline lens.

Optotype A standardized letter or other character, typically defined by features that subtend one-fifth of the height of the character, such as the horizontal bars, and the spaces between them, of the letter E.

Pinhole visual acuity Measurement of visual acuity as perceived through an occluder with pinhole apertures that reduce the impact of refractive error.

Presbyopia The loss of accommodation with increasing age.

Principal line of vision The line passing through the fixation target, perpendicular to the corneal surface.

Pupillary axis The line through the midpoint of the entrance pupil, perpendicular to the corneal surface.

Reduced schematic eye A simplified schematic eye model with a single refracting surface at the corneal apex.

Regular astigmatism A refractive error where the astigmatism is approximately constant across the optical aperture of the eye.

Snellen visual acuity The ability to identify small letters or other optotypes (presented at high contrast).

Spatial frequency The number of stripes or cycles of a periodic test target per degree of visual angle.

Visual axis The line connecting the fovea to the fixation target.

With-the-rule astigmatism Astigmatism with the greatest refractive power in the vertical meridian.

正视眼 在调节放松的条件下，无穷远处的物体聚焦在黄斑中心凹上的屈光状态。

入射光瞳 解剖学瞳孔经角膜所成的像。

Gullstrand 模型眼 Allvar Gullstrand 建立的精细模型眼。

远视 在调节放松的条件下，无穷远处的物体聚焦在视网膜之后的一种屈光状态。

不规则散光 通过眼光学孔径的散光明显变化的一种屈光不正。

调制传递函数 一种描述视觉刺激的对比度与在视网膜上的刺激物图像对比度之间的关系的函数，是空间频率的函数。.

近视 在调节放松的条件下，无穷远处的物体聚焦在视网膜之前的一种屈光不正。

光轴 角膜的光学中心和晶状体的光学中心的连线。

视标 一种标准化的字母或字符，其中由包含字符高度的 1/5 的特征，如字母 E 的 3 个水平条和 2 个间隔共同构成字母“E”的 1/5。

针孔视力 通过减弱屈光不正影响的针孔镜检测的视力。

老视 随着年龄增加，调节力逐渐丧失。

视觉主线 经过固定视标并垂直于角膜表面的连线。

瞳孔轴 经过入射光瞳的中点并垂直于角膜表面的连线。

简化眼 一种将角膜顶点作为单一屈光面的简化眼模型。

规则散光 通过眼光学孔径的散光几乎没有变化的一种屈光不正。

Snellen 视力 识别小字母或其他视标的能力（在高对比度下）。

空间频率 每度视角的周期测试视标的条纹数或周期数。

视轴 中心凹与固视目标的连线。

顺规散光 在垂直子午线上具有最大屈光力的散光。

Introduction

This chapter presents conceptual tools to aid in understanding the optics of the human eye. In addition, it covers the various methods used to measure the eye's ability to "see" and reviews the types of refractive errors of the eye. Treatment of refractive errors is discussed in Chapters 4, 5, and 6 of this volume.

Schematic Eyes

The major challenges to understanding the optics of the human eye lie in the complexities and "imperfections" of some of the eye's optical elements. Simplifications and approximations make models easier to understand but limit their ability to explain all the subtleties of the eye's optical system. As an example, the anterior surface of the cornea is frequently assumed to be spherical, but the actual anterior surface tends to flatten toward the limbus. Also, the center of the crystalline lens is usually decentered with respect to the cornea and the visual axis of the eye.

Many mathematical models of the eye's optical system are based on careful anatomical measurements and approximations. The model developed by Gullstrand (Fig 3-1, Table 3-1), a Swedish professor of ophthalmology, so closely approximated the human eye that he was awarded a Nobel Prize in 1911. Although very useful, this model is cumbersome for certain clinical calculations and is often simplified further.

EXAMPLE 3-1

What is the depth of the anterior chamber of the Gullstrand model eye?
Referring to Figure 3-1 or Table 3-1, the distance from the apex of the cornea to the front surface of the lens is 3.6 mm, while the thickness of the cornea is 0.5 mm, so the depth of the anterior chamber is 3.1 mm.

Because the principal points of the cornea and lens are fairly close to each other, a single intermediate point can substitute for them. In a similar fashion, the nodal points of the cornea and lens can be combined into a single nodal point located 17.0 mm in front of the retina. Thus, we can treat the eye as if it were a single refracting element, an ideal spherical surface separating 2 media of different refractive indices: 1.000 for air and 1.333 for the eye (Fig 3-2). This simplified model is known as the reduced *schematic eye.*

引言

本章介绍了帮助理解人眼光学的概念工具。另外，本章还涉及一些检测眼睛能“看”的多种方法，并复习了屈光不正的类型。屈光不正的治疗见第 4、5、6 章。

模型眼

了解人类眼球光学特性的主要问题是，人眼光学的复杂性和一些光学成分的“不完美”。简化和近似模型使我们更容易了解眼球，但却限制了对眼内光学系统所有的细微之处的解释能力。例如，角膜前表面被设定为球面，但实际上靠近角膜缘处趋于扁平。此外，晶状体中心通常是偏离角膜中心和视轴的。

许多眼光学系统的数学模型是基于精细的解剖测量的近似值。瑞典的眼科教授 Gullstrand 建立了一个非常接近人眼的模型（图 3–1、表 3–1），并因此在 1911 年获得了诺贝尔奖。尽管这个模型非常有用，但对于临床计算依然很繁琐，常常需要进一步简化。

例 3 –1

Gullstrand 模型眼的前房深度是多少？
参照图 3–1 或表 3–1，从角膜顶点到晶状体前表面的距离为 3.6mm，角膜厚度为 0.5mm，所以前房深度为 3.1mm。

因为角膜和晶状体的主点非常近，所以可用一个中间点来代替它们的主点。同样，角膜和晶状体的节点也可以归成一个，位于视网膜前 17mm。这样，我们可以将眼睛视为一个简单的屈光元素，有一个理想的球面，将 2 种不同折射率的介质分隔：空气折射率为 1.000，眼的折射率为 1.333（图 3–2）。这个简化的模型眼就是*简化眼*。

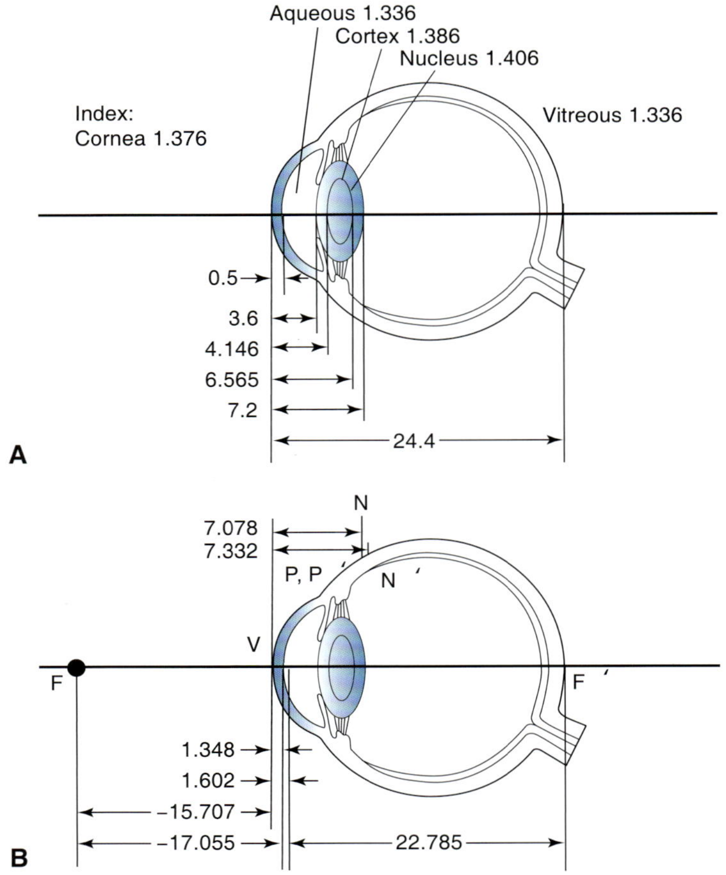

Figure 3-1 Optical constants of the Gullstrand eye. All values in millimeters. **A**, Refractive indices of the media and positions of the refracting surfaces. **B**, Positions of the cardinal points, which are used for optical calculations. *(Illustration by C. H. Wooley.)*

Using this reduced schematic eye, we can calculate the retinal image size of an object in space (such as a Snellen letter). This calculation utilizes the simplified nodal point, through which light rays entering or leaving the eye pass undeviated. The geometric principle of similar triangles can be used for the calculation of retinal image size if the following information is given: (1) the actual height of a Snellen letter on the eye chart, (2) the distance from the eye chart to the eye, and (3) the distance from the nodal point to the retina. The formula for this calculation is as follows:

$$\frac{\text{Retinal Image Height}}{\text{Snellen Letter Height}} = \frac{\text{Nodal Point to Retina Distance}}{\text{Chart to Eye Distance}}$$

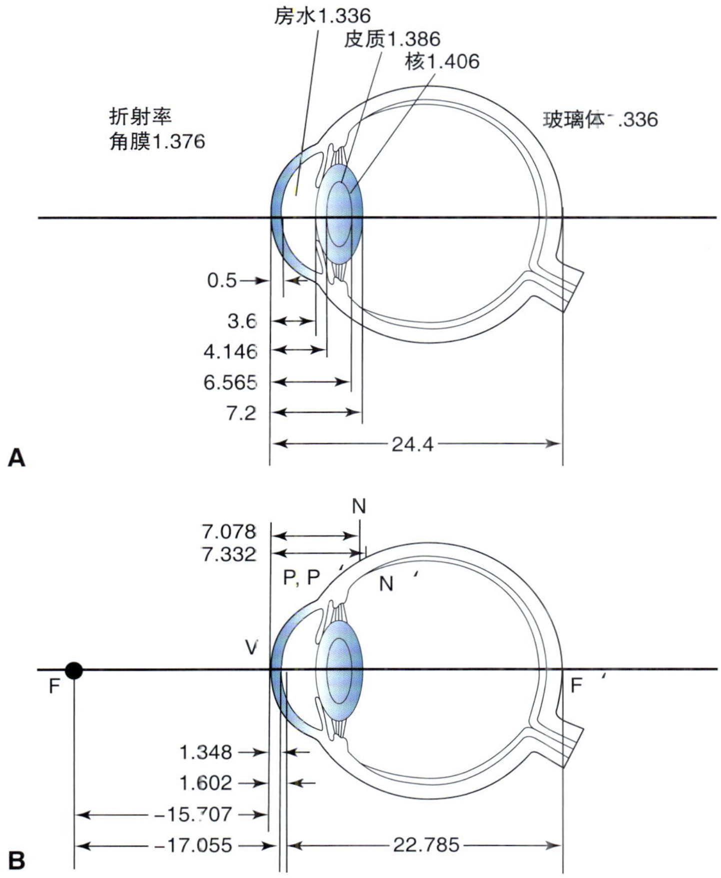

图 3–1　Gullstrand 眼的光学常数，所有单位为 mm。**A**. 屈光介质的折射率和屈光界面的位置。**B**. 用于光学计算的基点位置。*（译者注：资料来源见前页原文。）*

利用简化眼，可以计算空间物体（如 Snellen 视标）在视网膜成像的大小。计算利用简化的节点，经过节点的光线不改变方向。如果给出以下条件，可以应用相似三角形的几何原理计算视网膜成像大小：① Snellen 视力表上视标的实际高度，②眼睛到视力表的距离，③节点到视网膜的距离（假设为 17 mm）。计算公式如下：

$$\frac{\text{视网膜成像高度}}{\text{Snellen 视力表字母高度}} = \frac{\text{节点到视网膜距离}}{\text{视力表到眼睛的距离}}$$

Table 3-1 The Schematic Eye

	Accommodation Relaxed	Maximum Accommodation
Refractive index		
Cornea	1.376	1.376
Aqueous humor and vitreous body	1.336	1.336
Lens	1.386	1.386
Equivalent core lens	1.406	1.406
Position		
Anterior surface of cornea	0	0
Posterior surface of cornea	0.5	0.5
Anterior surface of lens	3.6	3.2
Anterior surface of equivalent core lens	4.146	3.8725
Posterior surface of equivalent core lens	6.565	6.5275
Posterior surface of lens	7.2	7.2
Radius of curvature		
Anterior surface of cornea	7.7	7.7
Posterior surface of cornea	6.8	6.8
Anterior surface of lens	10.0	5.33
Anterior surface of equivalent core lens	7.911	2.655
Posterior surface of equivalent core lens	−5.76	−2.655
Posterior surface of lens	−6.0	−5.33
Refracting power		
Anterior surface of cornea	48.83	48.83
Posterior surface of cornea	−5.88	−5.88
Anterior surface of lens	5.0	9.375
Core lens	5.985	14.96
Posterior surface of lens	8.33	9.375
Corneal system		
Refracting power	43.05	43.05
Position of first principal point	−0.0496	−0.0496
Position of second principal point	−0.0506	−0.0506
First focal length	−23.227	−23.227
Second focal length	31.031	31.031
Lens system		
Refracting power	19.11	33.06
Position of first principal point	5.678	5.145
Position of second principal point	5.808	5.255
Focal length	69.908	40.416
Complete optical system of eye		
Refracting power	58.64	70.57
Position of first principal point, P	1.348	1.772
Position of second principal point, P′	1.602	2.086
Position of first focal point, F	−15.707	−12.397
Position of second focal point, F′	24.387	21.016
First focal length	−17.055	−14.169
Second focal length	22.785	18.930
Position of first nodal point, N	7.078	NA[a]
Position of second nodal point, N′	7.332	NA
Position of fovea centralis	24.0	24.0
Axial refraction	−1.0	−9.6

[a] NA = not applicable.

表3–1　模拟眼

	放松调节时	最大调节时
折射率		
角膜	1.376	1.376
房水和玻璃体	1.336	1.336
晶状体	1.386	1.386
等效晶状体核	1.406	1.406
位置		
角膜前表面	0	0
角膜后表面	0.5	0.5
晶状体前表面	3.6	3.2
等效晶状体前表面	4.146	3.8725
等效晶状体后表面	6.565	6.5275
晶状体后表面	7.2	7.2
曲率半径		
角膜前表面	7.7	7.7
角膜后表面	6.8	6.8
晶体前表面	10.0	5.33
等效球镜的前表面	7.911	2.655
等效球镜的前表面	–5.76	–2.655
晶体后表面	–6.0	–5.33
屈光力		
角膜前表面	48.83	48.83
角膜后表面	–5.88	–5.88
晶状体前表面	5.0	9.375
晶状体核	5.985	14.96
晶体后表面	8.33	9.375
角膜系统		
屈光力	43.05	43.05
第一主点位置	–0.0496	–0.0496
第二主点位置	–0.0506	–0.0506
第一焦距	–23.227	–23.227
第二焦距	31.031	31.031
晶状体系统		
屈光力	19.11	33.06
第一主点位置	5.678	5.145
第二主点位置	5.808	5.255
焦距	69.908	40.416
全眼球光学系统		
屈光力	58.64	70.57
第一主点位置，*P*	1.348	1.772
第二主点位置，*P′*	1.602	2.086
第一焦点位置，*F*	–15.707	–12.397
第二焦点位置，*F′*	24.387	21.016
第一焦距	–17.055	–14.169
第二焦距	22.785	18.930
第一节点位置，*N*	7.078	NA[a]
第二节点位置，*N′*	7.332	NA
黄斑中心凹位置	24.0	24.0
轴性屈光度	–1.0	–9.6

[a]NA=不可用。

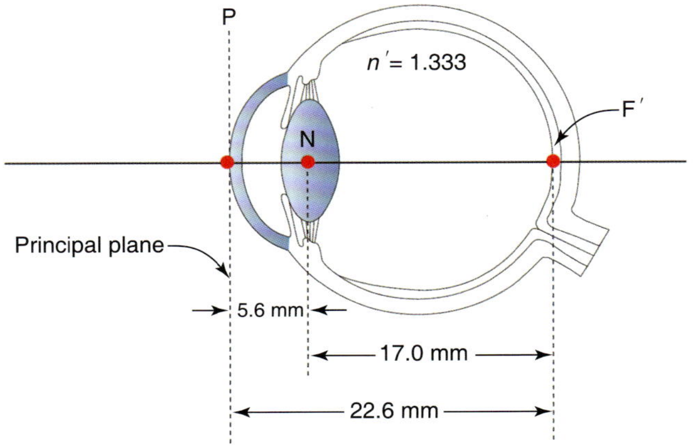

Figure 3-2 Dimensions of the reduced schematic eye, defined by the anterior corneal surface (P), the simplified nodal point of the eye (N), and the fovea (F′). The distance from the simplified nodal point to the fovea is 17.0 mm, and the distance from the anterior corneal surface to the nodal point is 5.6 mm. The refractive index for air is taken to be 1.000, and the simplified refractive index for the eye (n') is 1.333. The refractive power of this reduced schematic eye is 60.0D, with its principal plane at the front surface of the cornea. *(Illustration by C. H. Wooley.)*

Although the distance from the eye chart to the nodal point should be measured, it is much easier to measure the distance to the surface of the cornea. The difference between these measurements is 5.6 mm, which is usually insignificant. For example, if the distance between the nodal point and the retina is 17.0 mm, the distance between the eye chart and the eye is 20 ft (6000 mm), and the height of a Snellen letter is 60 mm, then the resulting image size on the retina is 0.17 mm.

Katz M, Kruger PB. The human eye as an optical system. In: Tasman W, Jaeger EA, eds. *Duane's Clinical Ophthalmology* [CD-ROM]. Vol 1. Philadelphia: Lippincott Williams & Wilkins; 2013:chap 33.

Important Axes of the Eye

Careful analysis of the orientation of the eye is frustrated by the imprecision of the alignment of the main optical elements. Ideally, one might imagine that the fixation target, the optical center of the cornea, the optical center of the lens, and the fovea should all fall on a single line, which one might envision as the "axis" of the eye. In fact, no 3 of these points typically lie on the same line. As a line is determined by 2 points, there are many choices, each of which determines a different "axis." The following are definitions of selected terms used to describe the various axes of the eye:

- The *principal line* of *vision* is the line passing through the fixation target, perpendicular to the corneal surface. (When the patient fixates a luminous target, the reflection in the cornea of the light source will lie on this line.)
- The *pupillary axis* is the line perpendicular to the corneal surface and passing through the midpoint of the entrance pupil. (The *entrance pupil* is the image of the pupil as seen through the cornea from the outside of the eye.) If an observer is aligned with a small light source, and centers the corneal reflection in the entrance pupil, he will be sighting along the pupillary axis. If the pupil is eccentric, this will not coincide with the principal line of vision. The *visual axis* is the line connecting the fixation target and the fovea.

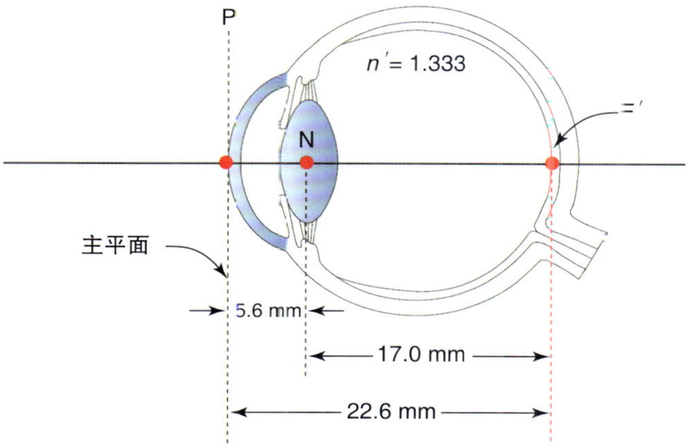

图 3–2　简化眼的参数包括了角膜前表面（P），简化节点（N）和中心凹（F′）。简化节点到中心凹的距离为 17.0 mm，角膜前表面到节点的距离为 5.6 mm。空气折射率为 1.000，简化眼折射率（n'）为 1.333，简化模型眼的屈光力为 60.0D，其主平面为角膜前表面。*（译者注：资料来源见前页原文。）*

我们可以计算视力表到节点的距离，但测量视力表到角膜表面的距离更为简便。通常 2 个测量方法的差距不大，大约为 5.6 mm。例如，假设节点到视网膜的距离是 17 mm，视力表到眼的距离是 20 ft（6 000 mm），视力表字母的高度是 60 mm，那么视网膜成像的高度为 0.17 mm。

Katz M, Kruger PB. The human eye as an optical system. In: Tasman W, Jaeger EA, eds. *Duane's Clinical Ophthalmology* [CD-ROM]. Vol 1. Philadelphia: Lippincott Williams & Wilkins; 2013:chap 33.

眼睛重要的轴线

由于眼球主要光学成分的排列不精确，无法进行眼睛的定位精细分析。理想情况下，人们可以想象固定目标、角膜的光学中心、晶状体的光学中心和黄斑中心凹都落在一条线上，可以把这条线想象成眼睛的“轴”。事实上，这些点中没有哪 3 个点位于同一条线上。而 2 点确定 1 条直线，所以有很多个选择，每个选择确定了不同的“轴”。下面描述眼睛各种轴的定义：

- *视觉主线*是指通过固视点，并垂直于角膜表面的直线（当患者固视发光目标时，光源在角膜的反射将位于这条线上）。
- *瞳孔轴*是通过入射光瞳的中点并垂直于角膜表面的线。（*入射光瞳*是从外透过角膜向眼内所看到的瞳孔的像。）如果观察者与小光源、入射光瞳的角膜反射中心对齐，观察者就对准了瞳孔轴。若瞳孔偏中心，将与视觉主线不吻合。*视轴*是注视目标与中心凹的连线。

- The *optical axis* is the line passing through the optical centers of the cornea and lens. This line typically does not pass through the center of the fovea.
- The *angle alpha* (α) is the angle between the visual axis and the optical axis. This angle is considered positive when the visual axis in object space lies on the nasal side of the optical axis.
- The *angle kappa* (κ) is the angle between the pupillary axis and the visual axis (Fig 3-3). The angle kappa is considered positive when the fovea lies temporal to pupillary axis, as is typically the case.

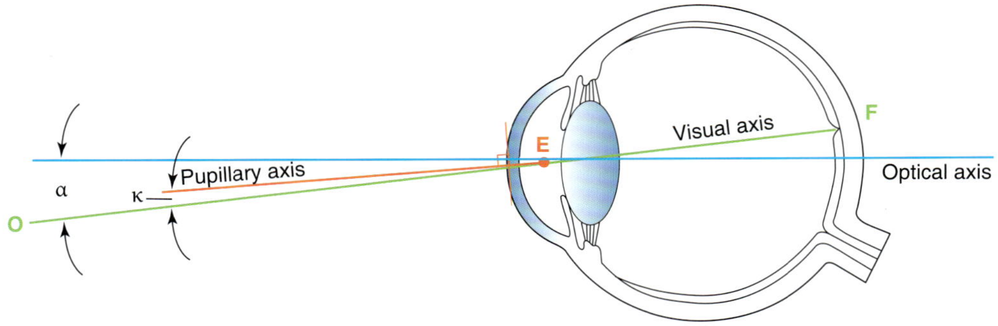

Figure 3-3 Angle kappa (κ). The pupillary axis (*red line*) is represented schematically as the line perpendicular to the corneal surface and passing through the midpoint of the entrance pupil (E). The visual axis (*green line*) is defined as the line connecting the fixation target (O) and the fovea (F). If all the optical elements of the human eye were in perfect alignment, these 2 lines would overlap. However, the fovea is normally displaced from its expected position. The angle between the pupillary axis and the visual axis (leader line) is called angle kappa (κ) and is considered positive when the fovea is located temporally, as is the usual case. Conditions that cause temporal dragging of the retina, such as retinopathy of prematurity, can lead to a large positive angle kappa. Clinically, this will present as pseudoexotropia. A large positive angle kappa may also mask a small-angle esotropia, which can be detected by the cover-uncover test. Angle alpha (α) is the angle between the optical axis and the visual axis of the eye and is con- sidered positive when the visual axis in object space lies on the nasal side of the optical axis, as is normally the case. *(Courtesy of Neal H. Atebara, MD. Revised illustration based on a drawing by C. H. Wooley.)*

Pupil Size and Its Effect on Visual Resolution

The size of the blur circle on the retina generally increases as the size of the pupil increases. If a pinhole aperture is placed immediately in front of an eye, it acts as an artificial pupil, and the size of the blur circle is reduced correspondingly (Fig 3-4).

- *光轴*是穿过角膜和晶状体光学中心的轴线，通常这条线不经过黄斑中央凹。

- α *角*是光轴和视轴的夹角，固视时，视轴在光轴的鼻侧，夹角为正角。

- κ *角*是瞳孔轴和视轴的夹角（图 3–3），当中心凹位于瞳孔轴颞侧时，κ 角是正的，这是典型的情况。

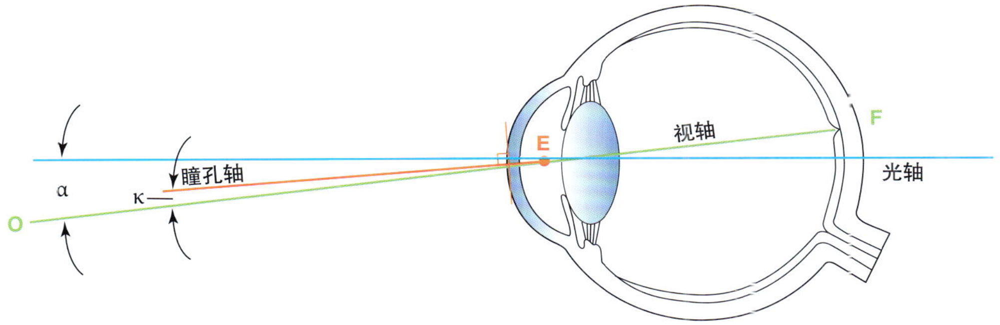

图 3–3 κ 角。瞳孔轴（*红线*）表示垂直于角膜表面通过入射瞳孔中心的轴线（E），视轴（*绿线*）表示注视点（O）和黄斑中心凹（F）的连线。如果人眼所有的光学成分都是完美的，这 2 条线就会重叠。然而，黄斑的位置常偏离。瞳孔轴和视轴（带箭头的线）的夹角即为 κ 角，因黄斑位于颞下方，κ 角为正角。临床上，向颞侧牵拉视网膜的条件下产生大的正 κ 角，如早产儿视网膜病变，形成假性外斜。大的正 κ 角也会掩盖小度数内斜，可以用遮盖 – 去遮盖检测。α 角是光轴和视轴的夹角，当视轴位于光轴的鼻侧时，夹角为正，此为正常情况。
（译者注：资料来源见前页原文。）

瞳孔大小和对视觉分辨率的影响

视网膜上弥散斑的大小一般随着瞳孔的扩大而增加。若将一个针孔迅速置于眼前，针孔就被作为一个人造瞳孔，弥散斑则相应减小（图 3–4）。

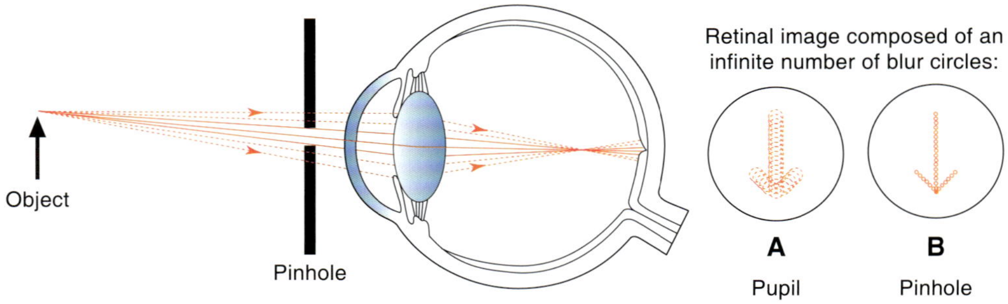

Figure 3-4 Light rays from each point on an object (upright arrow) form a blur circle on the retina of a myopic eye. The retinal image is the composite of all blur circles, the size of each being proportional to the diameter of the pupil (**A**) and the amount of defocus. If a pinhole is held in front of the eye, the size of each blur circle is decreased; as a result, the overall retinal image is sharpened (**B**). *(Courtesy of Neal H. Atebara, MD. Revised illustration based on a drawing by C. H. Wooley.)*

The pinhole is used clinically to measure *pinhole visual acuity*. If visual acuity improves when measured through a pinhole aperture, a refractive error is usually present. The most useful pinhole diameter for general clinical purposes (refractive errors between –5.00D and +5.00D) is 1.2 mm. If the pinhole aperture is made smaller, the blurring effects of diffraction around the edges of the aperture overwhelm the image-sharpening effects of the smaller aperture. For refractive errors greater than 5.00D, the clinician needs to use a lens that corrects most of the refractive error in addition to the pinhole.

After the best refractive correction has been determined, the pinhole can also be used with a dilated pupil. If visual acuity improves, optical irregularities, such as corneal and lenticular light scattering or irregular astigmatism, are likely to be present, given that the pinhole serves to restrict light to a relatively small area of the eye's optics. (This technique also can be used to identify optical causes of *monocular diplopia*.) If visual acuity worsens, macular disease must be considered, as a diseased macula is often unable to adapt to the reduced amount of light entering through the pinhole.

Because of the refractive effects of the cornea, the entrance pupil is about 13%–15% larger than the actual pupil and displaced somewhat anterior to the plane of the iris. This explains why the anterior chamber is actually deeper than it looks.

CLINICAL PROBLEMS 3-1

Why do persons with uncorrected myopia squint?
To obtain a pinhole effect (or rather a stenopeic slit effect). Better visual acuity results from smaller blur circles (or even smaller blur "slits").

Does pupil size affect the measured near point of accommodation?
Yes. With smaller pupil size, the eye's depth of focus increases, and objects closer than the actual near point of the eye remain in better focus.

Why are patients less likely to need their glasses in bright light?
One reason is that the bright light causes the pupil to constrict, allowing the defocused image to be less blurred on the retina.

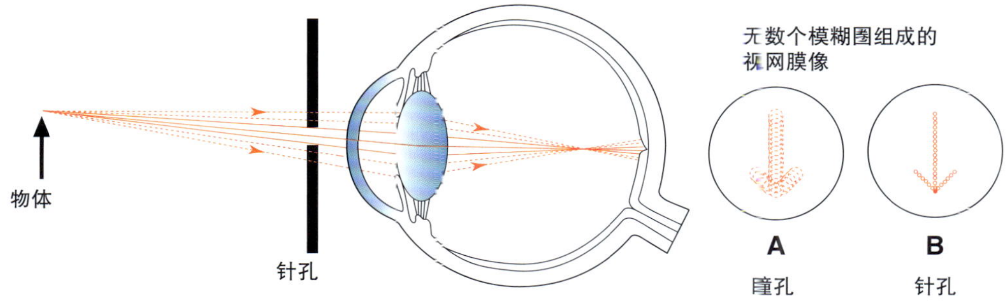

图 3–4　物体发出的每一条光线（向上箭头示）在近视的视网膜上形成一个弥散斑。视网膜成像是所有弥散斑的组合，弥散斑大小与瞳孔直径（**A**）和离焦量成比例。如果将一个针孔置于眼前，则每个弥散斑减小，使视网膜成像清晰（**B**）。*（译者注：资料来源见前页原文。）*

临床上利用针孔测量针*孔视力*。如果针孔视力有所改善，通常存在屈光不正。一般用于临床针孔测量的孔径为 1.2mm（屈光不正为 –5.00~+5.00D）。如果孔径变小，孔缘衍射的模糊效应会超过小孔径的成像清晰效果。若屈光度大于 5.00D，除了针孔之外，还需要用透镜矫正。

进行最佳屈光矫正后，针孔也可应用于散大的瞳孔。如果视力有所提高，可能存在角膜和晶状体的光散射或不规则散光等光学不规则，因为针孔将光限制在相对较小的眼睛内部的光学区域里。（可以用来判定光学原因引起的*单眼复视*）。如果视力下降，则须考虑黄斑疾病，因为病变的黄斑通常无法适应通过针孔减少的进光量。

由于角膜的折射效应，入射光瞳比实际瞳孔大 13%~15%，并且位于虹膜平面之前一点。这就解释了为什么前房深度比看上去的要深的问题。

临床问题 3–1

为什么未矫正的近视患者眯着眼?
眯眼可以获得针孔效果（或裂隙效果）。通过缩小的弥散斑（或更小的弥散“裂隙”）可以获得更好的视力。

瞳孔大小会影响调节近点的测量吗?
会。较小的瞳孔会增加景深，当物体靠近近点时其仍在焦点范围内。

为什么患者在光线明亮的时候很少需要配带眼镜?
明亮的光线可引起瞳孔收缩，使视网膜上离焦的像弥散斑减小是其原因之一。

EXAMPLE 3-2

Estimate the location of the entrance pupil. (assume the anatomical pupil lies in the same plane as the apex of the lens.) Using the Gullstrand model eye, the distance from the second principal plane of the cornea to the apex of the lens in mm is 0.0506 + 3.1 = 3.1506 mm. as the power of the corneal system is 43.05 diopters (D), the vergence equation gives 1.336/0.0031506 + 43.05 = 1/x, where 1.336 is the refractive index of the aqueous humor and vitreous body, *x* is the distance from the second principal plane to the image of the pupil (as seen by an external observer in air). this gives 1/*x* = 467.096, or *x* = 2.14 mm. thus, the entrance pupil and the external observer's view of the iris are about 1 mm closer to the observer than the anatomical pupil and the true iris plane.

Visual Acuity

Clinicians often think of visual acuity primarily in terms of Snellen acuity, but visual perception is a far more complex process than is encapsulated by this single measurement. Indeed, there are many ways to measure visual function. The following are definitions of terms used in the measurement of visual function:

- The *minimum legible threshold* refers to the point at which a patient's visual ability cannot further distinguish progressively smaller letters or forms from one another; Snellen visual acuity is the most common method of determining this threshold.
- The *minimum visible threshold* is the minimum contrast of a target at which the patient can distinguish the target from the background.
- The *minimum separable threshold* refers to the smallest visual angle formed by the eye and 2 separate objects at which a patient can discriminate them individually.
- *Vernier acuity* is defined as the smallest detectable amount of misalignment of 2 line segments.

Snellen visual acuity is measured with test letters or similar targets (optotypes) constructed such that each optotype as a whole is 5 times larger than the individual strokes or gaps that make up the optotype (eg, the horizontal lines, and the spaces between them, of the letter E, or the gap that differentiates a circle from the letter C). Letters of different sizes are designated by the distance at which the letter subtends an angle of 5 arcmin (Fig 3-5). The Snellen chart is designed to measure visual acuity in angular terms. However, the accepted convention does not specify visual acuity in angular measure; instead, it uses a notation in which the numerator is the *testing distance* (in feet or meters) and the denominator is the *distance at which a letter subtends the standard visual angle of 5 arcmin.* Thus, on the 20/20 line (6/6 in meters), the letters subtend an angle of 5 arcmin when viewed at 20 ft. In examination rooms with shorter distances than 20 ft (6 m), mirrors can be used to increase the viewing distance. On the 20/40 (6/12) line, the letters subtend an angle of 10 arcmin when viewed at 20 ft, or 5 arcmin when viewed at 40 ft. The "40" in the 20/40 letter (or the "12" in the 6/12 letter) refers to the viewing distance at which this letter subtends the "normal" visual angle of 5 arcmin. Table 3-2 lists conversions of visual acuity measurements for the various methods in use—the Snellen fraction, decimal notation (Visus), visual angle in minutes of arc, and *base-10 logarithm of the minimum angle of resolution* (logMAR). LogMAR is useful for averaging the results of multiple measurements of Snellen visual acuity.

例 3–2

判断入射光瞳的位置。(假设解剖学瞳孔与晶状体顶点位于同一平面。)使用 Gullstrand 模型眼，从角膜第二平面到晶状体顶点的距离是 0.0506 + 3.1 = 3.1506 mm，角膜系统的屈光力是 43.05D，聚散度方程是 1.336/0.0031506 + 43.05 = 1/*x*，其中 1.336 是房水和玻璃体的折射率，*x* 是第二主平面到瞳孔像的距离（与从外部空气中观察一样）。这样，1/*x* = 467.096，或 *x* = 2.14 mm。因此，入射光瞳和从外部看过去的虹膜要比解剖学瞳孔和真实瞳孔接近观察者 1mm。

视力

临床医生常认为 Snellen 视力就是视敏度，但是视知觉是一个极为复杂的过程，远不能用这单一的测量来概括。事实上有多种方法来测量视觉功能。下面是视觉功能测量的常用术语。

- *最小清晰度阈值*是指可识别的最小的字母或者图案视觉能力，是 Snellen 视力表最常用的测量方法。
- *最小可视阈值*是指可以区分目标与其背景的最小对比度。
- *最小分离阈值*是指可以辨别 2 个独立物体的最小视角。
- *游标视力*，是指两线段的最小可检出偏差量。

*Snellen 视力*用测试字母或相似的靶标（视标）检测，每个视标整体是组成视标的每个笔画或间隙的 5 倍（例如，E 字母的水平线和间隔，或 C 字母的环形缺口。）字母大小由 5 弧分视角在不同距离的大小决定（图 3–5）。Snellen 视力表通过检测视角来测量视力。但是常规的做法不是直接测量视角，而是用一个分式，其中分子为*测量距离*（单位为 ft 或 m），分母为*标准 5 弧分视角时的距离*。因此，20/20 行（6/6，以 m 为单位）的字母，当在 20ft 处观察时，对应 5 弧分的视角。如果检测室距离小于 20ft（6m），可用反光镜增加检测距离。对于 20/40（6/12）行字母，在 20ft 外观察是 10 弧分视角，在 40ft 处观察为 5 弧分视角。在 20/40 中的“40”（或 6/12 中的“12”）是指正常 5 弧分视角的检测距离。表 3–2 列出了不同视力测量方法的换算，包括 Snellen 分数、小数（Visus）、视角的分弧、*以最小分辨角的常用对数*（logMAR）。LogMAR 对于多次测量 Snellen 视力的结果进行平均是有用的。

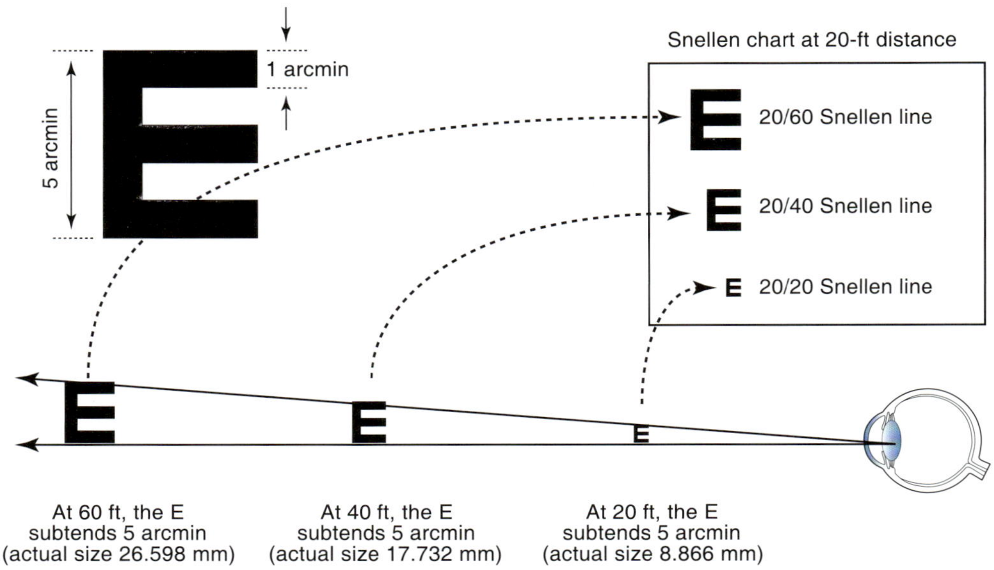

Figure 3-5 Snellen letters are constructed such that they subtend an angle of 5 arcmin when located at the distance specified by the denominator. For example, if a Snellen E is about 26 mm in height, it subtends 5 arcmin at 60 ft. Correspondingly, a 26-mm letter occupies the 20/60 line of the Snellen chart at the standard testing distance of 20 ft. *(Courtesy of Neal H. Atebara, MD. Revised illustration based on a drawing by C. H. Wooley.)*

Table 3-2 Visual Acuity Conversion Chart

Snellen Fraction					
Feet	Meters	4-Meter Standard	Decimal Notation (Visus)	Visual Angle Minute of Arc	LogMAR (Minimum Angle of Resolution)
20/10	6/3	4/2	2.00	0.50	−0.30
20/15	6/4.5	4/3	1.33	0.75	−0.12
20/20	**6/6**	**4/4**	**1.00**	**1.00**	**0.00**
20/25	6/7.5	4/5	0.80	1.25	0.10
20/30	6/9	4/6	0.67	1.50	0.18
20/40	6/12	4/8	0.50	2.00	0.30
20/50	6/15	4/10	0.40	2.50	0.40
20/60	6/18	4/12	0.33	3.00	0.48
20/80	6/24	4/16	0.25	4.00	0.60
20/100	6/30	4/20	0.20	5.00	0.70
20/120	6/36	4/24	0.17	6.00	0.78
20/150	6/45	4/30	0.13	7.50	0.88
20/200	6/60	4/40	0.10	10.00	1.00
20/400	6/120	4/80	0.05	20.00	1.30

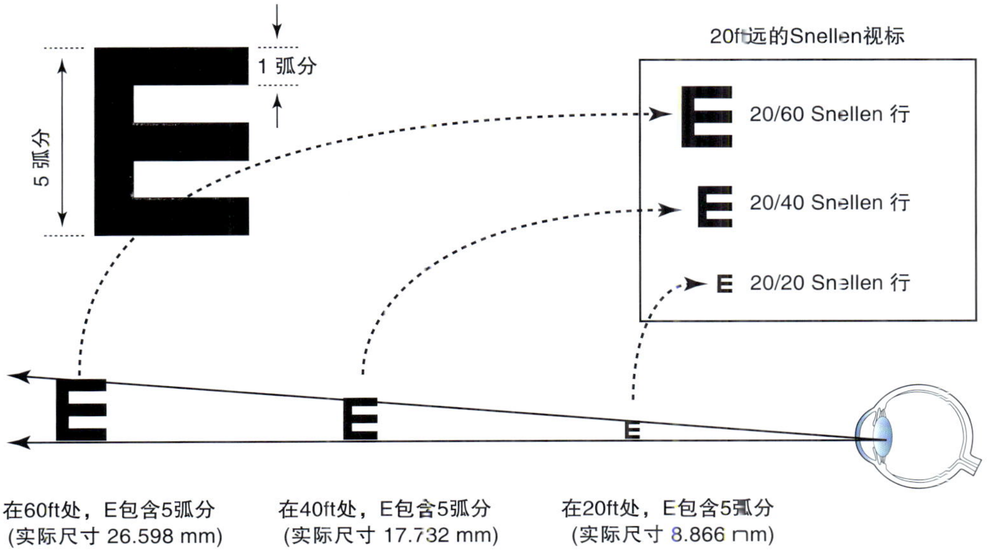

图 3-5　Snellen 视力表由分母在特定距离所视的 5 弧分视角的视标组成。例如，如果视标 E 高 26mm，它的 5 弧分视角应该距离 60ft。相应的，26mm 视标在 Snellen 视力表 20/60 一行，标准测试距离为 20ft。*（译者注：资料来源见前页原文。）*

表3-2　视力换算表

Snellen 分数 ft	Snellen 分数 m	Snellen 分数 4m标准	小数	弧分视角	LogMAR（分辨率最小角）
20/10	6/3	4/2	2.00	0.50	–0.30
20/15	6/4.5	4/3	1.33	0.75	–0.12
20/20	**6/6**	**4/4**	**1.00**	**1.00**	**0.00**
20/25	6/7.5	4/5	0.80	1.25	0.10
20/30	6/9	4/6	0.67	1.50	0.18
20/40	6/12	4/8	0.50	2.00	0.30
20/50	6/15	4/10	0.40	2.50	0.40
20/60	6/18	4/12	0.33	3.00	0.48
20/80	6/24	4/16	0.25	4.00	0.60
20/100	6/30	4/20	0.20	5.00	0.70
20/120	6/36	4/24	0.17	6.00	0.78
20/150	6/45	4/30	0.13	7.50	0.88
20/200	6/60	4/40	0.10	10.00	1.00
20/400	6/120	4/80	0.05	20.00	1.30

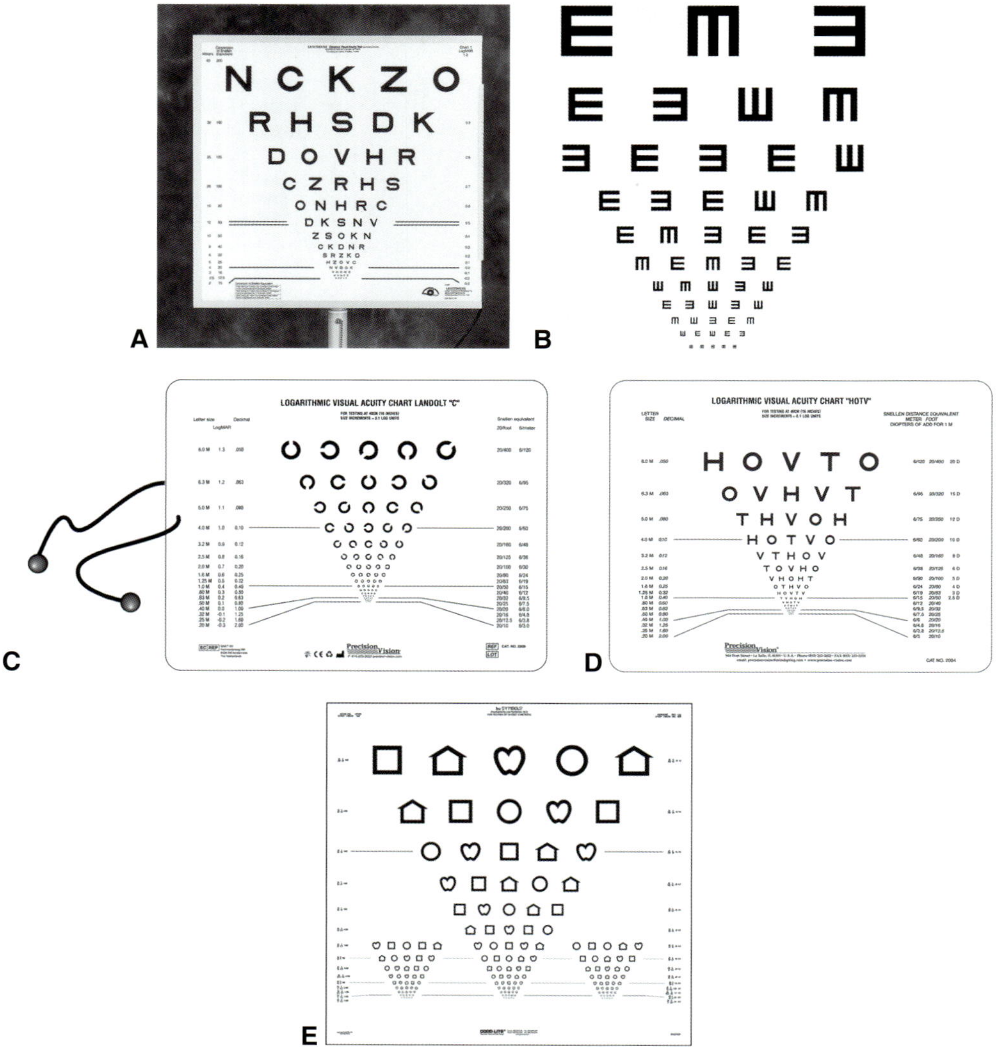

Figure 3-6 Modified Early Treatment Diabetic Retinopathy Study (ETDRS)-type eye charts with alternative optotypes. **A**, Visual acuity chart produced by the Lighthouse. The chart is intended for use at 20 ft (6 m) but can also be used at 10 ft (3 m) or 5 ft (1.5 m) with appropriate scaling. The optoptypes are Sloan letters. **B**, Tumbling E optotypes. **C**, Landolt C optotypes. **D**, HOTV optotypes. **E**, Lea symbols. *(Part A courtesy of Kevin M. Miller, MD; parts B–E courtesy of Precision Vision.)*

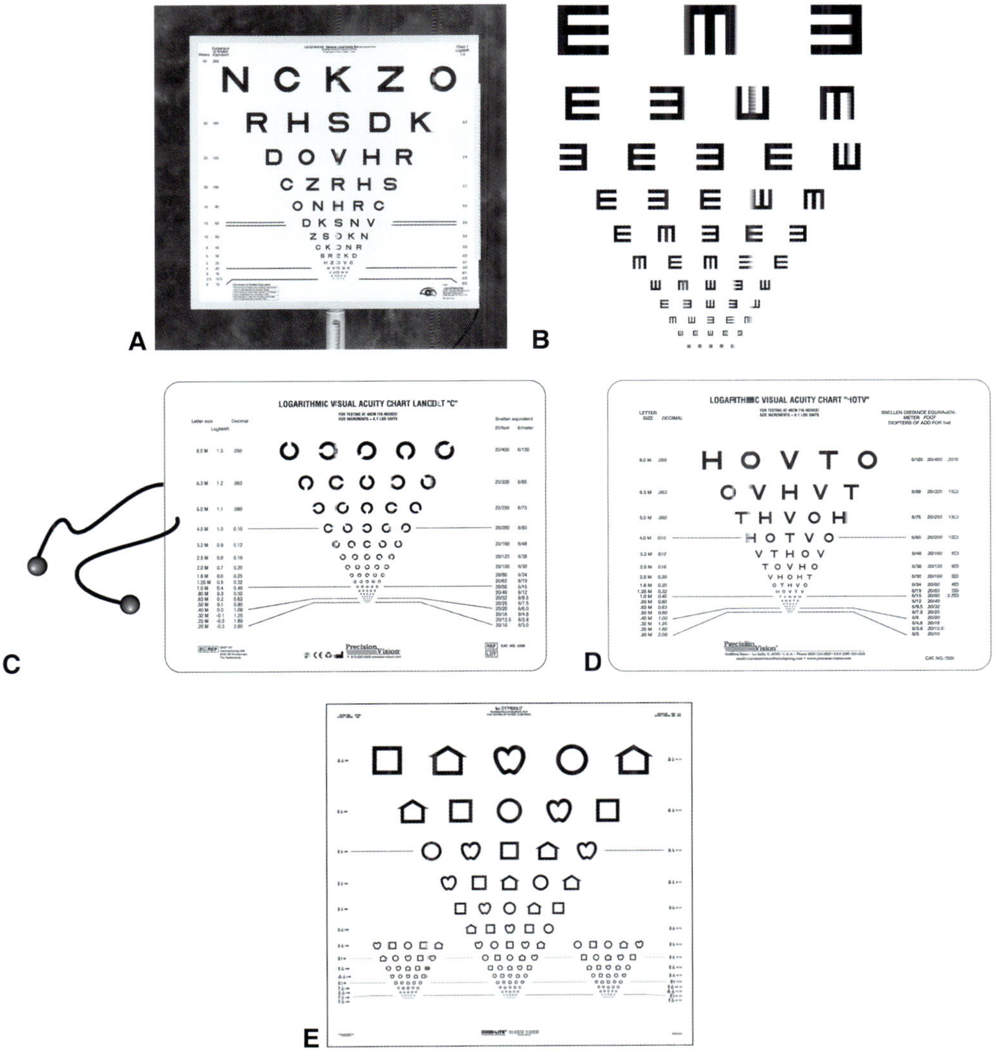

图 3-6　ETDRS（糖尿病视网膜病变早期治疗研究）修正视力表和替代视标。**A**.Lighthouse 视力表，可以用于 20ft（6m）的距离，也可适当缩小至 10ft（3m）或者 5ft（1.5m）。视标采用 Sloan 字母。**B**.Tumbling E 视标。**C**.Landolt C 视标。**D**.HOTV 视标。**E**.Lea 符号。*（译者注：资料来源见前页原文。）*

Though widely accepted, common Snellen eye charts are not perfect. The letters on different Snellen lines are not necessarily related to one another by size in any regular geometric or logarithmic sense. For example, the increase in letter size from the 20/20 line to the 20/25 line (an increase of 25%) differs from the increase from the 20/25 line to the 20/30 line (an increase of 20%). In addition, certain letters (such as C, D, O, and G) are inherently harder to recognize or to distinguish than others (such as A and J), partly because there are more letters of the alphabet with which they can be confused. For these reasons, alternative visual acuity charts have been developed and popularized in high-quality clinical trials (eg, the Early Treatment Diabetic Retinopathy Study [ETDRS] or Bailey-Lovie charts) (Fig 3-6). These charts feature careful choices of optotypes, uniform proportional(logarithmic) progression of optotype size from line to line, and the same number of optotypes on each line. Computer-based acuity devices that display optotypes on a monitor screen have also become popular because they allow presentation of a random assortment of optotypes and scrambling of letters, thereby eliminating problems associated with memorization by patients.

The original Snellen eye chart used ordinary typography font letters of various sizes. However, it is preferable to choose optotypes from simpler fonts that better present identifying features of 20% of the overall letter height, and to restrict the choice of letters to a subset of the alphabet that is as uniform in distinguishability as possible. A standard set of letters in a simple, sans-serif font, known as the *Sloan Letters* (C, D, H, K, N, O, R, S, V, and Z) is commonly used. (Note that the letter E is not a Sloan letter.) Alternative optotypes are available for patients with special needs (Fig 3-6 B–E). The tumbling E and Landolt C optotypes are suitable for preliterate patients. The 4-letter subset HOTV can be used with a reference sample to allow patients to point to the optotypes which they see, even if they cannot name the letters. Picture charts are often useful for small children. The carefully calibrated Lea symbols (circle, square, house, apple) are greatly preferable to the older traditional picture set (hand, horse, telephone, bird, birthday cake), because the former blur into indistinguishable circles with decreasing acuity, whereas the latter can often be recognized even after the smallest details can no longer be resolved.

Levi DM. Visual acuity. In: Levin LA, Nilsson SFE, Ver Hoeve J, Wu SM, eds. *Adler's Physiol- ogy of the Eye.* 11th ed. New York: Elsevier; 2011.

Contrast Sensitivity and the Contrast Sensitivity Function

Another important dimension in measuring visual function is contrast sensitivity—the sensitivity of an observer to differences in luminance between an object and the background. In general, the higher the contrast, the easier an optotype is to decipher. Over a broad range, the visual system is relatively insensitive to the absolute brightness of a visual stimulus, but is much more attuned to the contrast between adjacent surfaces. For example, the dark ink on a printed page reflects about 10% of the incident light. In comparison, the white paper background has a reflectance of perhaps 90%, regardless of the level of absolute illumination. Thus, when reading under bright sunlight, we still appreciate the printed text as black, even though the absolute brightness of the reflected light is greater than that reflected from white paper in dim illumination, as in twilight. If the brightness of an object (I_{min}) and the brightness of its background (I_{max}) are known, the following formula can be used to measure the degree of contrast between the object and its background:

虽然 Snellen 标准视力表的应用效果被广泛认同，但其并不完美。不同行的视标大小在几何或者对数上没有关联。例如，视标 20/20 到视标 20/25 大小的增大（增大 25%），不等于 20/25 到 20/30 大小的增大（增大 20%）。还有，某些字母本身（如 C、D、O、G）就比另一些字母（如 A、J）难辨认，出现过多也容易混淆。考虑到这些因素，开发出来一些替换视力表，并推广用于高质量的临床试验 [如糖尿病视网膜病变早期治疗研究（ETDRS），Bailey–Lovie 视力表]（图 3–6）。这些视力表特别注意选择视标、行与行视标递增比例（对数）一致，以及每一行视标数量一样多。计算机视力检测设备可以在屏幕上显示视标，随机分配视标，打乱字母顺序，消除记忆的问题。

最初的 Snellen 视标使用各种大小普通排版字体的字母。然而，更好是从更简单的字体中选择视标，这些字体能够更好地呈现出占整个字母高度 20% 的识别特征，并将字母的选择限制在尽可能一致的可识别性的字母表子集中。通常使用简单无衬线字体的标准字母集，称为 *Sloan 字母*（C、D、H、K、N、O、R、S、V 和 Z）。（请注意，字母 E 不是 Sloan 字母。）对于有特殊需要的患者，可以选择其他选项（图 3–6B–E）。“翻滚”E 和 Landolto C 型适合于不识字的患者。4 字母的 HOTV 可以与参考样本一起使用，即使患者无法说出这些字母，但可以指出所看到的视标。图画通常对儿童有用。仔细校准的 Lea 符号（圆、方形、房子、苹果）比传统的图集（手、马、电话、鸟、生日蛋糕）更可取，因为前者模糊成不易分辨的圆，而后者，即使最小的细节无法分辨，往往还是能识别。

Levi DM. Visual acuity. In: Levin LA, Nilsson SFE, Ver Hoeve J, Wu SM, eds. *Adler's Physiol- ogy of the Eye*. 11th ed. New York: Elsevier; 2011.

对比敏感度和对比敏感度函数

另一项重要的视觉功能测量是对比敏感度——观察者对物体和背景亮度差异的敏感度。一般来说，对比度越高，视标越容易认读。在一个较大的范围，视觉系统对视觉刺激的绝对亮度相对不敏感，而对相邻界面的对比度更加适应。例如，印刷纸上的黑字反射约 10% 的入射光，相比之下，无论绝对亮度是多少，纸的白背景反射率约是 90%。当我们在明亮的阳光下阅读时，即使反射光的绝对亮度大于白纸在昏暗的照明下（如黄昏）的反射光的绝对亮度，我们仍然会把印刷的文字看作是黑色的。如果已知物体的亮度（I_{min}）和背景亮度（I_{max}），以下公式可以测量该物体和背景之间的对比度：

$$\text{Contrast} = \frac{I_{max} - I_{min}}{I_{max} + I_{min}}$$

Thus, for typical printed matter, the contrast is about 80% (90% – 10%)/(90% + 10%). Snellen visual acuity is commonly tested with targets, either illuminated or projected charts, that *approximate* 100% contrast. Therefore, when we measure Snellen visual acuity, we are measuring, at approximately 100% contrast, the smallest optotype that the visual system can recognize. In everyday life, however, 100% contrast is rarely encountered, and most visual tasks must be performed in lower-contrast conditions.

To take contrast sensitivity into account when measuring visual function, we can use the *modulation transfer function* (*MTF*). Consider a target in which the light intensity varies from some peak value to zero in a sinusoidal fashion. The contrast is 100%, but instead of looking like a bar graph, it looks like a bar graph with softened edges. The number of light bands per unit length or per unit angle is called the *spatial frequency* and is closely related to Snellen acuity. For example, the 20/20 E optotype is composed of bands of light and dark, where each band is 1 arcmin. Thus, for a target at 100% contrast, 20/20 Snellen acuity corresponds roughly to 30 cycles per degree of resolution when expressed in spatial frequency notation. The relationship between spatial frequency and the contrast sensitivity at each spatial frequency constitutes the MTF.

In clinical practice, the ophthalmologist presents a patient with targets of various spatial frequencies and peak contrasts. A plot is then made of the minimum resolvable contrast target that can be seen for each spatial frequency. The minimum resolvable contrast is the *contrast threshold*. The reciprocal of the contrast threshold is defined as the *contrast sensitivity*, and the manner in which contrast sensitivity changes as a function of the spatial frequency of the targets is called the *contrast sensitivity function* (*CSF*) (Fig 3-7). Figure 3-8 shows a typical contrast sensitivity curve obtained with sinusoidal gratings. Contrast sensitivity can also be tested with optotypes of variable contrast (eg, the Pelli-Robson or Regan charts), which may be easier for patients to use. It is important to perform contrast sensitivity testing with the best possible optical correction in place. In addition, luminance must be kept constant when CSF is tested, because mean luminance affects the shape of the normal CSF. In low luminance, the low spatial frequency fall-off disappears and the peak shifts toward the lower frequencies. In brighter light, there is little change in the shape of the normal CSF through a range of luminance for the higher spatial frequencies. Generally, contrast sensitivity is measured at normal room illumination, which is approximately 30–70 lux.

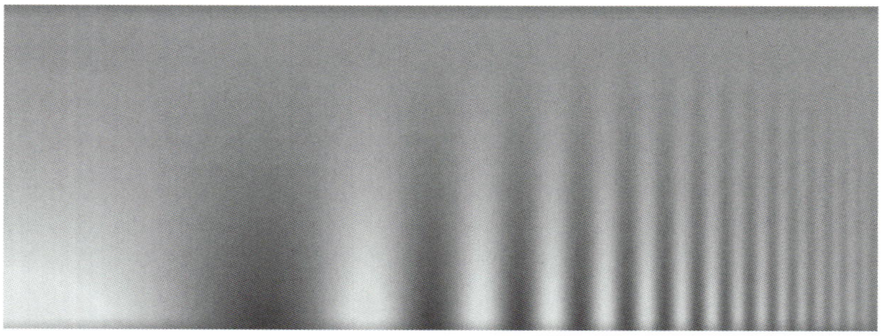

Figure 3-7 Campbell-Robson contrast sensitivity grating. In this example, the contrast diminishes from bottom to top, and the spatial frequency of the pattern increases from left to right. The pattern appears to have a hump in the middle at the frequencies for which the human eye is most sensitive to contrasts. *(Courtesy of Brian Wandell, PhD.)*

$$\text{对比度} = \frac{I_{max} - I_{min}}{I_{max} + I_{min}}$$

因此，标准的印刷品，对比度约为 80% (90%–10%)/(90% + 10%)。Snellen 视力表的视标，无论是照明还是投影，对比度都*接近* 100%。因此测量 Snellen 视力时，我们在测量对比度近 100% 时的视觉系统最小分辨视标。然而日常生活中，100% 对比度很少见，大多数的视觉行为是在低对比度下进行的。

考虑到对比敏感度，测量视功能的时候我们可以运用*调制传递函数*（*MTF*）。对于一个光强以正弦波的方式在峰值到 0 之间变化的物体，对比度为 100%。看上去像一个边缘柔化的条形图。每单位长度或单位角度的光带数称为*空间频率*，它与 Snellen 视力密切相关。例如，20/20 E 视标由明、暗光带组成，每一个光带为 1 弧分。因此，当为 100% 对比度、20/20 Snellen 视力时，对应的空间频率表达约为 30cpd 的分辨率。空间频率和每个空间频率的对比敏感度关系构成 MTF 去掉。

在临床实践中，眼科医生给患者出示一个不同的空间频率和最大对比度的视标。然后用每个空间频率可以看到的最小可分辨对比度视标绘制一个图。最小可分辨对比度就是对比度阈值，对比度阈值的倒数定义为*对比敏感度*，对比敏感度随空间频率变化的曲线称为*对比敏感度函数*（*CSF*）（图 3–7）。图 3–8 显示用正弦光栅获得的典型的对比敏感度曲线。对比敏感度也可以通过可变对比度的视标（如 Pellio – Robson 或 Regan 图表）来测试，这可能更便于患者使用。重要的是先进行最佳的屈光矫正，再进行对比敏感度的检查。另外，由于平均亮度影响 CSF 的形状，所以测定 CSF 时亮度必须保持不变。低亮度时，低空间频率衰减会消失，峰值转向较低的频率。在明亮的光线下，正常 CSF 通过一系列高空间频率的亮度，形状变化不大。一般来说，对比敏感度应在正常室内光线下测定，光照强度约为 30~70lx。

图 3–7　Campbell–Robson 对比敏感度光栅。如图，对比度从底部到顶部逐渐消失，对应的空间频率从左到右逐渐增加。在频率中间有一个“驼峰”，此时人眼的对比敏感度最强。*（译者注：资料来源见前页原文。）*

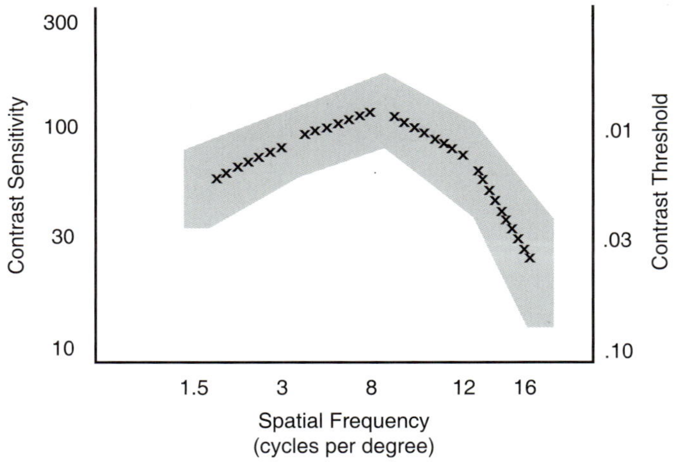

Figure 3-8 A typical contrast sensitivity curve is noted as x-x-x. The shaded area represents the range of normal values for 90% of the population. Expected deviations from normal due to specific diagnoses are noted in the text discussion. *(Developed by Arthur P. Ginsburg, PhD. Courtesy of Stereo Optical Company, Inc, Chicago.)*

Various physiologic and pathologic conditions of the eye affect contrast sensitivity. Any corneal pathology that causes distortion or edema can affect contrast sensitivity. Lens changes, particularly incipient cataracts, may significantly decrease CSF, even with a normal Snellen visual acuity. Retinal pathology may affect contrast sensitivity more (as with retinitis pigmentosa or central serous retinopathy) or less (certain macular degenerations) than it does Snellen visual acuity. Glaucoma may produce a significant loss in the mid-range of spatial frequencies. Optic neuritis may also be associated with a notch-type pattern of sensitivity loss. Amblyopia is associated with a generalized attenuation of the curve. Pupil size also has an effect on contrast sensitivity. With miotic pupils, diffraction reduces contrast sensitivity; with large pupils, optical aberrations may interfere with performance.

Impairments in contrast may be disqualifying in certain occupational situations, such as driving heavy vehicles. Recognition of these difficulties is often valuable in understanding the complaints of patients, who may have difficulty with certain visual tasks not with standing good Snellen acuity as measured with the standard high-contrast eyecharts.

Refractive States of the Eyes

In considering the refractive state of the eye, we can use either of the following approaches:

1. The *focal point* concept: The location of the image formed by an object at optical infinity through a nonaccommodating eye determines the eye's refractive state. Objects focusing at points anterior or posterior to the retina form a blurred image on the retina, whereas objects that focus on the retina form a sharp image.
2. The *far point* concept: The far point is the point in space that is conjugate to the fovea of the nonaccommodating eye; that is, the far point is where the fovea would be imaged if the light rays were reversed and the fovea became the object.

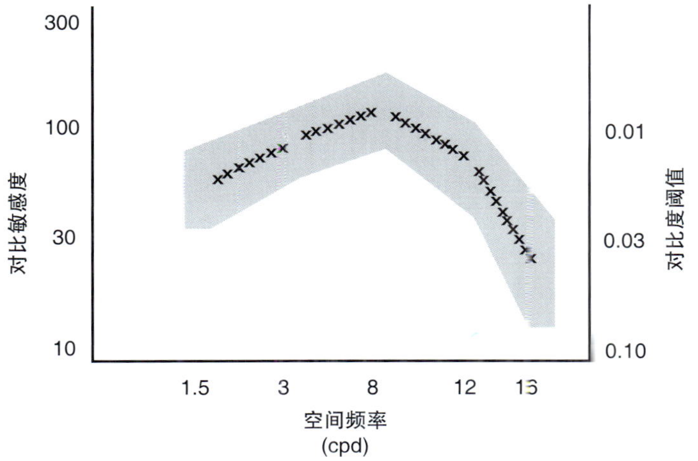

图 3-8　一个典型的对比敏感度曲线是以 x–x–x 为标记。阴影区域代表 90% 人群的正常值范围。有关偏离正常的特殊诊断见正文。*（译者注：资料来源见前页原文。）*

眼睛的生理和病理状态都会影响到对比敏感度。任何角膜病变的变形或水肿可以影响对比敏感度；晶状体改变，尤其是早期白内障，即使 Snellen 视力正常，也可能会严重降低对比敏感度函数（CSF）；相比 Snellen 视力，视网膜损伤可能更影响对比敏感度（如视网膜色素变性，或中心性浆液性视网膜病变），或者影响较小（如某些黄斑退行性变）。对比敏感度函数（CSF）和 Snellen 视力对青光眼的影响相近；视神经炎可能有切迹样缺损；弱视有广泛的曲线衰减。瞳孔大小也影响对比敏感度，瞳孔缩小时，衍射可以降低对比敏感度；瞳孔散大时，光学像差会干扰其性能。

对比敏感度损害可能会导致没有资格从事某些职业，比如驾驶重型车辆。这些有助于理解下面这种情况：这类患者尽管难以进行某项视觉工作，但用标准的高对比度视标测出的 Snellen 视力却仍然是正常的。

眼的屈光状态

关于眼的屈光状态，可以应用以下任一概念：

1. *焦点*概念：无调节时，无穷远处的物体所形成的像的位置决定了眼的屈光状态。物体聚焦在视网膜上，形成清晰像；聚焦在视网膜之前或之后，则形成模糊的像。

2. *远点*概念：远点是无调节眼中心凹与外界空间的共轭点，换句话说，中心凹作为物，光线由眼内射出，远点成为中心凹的像点。

Emmetropia is the refractive state in which parallel rays of light from a distant object are brought to focus on the retina in the nonaccommodating eye (Fig 3-9A). The far point of the emmetropic eye is at infinity, and infinity is *conjugate* with the retina (Fig 3-9B). *Ametropia* refers to the absence of emmetropia and can be classified by presumptive etiology as *axial* or *refractive*. In *axial ametropia*, the eyeball is either unusually long (*myopia*) or short (*hyperopia*). In refractive ametropia, the length of the eye is statistically normal, but the refractive power of the eye (cornea and/or lens) is abnormal, being either excessive (myopia) or deficient (hyperopia). *Aphakia* is an example of extreme refractive hyperopia unless the eye was highly myopic (>20.00D) before lens removal. An ametropic eye requires either a diverging or a converging lens to image a distant object on the retina.

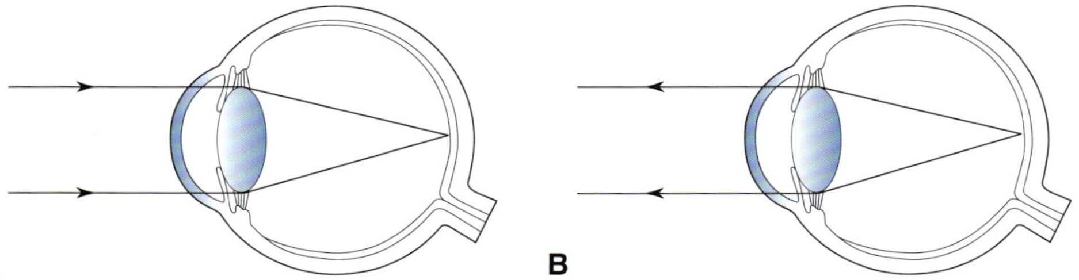

Figure 3-9 Emmetropia with accommodation relaxed. **A**, Parallel light rays from infinity focus to a point on the retina. **B**, Similarly, light rays emanating from a point on the retina focus at the far point of the eye at optical infinity. *(Illustration by C. H. Wooley.)*

Ametropias may also be classified by the nature of the mismatch between the optical power and length of the eye. In myopia, the eye possesses too much optical power for its axial length, and (with accommodation relaxed) light rays from an object at infinity converge too soon and thus focus in front of the retina (Fig 3-10A). This results in a defocused image on the retina; the far point of the eye is located in front of the eye, between the cornea and optical infinity (Fig 3-10B). In hyperopia, the eye does not possess enough optical power for its axial length, and (with accommodation relaxed) an object at infinity comes to a focus behind the retina, again producing a defocused image on the retina (Fig 3-11A); the far point of the eye (actually a virtual point rather than a real point in space) is located behind the retina (Fig 3-11B).

Astigmatism (*a* = without, *stigmos* = point) is an optical condition of the eye in which light rays from a point source on the eye's visual axis do not focus to a single point. Typically, light rays from a single object point are refracted to form 2 *focal lines*, perpendicular to each other. Each astigmatic eye can be classified by the orientations and relative positions of these focal lines (Fig 3-12). If 1 focal line lies in front of the retina and the other is on the retina, the condition is classified as *simple myopic astigmatism*. If both focal lines lie in front of the retina, the condition is classified as *compound myopic astigmatism*. If, in an unaccommodated state, 1 focal line lies behind the retina and the other is on the retina, the astigmatism is classified as *simple hyperopic astigmatism*. If both focal lines lie behind the retina, the astigmatism is classified as compound hyperopic astigmatism. If, in an unaccommodated state, one focal line lies in front of the retina and the other behind it, the condition is classified as *mixed astigmatism*. The orientations of the focal lines reflect, in turn, the strongest and weakest meridians of the net refracting power of the anterior segment refracting surfaces (the cornea and lens). These are referred to as the *principal axes*.

正视眼，是指来自远处物体的平行光线聚焦在无调节眼的视网膜上的屈光状态（图 3–9A）。正视眼的远点在无限远，并与视网膜*共轭*（图 3–9B）。*屈光不正*是指非正视眼，根据成因可分为*轴性*或*屈光性*。在*轴性屈光不正*中，眼球或过长（*近视*），或过短（*远视*）。在屈光性屈光不正中，眼轴长度正常，但眼的屈光力（角膜和/或晶状体）异常，过强（近视）或不足（远视）。*无晶状体眼*就是一个极端的屈光性远视，除非晶状体摘除前有高度近视（>20.00D）。屈光不正眼需用发散透镜或会聚透镜将远处物体成像在视网膜。

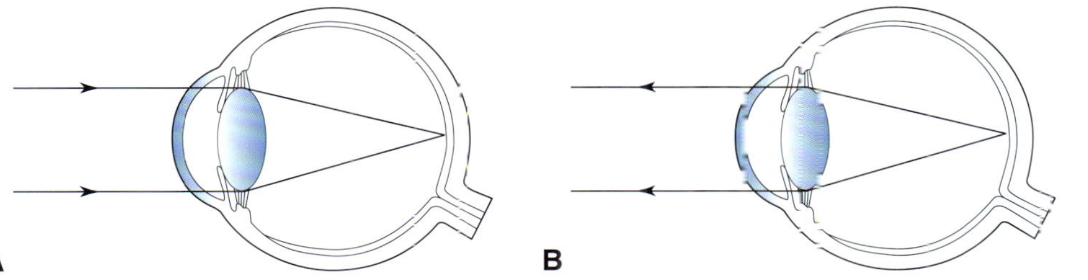

图 3–9　调节放松时的正视眼。**A**. 无限远的平行光线聚焦到视网膜的一点。**B** 同样，光线从视网膜聚焦的一点散发到无限远的远点。*（译者注：资料来源见前页原文。）*

屈光不正也可根据屈光力和眼轴的自然关系分类。在近视眼中，相对于眼轴来说，其屈光力过大，（在调节放松的情况下）来自无限远物体的光线会聚太靠前，从而聚焦于视网膜前（图 3–10A），这就形成了相对视网膜的离焦像，眼的远点位于眼前、角膜和光学上的无限远之间。（图 3–10B）。远视眼中，相对于眼轴来说，其屈光力不足，（在调节放松的情况下）远处的光线会聚于视网膜后，相对视网膜也成离焦像（图 3–11A），其远点（实际上是虚点，而不是空间中的真实点）位于视网膜后（图 3–11B）。

散光（*a* = 没有，stigmos= 点）是眼的视轴点光源发出的光线不能聚焦成单一点的光学状态。来自单一物点的光线折射后形成相互垂直的 2 条*焦线*。根据焦线的方向和焦线的相对位置进行分类（图 3–12），如果 1 条焦线位于视网膜前，另 1 条焦线在视网膜上，这种情况为*单纯近视散光*；如果 2 条焦线都位于视网膜前，则为*复性近视散光*。如果在无调节的状态下，1 条焦线位于视网膜后，而 1 条位于视网膜上，则为*单纯远视散光*；如果 2 条焦线位于视网膜后，则为复性远视散光。如果在无调节状态下，1 条焦线位于视网膜前，而另 1 条焦线位于视网膜后，则为混合散光。反过来，焦线的方向反映出前段屈光面（角膜和晶状体）总屈光力最强的子午线和最弱的子午线。这些称为主轴。

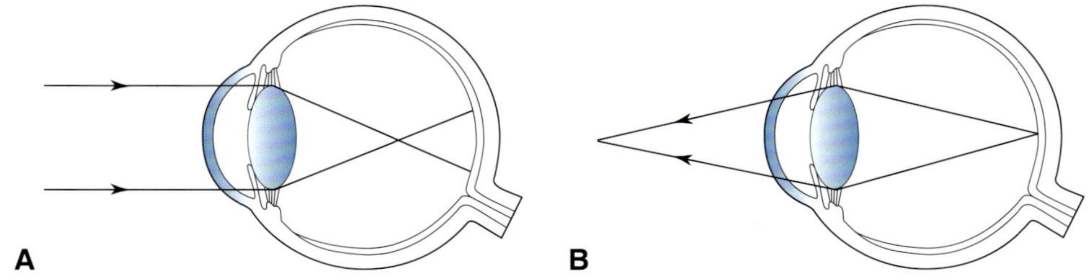

Figure 3-10 Myopia with accommodation relaxed. **A**, Parallel light rays from infinity focus to a point anterior to the retina, forming a blurred image on the retina. **B**, Light rays emanating from a point on the retina focus to a far point in front of the eye, between optical infinity and the cornea. *(Illustration by C. H. Wooley.)*

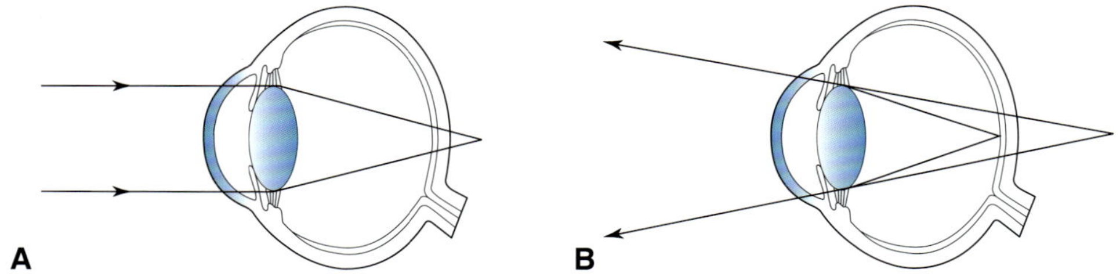

Figure 3-11 Hyperopia with accommodation relaxed. **A**, Parallel light rays from infinity focus to a point posterior to the retina, forming a blurred image on the retina. **B**, Light rays emanating from a point on the retina are divergent as they exit the eye, appearing to have come from a virtual far point behind the eye. *(Illustration by C. H. Wooley.)*

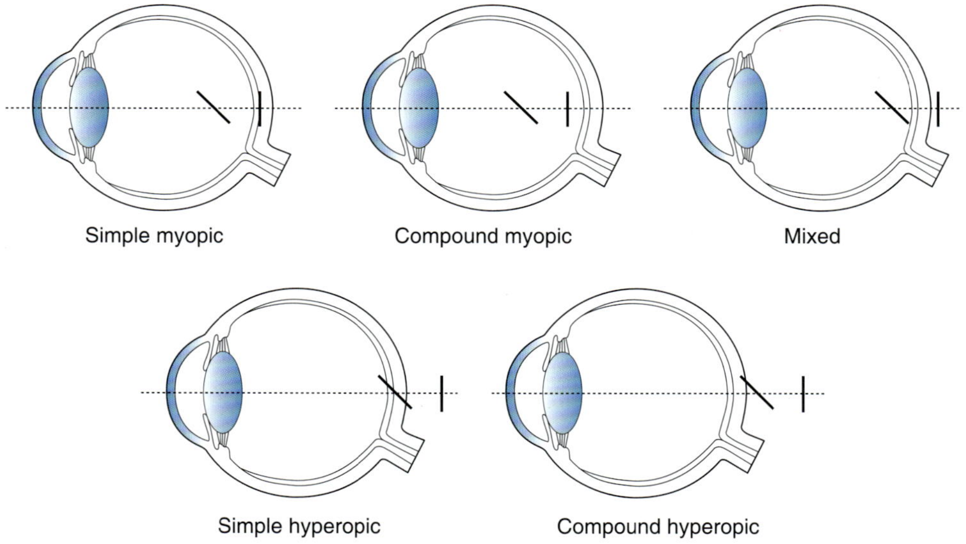

Figure 3-12 Types of astigmatism. The locations of the focal lines with respect to the retina define the type of astigmatism. The main difference between the types of astigmatism depicted in the illustration is the spherical equivalent refractive error. All of the astigmatisms depicted are with-the-rule astigmatisms—that is, they are corrected by using a plus cylinder with a vertical axis. If they were against-the-rule astigmatisms, the positions of the vertical and horizontal focal lines would be reversed.

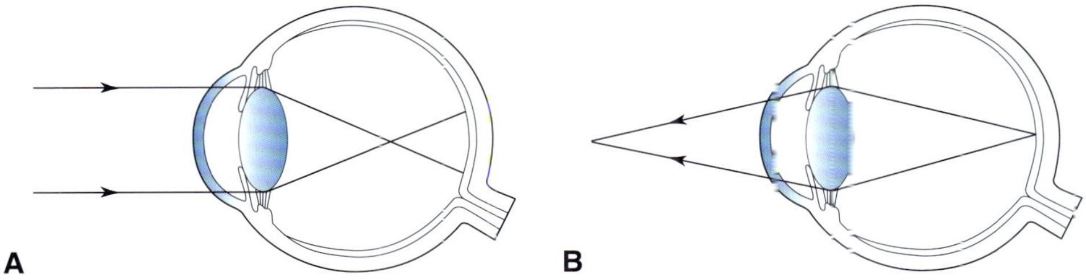

图 3-10　调节放松时的近视眼。**A**. 无限远处发出的平行光线聚焦于视网膜前，在视网膜上形成模糊的像。**B**. 视网膜上一点发出的光线会聚为眼前远点，位于角膜和无限远之间。

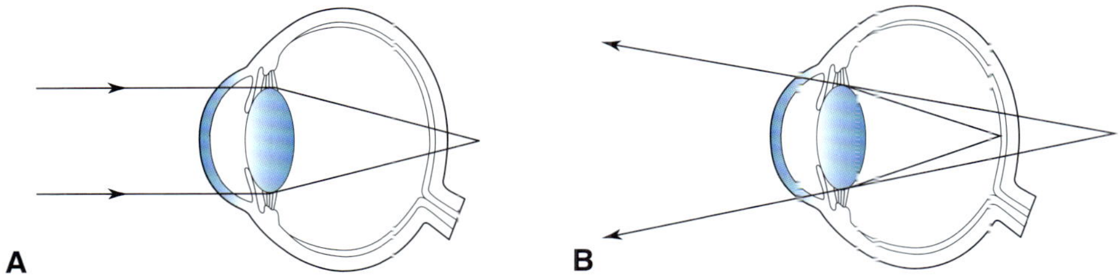

图 3-11　调节放松时的远视眼。**A**. 无限远处发出的平行光线聚焦于视网膜后，在视网膜上形成模糊的像。**B**. 视网膜上一点散发出的光线离开眼后发散，这束发散光似乎是从眼后一个虚的远点发出。*（译者注　资料来源见前页原文。）*

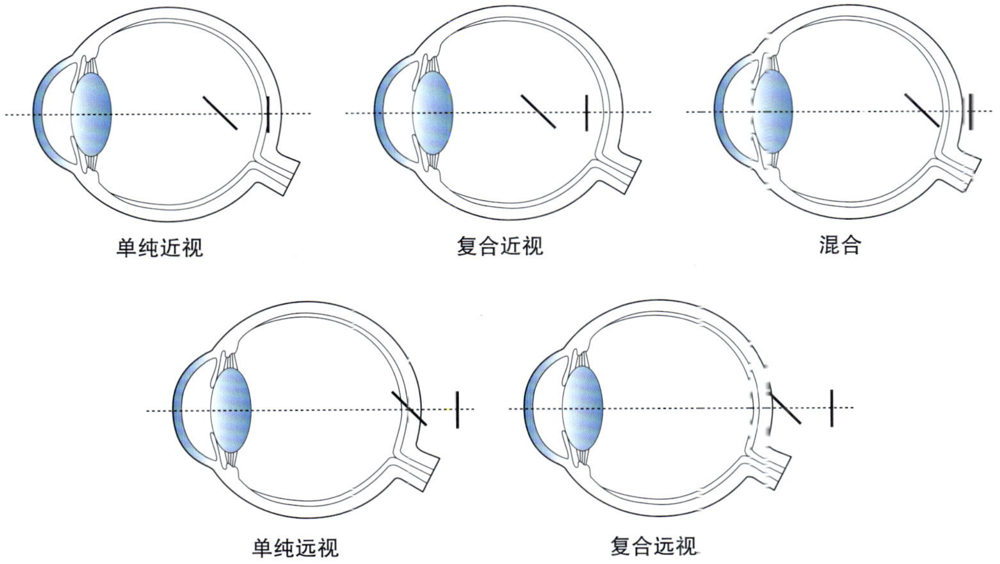

图 3-12　散光的类型。焦线相对于视网膜的位置决定了散光的类型。图中散光类型的主要区别为球面等效屈光不正。所有散光均为顺规散光——即，用垂直轴的正柱镜矫正。如为逆规散光，垂直焦线和水平焦线的位置则反转。

If the principal axes of astigmatism have constant orientation at every point across the pupil, and if the amount of astigmatism is the same at every point, the refractive condition is known as *regular astigmatism*. Regular astigmatism may be classified as *with-the-rule* or *against-the-rule astigmatism*. In *with-the-rule* astigmatism (the more common type in children), the vertical corneal meridian is steepest (resembling an American football or a rugby ball lying on its side), and a correcting plus cylinder is placed with the cylinder axis near 90°. In *against-the-rule* astigmatism (the more common type in older adults), the horizontal meridian is steepest (resembling a football standing on its end), and a correcting plus cylinder should be placed with the axis near 180°. The term oblique astigmatism is used to describe regular astigmatism in which the principal meridians do not lie at, or close to, 90° or 180°, but instead lie nearer 45° or 135°.

In *irregular astigmatism*, the orientation of the principal meridians or the amount of astigmatism changes from point to point across the pupil. Although the principal meridians are 90° apart at every point, it may sometimes appear by retinoscopy or keratometry that the principal meridians of the cornea, as a whole, are not perpendicular to one another. All eyes have at least a small amount of irregular astigmatism, and instruments such as corneal topographers and wavefront aberrometers can be used to detect this condition clinically. These *higher-order* aberrations in the refractive properties of the cornea and lens have been characterized by Zernike polynomials, which are mathematical shapes that approximate various types of irregular astigmatism more closely than the simple "football" model. These aberrations include such shapes as spherical aberration, coma, and trefoil. See Chapters 1 and 7 of this book and BCSC Section 13, *Refractive Surgery*, for further discussion.

Binocular States of the Eyes

The spherical equivalent of a refractive state is defined as the algebraic sum of the spherical component and half of the astigmatic component. *Anisometropia* refers to any difference in the spherical equivalents between the 2 eyes. Uncorrected anisometropia in children may lead to amblyopia, especially if 1 eye is hyperopic. Although adults may be annoyed by uncorrected anisometropia, they may be intolerant of initial spectacle correction. Unequal image size, or *aniseikonia*, may occur, and the prismatic effect of the glasses will vary in different directions of gaze, inducing *anisophoria* (disparate ocular alignment in different directions of gaze). Anisophoria may be more bothersome than aniseikonia for patients with spectacle-corrected anisometropias.

Even though aniseikonia is difficult to measure, anisometropic spectacle correction can be prescribed in such a manner as to reduce aniseikonia. Making the front surface power of a lens less positive can reduce magnification. Decreasing center thickness also reduces magnification. Decreasing vertex distance diminishes the magnifying effect of plus lenses as well as the minifying effect of minus lenses. These effects become increasingly noticeable as lens power increases. Contact lenses may provide a better solution than spectacles for some patients with anisometropia, particularly children, in whom fusion may be possible.

如果散光主轴在经过瞳孔的每个点有固定的方向，且每一点的散光程度相同，为规则散光。规则散光可分为*顺规散光*和*逆规散光*。*顺规散光*（儿童多见）的垂直角膜子午线最陡（类似于美式足球或横卧着的橄榄球），用 90° 轴的正柱镜矫正。*逆规散光*（多见于成人）的水平子午线最陡（类似于美式足球直立），用 180° 轴的正柱镜矫正。斜向散光，是指规则散光的主子午线不在 90° 或 180°，而在 45° 或 135°。

*不规则散光*是指主子午线的方向或散光的程度在瞳孔前后有所变化。尽管主子午线互为 90° 夹角，但有时用检影镜或角膜曲率计检查时，角膜子午线并不相互垂直。所有眼睛都有少量的不规则散光，临床上应用角膜地形图和波前相差仪可以检测。角膜和晶状体屈光特性中的*高阶*相差可以通过 Zernike 多项式来计算，这个数学模型相较于“足球模型”能更好地模拟不同类型的不规则散光，其中包括球差、彗差、三叶草。有关进一步的讨论，请参阅本书的第 1 章和第 7 章以及 BCSC 第 13 册《*屈光手术*》。

双眼视

屈光状态的等效球镜为球镜度数和 1/2 散光度数的代数和。*屈光参差*是指两眼屈光状态不一致。儿童未矫正的屈光参差会导致弱视，尤其是在一眼是远视的时候。虽然成人的屈光参差令人烦恼，但却无法忍耐初始的眼镜矫正。屈光参差导致成像大小不一，或*双眼不等像*，而且注视方向不同会引起眼镜产生不同的棱镜效应，导致不等*隐斜*（不同注视方向上双眼无法一致注视）。与戴眼镜矫正屈光参差的不等像相比，戴眼镜产生的不等隐斜更令患者烦恼。

尽管双眼不等像很难测量，但可以用一种方式开具处方屈光参差眼镜矫正来减小双眼不等像。减少镜片前表面的正焦度可以减少放大率，降低镜片中心厚度也可以减少放大率。减少顶点距，可以减少正镜片的放大效应和负镜片的缩小效应。随着镜片焦度的增加，这些效应更显著。接触镜比框架眼镜可以更好地解决屈光参差问题，尤其是对于儿童，儿童可能形成融合。

Unilateral aphakia is an extreme example of hyperopic anisometropia arising from refractive ametropia. In the adult patient, spectacle correction produces an intolerable aniseikonia of about 25%; contact lens correction produces aniseikonia of about 7%, which is usually tolerated. If necessary, the clinician may reduce aniseikonia still further by adjusting the powers of contact lenses and simultaneously worn spectacle lenses to provide the appropriate minifying or magnifying effect via the Galilean telescope principle. With the near-universal adoption of intraocular lenses for the correction of aphakia, this problem is now rarely encountered. For further information on the correction of aphakia, see Chapter 6.

Accommodation and Presbyopia

Accommodation is the mechanism by which the eye changes refractive power by altering the shape and position of its crystalline lens. The changes in lens geometry that create this alteration were first described by Helmholtz. The posterior focal point is moved forward in the eye during accommodation (Fig 3-13A). Correspondingly, the far point moves closer to the eye (Fig 3-13B). *Accommodative effort* occurs when the ciliary muscle contracts in response to parasympathetic stimulation, thus allowing the zonular fibers to relax. The outward-directed tension on the lens capsule is decreased, and the lens becomes more convex, possibly in response to a pressure gradient pressing the lens forward against a "sling" formed by the zonular fibers and the anterior lens capsule ("catenary suspension"). *Accommodative response* results from the increase in lens convexity (primarily the anterior surface) and the net forward displacement of the lens. It may be expressed as the *amplitude of accommodation* (in diopters) or as the *range of accommodation*, the distance between the far point of the eye and the nearest point at which the eye can maintain focus (*near point*). It is evident that as the lens loses elasticity from the aging process, the accommodative response wanes, a condition called *presbyopia* (Greek, "old eyes") even though the amount of ciliary muscle contraction (or accommodative effort) is virtually unchanged. For an eye with presbyopia, the amplitude is a more useful measurement for calculating the power requirement of the additional eyeglass lens. For appraising an individual's ability to perform a specific visual task, the range is more informative.

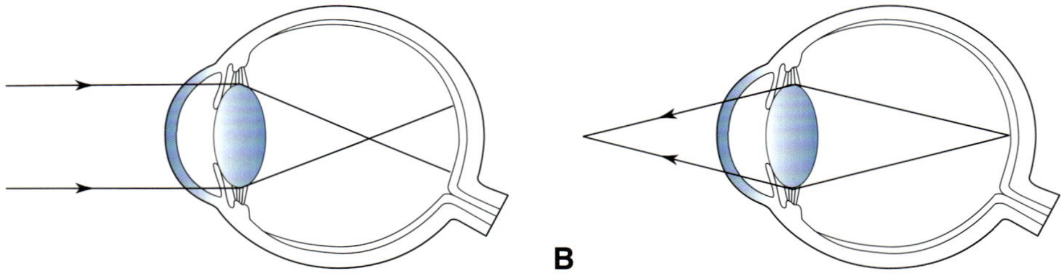

Figure 3-13 Emmetropia with accommodation stimulated. **A**, Parallel light rays now come to a point focus in frontof the retina, forming a blurred image on the retina. **B**, Light rays emanating from a point on the retina focus to a near point in front of the eye, between optical infinity and the cornea. *(Illustration by C. H. Wooley.)*

Coleman DJ, Silverman RH, Lloyd H, Physiology of accommodation and role of the vitreous body. In: Sebag J, ed. *Vitreous: in Health and Disease*. New York: Springer; 2014.

*单眼无晶状体眼*是屈光不正的极端的远视屈光参差状态。在成年患者中，人们无法耐受框架镜产生的 25% 的双眼不等像，由于接触镜矫正减小约 7% 的双眼不等像，所以可被接受。利用 Galileo 望远镜原理，通过调整接触镜的屈光力，同时配带框架镜，可以减少或增加放大效应。由于普遍采用人工晶体矫正无晶状体，所以现在很少遇到这个问题。有关无晶状体的矫正，请参阅第 6 章。

调节和老视

调节是通过改变晶状体的形状和位置，改变眼的屈光力。Helmholtz 首先描述了这种晶状体几何形状改变。调节发生时，后焦点向眼部移动（图 3–13A），相应的，远点更接近眼（图 3–13B）。当睫状肌在副交感神经刺激下收缩时，悬韧带放松，产生*调节*。晶状体向外的拉力降低，产生了一个压力梯度，该压力沿着由悬韧带和前晶状体囊（悬链线）形成的“悬带”的反方向压迫晶状体朝前，晶状体变得更凸。*调节反应*是由于晶状体凸度（主要指晶状体前表面）增加，以及晶状体位置的净前移。可以表示为*调节幅度*（*D*）或*调节范围*，即能保持聚焦（近点）的最近点与远点的距离。随着年龄的增长，晶状体失去弹性，即使睫状肌收缩（或调节效应）不变，调节反应仍会衰减，即*老视*（希腊语为“老眼睛”）。对于老视眼，调节幅度用于计算附加镜所需的镜片度数，调节范围能更好地评价一个人特定的视觉功能。

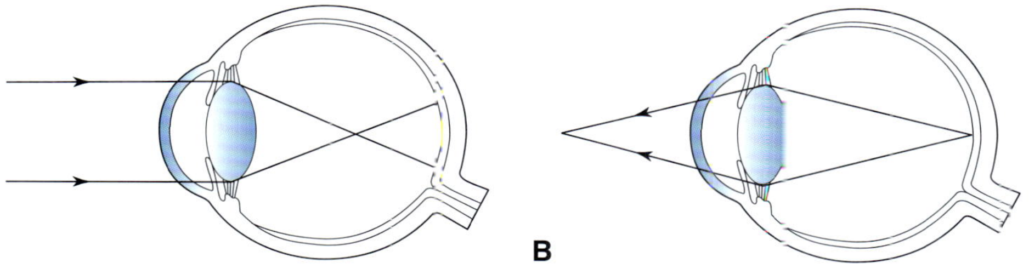

图 3–13 调节刺激的正视眼。**A**. 平行光线现在到达视网膜前方的焦点，在视网膜上形成模糊图像。**B**. 从视网膜上的一个点发出的光线聚焦到眼睛前方的近点，在光学无限远和角膜之间。*（译者注：资料来源见前页原文。）*

Coleman DJ, Silverman RH, Lloyd H, Physiology of accommodation and role of the vitreous body. In: Sebag J, ed. *Vitreous: in Health and Disease*. New York: Springer; 2014.

Epidemiology of Refractive Errors

An interplay among corneal power, lens power, anterior chamber depth, and axial length determines an individual's refractive status. All 4 elements change continuously as the eye grows. On average, babies are born with about 3.00D of hyperopia. In the first few months of life, this hyperopia may increase slightly, but it then declines to an average of about 1.00D of hyperopia by the end of the first year because of marked changes in corneal and lenticular powers, as well as axial length growth. By the end of the second year, the anterior segment attains adult proportions; however, the curvatures of the refracting surfaces continue to change measurably. One study found that average corneal power decreased 0.10–0.20D and lens power decreased about 1.80D between ages 3 years and 14 years.

From birth to age 6 years, the axial length of the eye grows by approximately 5 mm; thus, one might expect a high prevalence of myopia in children. However, most children's eyes are actually emmetropic, with only a 2% incidence of myopia at 6 years. This phenomenon is due to a still-undetermined mechanism called *emmetropization*. During this period of eye growth, a compensatory loss of 4.00D of corneal power and 2.00D of lens power keeps most eyes close to emmetropia.

Figure 3-14 shows the distribution of refractive errors in a large population based study. Figure 3-15 shows the effects of age on the prevalence of refractive errors.

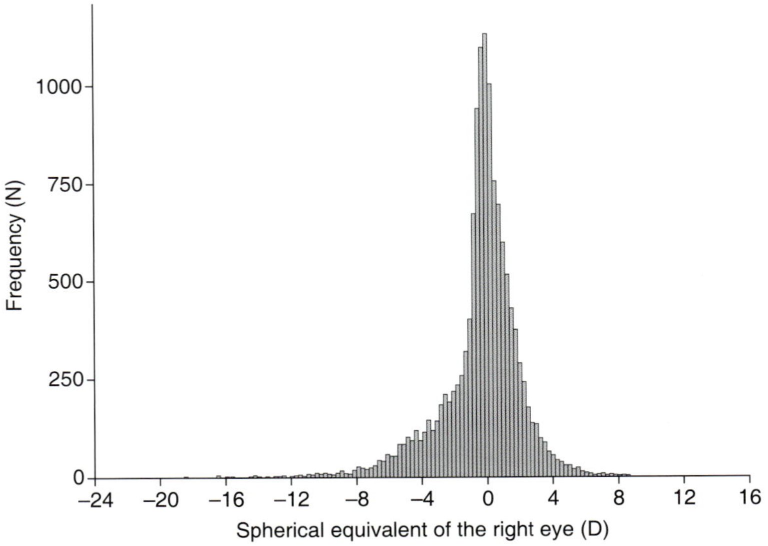

Figure 3-14 Distribution of refractive errors for adults from a population-based survey. The distribution is more sharply peaked than a normal distribution, which suggests the presence of a process of emmetropization. *(Reproduced with permission from Wolfram C, Höhn R, Kottler U, Wild P, et al. Prevalence of refractive errors in the European adult population: the Gutenberg Health Study [GHS]. Br J Ophthalmol. 2014;98(7):857–861.)*

屈光不正的流行病学

角膜屈光力、晶状体屈光力、前房深度及眼轴长度之间的相互作用决定了个体的屈光状态。随着眼球的发育生长，4 个屈光成分不断改变。平均而言，婴儿出生时应具有 + 3.00D 远视。在刚出生的几个月里，远视略有增加；但是年满 1 岁时，平均降至约 +1.00D 远视，这是由于角膜和晶状体屈光力明显改变，以及轴长度显著增长导致的结果。2 岁时，眼前段达到成人比例，但屈光表面的曲率继续改变。一项研究发现，在 3~14 岁之间，平均角膜屈光力下降 0.10~0.20D、晶状体屈光力下降约 1.80D。

从出生到 6 岁，眼轴长度增长约 5mm；因此，人们可能认为儿童近视的患病率很高。但事实是，大多数孩子呈现正视，6 岁时只有 2% 的近视发病率。这种现象是由于尚未明了的*眼正视化*的发育机制控制的。在眼轴生长的同时，伴有 4.00D 角膜屈光力和 2.00D 晶状体屈光力的补偿性减小，保持大多数眼睛呈现为正视。

图 3–14 显示了大样本人群的调查中的屈光不正分布。图 3–15 显示了年龄对屈光不正患病率的影响。

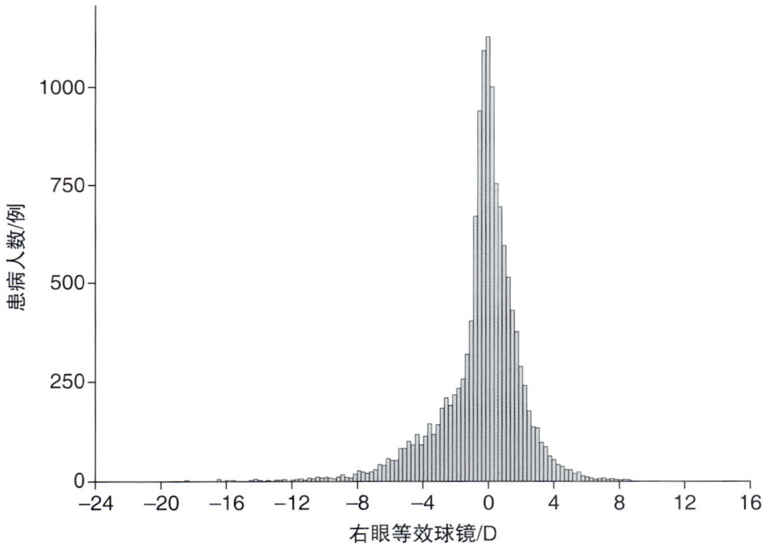

图 3–14 基于人群调查的成人屈光不正的分布。比正常正态分布更尖锐，这表明存在一个正视化过程。
（译者注：资料来源见前页原文。）

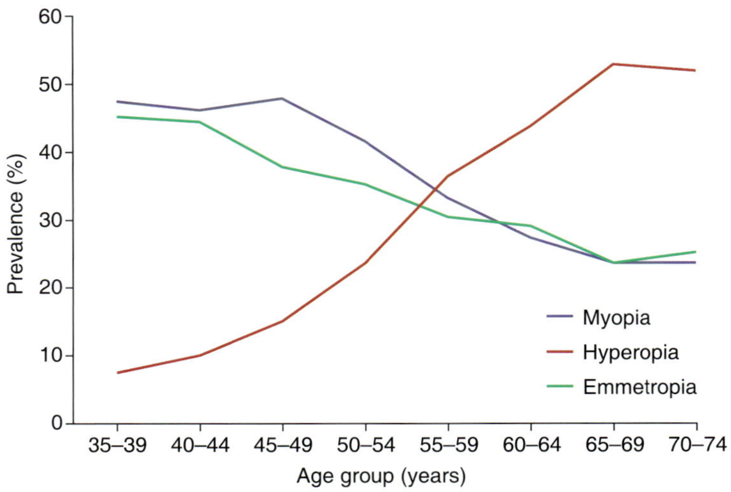

Figure 3-15 Changes in prevalence of refractive errors with age in a population-based survey. *(Reproduced with permission from Wolfram C, Höhn R, Kottler U, Wild P, et al. Prevalence of refractive errors in the Euro- pean adult population: the Gutenberg Health Study [GHS]. Br J Ophthalmol. 2014;98(7):857–861.)*

Prevent Blindness America; National Eye Institute. Vision Problems in the U.S.: Prevalence of Adult Vision Impairment and Age-Related Eye Disease in America. Available at www.visionproblemsus.org. Accessed October 4, 2017.

Wolfram C, Höhn R, Kottler U, Wild P, Blettner M, Bühren J, Pfeiffer N, Mirshahi A. Preva- lence of refractive errors in the European adult population: the Gutenberg Health Study (GHS). *Br J Ophthalmol.* 2014;98(7):857–61.

Developmental Myopia

Myopia increases steadily with increasing age. In the United States, the prevalence of myopia has been estimated at 3% among children aged 5–7 years, 8% among those aged 8–10 years, 14% among those aged 11–12 years, and 25% among adolescents aged 12–17 years. In particular ethnic groups, a similar trend has been demonstrated, although the percentages in each age group may differ. Ethnic Chinese children have much higher rates of myopia at all ages. A national study in CHINA Taiwan found the prevalence was 12% among 6-year-olds and 84% among adolescents aged 16–18 years. Similar rates have been found in Singapore and Japan.

Different subsets of myopia have been characterized. *Juvenile-onset myopia*, defined as myopia with an onset between 7 years and 16 years of age, is due primarily to growth in axial length. Risk factors include *esophoria*, against-the-rule astigmatism, premature birth, family history, and intensive near work. In general, the earlier the onset of myopia is, the greater is the degree of progression. In the United States, the mean rate of child- hood myopia progression is reported at about 0.50D per year. In approximately 75% of teenagers, refractive errors stabilize at about age 15 or 16. In those whose errors do not stabilize, progression often continues into the 20s or 30s.

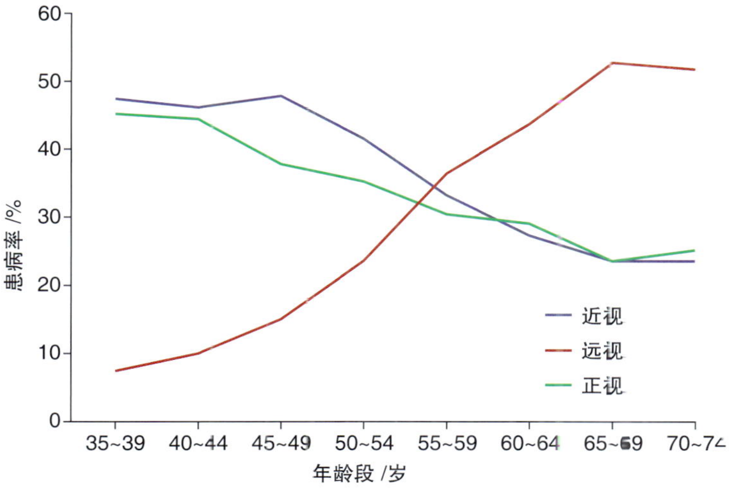

图 3-15　基于人群调查的随年龄增长屈光不正患病率的变化。*（译者注：资料来源见前页原文。）*

Prevent Blindness America; National Eye Institute. Vision Problems in the U.S.: Prevalence of Adult Vision Impairment and Age-Related Eye Disease in America. Available at www.visionproblemsus.org. Accessed October 4, 2017.

Wolfram C, Höhn R, Kottler U, Wild P, Blettner M, Bühren J, Pfeiffer N, Mirshahi A. Preva- lence of refractive errors in the European adult population: the Gutenberg Health Study （GHS）. Br J Ophthalmol, 2014,98（7）:857–61.

发育性近视

随着年龄的增长，近视比例也持续增加。在美国，5~7 岁儿童的近视眼患病率约占 3%，8~10 岁约占 8%，11~12 岁约占 14%，12~17 岁青少年约占 25%。在特定的种族中，虽然每个年龄组中的近视比例可能有所不同，但趋势是相似的。所有年龄段中，华裔儿童有更高的近视率。中国台湾地区的一项研究发现，6 岁儿童患病率为 12%，16~18 岁的患病率约为 84%。类似新加坡和日本的发病率。

不同类型近视有其特征。*青少年近视*主要是由于眼轴的增长，发病年龄在 7~16 岁之间。危险因素包括*内隐斜*、逆规散光、早产儿、家族史和大量视近工作等。一般来说，近视发病越早，进展的近视度数越高。美国儿童的近视进展每年约 0.50D，75% 的青少年的屈光不正在 15~16 岁趋于稳定，不稳定进展可以持续到 20~30 岁。

Adult-onset myopia begins at about 20 years of age, and extensive near work is a risk factor. A study of cadets at the United States Military Academy found myopia requiring corrective lenses in 46% at entrance, 54% after 1 year, and 65% after 2 years. The probability of myopic progression was related to the degree of initial refractive error. It is estimated that as many as 20%–40% of patients with low hyperopia or emmetropia who have extensive near-work requirements become myopic before age 25, compared with less than 10% of persons without such demands. Older Naval Academy recruits have a lower rate of myopia development than younger recruits over a 4-year curriculum (15% for 21-year-olds versus 77% for 18-year-olds). Some young adults are at risk for myopic progression even after a period of refractive stability. It has been theorized that persons who regularly perform considerable near work undergo a process similar to emmetropization for the customary close working distance, resulting in a myopic shift.

While there is no strict cut-off, myopic eyes with a spherical equivalent refractive error of -6.00D or greater, or an axial length of 26.5 mm or more are said to have "high myopia," and represent about 2% of the adult population. These eyes are at increased risk of retinal detachment, glaucoma, and choroidal neovascularization.

The etiologic factors concerning myopia are complex, involving both genetic and environmental factors. Regarding a genetic role, identical twins are more likely to have a similar degree of myopia than are fraternal twins, siblings, or parent and child. Identical twins separated at birth and having different work habits do not show significant differences in refractive error. Some forms of severe myopia suggest dominant, recessive, and even sex-linked inheritance patterns. However, studies of ethnic Chinese in CHINA Taiwan show an increase in the prevalence and severity of myopia over the span of 2 generations, a finding that implies that genetics alone are not entirely responsible for myopia. Some studies have reported that near work is not associated with a higher prevalence and progression of myopia, especially with respect to middle-distance activities such as tasks involving video displays. Higher educational achievement has been strongly associated with a higher prevalence of myopia. Poor nutrition has been implicated in the development of some refractive errors as well. Studies from Africa, for example, have found that children with malnutrition have an increased prevalence of high ametropia, astigmatism, and anisometropia. Participation in sports and time spent outdoors both appear to protect against juvenile myopia.

Sankaridurg PR, Holden BA. Practical applications to modify and control the development of ametropia. *Eye (Lond)*. 2014;28(2):134–141.

Developmental Hyperopia

Less is known about the epidemiology of hyperopia than that of myopia. There appears to be an increase in the prevalence of adult hyperopia with age that is separate from the development of nuclear sclerotic cataracts. Nuclear sclerosis is usually associated with a myopic shift. In whites, the prevalence of hyperopia increases from about 20% among those in their 40s to about 60% among those in their 70s and 80s. In contrast to myopia, hyperopia has been associated with lower educational achievement.

*成人近视*约在 20 岁发病，大量视近工作是危险因素。对美国陆军军官学校西点军校的一项研究发现，学员入校时近视率为 46%，1 年后为 54%，2 年后为 65%。近视进展与初始近视程度有关。据估计，存在轻度远视或正视者，由于大量视近工作，多达 20%~40% 于 25 岁之前呈轻度远视或正视的学员，25 岁前发生近视。而不近距离工作时，只有不到 10% 的人发生近视。经过 4 年课程的学习，年龄较大的海军学院新兵的近视发生率低于年龄较轻的新兵（21 岁的学员为 15%，而 18 岁的学员为 77%）。即使年轻人的屈光状态已经稳定了一段时间，也仍有近视进展的风险。据推断，长时间视近会导致一个类似正视化的过程，并导致近视化漂移。

虽然没有严格的界定，但等效球镜大于等于 -6.00D，或眼轴长大于等于 26.5 mm 的近视眼被称为“高度近视”，约占成人的 2%。这些眼睛患视网膜脱离、青光眼和脉络膜新生血管的风险增加。

关于近视的病因十分复杂，包括遗传因素和环境因素。关于遗传的作用，与异卵双胞胎的兄弟姐妹或父母子女相比较，同卵双胞胎近视程度更相似。出生后即被分开的同卵双胞胎，即使有不同的工作习惯，也不会有显著的屈光差异。一些重度近视的类型提示有显性、隐性或性连锁遗传的因素。但是，对中国台湾地区华人的研究显示，仅经历 2 代，就发生近视的患病率和严重程度增加，意味着遗传本身并不完全是近视的成因。一些研究报道，视近工作与近视的高患病率和进展也不相关，特别是中距离的工作，如视频显示终端。高等教育与近视的高患病率有密切关系。营养不良也与一些屈光不正的发展密切相关。例如，对非洲人员的研究发现，营养不良的儿童高屈光不正、散光和屈光参差的患病率增加。参加体育运动和户外活动都可以防止青少年近视。

Sankaridurg PR, Holden BA. Practical applications to modify and control the development of ametropia. *Eye*（*Lond*）. 2014;28(2):134–141.

发育性远视

对远视的流行病学了解比起近视来说相对较少。随着年龄的增长，成人远视的患病率似乎有所增加，这与核硬化白内障的发展无关。核硬化通常伴随着近视化漂移。在白种人中，远视的患病率增加，40 岁占 20%，而 70~80 岁占 60%。与近视相反，远视与低教育水平相关。

Prevention of Refractive Errors

Over the years, many treatments have been proposed to prevent or slow the progression of myopia. Because accommodation is a postulated mechanism for the progression of myopia, optical correction through the use of bifocal or multifocal spectacles or the removal of distance spectacles when performing close work has been recommended to reduce the progression of myopia. Administration of atropine eyedrops also has long been proposed because it inhibits accommodation, which may exert forces on the eye that result in axial elongation. Studies have suggested a protective effect of low-dose atropine (eg, 0.01% eye drops), even in the absence of evident cycloplegia. Use of a drug that lowers intraocular pressure has been suggested as an alternative pharmacologic intervention; this approach works presumably by reducing internal pressure on the eyewall. It has also been postulated that use of rigid contact lenses could slow the progression of myopia in children. Visual training purported to reduce myopia includes convergence exercises and those that incorporate changes in near–far focus.

The need to correct refractive errors depends on the patient's symptoms and visual needs. Patients with low refractive errors may not require correction, and small changes in refractive corrections in asymptomatic patients are not generally recommended. Correction options include spectacles, contact lenses, or surgery. Various occupational and recreational requirements, as well as personal preferences, affect the specific choices for any individual patient.

Morgan IG, He M. An Important Step Forward in Myopia Prevention: Low-Dose Atropine.*Ophthalmology*. 2016;123(2):232–3.

Chapter Exercises

Questions

3.1 Using the reduced schematic eye and the concept of the nodal point, what is the retinal image height of an 18-mm 20/40 Snellen letter at a distance of 20 ft (6 m)?

a.0.5 mm
b.0.05 mm
c.1 mm
d.0.1 mm

3.2 What is the approximate angle (in arcmin) subtended by the 20/40 Snellen letter at a distance of 20 ft (6 m)?

a.1 arcmin
b.2 arcmin
c.5 arcmin
d.10 arcmin
e.40 arcmin

屈光不正的预防

多年来，提出了许多预防或减缓近视进展的治疗方法。由于调节是近视进展的可能机制，人们利用双焦镜、多焦镜或视近时摘掉眼镜等视力矫正方法来减缓近视的进展。长期以来一直提出给予阿托品滴眼液，因为它抑制调节，而调节可能作用于眼球，使眼轴增长。研究表明，即使没有明显的睫状肌麻痹，低浓度阿托品（例如，0.01%的滴眼液）也具有保护作用。降眼压的药物作为一类替代的药物干预方案，可能与减少眼球内部对球壁的压力相关。硬性接触镜的使用可能会减缓儿童近视眼的进展。近 – 远聚焦练习和集合练习等视觉训练旨在减轻近视。

屈光不正的矫正取决于患者的症状和视力需求。屈光不正低的患者可能不需要矫正，无症状患者一般不需要矫正。矫正方案包括框架镜，接触镜或手术。职业、娱乐需求以及个人喜好，会影响患者的具体选择。

Morgan IG, He M. An Important Step Forward in Myopia Prevention: Low-Dose Atropine.Ophthalmology. 2016;123(2):232–3.

章节练习

问题

3.1　使用简化模型眼和节点的概念，在 20ft（6m）距离处，18mm 高的 20/40 Snellen 视力表字母的视网膜成像高度是多少？

a. 0.5mm
b. 0.05mm
c. 1mm
d. 0.1mm

3.2　在 20ft（6m）距离处，20/40 Snellen 字母对应的大致视角是多少？

a. 1 弧分
b. 2 弧分
c. 5 弧分
d. 10 弧分
e. 40 弧分

3.3 What is the relative size of target lights in a Goldmann perimeter (with a radius of 33 cm) relative to their corresponding retinal image?
a.same
b.5 times larger
c.10 times larger
d.20 times larger

3.4 Describe the location of the far point of an emmetropic eye with relaxed accommodation. Do the same for a myopic eye and a hyperopic eye.

3.5 In an eye with mixed astigmatism, where are the focal lines located?
a.Both are in front of the retina.
b.One is in front of the retina, the other is on the retina.
c.One is in front of the retina, the other is behind the retina.
d.One is located on the retina, the other is behind the retina.

3.6 A patient with myopic vision is wearing eyeglasses that were prescribed incorrectly with an over-minus of 1.00D. When he wears them, his near point of accommodation is 20 cm. What is his amplitude of accommodation?
a.none
b.1.00D
c.5.00D
d.6.00D

Answers

3.1. **b.** Utilizing the concepts of the nodal point and similar triangles, retinal image size is related to Snellen letter height (18 mm), the distance from the eye to the eye chart (6 m), and the distance from the nodal point to the retina (17 mm), as follows:

$$\frac{\text{Retinal Image Height}}{\text{Snellen Letter Height}} = \frac{\text{Retinal Image Distance From Nodal Point}}{\text{Snellen Letter Distance From Nodal point}} = \frac{17\text{ mm}}{6000\text{ mm}}$$

This implies

$$\text{Retinal Image Height} = \frac{18\text{mm} \times 17\text{mm}}{6000\text{ mm}} = 0.05\text{ mm}$$

The retinal image height of a 20/20 letter is half of this, about 0.025 mm.

3.2. **d.** Snellen letters are constructed such that they subtend an angle of 5 arcmin when located at the distance specified by the denominator (here, 40 ft). At a distance of 20 ft, the angle subtended by a 20/40 Snellen letter is twice that at 40 ft, or 10 arcmin.

3.3. **d.** The concept of the nodal point is applicable for the Goldmann perimeter, in which the target lights are located at 33 cm (330 mm) from the cornea. Because this distance is approximately 20 times greater than the 17-mm distance from the nodal point to the retina, the target lights in the perimeter are approxi- mately 20 times larger than their corresponding retinal images.

3.3 相对比视网膜成像，Goldmann 视野计（半径为 33 cm）目标光的相对大小是多少？
a. 一样
b. 5 倍大
c. 10 倍大
d. 20 倍大

3.4 在调节放松的状态下描述正视眼远点的位置。用同样的方法描述近视眼和远视眼的远点位置。

3.5 混合散光眼，焦线位于何处？
a.2 个都在视网膜前面。
b. 一个在视网膜前面，另一个在视网膜上。
c. 一个在视网膜前面，另一个在视网膜后面。
d. 一个位于视网膜上，另一个位于视网膜后面。

3.6 近视眼患者配了一副超过矫 1.00D 的错误处方眼镜。当他戴着这副眼镜时，他的调节近点是 20cm。他的调节幅度是多少？
a. 没有
b.1.00D
c. 5.00D
d. 6.00D

答案

3.1 **b**. 利用节点和相似三角形的概念，视网膜成像大小与 Snellen 视力表字母高度（18 mm），眼睛到视力表的距离（6 m）以及从节点到视网膜的距离（17mm）有关，如下：

$$\frac{\text{视网膜成像高度}}{\text{Snellen视力表字母高度}} = \frac{\text{节点到视网膜距离}}{\text{视力表到眼睛的节点距离}} = \frac{17\ \text{mm}}{6000\ \text{mm}}$$

这意味着

$$\text{视网膜成像高度} = \frac{18\text{mm}\times 17\text{mm}}{6000\ \text{mm}} = 0.05\ \text{mm}$$

20/20 字母高度在视网膜上的成像高度就是这个的一半，也就是大约 0.025mm。

3.2 **d**. Snellen 视力表由特定距离（这里是 40ft）所视的 5 弧分视角的视标组成。在 20ft 的距离处，20/40 字母在 Snellen 视力表所对的视角是 40ft 视角的 2 倍或为 10 弧分。

3.3 **d**. 节点的概念适用于 Goldmann 视野计，其中目标光位于离角膜 33cm（330mm）处。因为该距离约是节点到视网膜 17mm 距离的 20 倍，所以周边的目标光大约是其相应视网膜成像的 20 倍。

3.4. The far point of an emmetropic eye is located at optical infinity. For a myopic eye, the far point is located at a finite distance in front of the cornea. For a hy- peropic eye, the far point is located behind the retina.

3.5. **c.** One focal line is in front of the retina, the other is behind the retina. The circle of least confusion may be located very close to the retina (see Chapter 1), allowing such patients to see reasonably well even without optical correction if the magnitude of the astigmatism is not great.

3.6. **d.** The patient's amplitude of accommodation is 6.00D, because it takes 1.00D of accommodation to focus to infinity and an additional 5.00D of accommoda- tion to focus to the false near point at 20 cm.

3.4　正视眼的远点位于光学无限远处。对于近视眼，远点位于角膜前有限距离处。对于远视眼，远点位于视网膜后面。

3.5　**c**. 1 条焦线位于视网膜前方，另 1 条位于视网膜后方。最小弥散圈可能位于非常靠近视网膜的位置（见第 1 章），如果散光的幅度不大，即使没有光学矫正，这样的患者也可以看得清楚。

3.6　**d**. 患者的调节幅度为 6.00D，因为他需要 1.00D 调节注视无限远和额外的 5.00D 调节注视到 20cm 处的虚近点。

（翻译 冯坤 代秋楠 李易 // 审校 李易 石一宁）

CHAPTER 4

Clinical Refraction

This chapter includes related videos, which can be accessed by scanning the QR codes provided in the text or going to www .aao .org /bcscvideo section03.

Highlights

- terminology associated with clinical refraction
- proper use of the retinoscope
- use of the astigmatic dial for astigmatism determination
- use of the Jackson cross cylinder and the refractor (phoropter) as well as trial frame in determining the spherocylindrical correction of the eye
- how to identify and treat induced prism in spectacle corrections
- effective power changes that occur due to changes in lens vertex distance
- management of a dissatisfied patient with new spectacles

Glossary

Amplitude of accommodation A measurement of the ability of an eye to focus at near, assuming the eye is optically corrected for distance.

Autorefractor A computer controlled instrument for determining the refractive error of the eye.

Image displacement Change in apparent position of an object seen through a particular spectacle lens due to induced prismatic effect.

Image jump Sudden movement of an image when gaze is shifted across the border between the distance and the near portion of a spectacle lens.

Jackson cross cylinder Combination of 2 equal but opposite power cylinders used in the determin -ation of power and axis of refractive astigmatism.

Meridional aniseikonia Unequal magnification of retinal images in different meridians.

Oblique (marginal) astigmatism Astigmatism induced by the tilting of a spherical lens or by viewing through the periphery of a spherical lens.

第 4 章

临床验光学

本章包括相关的视频，您可以通过登录 www .aao .org /bcscvideo secticn03 扫描 QR 码来获取这些视频。

重点

- 临床屈光学相关的专业术语
- 检影镜的正确使用
- 使用散光表盘检测散光
- 使用 Jackson 交叉柱镜（JCC）在综合验光仪和试镜架上精确球柱镜

- 框架眼镜诱发性棱镜的鉴别和处理
- 镜眼距改变导致有效屈光度改变
- 新配框架眼镜不满意的处理

术语

调节幅度 在视远屈光矫正状态下，眼睛视近聚焦能力的一种检测。

电脑验光仪 一种用来测定眼睛屈光不正状态的电脑设备。

像位移 由于棱镜效应，透过特定镜片所看到物体位置明显改变的现象。

像跳 当注视点在眼镜的远近区域边界切换时，所引起像位置突然跳跃的现象。

Jackson 交叉柱镜 由两个度数相同而光度相反的柱镜组成的联合柱镜，用于精确散光的光度和轴位。

子午线不等像 由于各子午线放大率不等所成视网膜像。

斜向散光 由于球镜倾斜或者光线透过球镜边缘形成的散光。

Phoropter (refractor) An instrument containing a collection of spherical and cylindrical lenses for the performance of retinoscopy and manifest refraction. The instrument also commonly includes the Jackson cross cylinder, Risley prisms, and other accessories.

Prentice rule Each centimeter of lens decentration induces 1 prism diopter (Δ) of prism for each diopter of power of the lens.

Presbyopia Functional loss of accommodation with aging.

Retinoscopy A manual objective method of determining and evaluating the refractive status of an eye through the observation of the movement of a retinal reflex created by a beam of light through the pupil and the optical system of the eye.

Slab-off prism (bicentric grinding) Creation of base-up prism in the area of a bifocal to correct induced prismatic effect in downgaze through the bifocal reading segment.

Vertex distance The distance from the back surface of a spectacle or contact lens to the anterior surface of the cornea.

Introduction

The process of clinical refraction represents one of the practical applications of geometric optics. Refraction is a critical component in an ophthalmic examination. It allows the determination of the best corrected vision of the eye. This determination is often necessary in determining the diagnosis and recommended treatment course. The refraction is necessary in determining visual correction with spectacles, contact lenses, lens implants, and refractive corneal surgery. Other techniques, such as the pinhole, corneal topography and tomography, and various forms of autorefraction are valuable but, as yet, have not replaced manifest refraction in the ophthalmic examination.

Minus Cylinder and Plus Cylinder Terminology

The terms *minus cylinder* and *plus cylinder* are used in various ways in discussing refraction and prescription of eyeglasses. These include the measurement of refraction using the phoropter (refractor), the writing of the prescription for glasses, and the fabrication of spectacles with astigmatism correction.

The phoropter is made with both plus and minus spherical lenses. For simplicity, the cylinder component is made up by lenses of only one type—either plus cylinder lenses or minus cylinder lenses. (Trial lens sets may be ordered as minus cylinder–plus cylinder, or both.) There is no consensus as to which type is preferable. In some communities, optometrists tend to prefer phoropters with minus power and ophthalmologists tend to prefer plus power. Minus cylinder phoropters may have potential advantages in the fitting of contact lenses. Minus cylinder phoropters are also useful in determining astigmatism using the asigmatic (clock) dial technique. In contrast, the axis of the plus cylinder may indicate the position of a tight suture in an eye with a penetrating keratoplasty. Plus cylinder equipment is also more natural for purposes of retinoscopy and is often selected by pediatric ophthalmologists for that reason.

综合验光仪 一种将球柱镜片组合在一起可进行视网膜检影和主观验光的仪器。该仪器号包含 Jackson 交叉柱镜和 Risley 棱镜等其它辅助功能。

Prentice 法则 在透镜上 1 个屈光度（D）偏移 1cm 产生 1 个棱镜度（Δ)。

老视 随着年龄增长调节功能逐渐丧失。

检影 一种手动操作的客观验光法，通过瞳孔和屈光系统观察视网膜反射光带的位移情况来判断和评估屈光状态。

削薄棱镜（双中心磨削） 用以矫正当眼睛注视下转通过双光镜阅读子片是产生的基底向上的诱导棱镜效应。

顶点距离 框架眼镜镜片或者接触镜镜片后表面到角膜前表面的距离。

引言

临床上验光过程是几何光学的实际应用之一。验光是眼科检查中的重要组成部分，它可以判定人眼的最佳矫正视力，而最佳矫正视力在确诊病情和推荐治疗方案中起到关键作用。验光也是框架眼镜、角膜接触镜、人工晶体植入和角膜屈光手术等各种矫正方案必须的检查。而在眼科检查中的其它检查，如小孔镜、角膜地形图、断层扫描以及各种电脑验光仪也非常重要，但是仍不能代替主观验光。

负柱镜和正柱镜专业术语

*负柱镜*和*正柱镜*一词用于各种验光和给镜处方讨论中。主要包括综合验光仪的验光检查、眼镜处方的书写和带有散光矫正的眼镜加工。

综合验光仪同时包含了正球镜和负球镜两组透镜。为了方便起见，柱镜部分是仅由一种类型的透镜——正柱镜或负柱镜组成的。（镜片箱可能按照负柱镜 - 正柱镜，或两者均有的顺序摆放。）对于哪种类型更为合适，目前并没有达成共识。在某些地区，视光师多用负柱镜综合验光仪，而眼科医生多用正柱镜综合验光仪。负柱镜综合验光仪在验配接触镜时有优势，在用散光表盘技术确定散光时也很有用；而正柱镜可提示穿透性角膜移植术后缝线过紧的轴位，检影时自然影动，这也是儿科眼科医生最常选择正柱镜的原因。

CLINICAL EXAMPLE 4-1

This example demonstrates converting from plus to minus cylinder notation. The rule of thumb for this calculation is to add the cylinder power to the sphere power to find the new sphere power. Change the sign of the cylinder power but the magnitude of the power remains the same. Change the axis of the cylinder by 90°. This works when converting from plus to minus notation and also from minus to plus.

Take, for example, the following plus cylinder notated refraction:
−3.00 +4.00 × 180°

Sphere power: −3.00D
Cylinder power: +4.00D
Axis of the cylinder: 180°

In the conversion to minus cylinder the following transformations occur:

The cylinder power is added to the sphere power: +4.00 + (−3.00) = +1.00D
The sign of the cylinder power is changed: +4.00 becomes −4.00D
The axis of the cylinder is changed by 90°: 180° becomes 90°
Resultant minus cylinder notation: **+1.00 −4.00 × 90°**

The prescription for a spectacle correction may be written in either minus cylinder or plus cylinder format. Normally this is determined by the type of phoropter used to perform the refraction, so as to minimize the possibility of a transcription error; however, this is not necessary. Either form may be easily converted to the other (Clinical Example 4-1).

In the fabrication of spherocylindrical spectacle lenses, the cylindrical component may be placed on the anterior surface (plus or front cylinder) or the posterior surface (minus or back cylinder) of the lens. Current preferred practice is for lenses to be fabricated in minus (back) cylinder format regardless of what type of phoropter is used or how the prescription is written. This decreases the meridional magnification.

Exam Room Length

The room in which the refraction is carried out is important in achieving satisfactory results. For optical purposes, a 20-foot (6-M) distance from the patient to the vision chart approximates infinity (−0.17 diopters [D]). Many exam rooms are much shorter than this. If the vision chart is placed so that the distance to the patient is only 10 ft (3.05 m) the refraction will be overplussed by 0.33 D. Mirrors are used to extend the viewing distance to the standard 20 ft (6.09 m) in such rooms. Some patients (including many children) are not able to effectively fixate into a mirror and need to be examined in longer rooms or hallways. They may also tend to accommodate in a short room, even if it has a mirror to optically extend it. Simply correcting for the shorter working distance by decreasing the plus or increasing the minus in the measured refraction is not recommended because proper accommodative fogging techniques cannot be performed in such a situation.

临床案例 4–1

这个例子是显示如何将正柱镜转换为负柱镜。经验计算方法是：将柱镜焦度加到球镜焦度上，以获得新的球镜焦度；改变柱镜焦度的符号，但是焦度的值不变，改变柱镜的轴位为 90°。这可以用于将正柱镜符号转换为负柱镜，或将负柱镜转换为正柱镜。

例如，以下为正柱镜符号表示的屈光状态：

–3.00 +4.00 × 180°

球镜屈光度：–3.00 D
柱镜屈光度：+4.00 D
柱镜的轴位：180°

将其转换为负柱镜的过程如下：

将柱镜屈光度加入球镜屈光度中：+4.00 +（–3.00）= +1.00D
转换柱镜屈光度的符号：+4.00 变为 –4.00D
柱镜的轴位变为 90°：180° 变为 90°
转换后的负柱镜表示：**+ 1.00 –4.00 × 90°**

眼镜处方可以书写为负柱镜或正柱镜，这是由进行验光检查的综合验光仪决定的，以降低抄写错误。然而，这也不是必需的。2 种方式很容易被转换（临床案例 4–1）。

在球柱镜镜片的制作过程中，柱镜可放置于镜片的前表面（正柱镜或前柱镜）或后表面（负柱镜或后柱镜）。无论有多少类型的综合验光仪，或多种处方书写方式，当前最常用的方法是将镜片加工为负（后）柱镜的形式。这样可以减少子午线上的放大率。

检查室的距离

验光室对于获得满意的验光结果非常重要。从光学角度，患者至视力表的距离为 20ft（6 m），接近无穷（–0.17 D）。许多检查室比这个标准距离更短。如果视力表放置在距离患者 10ft（3.5 m）处，验光结果将增加 0.33 D。所以，很多检查室常常用镜子将检查距离增加至标准的 20ft（6.09 m）。一些患者（包括儿童）不能有效地固视镜子中的视标，他们需要在一个更长的房间或过道中接受检查。即使有镜子增加光程，他们在较小的房间内也需要调节。在进行屈光检查时，不建议仅通过减少正度数或者增加负度数来修正较短的工作距离，因为在这种状态下不能进行适当的调节雾视技术。

Objective Refraction Technique: Retinoscopy

Although autorefractors are easily accessible, retinoscopy remains an important skill and tool for the ophthalmologist to objectively determine the spherocylindrical refractive error of the eye. A *retinoscope* can also help the examiner detect optical aberrations, irregularities, and opacities, even through small pupils. Retinoscopy is especially useful for examinations of infants, children, and adults unable to communicate.

Most retinoscopes in current use employ the streak projection system developed by Copeland. The illumination of the retinoscope is provided by a bulb with a straight filament that forms a streak in its projection, or by means of a slit-shaped aperture. The light is reflected from a mirror that is either half silvered (Welch Allyn, Heine models) or totally silvered around a small circular aperture (Copeland instrument) (Fig 4-1). The filament light source (or the slit aperture) can be moved in relation to a convex lens in the system using the sleeve of the retinoscope. If the light is slightly divergent, it appears to come from a point behind the retinoscope, as if the light were reflected off a flat mirror (ie, a *plane mirror setting*) (Fig 4-2).

Alternatively, when the distance between the convex lens and the filament is increased by moving the sleeve on the handle, convergent light is emitted. In this situation, the image of the filament appears between the examiner and the patient, as if the light were reflected off a concave mirror (Fig 4-3).

Retinoscopy may be performed with either a concave mirror setting or a plane mirror setting, determined by the sleeve of the scope. Retinoscopy is usually performed using the plane mirror setting so that light is parallel (or slightly divergent) as it enters the pupil of the patient's eye. We restrict our discussion to the plane mirror effect; in the concave mirror effect, the direction of motion is opposite that of the plane mirror effect. One use of the concave setting is to sharpen the reflex while determining the axis of astigmatism. Using the concave setting during power determination (of sphere or cylinder) may lead to false end points (neutrality). Not all retinoscopes employ the same sleeve position for the plane mirror setting. For example, the original Copeland retinoscope is in plane position with the sleeve up; the Welch Allyn (or Heine) instrument is in plane position with the sleeve down. The axis of the streak is rotated with the sleeve.

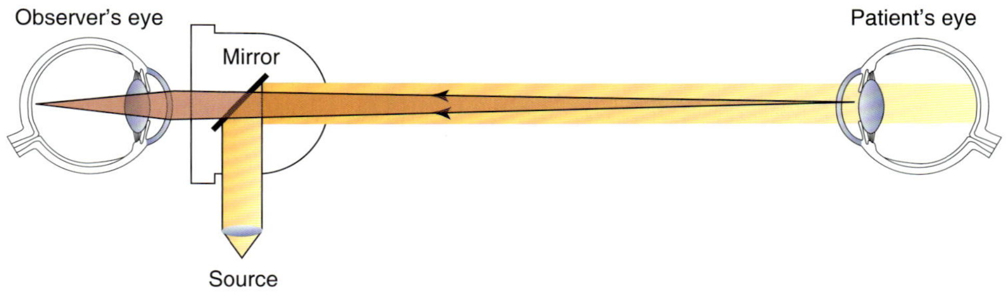

Figure 4-1 Retinoscope: Illumination system: Light path from light source through patient's pupil to retina. Observation system: Light path from patient's pupil, through mirror to observer's retina. *(Illustration by C. H. Wooley.)*

客观验光技术：检影镜

尽管自动验光仪使用方便，对于眼科医生客观确定眼的球柱镜屈光不正来说，检影技术仍然是一项重要的技术和工具。通过小瞳孔，*检影镜*可以帮助检查者发现光学像差、不规则像和屈光间质混浊。检影镜对于婴儿、儿童或无法交流的成人检查也非常有用。

目前使用的很多检影镜都是 Copeland 发明的带状投射系统。检影镜的照明由一个具有线状灯丝的灯泡提供，它投照时形成带状光；或者通过一个裂隙孔径提供带状光。光线被镜面反射，镜面可以是半镀银（Welch Allyn 仪器或 Heine 仪器），或是全镀银的，全镀银要留有 1 个小圆孔，光从孔的周围镜面反射（Copeland 设备）。（图 4–1）。灯丝光源（或裂隙孔径）可以用检影镜的套管相对于系统中的凸透镜移动。如果光线有轻度发散，好似来自检影镜后方的一个点，光线就像从镜面反射回来一样（如*平面镜*）（图 4–2）。

此外，当通过移动手柄上的套管使凸透镜和灯丝之间的距离增加时，可发出会聚光。在这种情况下，灯丝的影像出现在检查者和患者之间，就像光线是从一个凹面镜反射回来的（图 4–3）。

检影镜可被设置为凹面镜系统或平面镜系统，这取决于套管的移动范围。检影镜常常使用平面镜系统，所以当光线通过患者的瞳孔时是平行的（或轻度发散）。在这里我们仅讨论平面镜效果。在使用凹面镜时，影动方向与平面镜效应是相反的。凹面镜的其中一项用途是当确定散光轴位时，使反射变得更加清晰。使用凹面镜系统进行焦度检查时（球镜或柱镜），可能导致错误终点（中和）。不是所有使用平面镜系统的检影镜套管位置都是一样的。例如，最早的 Copeland 检影镜套管向上移动时是平行光；Welch Allyn（或 Heine）仪器套管向下移动时是平行光。光带的轴可随套管而转动。

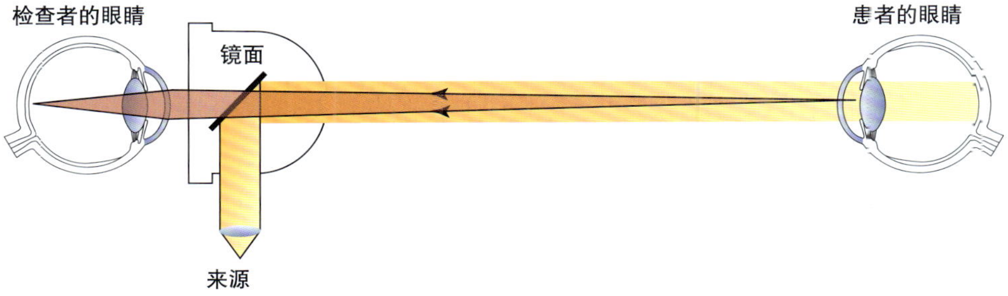

图 4–1　检影镜：照明系统：光源系统发出的光线通过患者的瞳孔到达视网膜。观察系统：光线从患者的瞳孔通过镜面观察视网膜。*（译者注：资料来源见前页原文。）*

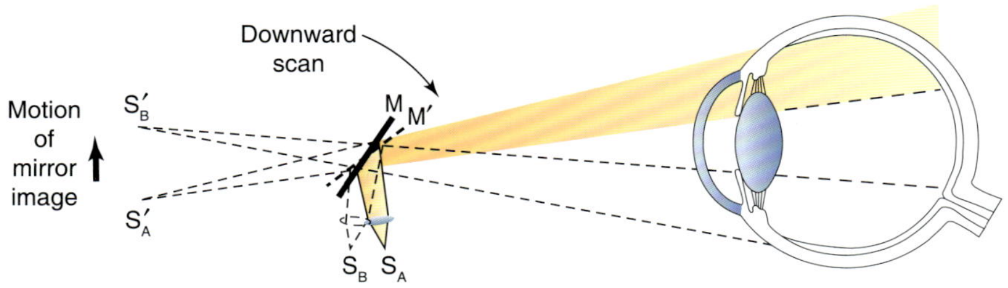

Figure 4-2 Illumination system: position of source (S) with plane mirror (M) effect.

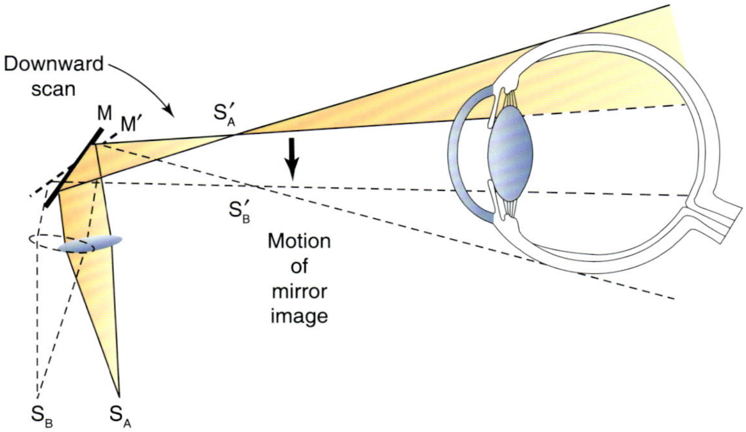

Figure 4-3 Illumination system: position of source with concave mirror effect.

Positioning and Alignment

Ordinarily, the examiner uses his or her right eye to perform retinoscopy on the patient's right eye, and the left eye for the patient's left eye. Doing so prevents the examiner's head from moving into the patient's line of sight and thus inadvertently stimulating accommodation. If the examiner looks directly through the optical centers of the trial lenses while performing retinoscopy, reflections from the lenses may interfere. In general, if the examiner is too far off-axis, unwanted spherical and cylindrical errors may occur. The optimal alignment is just off center, where the lens reflections can still be seen between the center of the pupil and the lateral edge of the lens. Video 4-1 demonstrates the basics of retinoscopy.

VIDEO 4-1 Retinoscopy: basics.
Animation developed by Thomas F. Mauger, MD.
Access all Section 3 videos at www .aao .org /bcscvideo _section03.

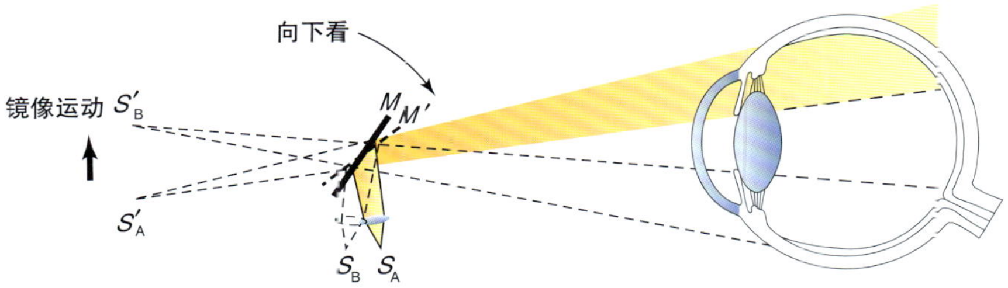

图 4–2　照明系统：平面镜（*M*）效果的光源位置（*S*）。

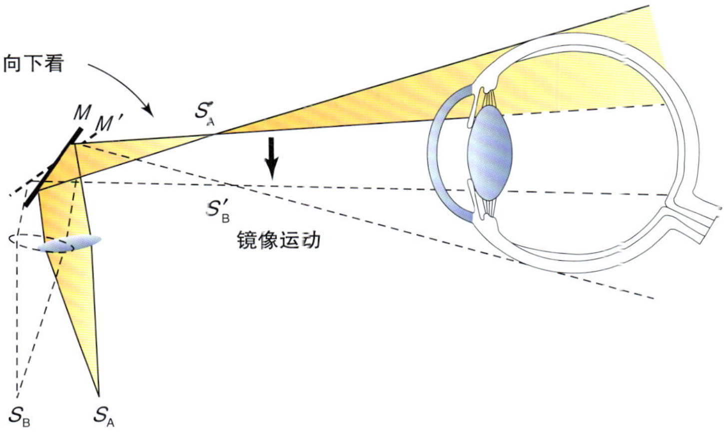

图 4–3　照明系统：凹面镜效果的光源位置。

姿势和校准

一般情况下，检查者用他 / 她的右眼通过检影镜观察患者的右眼，左眼观察左眼。这样可以避免检查者的头挡住患者的视线，刺激其产生调节。如果检查者在检影时直接通过试镜片的光学中心观看，从镜片反射回来的图像将会受到干扰。一般来说，如果检查者偏轴太远，将会导致不必要的球镜或柱镜误差。最佳位置是稍偏离中心，这时镜片的反射仍然可以通过瞳孔中心和镜片的边缘观察到。视频 4–1 演示了基本检影。

视频4–1　检影：基础。

由Thomas F. Mauger医学博士演示。

大家可通过网站www .aao .org /bcscvideo _section03获得第三册的所有视频。

Fixation and Fogging

Retinoscopy should be performed with the patient's accommodation relaxed. The patient should fixate at a distance on a nonaccommodative target. For example, the target may be a dim light at the end of the room or a large Snellen letter (20/200 or 20/400 size). Plus lenses may be introduced in front of the eye not being examined to aid in the relaxation of accommodation. Accommodating after fogging is performed will only further blur the image. Children typically require pharmacologic cycloplegia (such as cyclopentolate 1%).

The Retinal Reflex

The projected streak illuminates an area of the patient's retina, and this light returns to the examiner. By observing characteristics of this reflex, the examiner determines the refractive status of the eye. If the patient's eye is *emmetropic*, the light rays emerging from the patient's pupil are parallel to one another; if the eye is *myopic*, the rays are convergent (Fig 4-4); and if the eye is *hyperopic*, the rays are divergent. Through the peephole in the retinoscope, the emerging light is seen as a red reflex in the patient's pupil. If the examiner (specifically, the peephole of the retinoscope) is at the patient's far point, all the light leaving the patient's pupil enters the peephole and illumination is uniform. However, if the far point of the patient's eye is not at the peephole of the retinoscope, only some of the rays emanating from the patient's pupil enter the peephole, and illumination of the pupil appears incomplete.

If the far point is between the examiner and the myopic patient, the emerging rays will have focused and then diverged. The border between the dark and lighted portions of the pupil will move in a direction opposite to the motion (sweep) of the retinoscope streak (known as *against* movement) as it is moved across the patient's pupil. If the far point is behind the examiner, the light moves in the same direction as the sweep (known as *with* movement; Fig 4-5).

The state in which the light fills the pupil and apparently does not move is known as *neutrality* (Fig 4-6). At neutrality, if the examiner moves forward (in front of the far point), *with* movement is seen; if the examiner moves back and away from the far point, *against* movement is seen. The far point may be moved with placement of a correcting lens in front of the patient's eye.

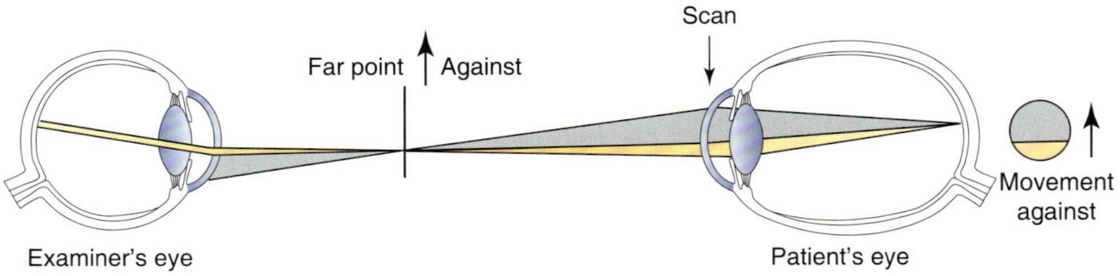

Figure 4-4 Observation system for myopia.

固视和雾视

检影时，患者应处于放松状态。患者应该注视远处的无调节目标。如该目标可以是房间另一端的微弱灯光或者一个大的 Sneller 字母（20/200 或 20/400 大小）。眼前所放置的正镜片不是为了检查，而是用于辅助调节放松。雾视后的调节仅会使图像更加模糊。儿童需要药物性睫状肌麻痹（如 1% 的环戊通）。

视网膜反光

投射光线照到的是患者视网膜的一个区域，该光线反射回检查者。通过观察该反射的特征，检查者可以确定该眼的屈光状态。如果患眼是*正视眼*，光线在患者瞳孔发出时是相互平行的；如果是*近视眼*，光线是会聚的（图 4–4）；如果是*远视眼*，光线是发散的。通过检影镜的窥孔，发出的光线在患者瞳孔区呈红色反射。如果检查者（特别是检影镜的窥孔）在患者的远点，所有离开患者的瞳孔的光线进入窥孔，其亮度是均匀的。但是，如果患者的远点不在检影镜的窥孔处，仅有一部分光线从患者的瞳孔发出进入窥孔，瞳孔区照明不完整。

如果远点位于检查者和近视眼患者之间，反射回的光线将先聚焦而后发散。当检影镜通过患者瞳孔区时，瞳孔的明暗部分的分界线将向检影镜的移动（扫动）方向的对侧运动（*逆动*）。如果远点在检查者后方，光线运动将与检影镜移动方向一致（*顺动*，图 4–5）。

当光线充满瞳孔并且明显不移动的状态称为*中和*（图 4–6）。中和状态时，如果检查者向前移动（在远点之前），*顺动*可见；如果检查者向后移动或者远离远点，*逆动*可见。在患者眼前放置矫正镜片，远点可能会移动。

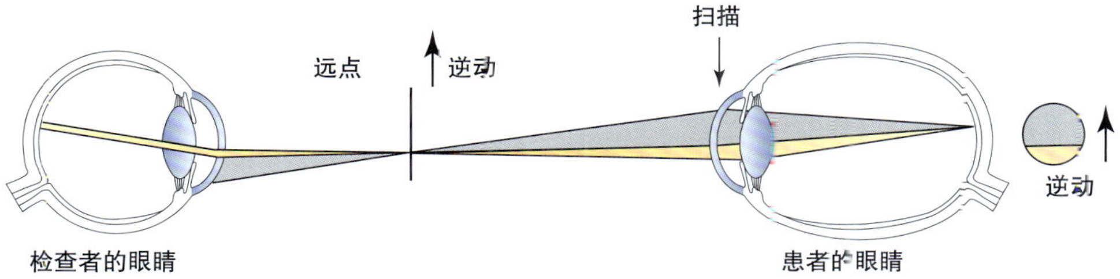

图 4–4　近视眼的观察系统

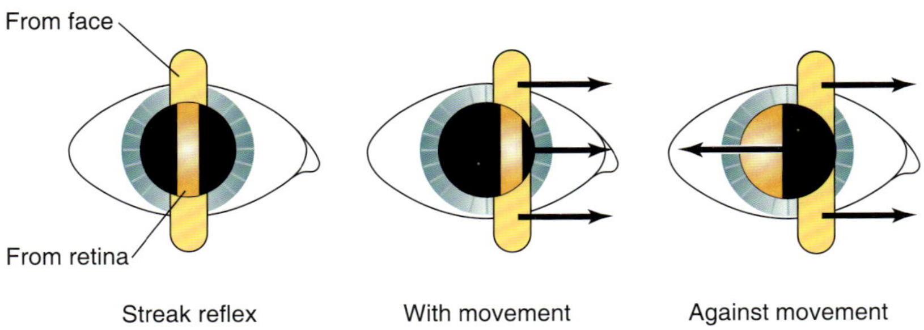

Figure 4-5 Retinal reflex movement. Note movement of the streak from face and from retina in with versus against movement. *(Illustration by C. H. Wooley.)*

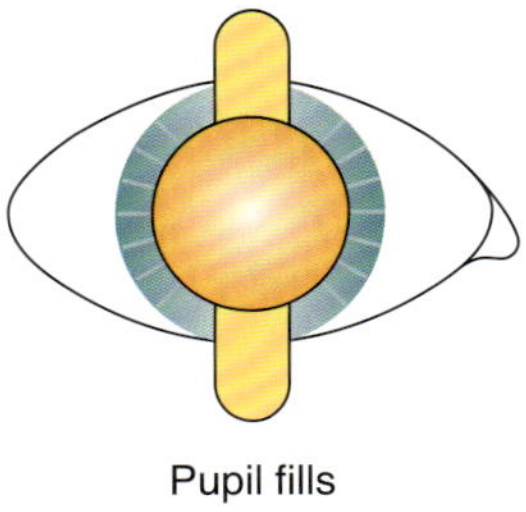

Figure 4-6 Neutrality reflex. Far point of the eye is conjugate with the peephole of the retinoscope. *(Illustration by C. H. Wooley.)*

Characteristics of the reflex

The moving retinoscopic reflex has 4 main characteristics (Fig 4-7):

1. *Speed.* The reflex seen in the pupil moves slowest when the far point is distant from the examiner (peephole of the retinoscope). As the far point is moved toward the peephole, the speed of the reflex increases. In other words, large refractive errors have a slow-moving reflex, whereas small errors have a fast reflex.
2. *Brilliance.* The reflex is dull when the far point is distant from the examiner; it becomes brighter as neutrality is approached.
3. *Width.* When the far point is distant from the examiner, the streak is narrow. As the far point is moved closer to the examiner, the streak broadens and, at neutrality, fills the entire pupil. This situation applies only to *with* movement reflexes.
4. *Regularity.* An irregular reflex indicates a media problem that should be further explored in examination.

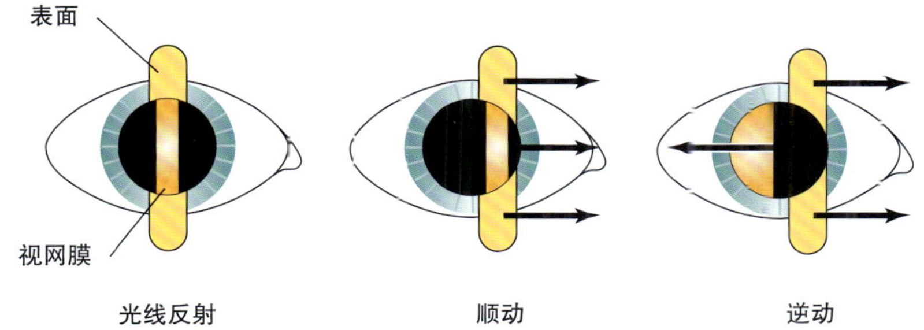

图 4–5　视网膜反光的移动。从面部到视网膜的顺动和逆动。*（译者注：资料来源见前页原文。）*

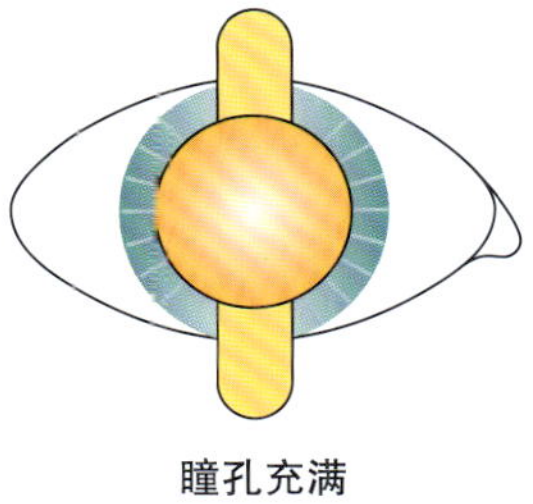

图 4–6　中和。眼的远点和检影镜的观察孔是共轭的。*（译者注：资料来源见前页原文。）*

反射的特点

检影镜反射光的移动具有 4 个主要特点（图 4–7）：

1. *速度：*当远点距离检查者（检影镜的观察孔）较远时，瞳孔区看到的反射光移动最慢；当远点移向窥孔时，反射光的移动速度加快。换句话说，高度屈光不正具有慢移动的反射光，而低度屈光不正具有快速度的反射光。

2. *亮度：*当远点距离检查者较远时，反射光较暗；接近中和时，反射光变亮。

3. *宽度：*当远点距离检查者较远时，反射光带是窄的；当远点向检查者靠近时，光带增宽；当中和状态时，充满整个瞳孔。这种状态仅适用于*顺动*反射光。

4. *规则性：*不规则的反射光提示应该进一步检查屈光间质问题。

The Correcting Lens

When the examiner uses the appropriate correcting lenses (with either loose lenses or a *phoropter*), the retinoscopic reflex is neutralized. In other words, when the examiner brings the patient's far point to the peephole, the reflex fills the patient's entire pupil (Fig 4-8). The power of the correcting lens (or lenses) neutralizing the reflex is determined by the refractive error of the eye and the distance of the examiner from the eye (the working distance). Theoretically, the working distance should be at optical infinity but this does not practically allow for changing lenses in front of the eye or seeing the retinal reflex. The dioptric equivalent of the *working distance* (ie, the inverse of the distance) must be subtracted from the power of the correcting lens to determine the actual refractive error of the patient's eye. Common working distances are 67 cm (1.50 D) and 50 cm (2.00 D), and many phoropters have a 1.50 D or 2.00 D "working-distance lens" for use during retinoscopy, which are then removed at the end of the retinoscopy (however, this lens can produce bothersome reflexes). If the examiner is not using the "built-in" working lens in the phoropter, he or she must algebraically subtract the appropriate amount of spherical power to move the neutralization point from the examiner to infinity (Clinical Example 4-2).

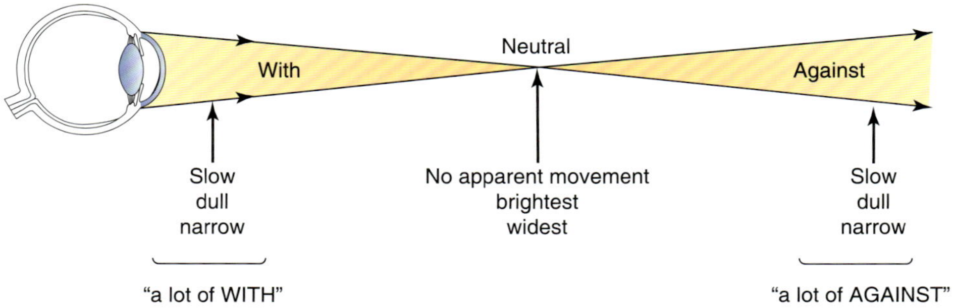

Figure 4-7 Characteristics of the moving retinal reflex on both sides of neutrality. The vertical arrows indicate the position of the retinoscope with regard to the point of neutrality. (*Illustration by C. H. Wooley.*)

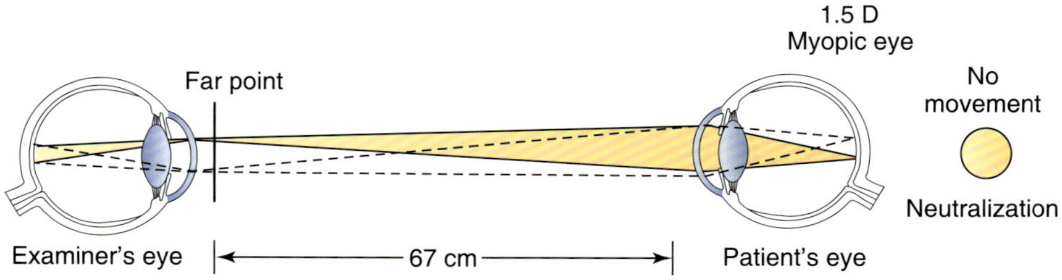

Figure 4-8 Observation system at neutralization.

For example, an examiner obtains neutralization with a total of +4.00 D over the eye (gross retinoscopy) at a working distance of 67 cm. Subtracting 1.50 D for the working distance yields a refractive correction of +2.50 D.

Any working distance may be used. If the examiner prefers to move closer to the patient for a brighter reflex, the working-distance correction is adjusted accordingly. Working without an explicit lens to correct for the working distance may allow the use of fewer lenses held in front of the eye, reducing distracting reflections from the lens surfaces.

矫正镜片

当检查者使用合适的矫正镜片（单独镜片或综合验光仪）时，检影镜的反射光都是中和状态的。换句话说，当检查者将患者的远点移向窥孔时，反射光将充满患者的整个瞳孔区（图 4–8）。矫正镜片的焦度（或一组镜片）是否中和反射光与患眼的屈光不正状态、检查者与患者的距离（工作距离）有关。理论上讲，工作距离应该在光学无穷远处，但实际中无法更换镜片或观察视网膜反射光。在确定最终屈光不正度数时，必须从总的屈光度中减去与*工作距离*等量的焦度（如距离的倒数）。工作距离通常是 67 cm（1.50 D）和 50 cm（2.00 D），很多综合验光仪具有一个 1.50 D 或 2.00 D 的“工作距离镜片”用于检影检查，在检影结束时移除（这种镜片会产生干扰性反光）。如果检查者未使用综合验光仪中的“内置”工作距离镜片，则必须减去适当的球镜焦度，将中和点移向无穷远处（临床病案 4–2）。

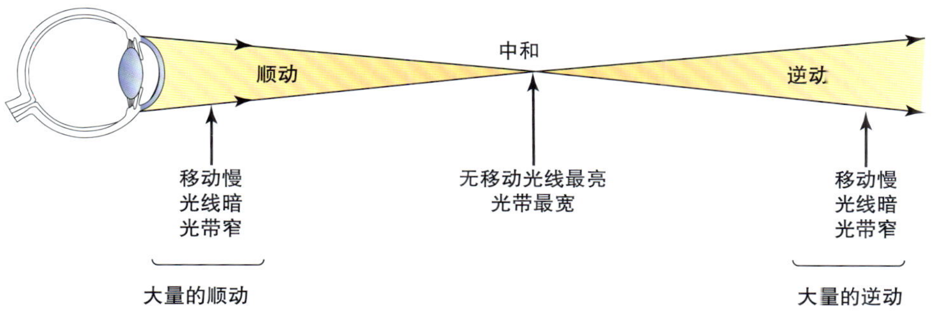

图 4–7　在中和两边的视网膜影动特点。垂直的箭头表示检影镜位于中和的位置。*（译者注：资料来源见前页原文。）*

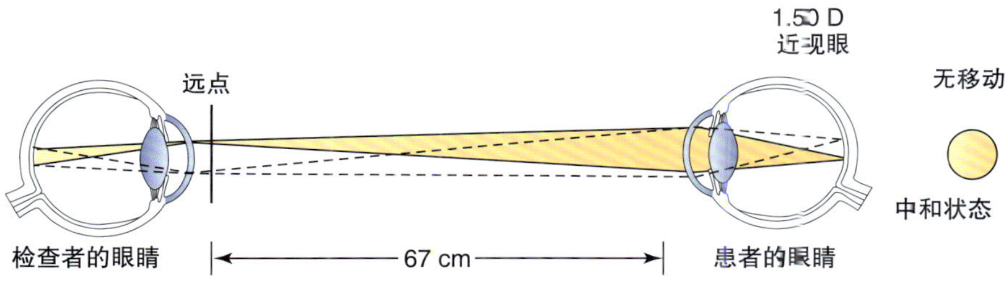

图 4–8　中和状态的观察系统。

例如，检查者在 67 cm 的工作距离，用 +4.00 D 屈光度获得中和状态。减去 1.50 D 的工作距离，屈光不正度数为 +2.50 D。

任何距离都可以作为工作距离。如果检查者习惯靠近患者以获取明亮的反射光，可以适当调整工作距离的矫正度数。未确定镜片矫正工作距离时，患眼前可以少放置镜片，以减少镜片表面的反射干扰光。

CLINICAL EXAMPLE 4-2

What happens if the correcting lens is not removed from the refractor at the conclusion of retinoscopy *and the subjective refraction is then performed?*

First the patient will be corrected for the focal length of the correcting lens if the retinoscopy is accurate. That would be 67 cm if the correcting (retinoscopy lens is +1.50). If the patient's vision following retinoscopy is very poor at distance suspect that the correcting lens is still in place.

If the subjective refraction is carried out, then 1 of 2 results may occur, depending on whether the retinoscopy lens built into the refractor was used or if the examiner simply dialed in +1.50 D of sphere.

If the built-in retinoscopy lens was used (and not removed before the subjective refraction) it will be −1.50 off due to having to correct for the +1.50D in the correcting lens as well as the patient's refraction.

If the +1.50 D was simply dialed into the refractor before starting retinoscopy and then not dialed out before the subjective refraction then the refraction should still be accurate (although difficult because of the +1.50 starting point error).

For this reason, many examiners choose to dial in the correcting lens rather than using the built-in retinoscopy lens in the refractor.

Finding Neutrality

In *against* movement, the far point is between the examiner and the patient. Therefore, to bring the far point to the peephole of the retinoscope, a minus lens is placed in front of the patient's eye. Similarly, in the case of *with* movement, a plus lens is placed in front of the patient's eye. This procedure gives rise to the simple clinical rule: If *with* movement is observed, add plus power (or subtract minus power); if *against* movement is observed, add minus power (or subtract plus power) (Fig 4-9).

Because it is easier to work with the brighter, sharper *with* movement image, one should "overminus" the eye and obtain a *with* reflex; then reduce the minus power (or add plus power) until neutrality is reached. Be aware that the slow, dull reflexes of high-refractive errors may be confused with the neutrality reflex. Media opacities may also produce dull reflexes.

Once neutrality is found, the lens to correct for the working distance must be removed, whether it is the built-in retinoscopy lens in the phoropter or by subtracting the appropriate correcting lens based on the working distance used.

Retinoscopy of Regular Astigmatism

Most eyes have some regular astigmatism. In such cases, light is refracted differently by the 2 principal astigmatic meridians. Let us consider how the retinoscope works in greater detail and apply it to astigmatism.

临床案例 4–2

如果在检影结束时矫正镜片未从验光仪移开会发生什么，下一步是否该进行主观验光？

如果检影镜结果准确无误，首先要修正矫正镜片的焦距，矫正距离是 67 cm（检影镜片是 +1.50 D）。如果检影后，患者远视力很差，应该考虑矫正镜片没有取出，仍在原位。

如果进行主观验光，可能发生下面 2 种结果之一，使用了验光仪中内置辅镜，或检查者置入了 +1.50 D 的球镜。

如果使用内置辅镜（并且在主观验光前没有移出），在矫正镜片和患者的验光中应用 −1.50 D 去矫正这 +1.50 D。

如果 +1.50 D 在检影之前加入验光仪中，并且在主观验光前没有取出，验光仍然是准确的（尽管有因为 +1.50 D 的初始检影有难度）。

也因此，许多检查者更喜欢在验光仪中加入矫正镜片，而不使用验光仪中的内置辅镜。

寻找中和点

在*逆动*中，远点位于检查者和患者之间。因此，要将远点移向检影镜的窥孔，应该在患者眼前放置负镜片。相似地，在*顺动*中，患者眼前放置正镜片。这个过程形成一个简单的临床规则：如果观察到*顺动*，加正度数（或去掉负度数）；如果观察到*逆动*，增加负度数（或减去正度数）。

因为明亮而清晰的*顺动*图像更容易观察，因此，检查者应该在患眼前“过负矫”以获得一个*顺动*的视网膜反射光，接着减少负度数（或增加正度数）达到中和。应该注意高度屈光不正时出现的缓慢的、昏暗的反射光可能干扰中和反射光的判断。屈光间质混浊同样可以产生暗的反射光。

一旦达到中和状态，用以矫正工作距离的修正镜片必须取出，无论是验光仪中的内置辅镜，还是根据工作距离减去适当的修正镜片。

规则散光的检影检查

大多数眼睛都会有些规则散光。在这种情况下，光线将在 2 条主散光子午线上发生不同的反射。我们来了解一下检影镜的具体操作和在散光中的应用。

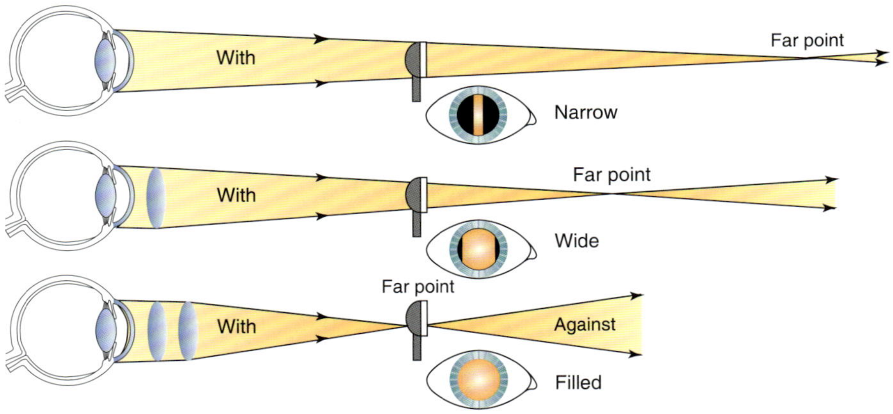

Figure 4-9 Approaching neutrality. Change in width of the reflex as neutrality is approached. Note that working distance remains constant, and the far point is pulled in with plus lenses.(*Illustration by C. H. Wooley.*)

Sweeping the retinoscope back and forth measures the power along only a single axis. Moving the retinoscope from side to side (with the streak oriented at 90°) measures the optical power in the 180° meridian. Power in this meridian is provided by a cylinder at the 90° axis. The convenient result is that the streak of the retinoscope is aligned with the axis of the correcting cylinder being tested. In a patient with regular astigmatism, one seeks to neutralize 2 reflexes, 1 from each of the principal meridians.

Finding the cylinder axis

Before the powers in each of the principal meridians can be determined, the axes of the meridians must be determined. Four characteristics of the streak reflex aid in this determination:

1. *Break.* A break is observed when the streak is not oriented parallel to 1 of the principal meridians. The reflex streak in the pupil is not aligned with the streak projected on the iris and surface of the eye, and the line appears broken (Fig 4-10). The break disappears (ie, the line appears continuous) when the projected streak is rotated to the correct axis.
2. *Width.* The width of the reflex in the pupil varies as it is rotated around the correct axis. The reflex appears narrowest when the streak, or *intercept*, aligns with the axis (Fig 4-11).
3. *Intensity.* The intensity of the line is brighter when the streak is on the correct axis.
4. *Skew.* Skew (oblique motion of the streak reflex) may be used to refine the axis in small cylinders. If the retinoscope streak is off-axis, it moves in a slightly different direction from that of the pupillary reflex (Fig 4-12). The reflex and streak move in the same direction when the streak is aligned with 1 of the principal meridians.

When the streak is aligned at the correct axis, the sleeve may be lowered (Copeland instrument) or raised (Welch Allyn instrument) to narrow the streak, allowing the axis to be determined more easily (Fig 4-13).

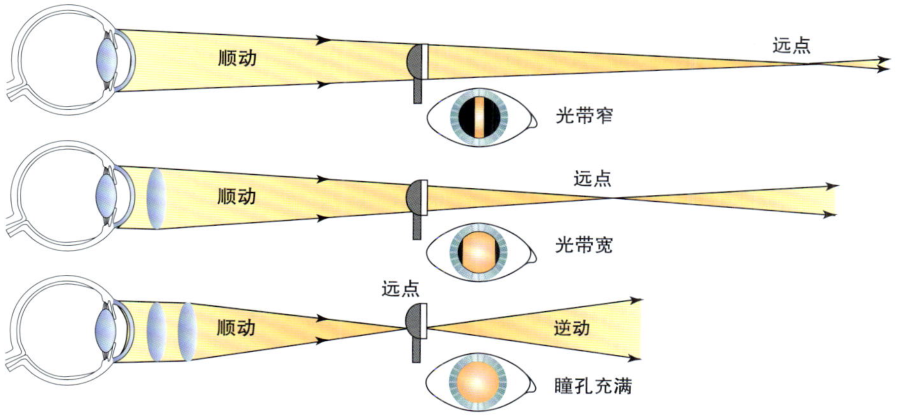

图 4–9　接近中和状态。改变反射光的宽度以达到中和。注意工作距离是一个常数，远点通过正镜片前移。*（译者注：资料来源见前页原文。）*

仅沿一个轴来回扫动检影镜检测屈光度。左右摆动检影镜（光带定在 90°）测定 180° 子午线的屈光力，90° 轴的柱镜可以测得这条子午线的屈光力。简言之，检影镜的光带和测得的矫正柱镜的轴位方向一致。如果患者是规则散光，应检测中和 2 个主子午线的反射光。

寻找柱镜轴位

在确定每条主子午线的屈光力之前，应该首先确定子午线的轴位。反射光带有 4 个特点：

1. *断裂*。断裂是指光带与主子午线不平行的现象。瞳孔内的反射光带与投射在虹膜和眼表面上的光带没成一条直线，出现断裂（图 4–10）。当投射光带被旋转至正确的轴位时，断裂消失（线出现连续）

2. *宽度*。当围绕着正确的轴位转动时，瞳孔区反射光的宽度变化。当光带或*套管*与轴位在 1 条直线上时（图 4–11），光带最窄。
3. *亮度*。当光带在正确轴位时，光带更为明亮。
4. *斜动*。斜动（光带反光斜向运动）可用于精确小柱镜的轴。如果检影镜的光带是偏离轴的，则检影镜的光带与瞳孔内反射光带运动的方向略有不同（图 4–12）。当光带与 1 条子午线一致时，反射光带运动方向与检影镜光带运动方向在一条直线。

当光带与正确的轴位相符时，通过降低（Copeland 检影镜）或升高（Welch Allyn 检影镜）套管，调整光带至其变窄，这样更容易确定轴位（图 4–13）。

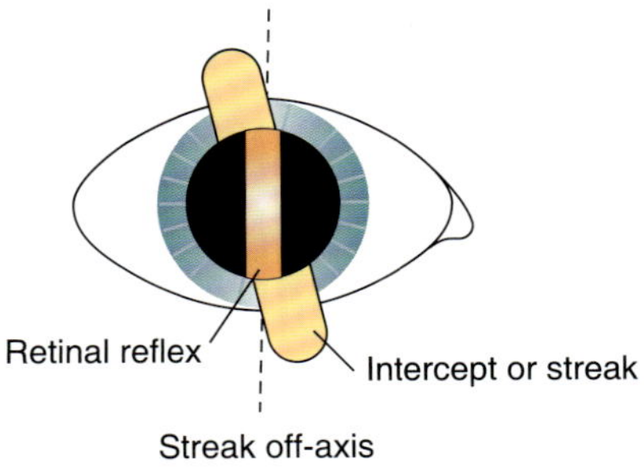

Figure 4-10 Break. The retinal reflex is discontinuous with the intercept when the streak is off the correct axis (dashed lines). *(Illustration by C. H. Wooley.)*

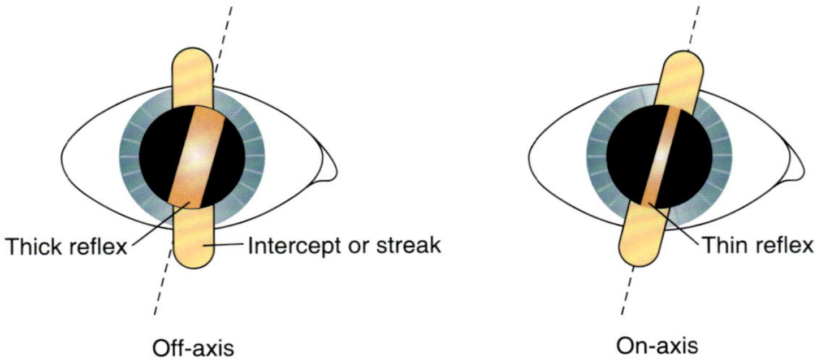

Figure 4-11 Width, or thickness, of the retinal reflex. The examiner locates the axis where the reflex is thinnest (dashed lines). *(Illustration by C. H. Wooley.)*

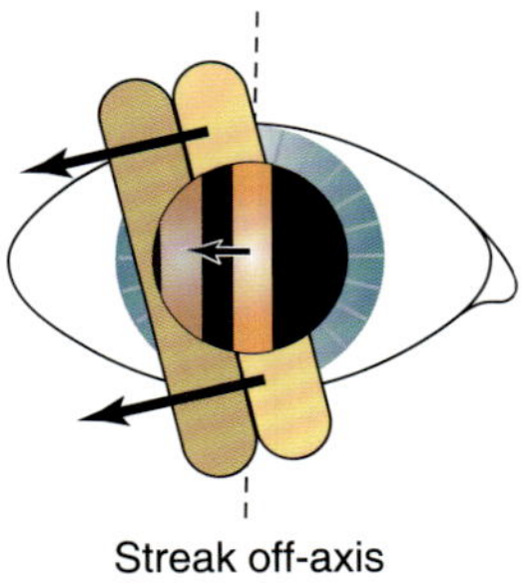

Figure 4-12 Skew. The *arrows* indicate that movements of the reflex (single *arrow*) and intercept (2 *arrows*) are not parallel. The reflex and intercept do not move in the same direction but are skewed when the streak is off axis. Dashed lines indicate the onaxis line. *(Illustration by C. H. Wooley.)*

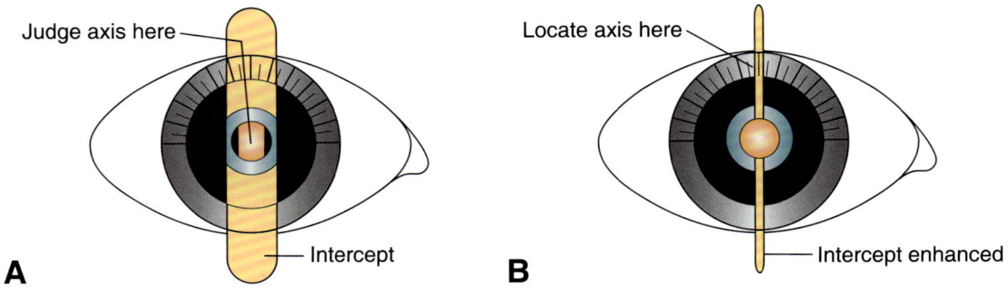

Figure 4-13 Locating axis on the protractor. **A**, First, determine the astigmatic axis. **B**, Second, adjust the sleeve to enhance the intercept until the filament is observed as a fine line pinpointing the axis. *(Illustration by C. H. Wooley.)*

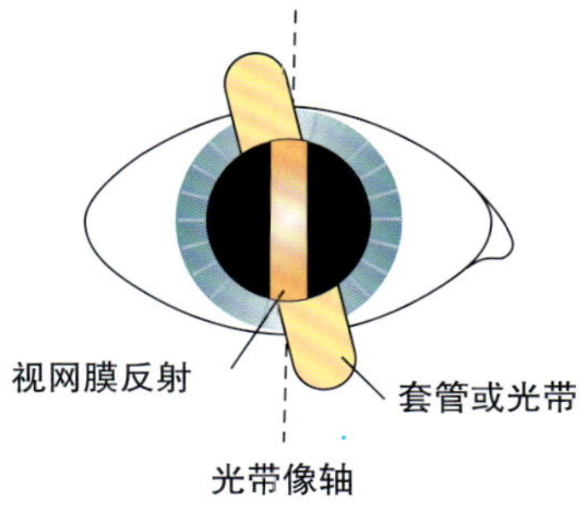

图 4–10　断裂。当光带偏离正确的轴位时视网膜反射光连续性中断（虚线）。*（译者注：资料来源见前页原文。）*

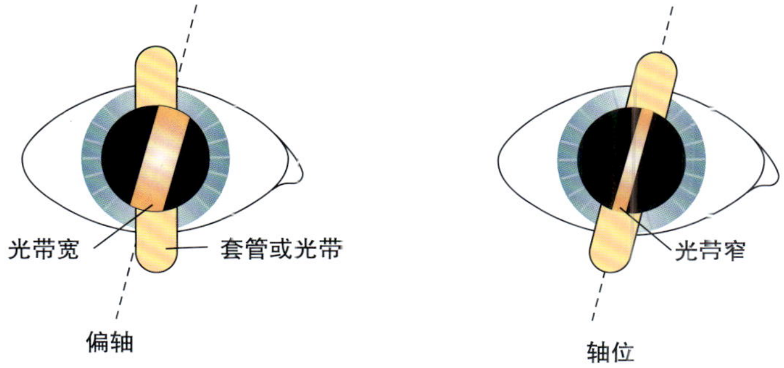

图 4–11　光带的宽度或厚度。检查者确定的轴位部分反射光是最窄的（虚线）。*（译者注：资料来源见前页原文。）*

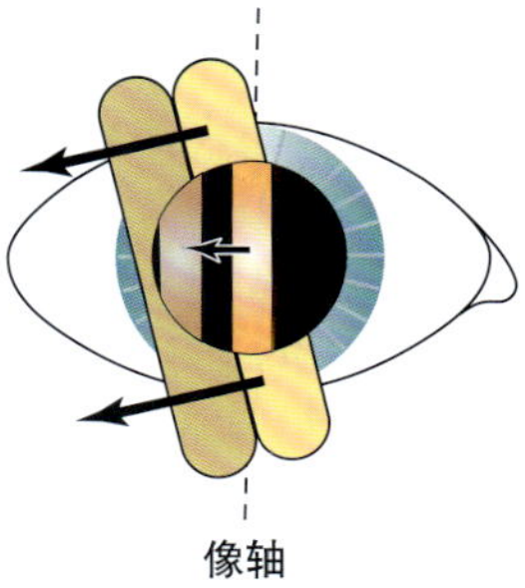

图 4–12　斜动。*箭头*表示反射光的移动方向（单个*箭头*）和拦截（2 个*箭头*）是不平行的。当光带偏离轴时，反射光和拦截移动方向不同，是偏斜的。虚线表示在轴线上。*（译者注：资料来源见前页原文。）*

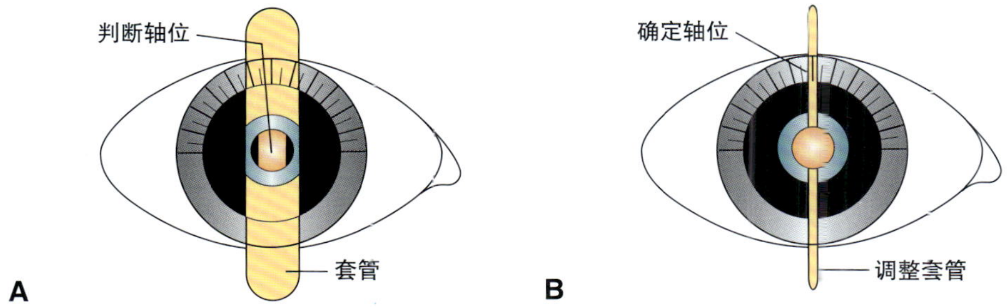

图 4–13　在验光仪上确定轴位。**A**. 先确定散光轴位。**B**. 调整套管，增加光带亮度，直至细线状的灯丝准确指向轴位。*（译者注：资料来源见前页原文。）*

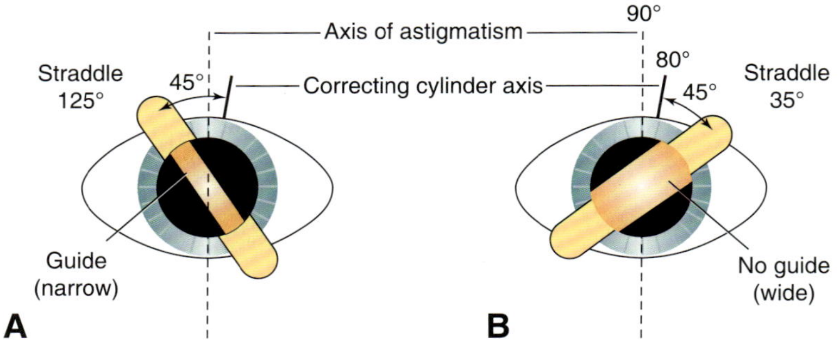

Figure 4-14 Straddling. The straddling meridians are 45° off the correcting cylinder axis, at roughly 35° and 125°. As the examiner moves back from the eye while comparing the meridians, the reflex at 125° remains narrow. (**A**) at the same distance that the reflex at 35° has become wide. (**B**) This dissimilarity indicates an axis error; the narrow reflex (**A**) is the guide toward which the examiner must turn the correcting cylinder axis. *(Illustration by C. H. Wooley.)*

This axis can be confirmed through a technique known as *straddling*, which is performed with the estimated correcting cylinder in place (Fig 4-14). The retinoscope streak is turned 45° off-axis in both directions, and if the axis is correct, the width of the reflex should be equal in both off-axis positions. If the axis is not correct, the widths are unequal in these 2 positions. The axis of the correcting plus cylinder should be moved toward the narrower reflex and the straddling repeated until the widths are equal.

Finding the cylinder power

After the 2 principal meridians are identified, the previously explained spherical techniques are applied to each axis:

- *With 2 spheres.* Neutralize 1 axis with a spherical lens; then neutralize the axis 90° away. The difference between these readings is the cylinder power.For example, if the 90°axis is neutralized with a +1.50 D sphere and the 180° axis is neutralized with a +2.25 D sphere, the gross retinoscopy is +1.50 +0.75 ×180. The examiner's working distance (ie, +1.50 D) is subtracted from the *sphere* to obtain the final refractive cor rection: plano +0.75 × 180.
- *With a sphere and cylinder.* Neutralize 1 axis with a spherical lens. To enable the use of *with* reflexes, neutralize the *less plus* axis first. Then, with this spherical lens in place, neutralize the axis 90° away by adding a plus cylindrical lens. The spherocylindrical gross retinoscopy is read directly from the trial lens apparatus.

It is also possible to use 2 cylinders at right angles to each other for this gross retinos-copy. Video 4-2 demonstrates the plus cylinder technique, and Video 4-3 demonstrates the minus cylinder technique.

VIDEO 4-2 Retinoscopy: plus cylinder technique.
Animation developed by Thomas F. Mauger, MD.'

VIDEO 4-3 Retinoscopy: minus cylinder technique.
Animation developed by Thomas F. Mauger, MD.'

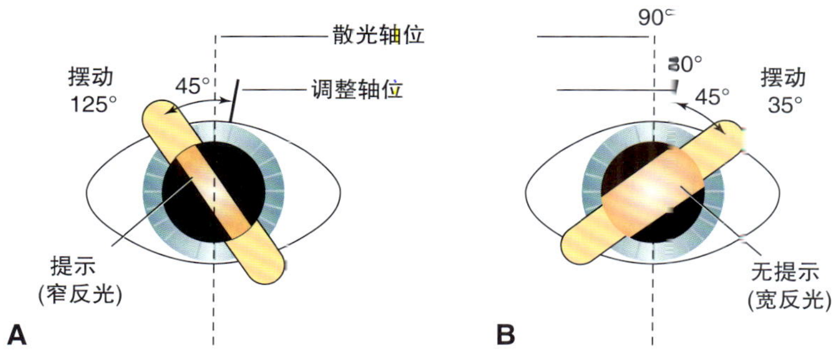

图 4–14　摆动技术。跨骑子午线偏离矫正轴位 45° 的位置，约在 35° 和 125° 。检查者从比较子午线的摆移回，125° 的反光带窄。（**A**）在同样的位置，35° 反光带变宽。（**B**）提示轴位错误　窄反光（**A**）时引导检查者转动 45° ，修正柱镜轴位。*（译者注：资料来源见前页原文。）*

这个轴可以通过一种称为*摆动*的技术来确认，该技术是在估计矫正柱镜轴的情况下进行的（图 4–14）。检影镜光带偏离轴两侧各转 45°，如果轴正确，在偏离轴 2 个位置反光宽度相等。如果轴位不正确，两边宽度不等。矫正的正柱镜轴位应该向窄影像移动，反复摆动调整，直到宽度一致。

确定柱镜度数

在 2 个主子午线确定后，前面讲到的球镜技术可应用在每个轴位上：

- *球球法*。用球镜中和 1 个轴位，再中和对应 90° 的另 1 个轴。2 个中和度数的差值就是柱镜度数。如 90° 轴位，用 +1.50 D 球镜中和；180° 轴位用 +2.25 D 球镜中和。总检影镜度数是 +1.50+0.75 × 180。检查者的工作距离（+1.50 D）从最终矫正度数中减去球镜：平光 +0.75 × 180。

- *球柱法*。用球镜中和 1 个轴位。利用反射光特点，先中和低度正镜轴向，偏移 90° 的轴向再添加正柱镜中和。球柱镜总共检影度数可直接从试镜片中读出。

也可通过 2 个柱镜在相互垂直的 2 个轴向进行联合视网膜检影。录像 4–2 演示的是正柱镜技术，录像 4–3 演示的是负柱镜技术。

录像 4–2 检影：正柱镜技术。
由 Thomas F. Mauger 医学博士演示。

录像 4-3 检影：负柱镜技术。
由 Thomas F. Mauger 医学博士演示。

Aberrations of the Retinoscopic Reflex

With irregular astigmatism, almost any type of aberration may appear in the reflex. Spherical aberrations tend to increase the brightness at the center or periphery of the pupil, depending on whether they are positive or negative.

As neutrality is approached, 1 part of the reflex may be myopic, whereas the other may be hyperopic relative to the position of the retinoscope. This situation produces a *scissors reflex*. Causes of the scissors reflex include keratoconus, irregular corneal astigmatism, corneal or lenticular opacities, and spherical aberration.

All of these aberrant reflexes, in particular spherical aberration, are more noticeable in patients with large scotopic pupils. When a large pupil is observed during retinoscopy, the examiner should focus on neutralizing the central portion of the light reflex.

Table 4-1 provides a summary of the technique of retinoscopy using a plus cylinder phoropter.

Corboy JM. *The Retinoscopy Book: An Introductory Manual for Eye Care Professionals.* 5th ed.Thorofare, NJ: Slack; 2003.

Wirtschafter JD, Schwartz GS. Retinoscopy. In: Tasman W, Jaeger EA, eds. *Duane's Clinical Ophthalmology* [CD-ROM]. Vol 1. Philadelphia: Lippincott Williams & Wilkins; 2006.

Pseudoneutralization

As noted above, in general, with reflexes are brighter, sharper, and easier to perceive and interpret than against reflexes. In particular, the reflex in severely myopic eyes is seldom recognizable as an against reflex—rather, one sees only a dull, motionless illumination of the entire pupil. This is referred to as *pseudoneutralization*. This is best handled by reversing the sleeve of the retinoscope (to the maximal sleeve-up position for Welch-Allyn type retinoscopes; maximal sleeve-down position for Copeland retinoscopes). This will convert the dull pseudoneutral reflex to a readily recognizable with reflex, but in this case, the with reflex must be neutralized by adding minus sphere power. As true neutrality is approached, return the retinoscope sleeve to the usual position. The reflex will revert to an against reflex as in typical myopic eyes. Continue to add minus sphere power until a with reflex is obtained, and then reduce the minus sphere so as to reach true neutrality from the with direction. Video 4-4 demonstrates pseudoneutralization.

VIDEO 4-4 Retinoscopy: pseudoneutralization.
Animation developed by Thomas F. Mauger, MD.

视网膜反光的像差

有不规则散光时，任何形式的像差都可以在反射光中观察到。无论是正片还是负片，球面像差倾向于在瞳孔中心或边缘增加亮度。

相对于视网膜检影镜，当接近中和点时，反射光带的一部分是近视，另一部分是远视。这种情况会产生*剪影*。产生剪影的原因包括有圆锥角膜、不规则角膜散光、角膜或晶状体混浊和球面像差。

所有像差反射，特别是球面像差多发生在大瞳孔。对大瞳孔进行视网膜检影时，应该注意中和反射光带的中心部分。

Corboy JM. *The Retinoscopy Book: An Introductory Manual for Eye Care Professionals.* 5th ed.Thorofare, NJ: Slack; 2003.

Wirtschafter JD, Schwartz GS. Retinoscopy. In: Tasman W, Jaeger EA, eds. *Duane's ClinicalOphthalmology* [CD-ROM]. Vol 1. Philadelphia: Lippincott Williams & Wilkins; 2006.

假中和

如上所述，一般情况下，与逆动反射相比，顺动反射明亮、清晰、更易于观察解释。特别是在高度近视眼中，逆动反射很难辨别，反而是看到占整个瞳孔暗的、不动的反射，这是*假中和*。最好的解决方法是反向转动检影镜（Welch-Allyn 型检影镜，套管上转到最大；Copeland 型检影镜，套管下转到最大）。这样将暗的假中和反射影转变为可见的顺动，需要用负球镜达到中和。到达中和后，调整检影镜至正常位置，反射光也呈近视的逆动影。继续加负球镜至顺动，再减少负球镜，从顺动方向达到中和。视频 4-4 演示了假中和。

录像 4-4 检影：假中和。
由 Thomas F. Mauger 医学博士演示。

Table 4-1 Retinoscopy Summary (Using a Plus Cylinder Phoropter)

1. Set the phoropter to 0.00 D sphere and 0.00 D cylinder. Use cycloplegia if necessary. Otherwise, fog the eyes or use a nonaccommodative target.
2. Hold the sleeve of the retinoscope in the position that produces a divergent beam of light. (If the examiner can focus the linear filament of the retinoscope on a wall, the sleeve is in the wrong position.)
3. Sweep the streak of light (the intercept) across the pupil perpendicular to the long axis of the streak. Observe the pupillary light reflex. Sweep in several different meridians.
4. Add minus sphere until the retinoscopic reflex shows *with* movement in all meridians. Add some extra minus sphere if uncertain. If the reflexes are dim or indistinct, consider high refractive errors and make large changes in sphere (–3.00 D, –6.00 D, –9.00 D, and so on).
5. Continue examining multiple meridians while adding plus sphere until the retinoscopic reflex neutralizes in 1 meridian. (If all meridians neutralize simultaneously, the patient's refractive error is spherical; subtract the working distance to obtain the net retinoscopy.)
6. Rotate the streak 90° and position the axis of the correcting plus cylinder parallel to the streak. A sweep across this meridian reveals additional *with* movement. Add plus cylinder power with axis parallel to the streak until neutrality is achieved.
7. Refine the correcting cylinder axis by sweeping 45° to either side of it. Rotate the axis of the correcting plus cylinder a few degrees toward the "guide" line, the brighter and narrower reflex. Repeat until both reflexes are equal.
8. Refine the cylinder power by moving in closer to the patient to pick up *with* movement in all directions. Back away slowly, observing how the reflexes neutralize. Change sphere or cylinder power as appropriate to make all meridians neutralize simultaneously.
9. Subtract the dioptric equivalent of the working distance. For example, if the working distance is 67 cm, subtract 1.50 D (1/0.67).
10. Record the streak retinoscopy findings and, when possible, check the patient's visual acuity with the new prescription.

Subjective Refraction Techniques

In subjective refraction techniques, the examiner relies on the patient's responses to determine the refractive correction. If all refractive errors were spherical, subjective refraction would be easy. However, determining the astigmatic portion of the correction is more complex, and various subjective refraction techniques may be used. The Jackson cross cylinder is the most common instrument used in determining the astigmatic correction. However, we begin by discussing the astigmatic dial technique because it is easier to understand.

Astigmatic Dial Technique

An astigmatic dial is a test chart with radially arranged lines that may be used to determine the axes of astigmatism. A pencil of light from a point source is refracted by an astigmatic eye as a conoid of Sturm. The spokes of the astigmatic dial that are parallel to the principal meridians of the eye's astigmatism are imaged as sharp lines, which correspond to the focal lines of the conoid of Sturm.

Figure 4-15A shows an eye with compound hyperopic astigmatism and how it sees an astigmatic dial. In this example, the vertical line of the astigmatic dial is the blackest and sharpest because the vertical focal line of each conoid of Sturm is closer to the retina than the horizontal focal line is. By accommodating, however, the patient might pull both focal lines forward. To avoid accommodation, fogging is used. Sufficient plus sphere is placed before the eye to pull both focal lines into the vitreous, creating compound myopic astigmatism (Fig 4-15B).

表4–1 视网膜检影小结（使用正柱镜综合验光仪）

1. 将综合验光仪设在0.00 D球镜和0.00 D柱镜。如果需要可以使用睫状肌麻痹剂。另外,可以采用雾视或无调节视标。
2. 握住检影镜，使检影镜套管处于发出发散光的位置（如果检查者可以在墙上聚焦检影镜的线状灯丝，那么镜筒的位置就不对）。
3. 垂直于光带长轴扫动穿过瞳孔的光带。观察瞳孔的光反射。在不同子午线扫动。
4. 增加负球镜，直到检影的反光在所有子午线上*顺动*。如果不确定，再添加一点负镜片。如果反光弱或不清楚,考虑高度屈光不正,可改较大球镜度数（–3.00 D，–6.00 D，–9.00 D，等等）。
5. 继续检查多个子午线,同时增加正球镜,直到检影反光在1条子午线上中和（如果所有子午线同时中和，那么屈光不正是球镜的，减去工作距离，得到最终检影结果）。
6. 旋转光带 90°，确定矫正正柱镜的轴位与光带平行。沿该子午线摆动，如果还有*顺动*，增加正柱镜度数直到中和。
7. 在轴位两侧45° 摆动,精确确定柱镜轴位，朝着更亮、更窄“指导”线将正柱镜矫正轴旋转几度。反复多次，直到2条反射光带相等。
8. 通过移近患者在各个方向获得*顺动*来精确柱镜度数。慢慢后退，观察反射光中和。改变球镜或柱镜度数，使所有子午线同时中和。
9. 减去工作距离（换算为屈光度）。如果工作距离为67 cm,减去1.50 D(1.00/0.67)。
10. 记录带状检影结果, 如果可以，用新处方检查患者视力。

主观验光技术

在主观验光技术中，检查者依赖患者的反应确定屈光矫正。如果所有屈光不正是球镜，主观验光较简单。然而，散光的矫正较复杂，可采用多种主观验光技术。Jackson 交叉柱镜是最常用的确定散光矫正的设备。我们首先讨论散光表技术，因为它相对较容易理解。

散光表盘技术

散光表盘是个放射状排列线的测试图标，用于确定散光轴位。点光源经散光眼，形成 Sturm 光锥。散光表盘上，平行于眼散光主子午线的放射线成像为清晰线，即为 Sturm 光锥的焦线。

图 4–15A 展示了复性远视散光眼如何看散光表盘。散光表盘的垂直线是最黑、最清晰的，因为Sturm 光锥的垂直焦线比水平焦线更接近视网膜。通过调节，将2条焦线前推。为避免调节，使用雾视法，眼前加足够的正球镜，将两条焦线移到玻璃体之内，形成复性近视散光（如图 4–15B）。

The focal line closest to the retina can then be identified with certainty because it is now the blackest and sharpest line of the astigmatic dial. (In the example in Fig 4-15B, this is the horizontal line on the dial.) Note that the terms *blackest* and *sharpest* are more easily understood by patients and should be used in place of the word *clearest*.

After the examiner locates the principal meridians of the astigmatism, the conoid of Sturm can be collapsed by moving the anterior focal line back toward the posterior focal line. This task can be accomplished by adding a minus cylinder with an axis parallel to the anterior focal line (perpendicular to the blackest and sharpest line). It is helpful to remember the "rule of 30": place the correcting minus cylinder axis along the meridian equal to 30 times the "clock-hour" of the sharpest, blackest line on the dial (reading between 0 and 6). In Figure 4-15C, the vertical focal line has been moved back to the position of the horizontal focal line and collapsed to a point by the addition of a minus cylinder with an axis at 90°. Note that $90 = 30 \times 3$, the clock-hour of the (horizontal) darkest line. Notice that the minus cylinder is placed with its axis *perpendicular* to the blackest meridian on the astigmatic dial. Also note that as the conoid of Sturm is collapsed, the focal lines disappear into a point focus.

All of the lines of the astigmatic dial now appear equally black but still are not in perfect focus, because the eye remains slightly fogged to control accommodation. At this point, a visual acuity chart is used; plus sphere is removed until the best visual acuity is obtained (Fig 4-15D).

In summary, the following steps are used in astigmatic dial refraction:

1. Obtain best visual acuity using spheres only.
2. Fog the eye to about 20/50 by adding plus sphere.
3. Note the blackest and sharpest line of the astigmatic dial.
4. Add minus cylinder with axis *perpendicular* to the blackest and sharpest line until all lines appear equal.
5. Reduce plus sphere (or add minus) until best acuity is obtained with the visual acuity chart.

最靠近视网膜的焦线可以被确定，因为它现在是散光表盘上最黑、最清晰的线。（图 4–15B 这是散光盘上的水平线）“*最黑*”“*最清晰*”的线这一表述是*最为清晰*的用词，患者也易于理解。

当检查者确定散光主子午线后，通过将前焦线移向后焦线，使 Sturm 光锥收拢。这项工作通过加负柱镜来完成，柱镜轴平行于前焦线（垂直于最黑和最清晰的线）。记住“30 倍法则”：矫正的负柱镜轴的子午线等于 30 倍的散光表盘上最清晰最黑线的钟点数（0~6 之间的读书）。在图 4–15C，通过加 90° 轴的负柱镜，使垂直焦线向后移至水平焦线，并且收拢成一个点。轴为 90 = 30 × 3，3 是最黑线（水平）的钟点数。需要注意的是使用负柱镜矫正时，负柱镜的轴应*垂直*散光盘上最黑子午线。还要注意，当 Sturm 光锥被收拢，焦线成为焦点。

散光表盘中所有的子午线亮度黑色相同，但是仍然没有完全聚焦，因为控制调节的雾视正镜尚未取出。之后，通过视力表，取出正球镜，直到获得最好的视力。（图 4–15D）

总体来说，散光表盘验光步骤如下：

1. 仅使用球镜获得最佳矫正视力。
2. 增加正球镜，雾视到 20/50。
3. 找到散光表中最黑、最清晰的线。
4. 以*垂直*于最黑和最清晰的线为轴，加负柱镜，直到所有的线一样清晰。

5. 减少正球镜（或增加负球镜），直到获得最好视力。

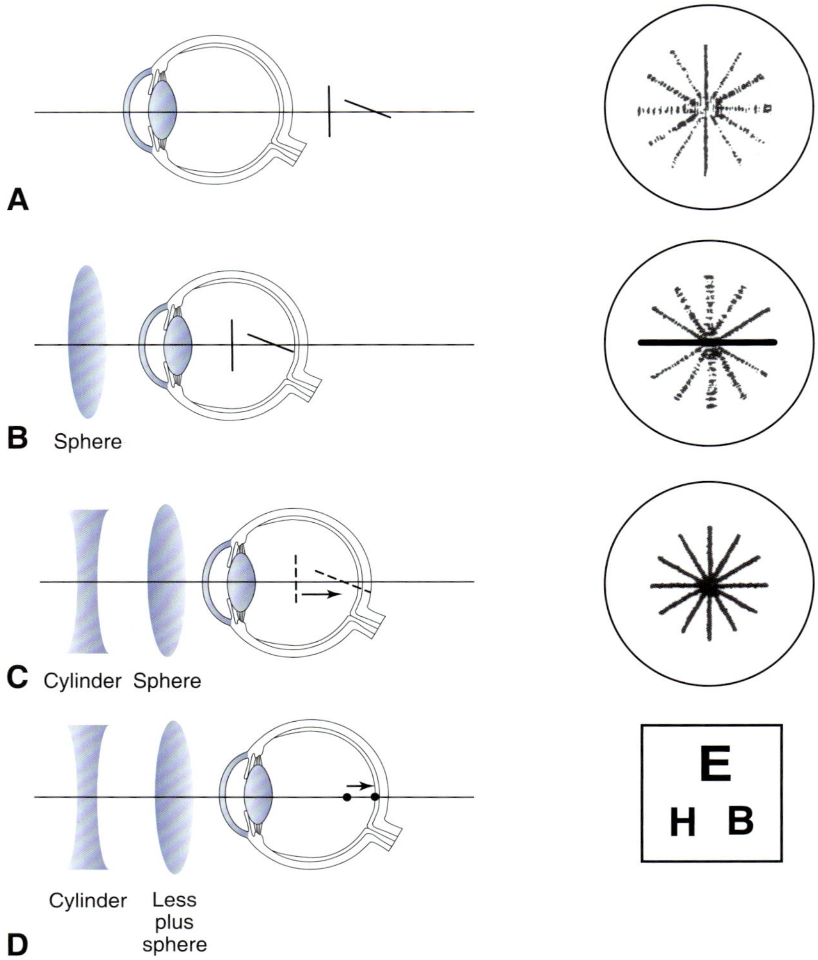

Figure 4-15 Astigmatic dial technique. **A,** Conoid of Sturm and retinal image of an astigmatic dial as viewed by an eye with compound hyperopic astigmatism. **B,** Fogging to produce compound myopic astigmatism. **C,** The conoid of Sturm is collapsed to a single point. **D,** Minus sphere is added (or plus sphere subtracted) to produce a sharp image, and a visual acuity chart is used for viewing.

Astigmatic dial refraction can also be performed with plus cylinder equipment, but this technique must be used in a way that simulates minus cylinder effect. All of the above steps remain the same except for step 4, which becomes "Add *plus* cylinder with the axis *parallel* to the blackest and sharpest line." As each 0.25 D of plus cylinder power is added, change the sphere simultaneously by 0.25 D in the minus direction. Doing so simulates minus cylinder effect exactly by moving the anterior focal line posteriorly without changing the position of the posterior focal line.

Michaels DD. *Visual Optics and Refraction: A Clinical Approach.* 3rd ed. St Louis: Mosby; 1985:319–322.

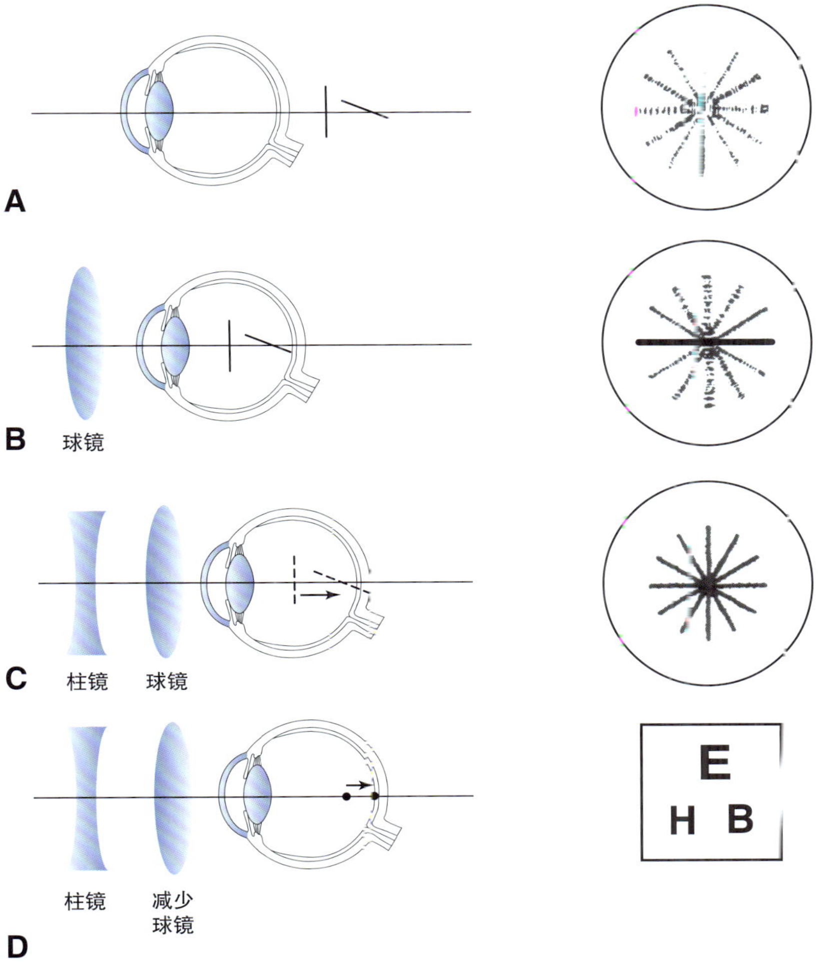

图 4-15　散光表盘技术。**A**. 复性远视散光眼观看时的 Sturm 光锥和散光表盘的视网膜像。**B**. 雾视形成复性近视散光。**C**. 光锥被收拢成一个点。**D**. 增加负球镜（或减少正球镜），形成清晰像。

散光表盘验光可以加正柱镜，但必须用于模拟负柱镜效应。除了第 4 步，其他步骤与上述相同。以"*平行*于最黑和最清晰的线为轴，增加*正*柱镜"。正柱镜以 0.25D 的速度递加，同时负球镜加 0.25D。这样，可以不改变后焦线的位置而将前焦线向后移动，模拟负柱镜效应。

Michaels DD. Visual Optics and Refraction: A Clinical Approach. 3rd ed. St Louis: Mosby; 1985:319–322.

Stenopeic Slit Technique

The stenopeic slit is an opaque trial lens with an oblong slit whose width forms a pinhole with respect to vergence perpendicular to the slit (Fig 4-16). If an examiner is unable to decipher the astigmatism by performing the usual retinoscopy because of the subject eye's irregular astigmatism or unclear media, he or she may neutralize the refractive error with spherical lenses and the slit at various meridians to find a spherocylindrical correction. This correction can then be refined subjectively. This process is especially useful for patients with small pupils, lenticular or corneal opacities, and/or irregular astigmatism. If the subject can accommodate, fog and unfog using plus sphere to find the most plus power accepted. Then turn the slit until the subject says the image is sharpest. If, for example, –3.00D sphere is best there, when the slit is oriented vertically, this finding indicates –3.00 D at 90° in a power cross. If the best sphere with the slit oriented horizontally is –5.00 D, then the result is –3.00 –2.00 × 90. It is helpful to think of the "axis" of the stenopeic slit as a thin line perpendicular to the orientation of the slit.

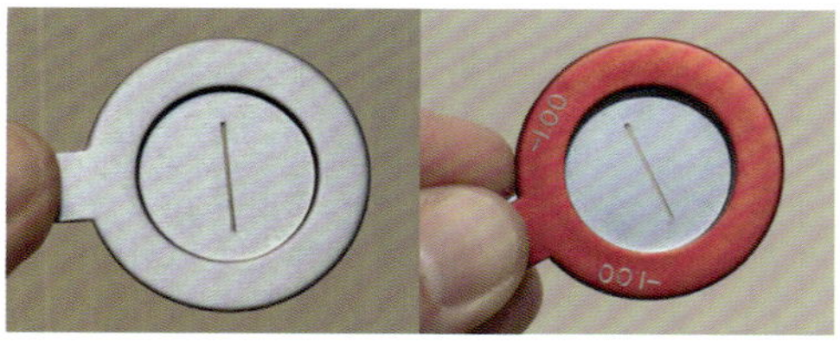

Figure 4-16 Stenopeic slit. The image on the right demonstrates the placement of a spherical lens in front of the stenopeic slit in order to determine the best visual acuity. *(Courtesy of Tommy Korn, MD.)*

Cross Cylinder Technique

The cross cylinder technique to measure astigmatism was described by Edward Jackson in 1887. In Jackson's words, the cross cylinder lens is probably "far more useful, and far more used" than any other lens in clinical refraction. Every ophthalmologist should be familiar with the principles involved in its use. Although the cross cylinder is usually used to *refine* the cylinder axis and power of a refraction that has already been obtained, it can also be used for the entire astigmatic refraction.

A cross cylinder is a lens with a spheroequivalent power of zero but with mixed astigmatism of equal amounts. Common cross cylinders are: – 0.50 +1.00 × 090 or – 0.25 +0.50 × 090. They are mounted so that they can be rotated about their axis (90° or 180°) or at a point halfway between the axis (45° or 135°).

The first step in cross cylinder refraction is to adjust the sphere to yield the best visual acuity with accommodation relaxed. Begin by selecting a starting point: this may be the current prescription, the retinoscopy, or autorefraction findings. Dial this into a trial frame or phoropter. Fog the eye to be examined with plus sphere while the patient views a visual acuity chart; then decrease the fog until the best visual acuity is obtained. If astigmatism is present, decreasing the fog places the circle of least confusion on the retina, creating a mixed astigmatism. Then use test figures that are 1 or 2 lines larger than the patient's best visual acuity. At this point, introduce the cross cylinder, first for refinement of cylinder axis and then for refinement of cylinder power.

裂隙技术

裂隙片是个不透明的试镜片，其中有格长方形裂隙，裂隙宽度形成针孔，限制垂直于裂隙的光束（图 4–16）。由于患者眼的规则散光或屈光介质混浊的原因，如果检查者通过常规的检影镜不能检测散光，可用球镜和裂隙片，在不同子午线中和屈光不正，得到球柱的矫正度数。然后，精确主观验光。这种方法特别适于小瞳孔、晶状体或角膜混浊、和 / 或不规则散光的患者。如果患者能调节，加正球镜至可接受的最大正球镜度数雾视和去雾视。然后，转动裂隙片，直到患者看到最清晰的像。例如，缝隙在竖直位置时，–3.00 D 的球镜最佳，在焦度十字表示中为 –3.00 D 在 90°。如果缝隙在水平位置时最佳球镜为 –5.00 D，则结果为 –3.00 –2.00 ×90。裂隙片的“轴”是垂直于缝隙方向的细线。

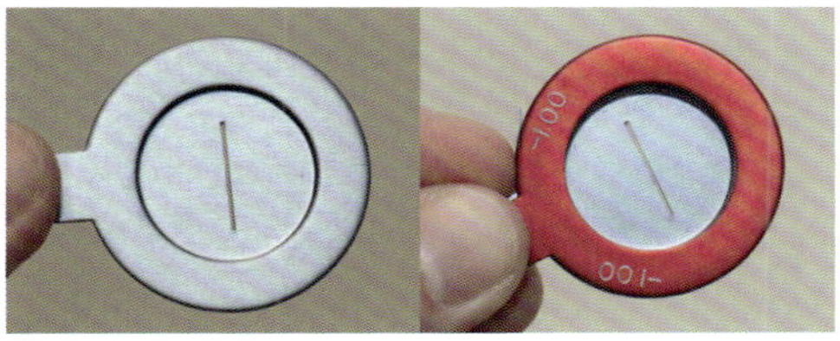

图 4–16　裂隙镜片。右侧的图显示，球镜置于裂隙镜片前，以得到最佳视力。*（译者注：资料来源见前页原文。）*

交叉柱镜技术

1887 年，Edward Jackson 提出用于测量散光的交叉柱镜技术。Jackson 交叉柱镜可以用 Jackson 的一句话概括，即“越有用，用得越多”。在临床验光中，Jackson 交叉柱镜比其他透镜应用得更广泛。每个眼科医生都应该熟悉其使用原则。交叉柱镜常用于*精准确定*散光轴位和精细验光，也可用于散光验光的全过程。

交叉柱镜是个球镜等效度数为 0 的镜片，具有等量的混合散光。常用的交叉柱镜是：–0.50+1.00×090 或 –0.25+0.50×090。交叉柱镜被安装成绕它们的轴 (90° 和 180°) 或绕轴 (45° 或 135°) 之间一半的一个点旋转。

交叉柱镜验光第一步，是在放松的状态下调整球镜至最佳视力。这种情况下，可以选择开始：让患者根据现有的验光处方进行检影或在自动验光仪上获得测量值。把相应度数的试镜片插入试镜架或在综合验光仪上拨入相应度数。注视视力表，加正球镜进行雾视法检查，然后降低雾视，直到视力最佳。如果存在散光，降低雾视，让最小弥散圈落在视网膜上，并形成混合散光。使用大于患者最佳视力 1~2 行的视标，此时使用交叉柱镜，先精准确定柱镜轴位，再精准确定散光度数。

If the starting point refraction contains no cylindrical component, the cross cylinder may be used to check for the presence of astigmatism in the following manner. The cross cylinder is first placed at 90° and 180°. If a preferred flip position is found, cylinder is added with the axis parallel to the respective plus or minus axis of the cross cylinder until the 2 flip choices are equal. If no preference is found with the cross cylinder axes at 90° and 180°, then check the axes at 45° and 135° before assuming that no astigmatism is present. Once any cylinder power is found, axis and power should be refined in the usual manner.

Another method of determining the presence of astigmatism is to dial 0.50 D of cylinder into the phoropter (while preserving the spherical equivalent with a compensatory 0.25 D change in the sphere). Ask the patient to slowly rotate the cylinder axis once around using the knob on the phoropter. If the patient finds a preferred position, it becomes the starting point for the cross cylinder refinement. If doing so has no effect, there may be no clinically significant astigmatism. Keratometry or corneal topography may be helpful if the examiner suspects that astigmatism may still be present.

Always refine cylinder axis before refining cylinder power. This sequence is necessary because the correct axis may be found in the presence of an incorrect power, but the full cylinder power is found only in the presence of the correct axis. The axis may be rechecked after the power is determined and is more important in higher levels of astigmatism power.

Refinement of cylinder axis involves the combination of cylinders at oblique axes. When the axis of the correcting cylinder is not aligned with that of the astigmatic eye's cylinder, the combined cylinders produce residual astigmatism with a meridian roughly.45° away from the principal meridians of the 2 cylinders. To refine the axis, position the principal meridians of the cross cylinder 45° away from those of the correcting cylinder (if using a handheld Jackson cross cylinder, the stem of the lens handle will be parallel to the axis of the correcting cylinder). Present the patient with alternative flip choices, and select the choice that is the blackest and sharpest to the patient. Then rotate the axis of the correcting cylinder toward the corresponding plus or minus axis of the cross cylinder (plus cylinder axis is rotated toward the plus cylinder axis of the cross cylinder, and minus cylinder axis is rotated toward the minus cylinder axis of the cross cylinder). Low-power cylinders are rotated in increments of 15°; high-power cylinders are rotated by smaller amounts, usually 5°, but can be as small as 1° for very high astigmatism. Repeat this procedure until the flip choices appear equal.

To refine cylinder power, align the cross cylinder axes with the principal meridians of the correcting lens (Fig 4-17). The examiner should change cylinder power according to the patient's responses; the spherical equivalent of the refractive correction should remain constant to keep the circle of least confusion on the retina. Ensure that the correction remains constant by changing the sphere half as much and in the opposite direction as the cylinder power is changed. In other words, for every 0.50 D of cylinder power change, change the sphere by 0.25 D in the opposite direction. Periodically, the sphere power should be adjusted for the best visual acuity.

如果验光没有先进行散光矫正，交叉柱镜的使用步骤如下：交叉柱镜首先置于 90° 和 180° 位置。如果发现有较为清晰的翻转位置，加柱镜，柱镜轴平行于交叉柱镜的正轴或负轴，直至 2 个翻转面相同。如果交叉柱镜在 90° 和 180° 没有改变，放在 45° 和 135° ，确定散光是否存在。只要柱镜度数确定，可用上述方法精细确定轴位和度数。

确定散光的另一种方法是综合屈光仪调整 0.50 D 的柱镜（同时球镜补偿 0.25 D，以保持等效球镜不变）。让患者慢慢旋转综合验光仪上的柱镜轴位旋钮。如果患者发现清晰位置，此点作为调整交叉柱镜的起点。如果没有变化，则没有临床意义上的散光。如果检查者考虑有散光存在，还可用角膜曲率计或角膜地形图验证。

在精确柱镜度数之前，首先应精确柱镜轴位。这个顺序是必要的，因为准确的轴可能会在未矫正的度数下找到，但是精确柱镜度数只会在准确的轴下找到。在确认柱镜度数后，还应再次检测轴位，这对于高度散光尤为重要。

精确柱镜轴位还包括斜轴位的柱镜联合。当矫正柱镜轴位与散光眼的轴位不一致时，联合柱镜在 2 个柱镜主轴位偏 45° 子午线上产生残余散光。用交叉柱镜精确轴位，主子午线偏离矫正柱镜 45° （手持 Jackson 交叉柱镜的手柄平行于矫正柱镜轴位）。翻转镜片，患者选择最黑、最清晰的一面。对应于交叉柱镜的正镜或负镜轴位，旋转矫正柱镜的轴位（正柱镜轴位向正交叉柱镜的正柱镜轴位旋转，负柱镜轴位向负交叉柱镜的柱镜轴位旋转）。低度数柱镜以 15° 旋转递增；高度数柱镜以 5° 旋转递增，甚至更小度数 1° 递增。反复操作这一步骤，直到翻转两面所看到的像一致。

精确柱镜度数，使交叉柱镜轴位与矫正镜的主子午线轴位一致（图 4-17）。根据患者的反应，检查者改变柱镜度数，屈光矫正的等效球镜应始终保持最小弥散圈落在患者视网膜上。当改变柱镜度数时，球镜以柱镜度数的一半、符号相反的度数改变，以确保矫正不变。换句话说，每个柱镜变化 0.50 D，将在球镜符号相反变化 0.25 D。不断地调整球镜度数到最佳视力。

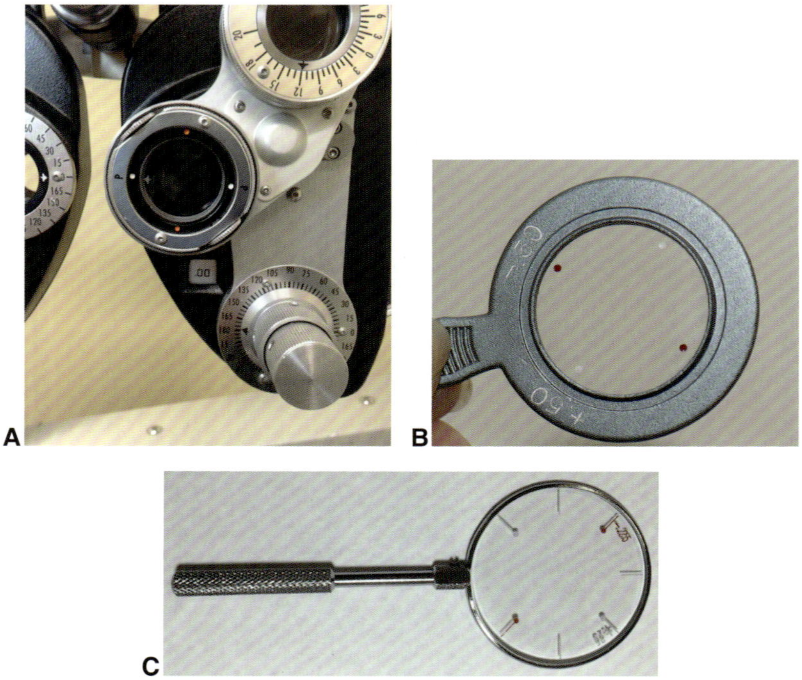

Figure 4-17 Jackson cross cylinder. **A,** In the phoropter. **B,** Manual trial lens. **C,** Rotating manual trial lens. *(Parts A and C courtesy of Thomas F. Mauger, MD. Part B courtesy of Tommy Korn, MD.)*

Continue to refine cylinder power until the patient reports that both flip choices appear equal. At that point, the 2 flip choices produce equal and opposite mixed astigmatism, blurring the visual acuity chart equally.

If the examiner is planning on prescribing for astigmatism at an axis different from that measured with the cross cylinder (ie, 90° or 180° instead of an oblique axis) the cross cylinder can be used to measure the cylinder power at the new axis.

Remember to use the proper-power cross cylinder for the patient's visual acuity level. For example, a ±0.25 D cross cylinder is commonly used with visual acuity levels of 20/30 and better. A high-power cross cylinder (±0.50 D or ±1.00 D)allows a patient with poorer vision to recognize differences in the flip choices.

The patient may be confused with prior choices during cross cylinder refinement. Giving different numbers to subsequent choices avoids this problem: ***"Which is better, 1 or 2, 3 or 4?"*** and so forth. If the patient persists in choosing either the first or second number, reverse the order of presentation to check for consistency.

Table 4-2 summarizes the cross cylinder refraction technique. Also see Part 2 of the Quick-Start Guide.

Guyton DL. *Retinoscopy: Minus Cylinder Technique, 1986; Retinoscopy: Plus Cylinder Technique,1986; Subjective Refraction: Cross-Cylinder Technique, 1987.* Reviewed for currency, 2007.Clinical Skills DVD Series [DVD]. San Francisco: American Academy of Ophthalmology.

Jackson E. A trial set of small lenses and a modified trial size frame. *Trans Am Ophthalmol Soc.* 1887;4:595–598.

Wunsh SE. The cross cylinder. In: Tasman W, Jaeger EA, eds. *Duane's Clinical Ophthalmology on CD-ROM.* Vol 1. Philadelphia: Lippincott Williams & Wilkins; 2006.

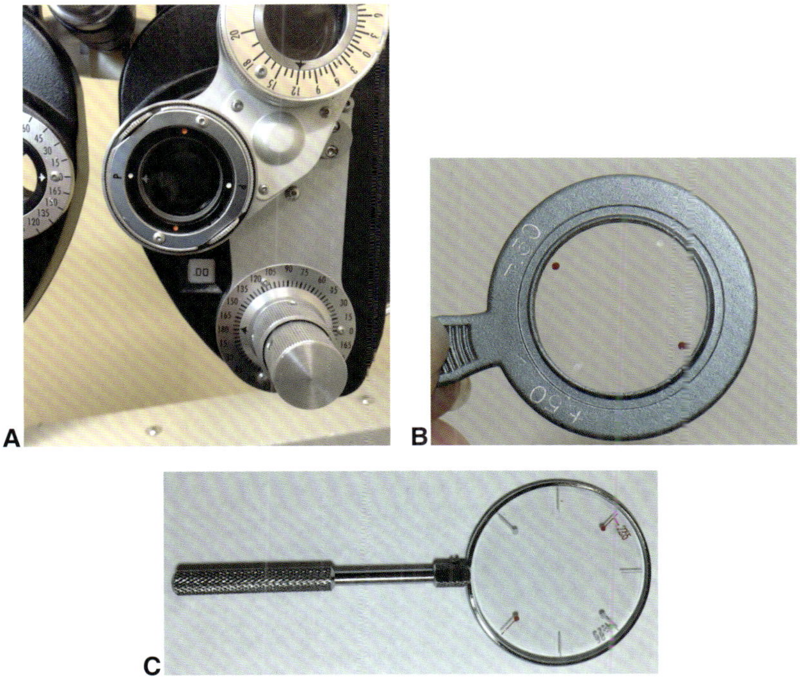

图 4–17　Jackson 交叉柱镜。**A**. 在综合验光仪上。**B**. 手持试镜片。**C**. 旋转手持试镜片。*（译者注：资料来源见前页原文。）*

继续精确柱镜度数，直到患者回复翻转两面一样清晰。这时，2 个翻转面产生相等且相反的混合散光，视力表的模糊程度一致。

如果检查者的处方散光与交叉柱镜检测的柱镜轴位不同（即是 90° 和 180° ，而不是斜轴），交叉柱镜可以在新轴位测量柱镜度数。

注意根据患者视力水平选择合适的交叉柱镜度数。例如，± 0.25 D 交叉柱镜用于 20/30 或更好的视力水平，高度交叉柱镜（ ± 0.50 D 或 ± 1.00 D）用于视力较差的患者，便于翻转时分辨区别。

在进行交叉柱镜检查的过程中，患者可能会对之前的选择感到困惑。用不同数字做接下来的选择会避免这一问题：***“哪一个更好，1 还是 2，3 还是 4？”*** 如果患者一直选择第 1 个或第 2 个数字，就颠倒检查顺序。

表 4–2 总结了交叉柱镜验光技术。也可查阅第 2 部分的《快速入门指南》。

Guyton DL. *Retinoscopy: Minus Cylinder Technique, 1986; Retinoscopy: Plus Cylinder Technique,1986; Subjective Refraction: Cross-Cylinder Technique, 1987.* Reviewed for currency, 2007.Clinical Skills DVD Series [DVD]. San Francisco: American Academy of Ophthalmology.

Jackson E. A trial set of small lenses and a modified trial size frame. *Trans Am Ophthalmol Soc.*1887;4:595–598.

Wunsh SE. The cross cylinder. In: Tasman W, Jaeger EA, eds. *Duane's Clinical Ophthalmology on CD-ROM.* Vol 1. Philadelphia: Lippincott Williams & Wilkins; 2006.

Table 4-2 Cross Cylinder Refraction Summary

1. Adjust sphere to the most plus or least minus that gives the best visual acuity.
2. Use test figures that are 1 or 2 lines larger than the patient's best visual acuity.
3. If cylindrical correction is not already present, look for astigmatism by testing with the cross cylinder at axes 90° and 180°. If none is found there, test at 45° and 135°.
4. Refine axis first. Position the cross cylinder axes 45° from the principal meridians of the correcting cylinder. Determine the preferred flip choice, and rotate the cylinder axis toward the corresponding axis of the cross cylinder. Repeat until the 2 flip choices appear equal.
5. Refine cylinder power. Align the cross cylinder axes with the principal meridians of the correcting cylinder. Determine the preferred flip choice, and add or subtract cylinder power according to the preferred position of the cross cylinder. Compensate for the change in position of the circle of least confusion by adding half as much sphere in the opposite direction each time the cylinder power is changed.
6. Refine sphere, cylinder axis, and cylinder power until no further change is necessary.

Refining the Sphere

After cylinder power and axis have been determined using either the astigmatic dial technique or the cross cylinder method, the final step of determining monocular refraction is to refine the sphere. The endpoint in the refraction is the strongest plus sphere, or weakest minus sphere, that yields the best visual acuity. The following discussion briefly considers some of the methods used.

When the cross cylinder technique has been used to determine the cylinder power and axis, the refractive error is presumed to a single point. Add plus sphere in+0.25 D increments until the patient reports decreased vision. If no additional plus sphere is accepted, add minus sphere in –0.25 D increments until the patient achieves the most optimal visual acuity.

Using accommodation, the patient can compensate for excess minus sphere. Therefore, it is important to use the least minus sphere necessary to reach the best visual acuity. In effect, accommodation creates a reverse Galilean telescope, whereby the eye generates more plus power as minus power is added to the trial lenses before the eye. As this minus power increases, the patient observes that the letters appear smaller and more distant (but also "darker," which the patient may misinterpret as "clearer").

The patient should be told what to look for. Before subtracting each 0.25 D increment, tell the patient that the letters may appear sharper and brighter or smaller and darker, and ask the patient to report any such change. Reduce the amount of plus sphere only if the patient can actually read more letters.

If the astigmatic dial technique has been used and the astigmatism is neutralized (ie, if all the lines on the astigmatic dial are equally sharp or equally blurred), the eye should still be fogged; additional plus sphere only increases the blur. Therefore, use minus sphere to reduce the sphere power until the best visual acuity is achieved. Again, the examiner should be careful not to add too much minus sphere.

To verify the spherical endpoint, the *duochrome* test (also known as the *red-green* or *bichrome test*) is used (Fig 4-18). A split red-green filter makes the background of the visual acuity chart appear vertically divided into a red half and a green half. Because of the chromatic aberration of the eye, the shorter (green) wavelengths are focused in front of the longer (red) wavelengths. The eye typically focuses near the midpoint of the spectrum, between the red and green wavelengths. With optimal spherical correction, the letters on the red and green halves of the chart appear equally sharp. The commercial filters used in the duochrome test produce a chromatic interval of approximately 0.50D between the red and green wavelengths. When the image is clearly focused in white light, the eye is 0.25 D myopic for the green letters and 0.25 D hyperopic for the red letters.

表4—2 交叉柱镜验光总结

1. 调整球镜至最大正镜或最小负镜以获得最佳视力
2. 选1行或2行大于患者的最佳视力的测试视标
3. 如果没有进行柱镜矫正,可用90° 或 180° 交叉柱镜查找散光。如果还没有发现,再用45° 和135° 交叉柱镜测试
4. 先精确轴位。将交叉柱镜轴置于偏离矫正柱镜主子午线45° 的位置。确定较清晰交叉柱镜翻转面，并旋转柱镜轴位与交叉柱镜使其一致。重复操作直到2个翻转面清晰度一致
5. 精确柱镜度数。矫正柱镜主子午线与交叉柱镜轴位一致。确定较清晰翻转面, 根据交叉柱镜轴位，加或减柱镜度数。为补偿最小弥散圈位置的改变,当每次柱镜度数改变时，增加符号相反、柱镜度数一半的球镜度数
6. 精细确定球镜、柱镜轴位、柱镜度数，直到没有改变为止

精确球镜

散光表盘或交叉柱镜法确定柱镜度数和轴位后，单眼验光的最后一步是精确球镜。验光终点是获得最佳视力的最大正球镜或最小负球镜度数。我们将简明介绍一些方法。

当交叉柱镜技术用于确定柱镜度数和轴位时，屈光不正假设为一个点。以 +0.25 D 递增，直到患者视力下降为止。如果正球镜不再接受，再以 –0.25 D 递增，直到患者达到最佳视力。

使用调节时，患者可以补偿额外的负球镜。因此，使用最小负球镜达到最佳视力是非常重要的。调节产生一个反 Galileo 望远镜效应，即当在眼前增加负镜片时，眼睛产生更多的正度数。当负度数增加，患者观察字母变小并更远（可能“更暗”，患者可能误解为“更清晰”）。

必须告知患者应该看什么。在每递减 0.25 D 之前，告知患者字母可能更清晰或更小、更暗，并请患者说出发生的变化。当患者可以准确地读出更多视标时再减少正球镜。

如果已经使用了散光表盘，并中和散光（即散光表所有线都同样清晰或同样模糊），应该继续雾视，直至增加正球镜会加重模糊。因此，用负球镜减少球镜度数，直到获得最佳视力。检查者应注意不要增加过多负球镜。

确定球镜终点，使用*双色测试*（也称作*红绿测试或双色测试*）（图 4–18）。红绿分离镜片让视力表背景平分为一半绿一半红。因为眼睛存在色差，短波长（绿色）聚焦在长波长（红色）之前。眼睛聚焦在光谱中点附近，在红色和绿色之间。最理想的球镜矫正是视标在红色和绿色上同等清晰。商业滤光片用于红绿测试时在红、绿波长之间产生大约 0.50 D 屈光度。当像以白光清晰聚焦时，绿色视标产生 0.25 D 近视，红色视标产生 0.25 D 远视。

Each eye is tested separately for the duochrome test, which is begun with the eye slightly fogged (by 0.50 D) to relax accommodation. The letters on the red side should appear sharper; the clinician should add minus sphere until the 2 sides appear the same. If the patient responds that the letters on the green side are sharper, the patient is over- minused, and more plus power should be added. When in doubt, it is preferable to err on the side of the more-plus or less-minus alternative ("leave 'em in the red"). Some clinicians use the RAM–GAP mnemonic—"*red* add *minus*; *green* add *plus*"—to recall how to use the duochrome test.

Because this test is based on chromatic aberration and not on color discrimination, it is used even with color-blind patients (although it may be necessary to identify the sides of the chart as left and right rather than red and green). An eye with overactive accommodation may still require too much minus sphere in order to balance the red and green. Cycloplegia may be necessary. The duochrome test is not used with patients whose visual acuity is worse than 20/30 (6/9), because the 0.50D difference between the 2 sides is too small to distinguish.

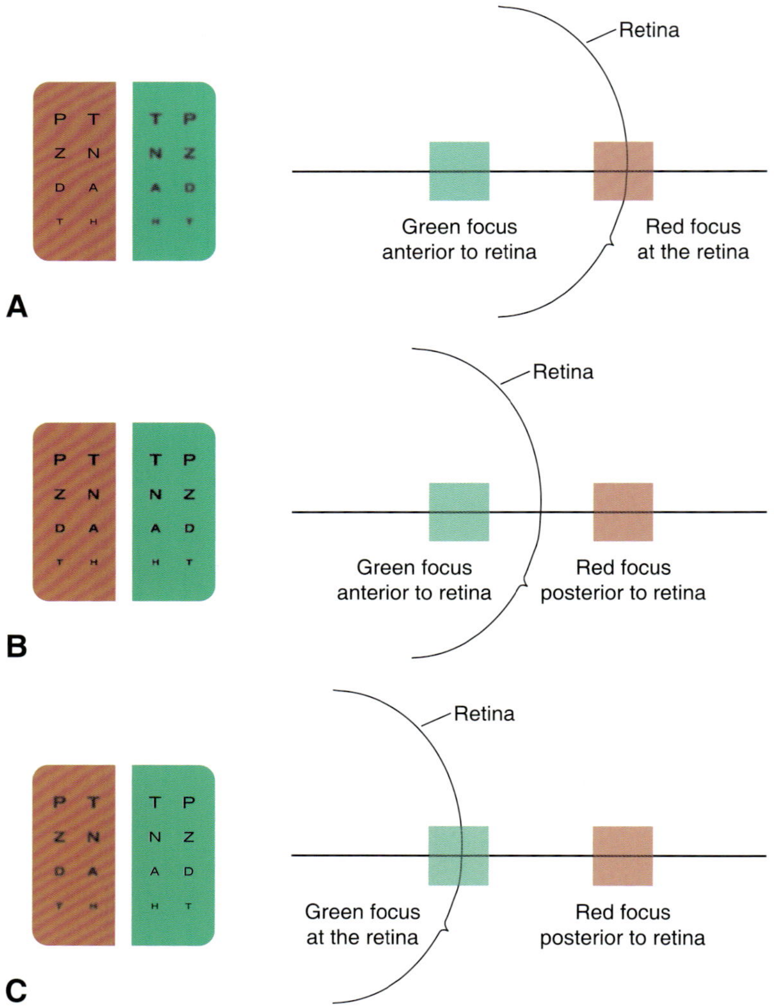

Figure 4-18 Diagram of duochrome test. **A**, Starting point with eye blurred using excess plus power—red letters should be clearer. **B**, Decreasing plus power (or increasing minus) until both sides of the chart have equal clarity. **C**, Continuing to decrease plus (increase minus) power until the green side of the chart is clearer. *(Illustration developed by Thomas F. Mauger, MD.)*

每只眼睛分别进行双色测试。首先雾视放松调节（0.50D）。当视标在红色一侧更清楚时，增加负球镜，直至两边同样清晰。如果视标在绿色这边更清晰，表示负度数太多或需增加正度数。当有怀疑时，宁可多正或少负（“留在红区”）。可以用 RAM-GAP 记忆——*红增负*，*绿增正*来记住怎样使用双色实验。

因为这个测试是基于色差而不是颜色识别，所以色盲患者也可以检测（尽管可能有必要确定双色视标的左边和右边，而不是红色和绿色）。过度调节反应时需要更多负球镜来平衡红绿色差。可能还需要睫状肌麻痹。视力低于 20/30（6/9）的患者不用进行双色检测，因为 0.5CD 在两色之间不易区分。

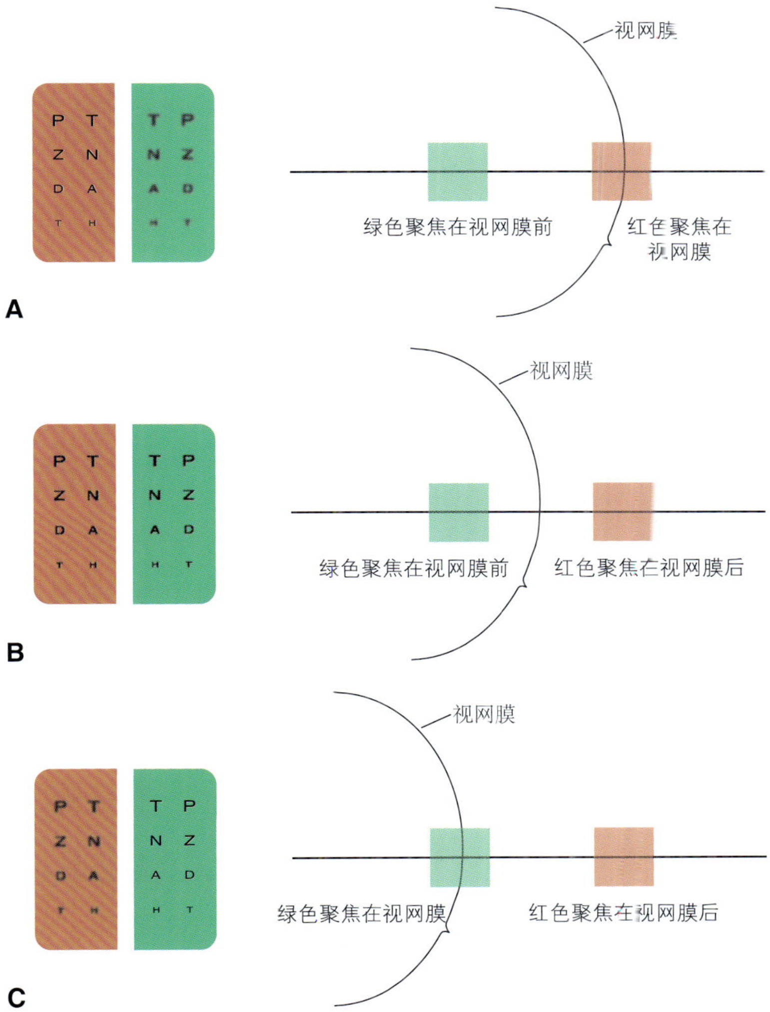

图 4–18　双色检测。**A**. 加正镜片使视力模糊，红色清楚，作为初始点。**B**. 减少正镜片（或增加负镜片），直到两侧一样清楚。**C**. 继续减少正镜片（增加负镜片），直到绿色清楚。*（译者注：资料来源见前页原文。）*

Binocular Balance

The final step of subjective refraction is to make certain that accommodation has been relaxed equally in both eyes. Several methods of binocular balance are commonly used. Most require that the corrected visual acuity be nearly equal in both eyes.

Alternate occlusion

When the endpoint refraction is fogged using a +0.75 D sphere before each eye, the visual acuity should be reduced to 20/40–20/50 (6/12–6/15). Alternately cover the eyes and ask the patient if the chart is equally blurred. If the eyes are not in balance, plus sphere should be added to the better seeing eye until balance is achieved.

In addition to testing for binocular balance, the fogging method also provides information about appropriate sphere power. If either eye is overminused or underplussed, the patient should read smaller (better than 20/40) letters than expected. In this case, the refraction endpoints should be reconsidered.

Prism dissociation

The most sensitive test of binocular balance is prism dissociation (Fig 4-19). For this test, the refractive endpoints are fogged with+0.75 to+1.00 D spheres, and vertical prisms of 4 or 6 prism diopters (Δ) are placed before 1 eye (or divided equally between the 2 eyes) using the Risley prisms in the phoropter (or in a trial lens frame). Some phoropters have a built-in 6Δ setting for this test. Use of the prisms causes the patient to see 2 charts, 1 above the other. A single line, usually 20/40 (6/12), is isolated on the chart; the patient sees 2 separate lines simultaneously, 1 for each eye. The patient can readily identify differences between the fogged images in the 2 eyes of as little as 0.25 D sphere. In practice, +0.25 D sphere is placed before 1 eye and then before the other. In each instance, if the eyes are balanced, the patient reports that the image corresponding to the eye with the additional +0.25 D sphere is blurrier. After a balance is established between the 2 eyes, remove the prism and reduce the fog binocularly until the best visual acuity is obtained.

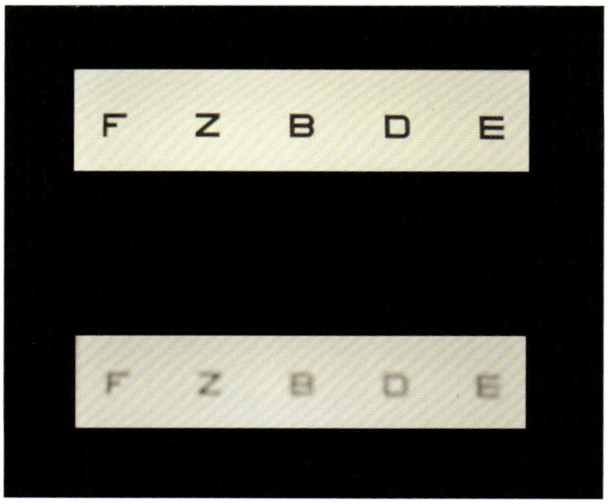

Figure 4-19 Binocular balancing by prism dissociation from patient perspective. *(Courtesy of Tommy Korn, MD.)*

双眼视平衡

主观验光的最后一步是确定两眼调节同时放松。双眼视平衡有很多方法，最重要的是双眼矫正视力接近一致。

交替遮盖

当每只眼 +0.75 D 球镜雾视时达到验光终点，视力可能降低到 20/40~20/50（6/12~6/15）。交替遮盖眼睛并询问患者视标是否一样模糊。如果双眼不平衡，在较清晰的眼睛增加正球镜，直至达到平衡。

除了测试双眼视平衡以外，雾视法也可以给出球镜度数。如果一只眼的负度数过矫或正度数低矫，患者可以看到更小的视标（多于 20/40），就应重新确认验光结果。

棱镜分离

双眼平衡最敏感的测试方法是棱镜分离（图 4–19）。测试时，验光终点用 −0.75~+1.00D 的球镜雾视，使用综合验光仪的 Risley 棱镜（或试镜架）4Δ 或 6Δ 垂直棱镜度，置于一只眼前（或平分给两眼）。一些综合验光仪内置 6Δ。棱镜使患者看到 2 个视力表，一个位于另一个之上。在视力表上留出一行 20/40（6/12）视标，患者同时看到 2 行视标，一只眼看到一行视标。两眼雾视时，患者可辨别 0.25D 球镜差异的像。在验光时，+0.25 D 球镜分别置于每只眼前。如果双眼平衡，增加 +0.25D 的像出现模糊。两眼平衡后，移除棱镜，减少双眼雾视，直到达到最佳视力。

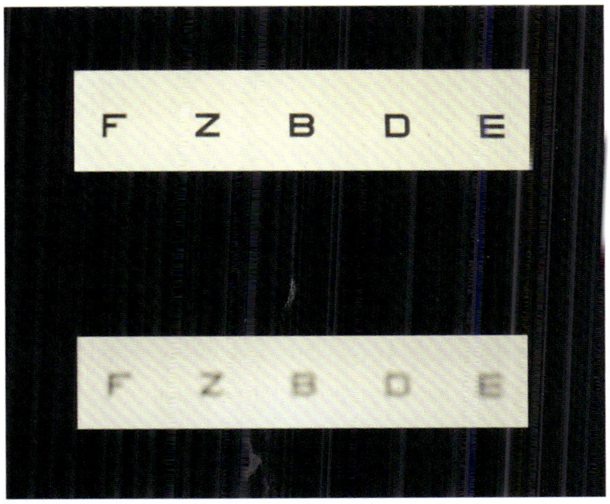

图 4–19　棱镜分离检测双眼平衡。*（译者注：资料来源见前页原文。）*

Cycloplegic and Noncycloplegic Refraction

Ideally, refractive error is measured with accommodation relaxed. The amount of habitual accommodative tone varies from person to person, and even within an individual it varies at times and decreases with age. Because determining this variable may not always be possible, cycloplegic drugs are sometimes used. The indication and appropriate dosage for a specific cycloplegic drug depend on the patient's age, accommodative amplitude, and refractive error.

A practical approach to obtaining satisfactory refraction is to perform a careful non-cycloplegic (or manifest) refraction, ensuring relaxed accommodation with fogging or other nonpharmacologic techniques. If the results are inconsistent or variable, a cycloplegic refraction should be performed. If the findings of these 2 refractions are similar, the prescription may be based on the manifest refraction. If there is a disparity, a postcycloplegic evaluation (performed at a time after the cycloplegic effects have abated, usually several days later) may be necessary. Most children require cycloplegic refraction because of their high amplitude of accommodation. For more details on the cycloplegic drugs used in adults and children, please refer to BCSC Section 2, *Fundamentals and Principles of Ophthalmology.*

Overrefraction

Phoropters may be used to refract the eyes of patients with highly ametropic vision. Variability in the vertex distance of the refraction (the distance from the back surface of the spectacle lens to the cornea) and other induced errors make prescribing directly from the phoropter findings unreliable.

Some of these problems can be avoided if highly ametropic eyes are refracted over the patients' current glasses (overrefraction). If the new lenses are prescribed with the same base curve and thickness (contributors to image size and aniseikonia) as the current lenses and are fitted in the same frames, many potential difficulties can be circumvented, including vertex distance error and pantoscopic tilt error (inducing effective refraction changes), as well as problems caused by oblique (marginal) astigmatism and chromatic aberration (if lens material remains the same). Overrefraction may be performed with loose lenses (using trial lens clips such as Halberg trial clips), with a standard phoropter in front of the patient's glasses, or with some automated refracting instruments.

If the patient is wearing spherical lenses, the new prescription is easy to calculate by combining the current spherical correction with the spherocylindrical overrefraction. If the current lenses are spherocylindrical and the cylinder axis of the overrefraction is not at 0° or 90° to the present correction, other methods previously discussed are used to determine the resultant refraction. Such lens combinations were often determined with a lensmeter used to read the resultant lens power through the combinations of the old glasses and the overrefraction correction. This procedure is awkward and prone to error because the lenses may rotate with respect to one another on transfer to the lensmeter. Manual calculation is possible but complicated. Programmable calculators can be used to perform the trigonometric combination of cylinders at oblique axes, but they may not be readily available in the clinic.

Overrefraction has other uses. For example, a patient wearing a soft toric contact lens may undergo overrefraction for the purpose of ordering new lenses. An overrefraction is especially useful for patients wearing rigid, gas-permeable, hard contact lenses for irregular corneal astigmatism or corneal transplants. This may be used to determine the amount of visual reduction that is caused by irregular astigmatism. Overrefraction can also be used in the retinoscopic examination of children.

睫状肌麻痹性与非睫状肌麻痹性验光

理论上，验光应在调节放松的状态下进行。习惯性调节张力的量因人而异，即使是同一个人，在不同的时间和年龄段也会有所不同。因为这种变化常无法确定，所以有时会用到睫状肌麻痹剂。根据患者的年龄、调节幅度和屈光不正程度，采用不同的睫状肌麻痹剂和不同的剂量。

仔细的非睫状肌麻痹（或主观）验光，用雾视法或其他非药物的方法达到调节放松状态，可以达到临床上满意的验光结果。如果验光结果不理想，或有变化，就需要进行睫状肌麻痹验光。如果这 2 种验光方法所获得的结果相似，则处方应以主观验光为基础；如果 2 种结果有差异，则需要睫状肌麻痹后进一步评估（在睫状肌麻痹作用消失稳定后，一般在几天后进行）。因为儿童具有很强的调节力，所以大多数儿童都需要睫状肌麻痹验光。有关成人和儿童使用的睫状肌麻痹药物的详细信息，请参阅 BCSC 第 2 册《*眼科基础与原理*》。

镜上验光

高度屈光不正的患者需用综合验光仪验光。验光的顶点距（眼镜后表面到角膜的距离）和其他误差导致直接用综合验光仪验光的结果不可靠。

如果在所配戴的眼镜上验光（镜上验光），可以避免上述高度屈光不正的验光问题。如果新配的眼镜与现在所配戴的眼镜基弧和厚度相同（产生成像大小和双眼不等像），并且用原有镜架，很多问题就可以避免了，包括镜眼距、前倾角（引发屈光改变）以及斜向（边缘）散光和色差（镜片材料也相同）所引起的问题。镜上验光常常被用于单独试镜片（使用镜片夹，例如 Halberg 试镜夹）、可以在患者眼镜前用标准综合验光仪或自动验光设备。

如果患者配戴的是球面镜片，通过镜上验光将现戴的球镜与球柱镜相结合后计算新的配镜处方比较容易。如果现在的眼镜为球柱镜，或镜上验光的柱镜轴位不在 0° 或 90°，那么可以用其他方法获得最终的屈光。例如组合透镜的度数可通过焦度计获取，该仪器可将旧镜片及镜上验光联合，得出新的光度。但这个仪器不准确，因为两镜片可能在检测时旋转导致测量误差，最终焦度也可以通过人工计算，但过程比较复杂。计算程序常常用三角函数对斜轴上柱镜组合计算，但不便于临床应用。

镜上验光还有其他的应用。例如，一个患者配戴软性复曲面接触镜，可以镜上验光后订购新镜。对于不规则角膜散光或角膜移植矫正的患者的硬性透氧性硬镜尤其有用。这可以确定不规则散光引起的视觉质量的降低。镜上验光还可用于儿童的检影检查。

Spectacle Correction of Ametropias

Ametropia is a refractive error; it is the absence of emmetropia. The most common method of correcting refractive error is through prescription of spectacle lenses.

Spherical Correcting Lenses and the Far Point Concept

The far point plane of the nonaccommodated eye is conjugate with the retina. For a simple lens (plus or minus sphere), distant objects (those at optical infinity) come into sharp focus at the *secondary focal point* (F_2) of the lens. To correct the refractive error of an eye, a correcting lens must place the image it forms (or its F_2) at the eye's far point. The image at the far point plane becomes the object that is focused onto the retina. For example, in a myopic eye, the far point lies somewhere in front of the eye, between it and optical infinity. In this case, the correct *diverging lens* forms a virtual image of distant objects at its F_2, coincident with the far point of the eye (Fig 4-20).

The same principle holds for the correction of hyperopia (Fig 4-21). However, because the far point plane of a hyperopic eye is behind the retina, a *converging lens* must be chosen with appropriate power to focus parallel rays of light to the far point plane.

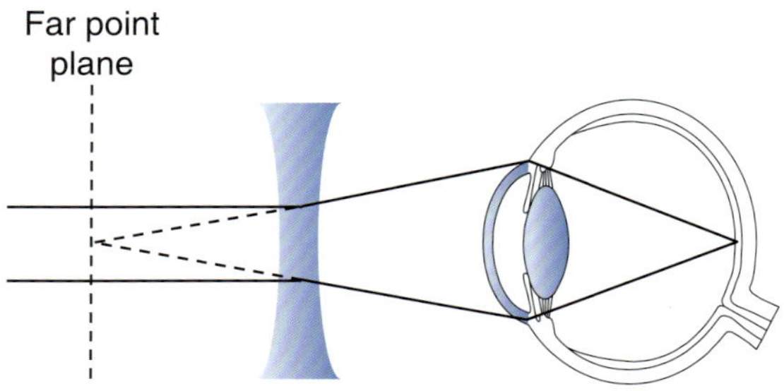

Figure 4-20 A diverging lens is used to correct myopia.

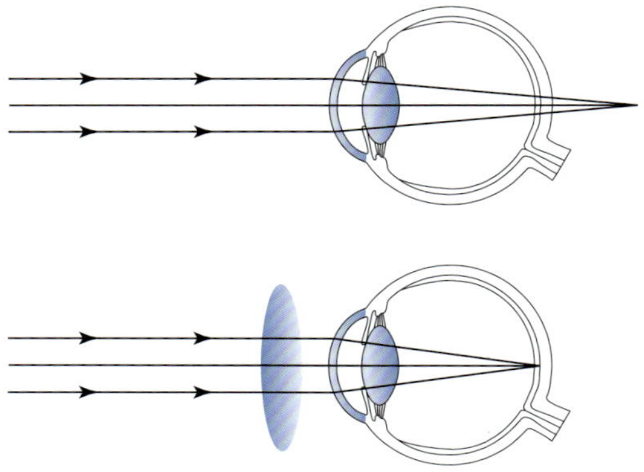

Figure 4-21 A converging lens is used to correct hyperopia.

The Importance of Vertex Distance

For any spherical correcting lens, the distance from the lens to its focal point is constant. Changing the position of the correcting lens relative to the eye also changes the relationship between the F_2 of the correcting lens and the far point plane of the eye. With high-power lenses, as used in the spectacle correction of aphakia or high myopia, a small change in the placement of the lens produces considerable blurring of vision unless the lens power is altered to compensate for the new lens position so that the secondary focal point of the lens coincides with the far point of the eye.

框架眼镜矫正屈光不正

屈光不正是屈光异常，为非正视眼。最常用的屈光不正矫正方法为配戴框架眼镜。

球镜矫正镜片和远点的概念

无调节眼的远点平面与视网膜共轭。对于一个单纯镜片（正球镜或负球镜），远距离的物体（光学上无限远）聚焦投射到镜片*第二焦点*（F_2）。若要矫正眼睛的屈光不正，矫正镜片必须将像（或说是 F_2）成在眼的远点处。位于远点平面的图像成为在视网膜成像的物体。例如，在近视眼时，远点位于眼前的某个地方，在眼睛与光学无限远之间。这时，矫正的*发散透镜*在它的 F_2 处形成一个远处物体的虚像。与眼的远点平面重合。

该原则同样适用于远视的矫正（图 4–21）。但是，因为远视的远点平面位于视网膜后，所以必须选取*会聚透镜*使平行光聚焦于远点平面。

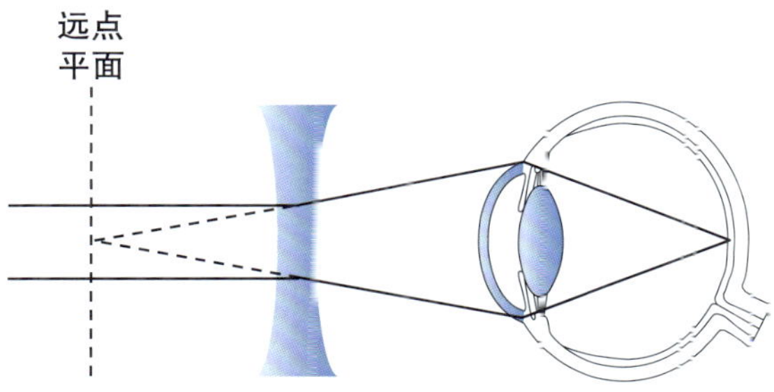

图 4–20　发散透镜用于矫正近视。

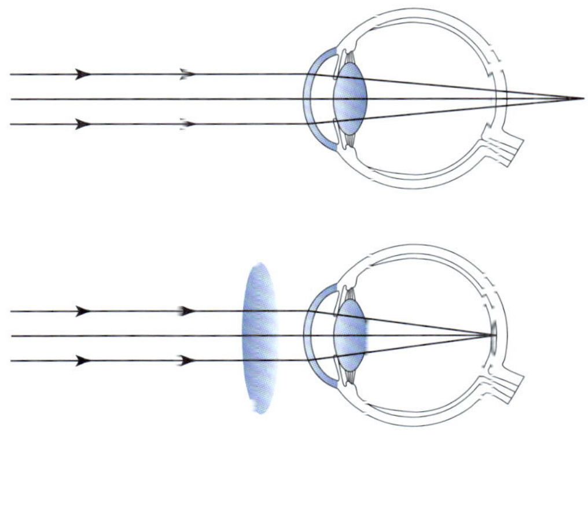

图 4–21　会聚透镜用于矫正远视。

顶点距的重要性

对于球面矫正镜片来说，从镜片到焦点的距离是一个常数。当改变矫正镜片与眼球的位置时，镜片第二焦点 F_2 与眼睛远点平面之间的关系也随之而变。高焦度镜片，像用于无晶体或高度近视的框架眼镜矫正，其镜片位置的微小改变可能导致明显视物模糊，需调整镜片焦度以抵偿新镜片的位置变化，以使镜片的第二焦点与眼睛的远点平面重合。

With refractive errors greater than ±5.00 D, the vertex distance must be accounted for in prescribing the power of the spectacle lens. A *distometer* (also called a *vertexometer*) is used to measure the distance from the back surface of the spectacle lens to the cornea with the eyelid closed (Fig 4-22A). Moving a correcting lens closer to the eye—whether the lens has plus or minus power—reduces its effective focusing power (the image moves posteriorly away from the fovea), whereas moving it farther from the eye increases its focusing power (the image moves anteriorly away from the fovea).

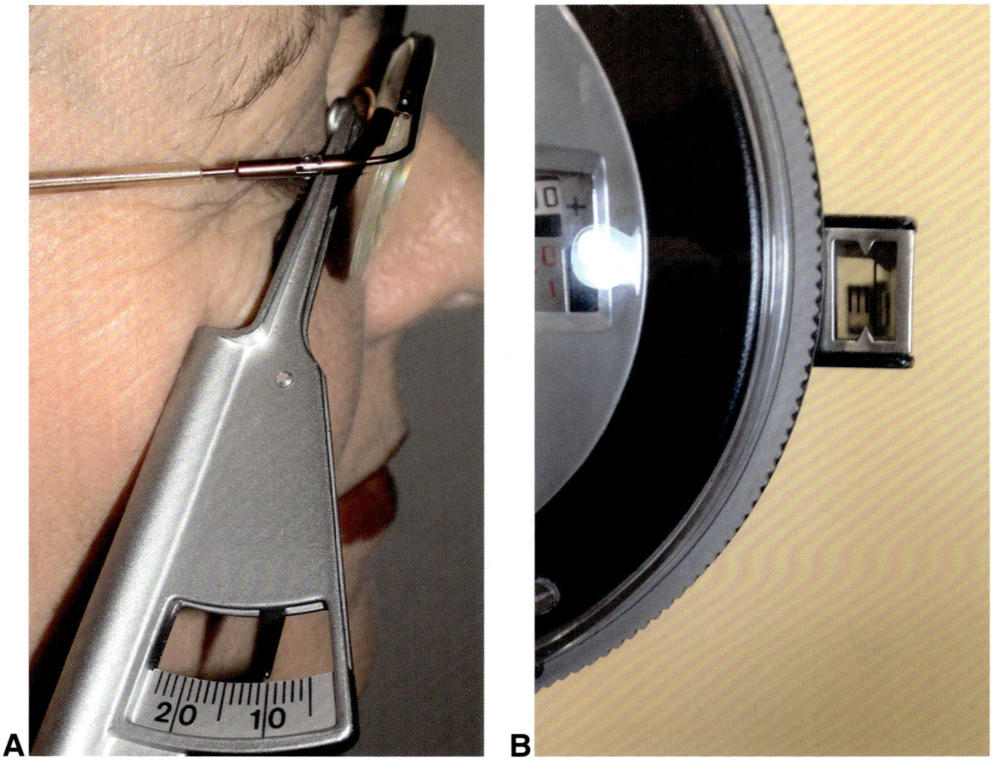

Figure 4-22 Measuring vertex distance. **A**, Vertexometer (distometer). **B**, Corneal alignment tool. *(Part A courtesy of Tommy Korn, MD; part B courtesy Thomas F. Mauger, MD.)*

For example, in Figure 4-23 the +10.00 D lens placed 10 mm in front of the cornea provides sharp retinal imagery. Because the focal point of the correcting lens is identical to the far point plane of the eye and because this lens is placed 10 mm in front of the eye, the far point plane of the eye must be 90 mm behind the cornea. If the correcting lens is moved to a new position 20 mm in front of the eye and the far point plane of the eye is 90 mm behind the cornea, then the focal length of the new lens must be 110 mm, requiring a +9.10 D lens for correction. A contact lens will need to have a power of 11.10 D. This example demonstrates the significance of vertex distance in spectacle correction of large refractive errors. Thus, the prescription must indicate not only the lens power but also the vertex distance at which the refraction was performed. The optician must recalculate the lens power as necessary for the actual vertex distance of the chosen spectacle–frame combination. Clinical Example 4-3 also demonstrates examples of vertex distance.

屈光不正大于 ±5.00 D 时，框架眼镜的处方必须考虑到顶点距的问题。*测距仪*（也称为*顶点测量仪*）用于测量眼镜片后面到眼睑闭合的角膜距离（图 4–22A）。将矫正镜片靠近眼球——无论镜片是正镜片还是负镜片——减弱的有效聚焦度（图像后移远离中央凹）；反之，如果将镜片远离眼球，会增加有效聚焦度（图像前移远离中央凹）。

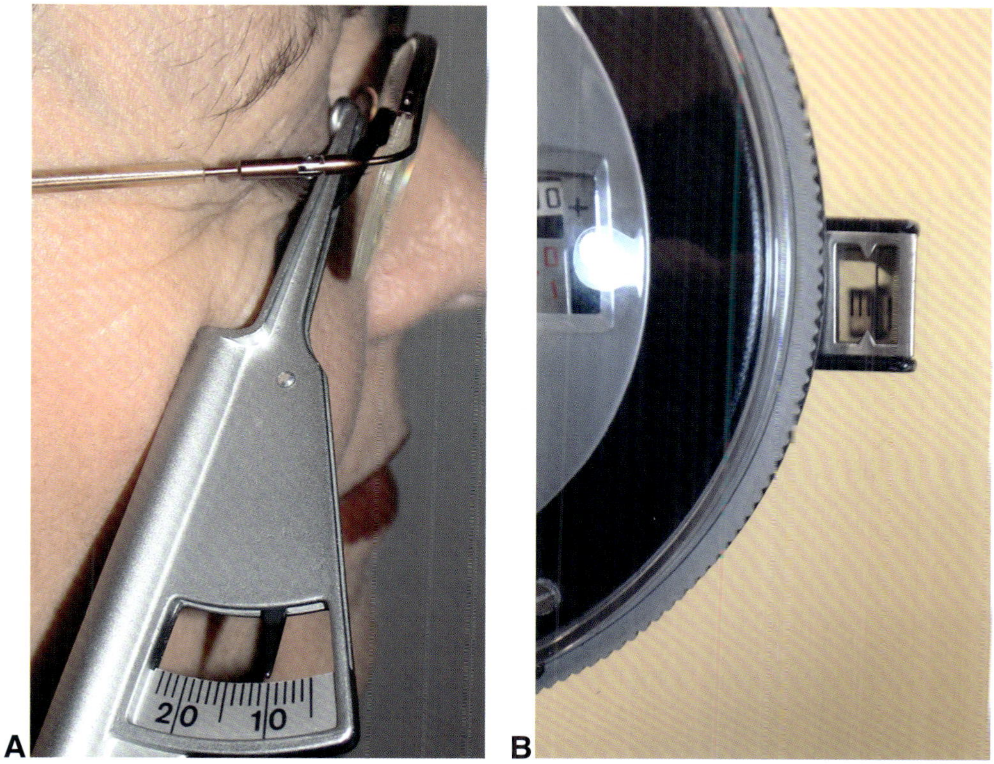

图 4–22　测量顶点距。**A**. 顶点测量仪。**B**. 角膜对齐工具。*（译者注：资料来源见前页原文。）*

例如，在图 4–23 中，将 +10.00 D 镜片置于角膜前 10 mm，可以提供清晰的视网膜图像。因为矫正镜片的第二焦平面为眼球的远点平面，而且这个镜片被置于眼球前 10 mm 处，所以眼球远点平面应该在角膜后 90 mm 处。如果矫正镜片被移动到眼球前 20 mm 的新位置，那么眼球的远点平面是 90 mm，新的镜片第二焦平面为 110 mm，就需要一个 +9.1D 的镜片来矫正；接触镜则需要 11.10 D 焦度。这显示了高度数屈光不正所需框架眼镜的顶点距的重要性。因此，配镜时除了考虑镜片焦度，还要考虑矫正镜片的顶点距。验光师根据所选择的框架眼镜（框架组合）的实际顶点距离，重新计算镜片焦度。临床案例 4–3 演示了顶点距的实例。

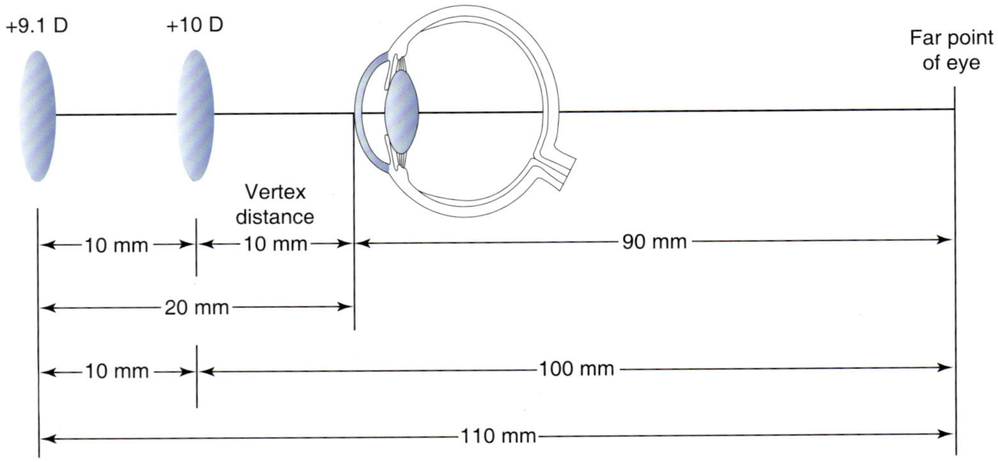

Figure 4-23 The importance of vertex distance in the correction of high refractive errors.

CLINICAL EXAMPLE 4-3

A +10D lens at a vertex distance of 10 mm corrects an eye for distance. A new frame is used and the vertex distance is now 15 mm. What should the power of the lens be to correct the eye for distance?

The far point is 1/10 = 0.1M (100 mm) behind the original lens. at the new vertex distance (15 mm), the lens needs to correct for a far point that is now 105 mm behind the lens. Therefore, the correcting lens power is 1/105 = +9.50 D.

A −10D lens that corrects an eye for distance with an original vertex distance of 10 mm that is changed to 15 mm will need to be changed to −10.50 D.

Note: If the glasses are simply moved out 5 mm without changing the lens power, the eye will be 0.50 D myopic. This is one reason that people with high spectacle corrections move their glasses down their nose to read.

Allowing for vertex distance with the phoropter is made easier due to 2 commonly found features. The first feature is that the lenses within the phoropter, even though found in different planes, have their power referenced to the back surface of the most posterior lens in the system. The second feature is that if the cornea of the eye is aligned at the zero mark on the corneal alignment tool (Fig 4-22B), the vertex distance equals that assumed for the phoropter (13.75 mm for the Reichert Phoroptor) and has an accompanying table with the proper conversion for each mm anterior or posterior that the cornea is positioned. The patient should be refracted in a trial frame or overrefracted in their current spectacles if the vertex distance varies significantly (>6 mm) from that assumed in the phoropter.

Cylindrical Correcting Lenses and the Far Point Concept

The far point principles used in the correction of hyperopia and myopia are also employed in the correction of astigmatism with spectacle lenses. However, in astigmatism, the required lens power must be determined separately for each of the 2 principal meridians.

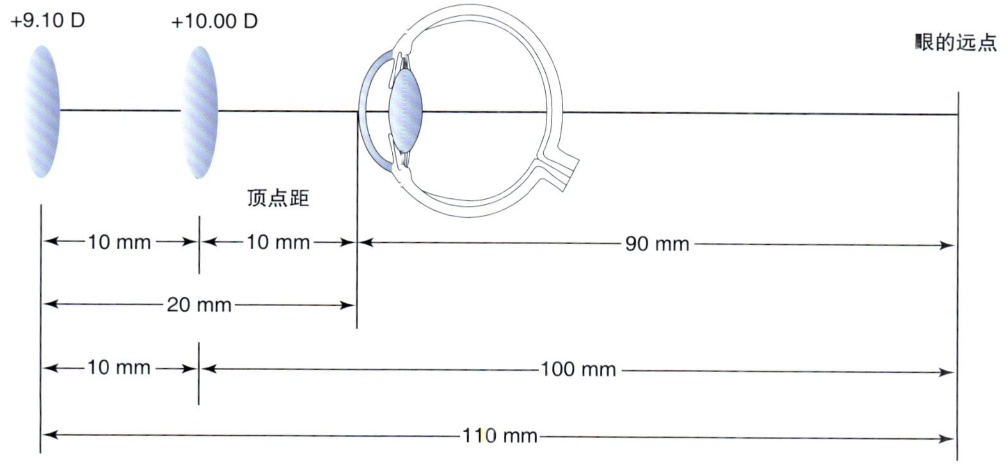

图 4–23　在高度屈光不正中顶点距的重要性。

临床案例 4–3

顶点距为 10 mm 的 +10.00 D 透镜。现在使用新框架的顶点距是 15 mm。透镜的焦度应该怎样变化来纠正顶点距离的改变？

远点位于原镜片后 1/10=0.1 m(100 mm)。在新的顶点距（15 mm），需要矫正的镜片其远点位于镜片后 105 mm。因此，矫正透镜焦度为 1/105 mm=+9.50 D。

–10.00 D 的矫正镜片，顶点距由原来的 10 mm 改为 15 mm，需要将透镜焦度更改为 –10.50 D。

注意：如果仅将眼镜移出 5 mm 而不改变镜片焦度，则形成 0.50 D 近视。这也是眼镜焦度高的人把眼镜从鼻子向下移可以阅读的原因之一。

由于以下这 2 个常见特征，综合验光仪的顶点距离更容易测量。第一个特征是，综合验光仪内的镜片，即使在不同平面，都能以系统中最后那个透镜的后表面为参考具有各自的焦度。第二个特征是，如果眼角膜对齐角膜对齐工具中的 0 标记（图 4–22B），顶点距等于验光仪的设定（Reichert 综合验光仪为 13.75 mm），并可以对于每 1mm 的角膜前移或后移进行矫正。如果顶点距离明显改变（＞6 mm），患者应戴试镜架验光或他们戴的眼镜上验光。

柱镜矫正镜片和远点概念

用于远视和近视矫正的远点原理，也可应用到框架镜散光矫正中。但在散光矫正时，须分别确定 2 条主子午线的焦度。

Cylinders in spectacle lenses produce both monocular and binocular distortion. The primary cause is *meridional aniseikonia*—that is, unequal magnification of retinal images in the various meridians. Although aniseikonia may be decreased by iseikonic spectacles, such corrections may be complicated and expensive, and most practitioners prefer to prescribe cylinders according to their clinical judgment. Clinical experience also suggests that adult patients vary in their ability to tolerate distortion, whereas young children always adapt to their cylindrical corrections.

The following guidelines may prove helpful in prescribing astigmatic spectacle corrections:

- For *children*, prescribe the full astigmatic correction at the correct axis.
- For *adults*, try the full correction initially. Give the patient a "walking-around" trial with trial frames before prescribing, if appropriate. (The experience of seeing the effects of motion is an important part of this process—just sitting in a chair with the proposed prescription in trial frames is not an adequate test.) Inform the patient about the need for adaptation. To reduce distortion, use minus cylinder lenses (now standard) and minimize vertex distance.
- Because spatial distortion from astigmatic spectacles is a binocular phenomenon, occlude 1 eye to verify that spatial distortion is the cause of the patient's difficulty.
- If necessary, reduce distortion by rotating the axis of the cylinder toward 180° or 90° (or toward the old axis) and/or reduce the cylinder power. Adjust the sphere to maintain spherical equivalent, but rely on a final subjective check to obtain the most satisfactory visual result.
- If distortion cannot be reduced sufficiently, consider contact lenses or iseikonic corrections.

For a more detailed discussion of the problem of, and solutions for, spectacle correction of astigmatism, see the reference.

Guyton DL. Prescribing cylinders: the problem of distortion. *Surv Ophthalmol.* 1977;22(3): 177–188.

Prescribing for Children

The correction of ametropia in children presents several special and challenging problems. In adults, the correction of refractive errors has 1 measurable endpoint: the best-corrected visual acuity. Prescribing visual correction for children often has 2 goals: providing a focused retial image and achieving the optimal balance between accommodation and convergence.

In some young patients, *subjective refraction* may be impossible or inappropriate, often because of the child's inability to cooperate with subjective refraction techniques. In addition, the optimal refraction in infants or small children (particularly those with esotropia) requires the *paralysis of accommodation* with complete cycloplegia. In such cases, objective techniques such as retinoscopy are the best way to determine the refractive correction. Moreover, the presence of *strabismus* may require modification of the normal prescribing guidelines.

框架镜中的柱镜可产生单眼和（或）双眼视物变形，主要的原因是*子午线不等像*。也就是说，在不同子午线上视网膜像放大率不等。尽管双眼不等像可以被双眼等像框架镜所矫正，但是这种矫正镜非常复杂和昂贵，而且很多医生喜欢根据临床经验开具柱镜处方。临床经验表明，成人对视物变形的耐受力不同，而儿童常能适应柱镜矫正。

以下指南有助于指导框架散光镜的配镜处方：

- 对于*儿童*来说，应选择在正确的轴位上足矫散光的配镜处方。
- 对于*成人*，开始可尝试足矫。在开配镜处方前，可以试戴镜架“四处走动”。如果有的话（患者活动时的配镜体验，是试戴的一个重要部分——坐着试戴是不够的），告知患者需要一个适应过程。为了减少变形，使用负柱镜（现行标准），并采用最小顶点距。
- 散光镜所引起的空间变形是双眼现象，遮挡一眼可以确定空间变形的原因。
- 必要时，可以通过转换柱镜的轴位至 180° 或 90°（或朝着原轴位）和（或）降低柱镜焦度。调整球镜以维持等效球镜，但需要取决于最终的主观检查，以获取最满意的视觉效果。
- 如果变形不能充分地减轻，可以考虑接触镜或等像镜矫正。

对于散光框镜矫正的详细探讨和解决方法见参考文献。

Guyton DL. Prescribing cylinders: the problem of distortion. *Surv Ophthalmol.* 1977;22(3):177–188.

儿童的验配处方

儿童屈光不正的矫正存在几个特殊而又具有挑战性的问题。成人屈光不正的矫正有 1 个可测量的终点，即最佳矫正视力。对于儿童视力的矫正有 2 个目标：提供可聚焦的视网膜像，达到最优的调节和聚散平衡。

在一些年幼患者中，*主观验光*不适宜实施，常常是因为儿童不能配合主观验光。另外，在婴幼儿（特别是有内斜视患儿）中，最好用完全的睫状肌麻痹，达到*调节麻痹*后验光。这种情况下，客观验光如检影是确定屈光状态的最好方法。而且，*斜视*的存在可能需要调整常规的验配处方原则。

Myopia

There are 2 types of childhood myopia: *congenital* (usually high) myopia and *developmental* myopia, which usually manifests itself between the ages of 7 and 10 years. Developmental myopia is less severe and easier to manage because the patients are older and refraction is less difficult. However, both forms of myopia are progressive; frequent refractions (every 6–12 months) and periodic prescription changes are necessary. The following are general guidelines for correction of significant childhood myopia:

- Cycloplegic refractions are mandatory. In infants, children with esotropia, and children with very high myopia (>10.00 D), atropine refraction may be necessary if tropicamide or cyclopentolate fails to paralyze accommodation in the office.
- In general, the full refractive error, including cylinder, should be corrected. Young children tolerate cylinder well.
- Some ophthalmologists undercorrect myopia, and others use bifocal lenses with or without atropine, based on the theory that accommodation hastens or increases the development of myopia. This topic remains controversial among ophthalmologists. (See BCSC Section 6, *Pediatric Ophthalmology and Strabismus.*)
- Intentional undercorrection of a child's myopic esotropia to decrease the angle of deviation is rarely tolerated.
- Intentional overcorrection of a myopic error (or undercorrection of a hyperopic error) may help control intermittent exodeviations. However, such overcorrection can cause additional accommodative stress.
- Parents should be educated about the natural progression of myopia and the need for frequent refractions and possible prescription changes.
- In older children, contact lenses may be desirable to avoid the problem of image minification that arises with high-minus lenses.

Hyperopia

The appropriate correction of childhood hyperopia is more complex than that of myopia for 2 reasons. First, children who are significantly hyperopic (>5.00 D) are more visually impaired than are their myopic counterparts, who can at least see clearly at near. Second, childhood hyperopia is more frequently associated with strabismus and abnormalities of the *accommodative convergence/accommodation (AC/A)* ratio (see BCSC Section 6, *Pediatric Ophthalmology and Strabismus*). The following are general guidelines for correcting childhood hyperopia:

- Unless there is esodeviation or evidence of reduced vision, it is not necessary to correct low hyperopia. Most children have very high amplitude of accommodation. As with myopia, significant astigmatic errors should be fully corrected.
- When hyperopia and esotropia coexist, initial management includes full correction of the cycloplegic refractive error. Reductions in the amount of correction may be appropriate later, depending on the amount of esotropia and level of stereopsis with the full cycloplegic correction in place.
- In a school-aged child, the full refractive correction may cause blurring of distance vision because of the inability to relax accommodation fully. Reducing the amount of correction is sometimes necessary for the child to accept the glasses. A short course of cycloplegia may help a child accept the hyperopic correction.

近视

儿童近视分为 2 类：*先天性*（常常是高度的）近视和*发育性*近视，通常在 7~10 岁显现出来。发育性近视一般不严重，较容易检查，因为孩子年龄越大，验光越容易。但是，这 2 种近视都是进行的；经常验光（6~12 个月 1 次）和定期更换眼镜非常必要。下面是儿童近视屈光矫正的指导原则：

- 必须进行睫状肌麻痹性验光。婴儿、内斜视的儿童和高度近视儿童（＞10.00 D），如果托比卡胺或环戊通不能充分麻痹睫状肌而放松调节，就必须用阿托品后验光。
- 一般来说，应给予全矫处方，矫正包括柱镜的全部屈光不正。幼儿能很好耐受柱镜矫正。
- 一些眼科医生主张近视欠矫，而其他医生使用或不使用阿托品给予双焦镜，这是基于“调节可以加速近视的发展”的理论。眼科医生对这个问题仍然存在争议。（见 BCSC 第 6 册《*小儿眼科与斜视*》。）
- 为减小斜视度，儿童近视内斜视的有意欠矫是不可取的。
- 近视的有意过矫（或远视欠矫），有助于控制间歇性外斜视。但是，这种过度矫正会导致额外的调节张力。
- 应该告诉父母关于近视的自然进展过程，以及经常进行验光并合理更换眼镜的必要性。
- 对于较大的儿童，可以使用接触镜，可以避免高度负镜片引起的像缩小问题。

远视

儿童远视适当矫正比近视矫正复杂，有 2 个原因。首先，高度远视（＞5.00 D）的儿童视力受损程度高于相同度数近视儿童，后者至少视近时是清晰的。其次，儿童远视常伴发斜视和*调节性集合 / 调节*（AC / A）比率异常（见 BCSC 第 6 册《*小儿眼科与斜视*》）。以下是儿童远视的矫正指南：

- 除非有内斜视或视力下降的证据，否则不需要矫正低度远视，因为大多数儿童的调节幅度很大。有近视和较大的散光时，应充分矫正。
- 当远视和内斜视并存时，初期治疗必须睫状肌麻痹验光全矫。以后是否减少矫正度数，取决于睫状肌麻痹全矫后，内斜度数和立体视水平。
- 在学龄期儿童中，由于不能完全放松调节，所以屈光不正的全矫可能引起视远模糊。必要时，减少矫正度数，可以帮助孩子接受眼镜。睫状肌麻痹剂的短期应用可以帮助孩子接受矫正远视镜。

Anisometropia

A child or infant with anisometropia is typically prescribed the full refractive difference between the 2 eyes, regardless of age, presence or amount of strabismus, or degree of anisometropia. Anisometropic amblyopia is frequently present and may require occlusion therapy. *Bilateral amblyopia* occasionally occurs when there is significant hyperopia, myopia, and/or astigmatism in both eyes. Refractive amblyopia is less common with bilateral myopia because these patients have clear near vision.

Clinical Accommodative Problems

See Chapter 3 for a discussion of the terminology and mechanisms of accommodation.

Presbyopia

Presbyopia is the gradual loss of accommodative response resulting from reduced elasticity of the crystalline lens. Accommodative amplitude diminishes with age. It becomes a clinical problem when the remaining accommodative amplitude is insufficient for the patient to read and carry out near-vision tasks comfortably. Fortunately, appropriate convex lenses can compensate for the waning of accommodative power.

Symptoms of presbyopia usually begin to appear in patients after 40 years of age. The age of onset depends on preexisting refractive error, depth of focus (pupil size), the patient's visual tasks, and other variables. Table 4-3 presents a simplified overview of age norms. The KAMRA corneal Inlay (AcuFocus Inc, Irvine, CA) has been approved by the United States Food and Drug Administration (FDA) for the correction of presbyopia through the use of pinhole optics. The inlay is 3.8 mm in diameter and has a 1.6-mm aperture.

Table 4-3 Average Accommodative Amplitudes for Different Ages

Age	Average Accommodative Amplitude[a]
8	14.0 (±2 D)
12	13.0 (±2 D)
16	12.0 (±2 D)
20	11.0 (±2 D)
24	10.0 (±2 D)
28	9.0 (±2 D)
32	8.0 (±2 D)
36	7.0 (±2 D)
40	**6.0 (±2 D)**
44	4.5 (±1.5 D)
48	3.0 (±1.5 D)
52	2.5 (±1.5 D)
56	2.0 (±1.0 D)
60	1.5 (±1.0 D)
64	1.0 (±0.5 D)
68	0.5 (±0.5 D)

[a] Up to age 40, accommodation decreases by 1 D for each 4 years. After age 40, accommodation decreases more rapidly. From age 48 on, 0.5 D is lost every 4 years. Thus, one can recall the entire table by remembering the amplitudes at age 40 and age 48.

屈光参差

儿童或婴儿屈光参差是指双眼之间的屈光差异，无论年龄、斜视是否存在或斜视数量，或者是屈光参差的程度如何。屈光参差性弱视经常出现，并需要遮盖治疗。当双眼都出现明显的远视、近视和（或）散光时，偶尔会出现*双眼弱视*。屈光性弱视在双眼近视中较少见，因为这些患者具有清晰的近视力。

临床调节问题

见第 3 章“人眼的光学相关术语和调节机制”。

老视

老视是由于晶状体弹性降低而导致调节力逐渐下降的过程。随着年龄增长，调节幅度逐渐减小。当剩余的调节幅度不足以完成阅读和近距离工作时，老视就成为一个临床问题。幸运的是，可用适合的凸透镜代偿所需的调节力。

老视的症状常在 40 岁以后发生。发病年龄取决于先前的屈光不正、焦深（瞳孔大小）、视觉工作和其他因素。表 4–3 简要概述了不同年龄的调节幅度值。KAMRA 角膜内置物（AcuFocus Inc，Irvine，CA）已经由美国食品和药物管理局（FDA）批准用于通过针孔镜来矫正老视。内置物直径为 3.8 mm，孔径为 1.6 mm。

表4–3　不同年龄人群调节幅度的平均值

年龄	调节幅度平均值[a]
8	14.0 (±2.00 D)
12	13.0 (±2.00 D)
16	12.0 (±2.00 D)
20	11.0 (±2.00 D)
24	10.0 (±2.00 D)
28	9.0 (±2.00 D)
32	8.0 (±2.00 D)
36	7.0 (±2.00 D)
40	**6.0 (±2.00 D)**
44	4.5 (±1.50 D)
48	3.0 (±1.50 D)
52	2.5 (±1.50 D)
56	2.0 (±1.00 D)
60	1.5 (±1.00 D)
64	1.0 (±0.50 D)
68	0.5 (±0.50 D)

[a] 40岁前，每4年调节降低1.00 D；40岁以后下降速度加快。从48岁起，每4年下降0.50 D。只需要记住40～48岁的调节幅度，整个表就都可以记住了。

Accommodative Insufficiency

Accommodative insufficiency is the premature loss of accommodative amplitude. This problem may manifest itself by blurring of near visual objects (as in presbyopia) or by the inability to sustain accommodative effort. The onset may be heralded by the appearance of asthenopic symptoms; the ultimate development is blurred near vision. Such "premature presbyopia" may signify concurrent or past debilitating illness, or it may be induced by medications such as tranquilizing drugs or the parasympatholytics used in treating some gastrointestinal disorders. In both cases, the condition may be reversible; however, permanent accommodative insufficiency may be associated with neurogenic disorders such as encephalitis or closed-head trauma. In some cases, the etiology may never be determined. These patients require additional reading plus power for near vision. The most common causes of premature presbyopia, however, are unrecognized (latent) hyperopia and overcorrected myopia.

Accommodative Excess

Ciliary muscle spasm, often incorrectly termed spasm of accommodation, causes accommodative excess. A ciliary spasm has characteristic symptoms: headache, brow ache, variable blurring of distance vision, and an abnormally close near point. Ciliary spasm may be a manifestation of local disease such as iridocyclitis; it may be caused by medications such as the anticholinesterases used in the treatment of glaucoma; or it may be associated with uncorrected refractive errors, usually hyperopia but also astigmatism. In some patients, ciliary spasm exacerbates preexisting myopia. Postcycloplegic refraction often helps de- termine the patient's true refractive error in such cases.

Ciliary spasm may also occur after prolonged and intense periods of near work. *Spasm of the near reflex* is a characteristic clinical syndrome often observed in tense or anxious persons who present with (1) excess accommodation, (2) excess convergence, and (3) miosis.

Accommodative Convergence/Accommodation Ratio

Normally, accommodative effort is accompanied by a corresponding convergence effort. For practical purposes, the AC/A ratio is ordinarily expressed in terms of prism diopters of deviation per diopter of accommodation. Using this type of expression, the normal AC/A ratio is 3:1–5:1.

The AC/A ratio is relatively constant in a particular patient, but it should be noted that there is some variability among individuals. For example, a patient with an uncorrected 1.00D of hyperopia may accommodate 1.00D for clear distance vision without exercising a convergence effort. Conversely, a patient with uncorrected myopia must converge without accommodative effort to fuse at the far point.

The AC/A ratio can be measured by varying the stimulus to accommodation in several ways. These methods are described in the following subsections.

Heterophoria method

The heterophoria method involves moving the fixation target. The heterophoria is measured at 6 m and again at 0.33 m .

$$\frac{\mathrm{AC}}{\mathrm{A}} = PD + \frac{\Delta n - \Delta d}{D}$$

where

PD = interpupillary distance in centimeters

调节不足

调节不足是调节幅度过早下降，常常表现为视近模糊（如同老视），或不能维持调节。视疲劳提示调节不足，最终导致视近模糊。这种“早老视”提示同时存在或既往患衰弱性疾病，也可能是由镇静药物或用于治疗某些胃肠道疾病的副交感神经阻断剂等药物引起的，这 2 种情况的早老视是可逆的。但是，永久性调节不足可能与神经系统功能紊乱有关，例如脑炎或闭合性颅脑损伤。有时无法确定病因。这些患者阅读时需要近附加镜。然而，早老视的最常见原因是未被诊断的（隐性）远视和过度矫正的近视。

调节过度

睫状肌痉挛，常常被误称为调节痉挛，可导致调节过度。睫状肌痉挛的特征性症状为头痛、前额痛、视远模糊和近点异常。睫状肌痉挛可能提示局部眼病，如虹膜睫状体炎；也可能是由于青光眼治疗中使用的胆碱酯酶抑制剂等药物所致；还可能与未矫正的屈光不正有关，如远视、散光。有时睫状肌痉挛可能加重已有的近视，经睫状肌麻痹后验光可确定患者的真实屈光状态。

睫状肌痉挛也可能发生在持续和紧张的近距离工作之后。*近反射痉挛*是一种特征性临床综合征，人在紧张或担心时，会同时发生过度调节、过度集合和瞳孔缩小。

调节性集合 / 调节比率

通常情况下，调节常常伴随着一个相应的集合努力。在临床上，AC/A 率通常用偏向的棱镜度每屈光度调节表示，用这种表达，正常的 AC/A 值为 3∶1~5∶1。

每个人的 AC/A 值是一个相对的常数，但个体之间存在一些差异。例如，一个远视患者存在 1.00 D 的欠矫，视远时可能需要 1.00 D 的调节，而没用集合。相反，未矫正的近视患者必须在没有调节的情况下进行集合，以便在远点融合。

AC/A 值可用不同途径的调节刺激量来表示，方法如下。

隐斜法

隐斜法是移动固视目标，测量 6 m 和 0.33 m 处的隐斜。

$$\frac{\mathrm{AC}}{\mathrm{A}} = PD + \frac{\Delta n - \Delta d}{D}$$

其中，

PD= 瞳距，以 cm 为单位。

Δn = near deviation in prism diopters
Δd = distance deviation in prism diopters
D = amount of accommodation in diopters

Sign convention:

Esodeviations: +
Exodeviations: -

Gradient method

The AC/A ratio can be measured in 1 of 2 ways with the gradient method. The first way is by *stimulating accommodation*. Measure the heterophoria with the target distance fixed at 6 m. Then remeasure the induced phoria after interposing a –1.00 D sphere in front of both eyes. The AC/A ratio is the difference between the 2 measurements.

The second way is by relaxing accommodation. With the target distance fixed at 0.33 m, measure the phoria before and after interposing +3.00 D spheres. The phoria difference divided by 3 is the AC/A ratio.

An abnormal AC/A ratio can place stress on the patient's fusional mechanisms at one distance or another, causing asthenopia or manifest strabismus. Abnormal AC/A ratios should be accounted for when prescribing corrective lenses.

Parks MM. Vergences. In: Tasman W, Jaeger EA, eds. *Duane's Clinical Ophthalmology on CD-ROM*. Vol 1. Philadelphia: Lippincott Williams & Wilkins; 2006.

Effect of Spectacle and Contact Lens Correction on Accommodation and Convergence

Both accommodation and convergence requirements differ between contact lenses and spectacle lenses.The effects become more noticeable as the power of the correction increases.

Let us first consider accommodative requirements (see Chapter 5). Recall that because of vertex distance considerations, particularly with high-power corrections, the dioptric power of the distance correction in the spectacle plane is different from that in the contact lens plane: for a near object held at a constant distance, the amount that an eye needs to accommodate depends on the location of the refractive correction relative to the cornea. Patients with myopia must accommodate more for a given near object when wearing contact lenses than when wearing glasses. For example, patients in their early 40s with myopia who switch from single-vision glasses to contact lenses may suddenly experience presbyopic symptoms. The reverse is true with patients with hyperopia; spectacle correction requires more accommodation for a given near object than does contact lens correction. Patients with spectacle-corrected high myopia, when presbyopic, need only weak bifocal add power or none at all. For example, a patient with high myopia who wears –20.00 D glasses needs to accommodate only approximately 1.00 D to see an object at 33 cm.

Now let us consider convergence requirements and refractive correction. Because contact lenses move with the eyes and spectacles do not, different amounts of convergence are required for viewing near objects. Spectacle correction gives a myopic patient a base-in prism effect when converging and thus reduces the patient's requirement for convergence. (Fortunately, this reduction parallels the lessened requirement for accommodation.) In contrast, a patient with spectacle-corrected hyperopia encounters a base-out prism effect that increases the requirement for convergence. This effect is beneficial in the correction of residual esotropia at near in patients with hyperopia and accommodative esotropia. These effects may be the source of a patient's symptoms on switching between glasses and contact lenses (see Clinical Example 5-2).

Δn= 近偏位，以 Δ 为单位。
Δd= 远偏位，以 Δ 为单位。
D= 调节量，以 D 为单位。
符号规则：内隐斜 +，外隐斜 –。

梯度法

AC/A 值可以通过 2 种梯度法来测量。第一种方法是通过*调节刺激量*来计算的。先观察 6 m 处的目标测量隐斜，然后通过在双眼前插入一个 –1.00 D 的球镜后，测量诱发的隐斜。AC/A 比是 2 次测量的差值。

第二种方法为*放松调节*。在眼前 0.33 m 处设置固定目标，在插入 +3.00 D 球镜前后分别测量隐斜度，用隐斜度差除以 3，即 AC/A 值。

AC/A 值异常说明了患者在某一距离的融合，可以导致视疲劳或显性斜视。配带矫正镜片时应考虑 AC/A 值异常。

Parks MM. Vergences. In: Tasman W, Jaeger EA, eds. *Duane's Clinical Ophthalmology on CD-ROM*. Vol 1. Philadelphia: Lippincott Williams & Wilkins; 2006.

框架镜和接触镜对调节和集合的影响

接触镜和框架镜对于调节和集合的需求是不同的，当矫正度数增加时，这种影响就变得更明显。

首先让我们了解一下调节需求量（见第 5 章）。考虑到顶点距离，特别是高度屈光矫正时，框架镜矫正的屈光力与接触镜的是不同的：对于放置在固定位置的近距离物体，一只眼睛的调节需求量取决于矫正镜片与角膜之间的距离。与框架镜相比，配戴接触镜的近视患者对固定近距离目标须动用更多的调节。例如，40 岁的近视眼患者，将单光眼镜换成接触镜时，可能突然出现老视症状；相同的情况在远视患者恰恰相反。与接触镜相比，框架镜矫正相对于给定的近距离物体需要更多的调节。配戴框架镜的高度近视患者出现老视时，仅需要少量的双焦镜，或完全不需要，如 –20.00 D 框架镜的高度近视患者，在看 33 cm 处的物体时，可能仅需要 1.00 D 的调节量。

现在，我们分析集合需求量与屈光矫正。因为接触镜是随着眼睛移动的，而框架眼镜是不随眼睛移动的，所以，对于接触镜和框架眼镜来说，视近所需要的集合量是不同的。近视眼患者集合时，框架眼镜产生一个底向内棱镜效应，从而减少集合需求量（集合量减少正好与调节需求量的降低平行发生）。相反的，远视的框架镜可产生一个底向外棱镜效应，因此增加集合需求量。这对于远视眼伴调节性内斜视患者而言，矫正视近时残余内斜视是有帮助的。这些效应可能是患者在框架眼镜和接触镜之间转换时出现症状的原因（见临床案例 5–2）。

Prescribing Multifocal Lenses

A multifocal lens has 2 or more refractive elements. The power of each segment is prescribed separately.

Determining the Add Power of a Bifocal Lens

The information necessary to prescribe bifocal lenses includes (1) an accurate baseline refraction, (2) the accommodative amplitude, and (3) the patient's social or occupational activities that require near-vision correction (eg, reading, sewing, or computer use).

Measuring accommodative amplitude

Any of the following tests can provide useful information for determining the accommodative amplitude: (1) the near point of accommodation with accurate distance refractive correction in place, (2) the accommodative rule (eg, with a Prince rule [Royal Air Force Rule]), and (3) the use of plus and minus spheres at near distance until the fixation target blurs. *Binocular amplitude of accommodation* is normally greater than the measurement for either eye alone by 0.50–1.00D.

Near point of accommodation A practical method for measuring the near point of accommoda -tion is to have the patient fixate on a near target (usually small print such as 5-point or Jaeger 2 type print) and move the test card toward the eye until the print blurs. If the eye is emmetropic (or rendered emmetropic by proper refractive correction), then the far point of the eye is at infinity and the near point can be converted into diopters of amplitude.

This method is subject to certain errors, including the apparent increased amplitude resulting from angular magnification of the letters as they approach the eye. In addition, if the eye is ametropic and not corrected for distance, the near point of accommodation cannot be converted into diopters of amplitude. In the following examples, each eye has 3 D of accommodative amplitude:

- A person with emmetropia would have a near point of 33 cm and a far point at optical infinity.
- A patient with an uncorrected 3.00D of myopia would have a near point at 16.7 cm because at the far point of 33 cm, no accommodation is needed.
- A patient with an uncorrected 3.00D of hyperopia would have a near point at infinity because all of the available accommodation is needed to overcome the hyperopia.

Accommodative rule Amplitude of accommodation can be measured with a device such as a Prince rule (Royal Air Force Rule) (Fig 4-24), which combines a reading card with a ruler calibrated in centimeters and diopters. Placing a+3.00D lens before the emmetropic (or accurately corrected ametropic) eye places the far point of accommodation at 33 cm, and the near point is also brought closer by a corresponding 3.00D. The amplitude is then determined by subtraction of the far point (in diopters) from the near point (in diopters).

Method of spheres Amplitude of accommodation may also be measured by having the patient fixate on a reading target at 40 cm. Accommodation is stimulated by the placement of successively stronger minus spheres before the eye until the print blurs; accommodation is then relaxed by the use of successively stronger plus lenses until blurring begins. The difference between the 2 lenses is a measure of accommodative amplitude. For example, if the patient accepts –3.00D to blur (stimulus to accommodation) and+2.50D to blur (relaxation of accommodation), the amplitude is 5.50D.

多焦点眼镜的配镜处方

多焦点眼镜通常有 2 个或更多的子片，应该分别给出每一子片的配镜处方。

双焦眼镜附加度的确定

双焦镜处方的必要信息包括：① 精确验光；② 调节幅度；③ 患者的社会活动或职业所需近视觉矫正（如阅读、针线活和电脑使用）。

测量调节幅度

以下的任一个测试都能为测定调节幅度提供有用的信息：①准确合适的远用屈光矫正下的调节近点，②调节法则 [如 Prince 尺 (英国皇家空军尺)]，③视近时正和负球镜的使用，直至固定的目标模糊。*双眼的调节幅度*通常比单眼大 0.50~1.00 D。

调节近点　临床测量调节近点的方法是，让患者盯住一个近距离的视标（小的打印的字体，例如 5 点或 Jaeger 2 号字体），并将测试卡向眼球移动，直至字体模糊为止。如果是正视（或屈光矫正的正视），眼的远点在无限远处，近点被转换为调节幅度的屈光度。

这种方法也会有一定的误差，包括随着移近眼，字母的视角放大，导致调节幅度的明显增大。另外，如果屈光不正未矫正，调节近点则不能转换为调节幅度的屈光度。在以下的例子中，每眼有 3.00 D 的调节幅度：

- 正视眼者有 33 cm 的近点和无限远的远点。
- 未矫正的 3.00 D 近视患者，近点在 16.7 cm 处，因为 33 cm 的远点处不需要任何调节。
- 未矫正的 3.00D 远视患者，近点在无限远处，因为所有可用的调节都需要克服远视。

调节法则　调节幅度可以测量，例如 Prince 尺 (英国皇家空军尺)（图 4–24），它将 1 个阅读卡片与 1 个用 cm 和 D 标注的尺子结合起来。在正视 (或精确矫正屈光不正) 眼前放置 1 个 +3.00 D 的镜片，将调节远点置于 33 cm 处，并且近点也被相应的 3.00 D 移近了。调节幅度通过远点（以 D 为单位）与近点（以 D 为单位）相减来确定。

球镜的方法　调节幅度也可以用固视位于眼前 40 cm 的阅读目标来测量。通过逐渐增加置于眼前的负球镜刺激调节，直至出现视物模糊，然后依次增加正镜放松调节，直至出现字体模糊。这两镜片之差就是调节幅度。例如，加至 –3.00 D 镜片（调节紧张）和 +2.50 D 镜片（调节放松）出现视物模糊，那么其调节幅度就是 5.50 D。

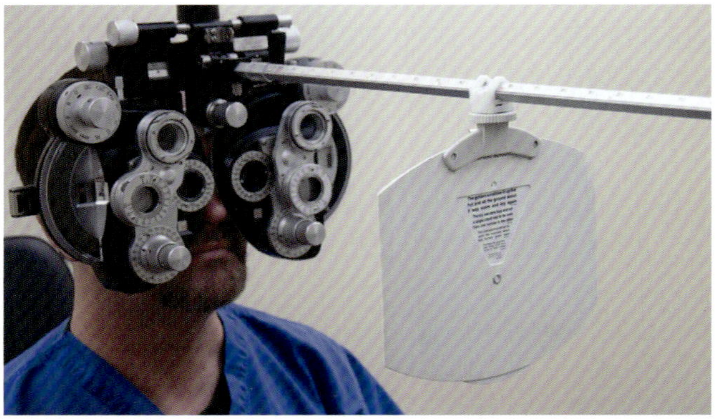

Figure 4-24 Prince rule. *(Courtesy of Tommy Korn, MD.)*

Range of accommodation

Determining the range of accommodation, like measuring the amplitude of accommodation, is valuable in ensuring that the prescribed bifocal add power meets the patient's visual needs. The range of accommodation measures the useful range of clear vision when a given lens is employed. For this purpose, a measuring tape, meter stick, or accommodation rule may be used.

Selecting an add power

Determine the amount of accommodation required for the patient's near-vision tasks. For example, reading at 40 cm would require 2.50 D of accommodation. From the patient's measured accommodative amplitude, allow one-half to be held in reserve. This reserve allows for some comfortable movement should the patient move the reading material either closer or farther away from the optimal reading distance. For instance, if the patient has 2.00 D of accommodation, 1.00 D may be comfortably contributed by the patient. (Some patients may use more than one-half of their available accommodation with comfort.) Subtract the patient's available accommodation (1.00 D) from the total amount of accommodation required (2.50 D); the difference (1.50 D) is the approximate additional plus lens power (add) needed.

Place a lens with this add power in front of the distance refractive correction, and measure the range of accommodation (near point to far point of accommodation in centimeters). Does this range adequately meet the requirements of the patient's near-vision activities? If the accommodative range is too close, reduce the add power in increments of 0.25 D until the range is appropriate for the patient's requirement. Because binocular accommodative amplitude is usually 0.50–1.00 D greater than the monocular measurement, using the binocular measurement generally guards against prescribing an add power that is too high.

Types of Bifocal Lenses

Most bifocal lenses currently dispensed are 1- piece lenses that are made by generating the different refracting surfaces on a single lens blank (Fig 4-25). One-piece round segment bifocal lenses have their segment on the concave surface. One-piece molded plastic bifocal lenses are available in various shapes, including (1) round top with button on convex surface, (2) flat top with button on convex surface, and (3) Franklin (executive) style with split bifocal.

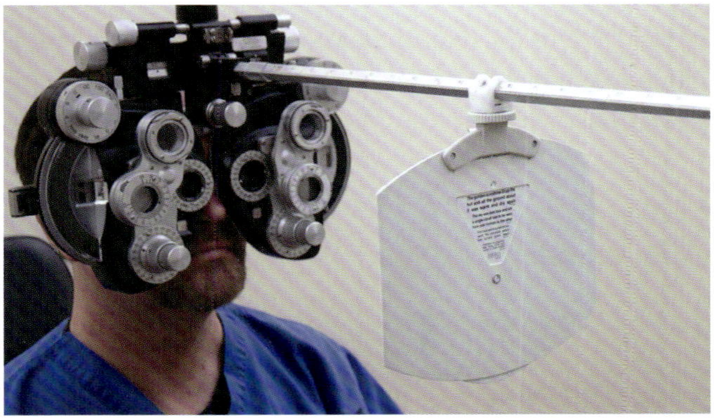

图 4-24　Prince 尺。*（译者注：资料来源见前页原文。）*

调节范围

确定调节范围，与测量调节幅度一样，确定验配双焦镜的附加度，以满足视觉需求。调节范围是给出镜片清晰视觉的有效范围。可以使用卷尺、米尺或调节尺测量。

附加光度的选择

确定患者视近所需的调节量。如在 40 cm 处阅读需要 2.50 D 的调节。根据患者的测量调节幅度，需要一半的调节量作为储备，当远近移动阅读材料时，该储备可以用于舒适的移动。例如，患者具有 2.00 D 的调节，则可以舒适地应用 1.00 D 的调节（有些患者可以使用超过一半的调节而无不适）。从所需调节总量（2.50 D）中减去患者可用调节（1.00 D），差值（1.50 D）是所需近似的附加正镜度数。

将这个附加度数加在远用屈光矫正前，并测量调节范围（以厘米为单位从调节近点到远点处）。该范围是否能满足患者近视觉活动的要求？如果调节范围太近，则以 0.25 D 递减附加度，直到该距离适合患者的要求。由于双眼调节幅度通常比单眼大 0.50~1.00 D，因此使用双眼测量可防止附加度过高。

双焦镜类型

目前大多数双焦镜片是单片式镜片，即在一个镜片毛坯上生成不同的屈光面（图 4-25）。单片式圆形双焦镜将子片作在凹面。单片式注塑双焦镜片有各种形状可供选择，包括：① 圆顶双焦镜；② 平顶双焦镜；③ Franklin E 型双焦镜。

With *fused bifocal lenses,* the increased refracting power of the bifocal segment is produced by fusing a button of glass that has a higher refractive index than the basic crown glass lens into a countersink in the crown glass lens blank. With all such bifocal lenses, the add segment is fused into the convex surface of the lens; astigmatic corrections, when necessary, are ground on the concave surface.

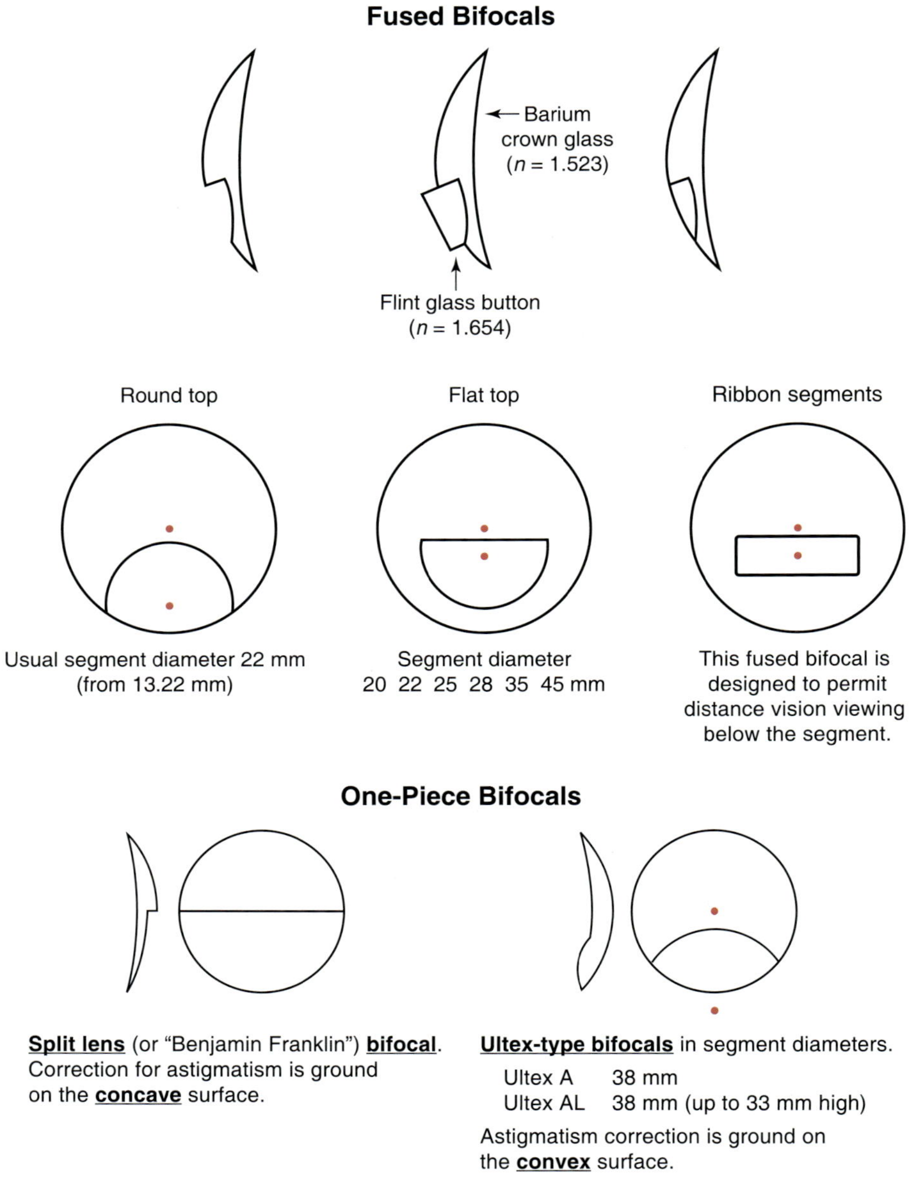

Figure 4-25 Bifocal lens styles. n = index of refraction.

熔合双焦镜片，是通过比母片折射率更高的材料如玻璃，（钻孔装埋）熔合母片（冕牌玻璃透镜毛坯），增加附加光折射能力，形成双焦点的双焦子片。对于所有熔合性双光镜，将高折材料添加融合到镜片的凸面中，必要时，在凹面上打磨矫正散光。

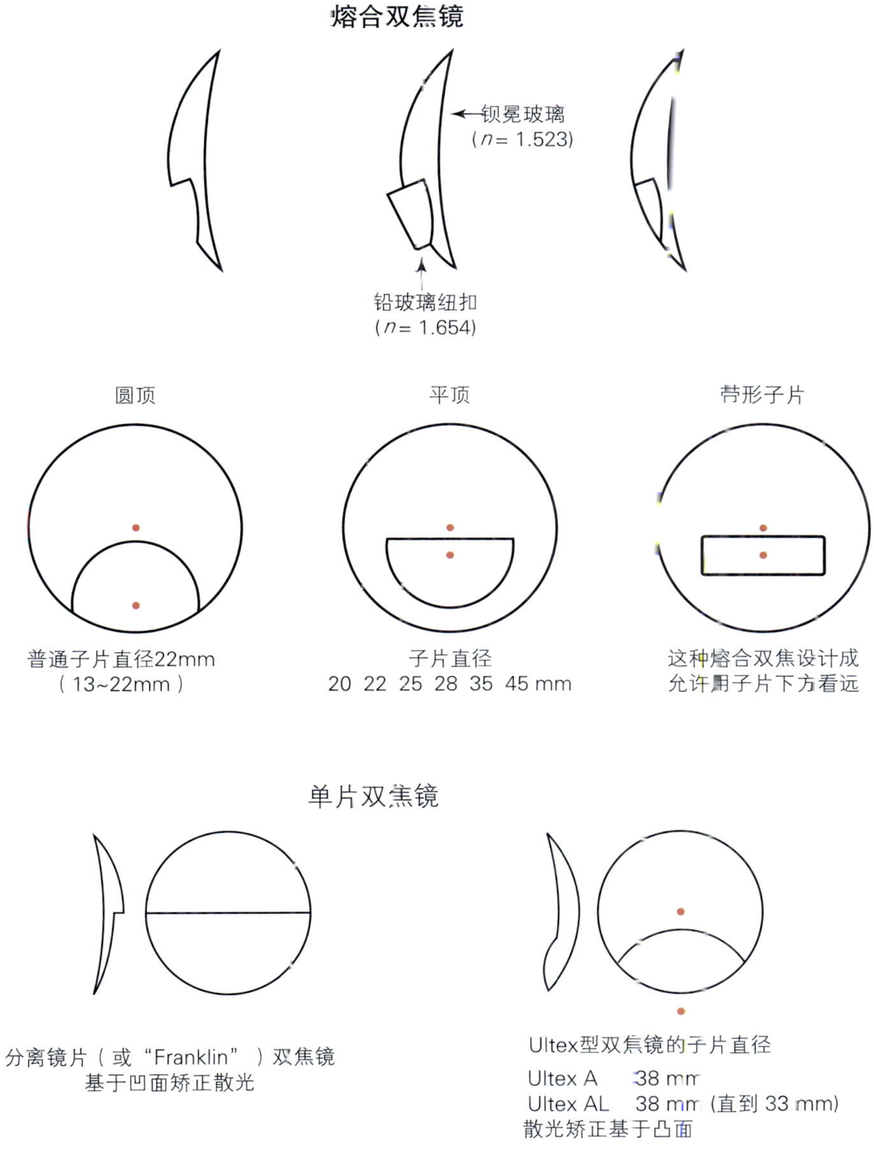

图 4–25 双焦镜片。n 为折射率。

Trifocal Lenses

A bifocal lens may not fully satisfy all the visual needs of an older patient with limited accommodation. Even when near and distant ranges are corrected appropriately, vision is not clear in the intermediate range, approximately at arm's length. The loss of intermediate-range vision may be exacerbated by a stronger bifocal add than is needed. This problem can be solved with trifocal spectacles, which incorporate a third segment of intermediate strength (typically one-half the power of the reading add) between the distance correction and the reading segment. The intermediate segment allows the patient to focus on objects beyond the reading distance but closer than 1 m (Clinical Example 4-4.) In contemporary practice, progressive addition lenses have supplanted trifocals in most instances.

CLINICAL EXAMPLE 4-4

This example demonstrates the advantage of trifocal lenses. Consider a patient with 1.00 D of available accommodation. He wears a bifocal lens with a+2.00 add. His accommodative range for each part of the spectacle lens is

Distance segment: Infinity to 100 cm
Bifocal segment: 50–33 cm

He now has a blurred zone between 50 and 100 cm. an intermediate segment, in this case+1.00 D (half the power of the reading segment), would provide sharp vision from 50 cm (using all of his available accommodation plus the+1.00D add) to 100 cm (using the add only).this trifocal lens combination therefore provides the following ranges:

Distance segment: Infinity to 100 cm
Intermediate segment: 100–50 cm
Near segment: 50–33 cm

Progressive Addition Lenses

Both bifocal and trifocal lenses have an abrupt change in power as the line of sight passes across the boundary between one portion of the lens and the next; image jump and diplopia can occur at the segment lines. Progressive addition lenses (PALs) avoid these difficulties by supplying power gradually as the line of sight is depressed toward the reading level. Unlike bifocal and trifocal lenses, PALs offer clear vision at all focal distances. Other advantages of PALs include lack of intermediate blur and absence of any visible segment lines.

The PAL form has 4 types of optical zones on the convex surface: a spherical distance zone, a reading zone, a transition zone (or *"corridor"*), and zones of peripheral distortion. The progressive change in lens power is generated on the convex surface of the lens by progressive aspheric changes in curvature from the top to the bottom of the lens. The concave surface is reserved for the cylinder of the patient's distance lens prescription, as in traditional minus cylinder lens designs.

However, there are certain drawbacks to PALs. Most notably, some degree of peripheral distortion is inherent in the design of all PALs. This peripheral aberration is caused by astigmatism resulting from the changing aspheric curves; these curves are most pronounced in the lower inner and outer quadrants of the lens. These distortions produce a "swimming" sensation with head movement.

三焦点镜片

双焦镜片可能无法完全满足调节有限的老年患者的所有视觉需求。即使矫正了近距离和远距离范围，但在中间范围内，大约在手臂的长度处视物仍不清楚。较强的双焦附加度使得中间视觉下降可能比实际存在的视觉下降严重。这个问题可用三焦点镜片来解决。三焦点镜片上包含了一个视远区与阅读区域之间的第三区域（通常是阅读附加度的一半）。中间区域允许患者聚焦点于阅读距离之外、靠近 1m 的物体（临床案例 4–4）。目前，渐进多焦点镜片已经取代了三焦点镜片。

临床案例 4–4

这个例子展示了三焦点镜片的优点。有 1.00 D 可用调节的患者，他戴着一个 +2.00 附加度的双焦镜。眼镜镜片各部分的调节范围是：

视远区：无限至 100 cm
视近区：50~33 cm

他现在有一个 50~100 cm 的模糊区域。在这种情况下，+1.00 D（阅读区一半的焦度）中间区将提供从 50 cm（使用所有可用的调节加 +1.00 D 附加）到 100 cm 的清晰视野（仅使用附加度）。因此，这个三焦镜组合提供以下调节范围

视远区：无限至 100 cm
中间区：100~50 cm
视近区：50~33 cm

渐进多焦点镜片

当视线穿过镜片的上下部分之间的分界线时，双焦镜和三焦镜都有一个度数的突变。像跳跃和复视可能发生在分界线。渐进多焦镜片（PALs）避免了这些困难，当视线压低至阅读水平线时，它逐渐地变化度数。与双焦和三焦镜片不同，渐进多焦点镜片可在所有焦距处提供清晰的视觉。渐进多焦点镜片的其他优点包括没有中间模糊和无任何视觉分界线。

渐进多焦点镜片在凸面上有 4 种类型的光学区域：球面视远区、阅读区、过渡区域（或“通道”），和周边变形区。通过从镜片顶部到底部的曲率的渐进的非球面变化，镜片凸面产生镜片焦度的渐进变化。与传统的负柱镜片设计一样，凹面保留用于患者的散光矫正。

但是，渐进多焦点镜片也有一些缺点。最显著的是，所有渐进多焦点镜片设计中都存在一定程度的外围失真。这种周边像差是由非球面弯曲变化引起的散光所致。这种曲面在镜片的下部内外象限中最为明显。这些变形产生头部运动时的“泳动”感觉。

The vertical meridian joining the distance and reading optical centers is free of surface astigmatism and provides the optimal visual acuity. To either side of this distortion-free vertical meridian, induced astigmatism and a concomitant degradation of visual acuity occur. If the lens is designed such that the peripheral distortions are spread out over a relatively wide portion of the lens, there is a concomitant decrease in the distortion-free principal zones. This effect is the basis of *soft-design PALs* (Fig 4-26). Conversely, a wider distortion-free zone for distance and reading means a more intense lateral deformity. This effect is the basis of hard-design PALs. If the transition corridor is lengthened, the distortions are less pronounced, but problems arise because of the greater vertical separation between the distance optical center and the reading zone. Therefore, each PAL design represents a series of compromises. Some manufacturers prefer less distortion at the expense of less useful aberration-free distance and near visual acuity; others opt for maximum acuity over a wider usable area, with smaller but more pronounced lateral distortion zones.

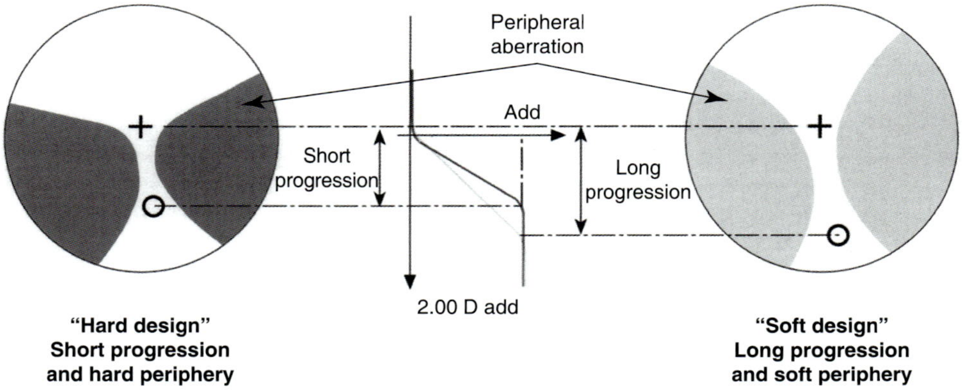

Figure 4-26 Comparison of hard–design and soft–design progressive addition lenses (PALs). These illustrations compare the power progression and peripheral aberration of these 2 PAL designs. *(From Wisnicki HJ. Bifocals, trifocals, and progressive-addition lenses. Focal Points: Clinical Modules for Ophthalmologists. San Francisco: American Academy of Ophthalmology; 1999, module 6.)*

Good candidates for progressive lenses may be patients with new presbyopia who have not experienced traditional lined bifocals or trifocals, those who only occasionally need intermediate vision, and those with strong aversions to lined lenses. Less successful candidates are those who are currently happy with other alternatives (lined bifocals/ trifocals or single vision correction), anisometropia, and those requiring prism or high adds, a large field of view, or multiple near-fixation lines of sight, or those who have very mobile/dynamic eye movements (sports). Personality may play a role in acceptance of these lenses, and those factors should be taken into consideration.

Fitting of these lenses is a critical process. Measurement of pupillary distance should be performed monocularly, as any asymmetry must be accounted for. Frame selection is important. The frame must have adequate vertical depth to allow the full progressive add to be present. The distance and near reference areas should be marked with the frame in place. Frames with adjustable nose pads allow future adjustment of the PAL position. A shorter back vertex distance will give greater binocular field of vision. Greater pantoscopic tilt gives increased near visual field but must be accounted for in the effective lens power.

连接视远与阅读光学中心的垂直子午线没有散光，并提供最佳视力。在无变形的垂直子午线的两侧，诱发散光都伴随视力降低。如果将镜片被设计成周边变形扩展到镜片的较宽部分，则无变形的主要区域同时减少。这种效果是*软设计 PAL* 的基础（图 4–26）。相反，用于视远和阅读的区域越宽，则两侧的变形越大。这种效果是硬设计 PAL 的基础。如果过渡通道延长，变形就不太明显，但由于视远区的光学中心与阅读区垂直间隔较大也会产生问题。因此，每个 PAL 设计都需要做一系列权衡。一些制造商倾向于减少变形，但以较小的无像差视远区和近视力区为代价；另一些人选择是在更宽的有效的面积内获得最佳视力，具有更小但更显著的两侧变形区。

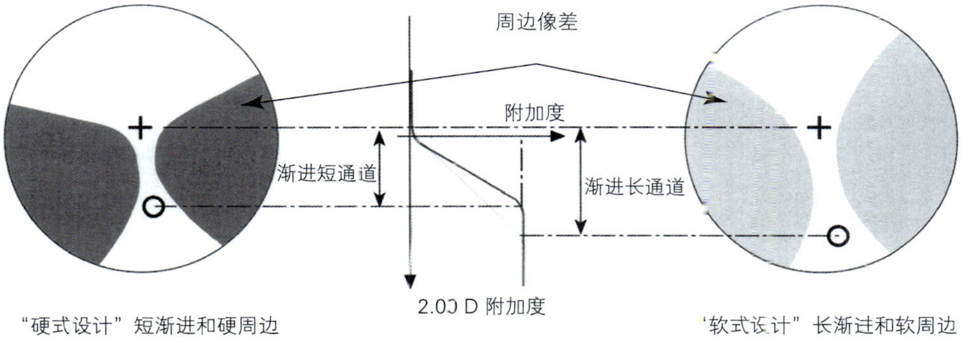

图 4–26　硬设计和软设计渐进镜片（PALs）的比较。本图比较了这 2 种 PAL 设计的中间带和周边像差。*（译者注：资料来源见前页原文。）*

渐进镜片的适宜人群是未有戴过双焦镜和三焦镜经验的新老视患者，偶尔需要中间视力的患者，以及排斥双焦镜片外形的患者。不适宜配戴的人群是乐于接受其他替代方案（双焦 / 三焦点镜片或单光）患者，屈光参差患者，以及需要棱镜矫正或高附加度患者，要求大视野者，有多个近注视视线者，或很多移动电话使用 / 动态的眼球运动（体育运动）者。个人性格在接受镜片过程中也起一定作用，应考虑。

这种镜片的安装是一个重要过程。应测量单眼瞳距，须考虑双眼不对称性。框架选择很重要，框架须具有足够的垂直深度，可以确保渐进通道的完整。视远与视近的参考区域应标记在眼镜框架内。采用可调整鼻托的框架，可以调整渐进片的位置。较短的后顶点距可以提供更大的双眼视野，较大的前倾角也可以增加近视野，但必须考虑有效的镜片焦度的因素。

PALs are readily available from −8.00 to+7.50 D spheres and up to 4.00 D cylinders; the available add powers are from+1.50 to+3.50 D. Some vendors also make custom lenses with parameters outside these limits. Prism can be incorporated into PALs.

The best candidates for PALs are patients with early presbyopia who have not previously worn bifocal lenses, patients who do not require wide near-vision fields, and highly motivated patients. Patients who change from conventional multifocal lenses to PALs should be advised that distortion will be present and that adaptation will be necessary. Small-frame PALs can reduce the usable reading zone to a small area at the bottom edge of the lens. Also, the differential magnification through the progressive zone can make computer screens appear trapezoidal. Progressive designs are also available for indoor use, with large zones devoted to computer monitor and reading distances (eg, 23 inches and 16 inches from the eye).

The Prentice Rule and Bifocal Lens Design

There are special considerations when prescribing lenses for patients with significant anisometropias.

Prismatic effects of lenses

All lenses act as prisms when one looks through the lens at any point other than the optical center. The amount of the induced prismatic effect depends on the power of the lens and the distance from the optical center. Specifically, the amount of prismatic effect (measured in prism diopters) is equal to the distance (in centimeters) from the optical center multiplied by the lens power (in diopters). This equation is known as the *Prentice rule*:

$$\Delta = hD$$

Where

Δ = prismatic effect (in prism diopters)
h = distance from the optical center (in centimeters)
D = lens power (in diopters)

Image displacement

When reading at near through a point below the optical center, a patient wearing spectacle lenses of unequal power may notice vertical double vision. With a bifocal segment, the gaze is usually directed 8–10 mm below and 1.5–3.0 mm nasal to the distance optical center of the distance lens (in the following examples, we assume the usual 8 mm down and 2 mm nasal). As long as the bifocal segments are of the same power and type, the induced, vertical prismatic displacement is determined by the powers of the distance lens alone.

If the lens powers are the same for the 2 eyes, the displacement of each is the same (Figs 4-27, 4-28). However, if the patient's vision is anisometropic, a phoria is induced by the unequal prismatic displacement of the 2 lenses (Figs 4-29, 4-30). The amount of *vertical phoria* is determined by subtracting the smaller prismatic displacement from the larger if both lenses are myopic or hyperopic (see Fig 4-29) or by adding the 2 lenses if the patient is hyperopic in 1 eye and myopic in the other (see Fig 4-30).

市场上已有 −8.00~+7.50 D 球镜和至 4.00 D 柱镜的渐进镜片，附加度为 +1.50~+3.50 D。某些供应商也能生产超出这些参数的定制镜片。棱镜可以植入渐进镜片中。

最适宜渐进镜片的患者是早期老视患者，他们没有配戴过双焦镜，对视近视野的需求不高，患者对渐进镜片也有很积极的态度。若从传统的多焦点镜改为渐进镜，应告知患者存在视物变形，并且需要有一个适应过程。小框渐进镜可将有用视近区域缩小至底部边缘的较小区域。此外，对渐进区的差异放大，使计算机屏幕呈现梯形。渐进镜也可用于室内，阅读区域加大，专用于计算机的中距离和阅读的近距离（例如距离眼睛 23 in 和 16 in，1in=2.54 cm）。

Prentice 法则和双焦设计

要特别注意有明显屈光参差的镜片处方。

镜片的棱镜效应

从镜片光学中心以外的任何位置通过时，都会产生棱镜效应。棱镜效应的量取决于镜片焦度和距光学中心的距离。具体而言，棱镜效应（以棱镜度 Δ 为单位测量）等于距光学中心的距离（以 cm 为单位）乘以镜片焦度（以 D 为单位）。这个公式称为 *Prentice 法则*：

$$\Delta = hD$$

其中 Δ 为棱镜效应（Δ），h 为距光学中心的距离（cm），D 为镜片焦度（D）。

像移位

当通过靠近光学中心下方的点处阅读时，配戴不等焦度镜片的患者可能出现垂直方向上的双眼复视现象。双焦镜的视近通过镜片的视远中心垂直向下 8~10 mm、水平鼻侧 1.5~3.0 mm（下面的例子中，假设垂直向下 8 mm 和水平鼻侧 2 mm）固视。如果双焦镜片具有相同焦度和折射率，则诱导的垂直棱镜效应仅由视远镜片的焦度决定。

如果患者双眼的镜片焦度相同，则每只眼睛的位移是相同的（图 4–27、图 4–28）。如果患者双眼有屈光参差，则 2 个镜片的不同棱镜位移会引起隐斜（图 4–29、图 4–30）。如果 *2 个镜片*都是近视或都是远视，则垂直隐斜量可以由从较大镜片棱镜度位移减去较小棱镜位移来确定（见图 4–29）；如果一只眼远视而另一只眼近视，则垂直隐斜量可以由 2 个镜片棱镜位移量相加来确定（见图 4–30）。

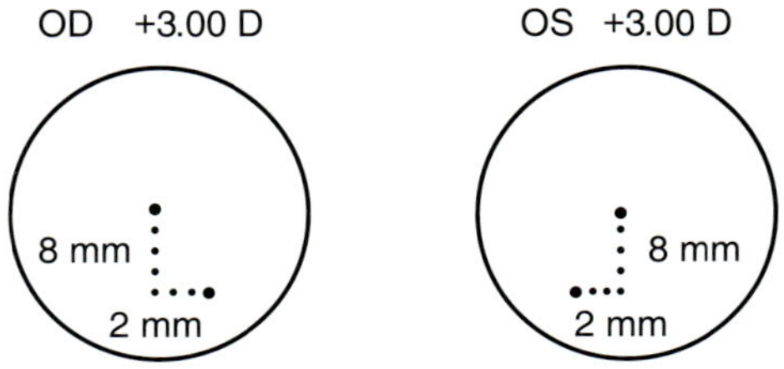

Vertical: 0.8 × +3.00 = 2.4Δ BU
Horizontal: 0.2 × +3.00 = 0.6Δ BO
BU = base of prism up
BO = base of prism out
} for each eye

Figure 4-27 Prismatic effect of bifocal lenses in isometropic hyperopia.

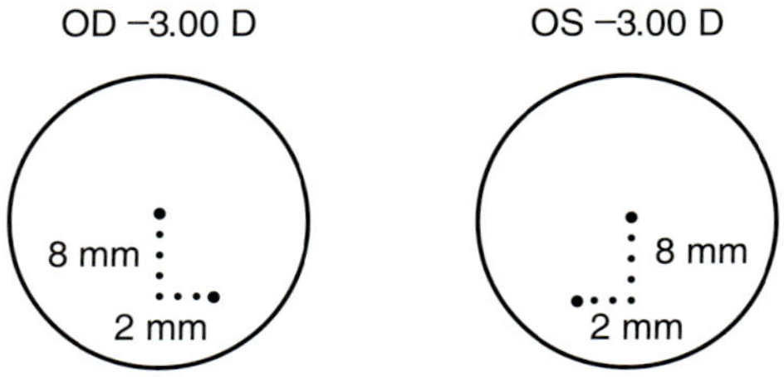

Vertical: 0.8 × −3.00 = 2.4Δ BD
Horizontal: 0.2 × −3.00 = 0.6Δ BI
BD = base of prism down
BI = base of prism in
} for each eye

Figure 4-28 Prismatic effect of bifocal lenses in isometropic myopia.

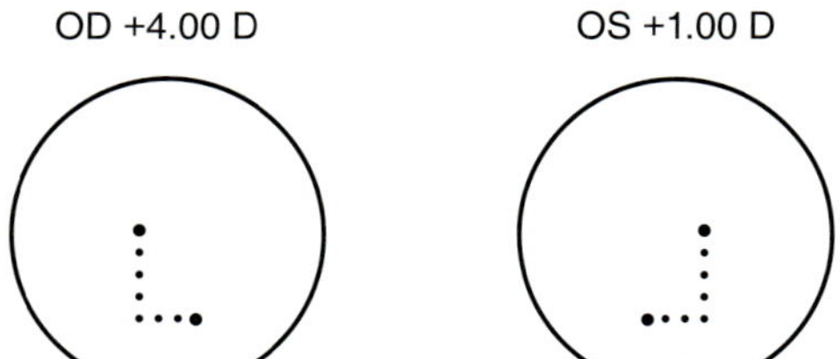

Vertical: OD 0.8 × 4 = 3.2Δ BU — OS 0.8 × 1 = 0.8Δ BU
Horizontal: OD 0.2 × 4 = 0.8Δ BO — OS 0.2 × 1 = 0.2Δ BO
Induced phoria: OD 3.2Δ – 0.8Δ = 2.4Δ BU
OD 0.8Δ BO + 0.2Δ BO = 1.0Δ BO

Figure 4-29 Prismatic effect of bifocal lenses in anisometropic hyperopia.

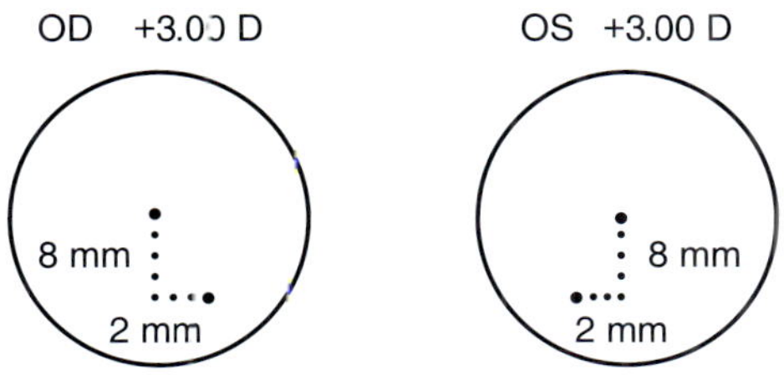

垂直移位: 0.8 × +3.00 = 2.40Δ BU
水平移位: 0.2 × +3.00 = 0.60Δ BO
BU = 底向上
BO = 底向外

} 每只眼

图 4–27　等量远视时双焦镜的棱镜效应。

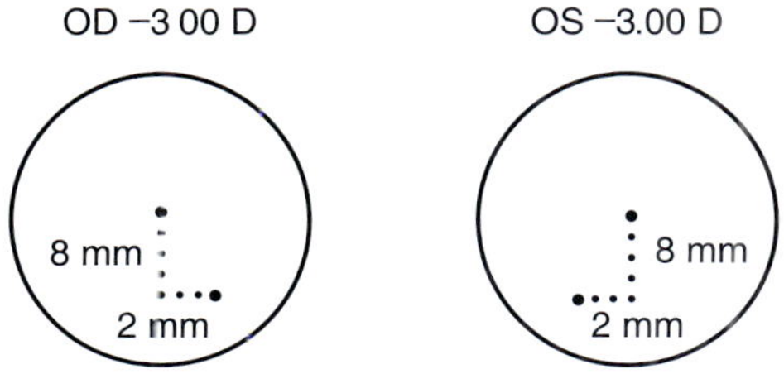

垂直移位: 0.8 × −3.00 = 2.40Δ BD
水平移位: 0.2 × −3.00 = 0.60Δ BI
BD = 底向下
BI = 底向内

} 每只眼

图 4–28　等量近视时双焦镜的棱镜效应。

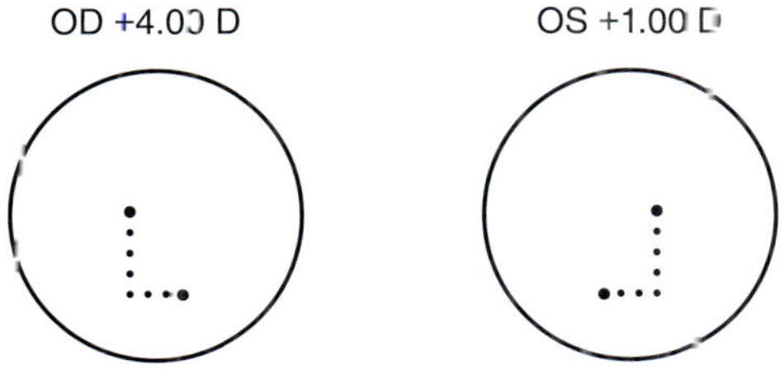

垂直移位: 右眼OD 0.8 × 4 = 3.20Δ BU　　左眼OS 0.8 × 1 = 0.80Δ BU
水平移位: 右眼OD 0.2 × 4 = 0.80Δ BO　　左眼OS 0.2 × 1 = 0.20Δ BO
诱发隐斜: 垂直右眼OD 3.20Δ − 0.80Δ = 2.40Δ BU
水平右眼OD 0.80Δ BO + 0.20Δ BO = 1.00Δ BO

图 4–29　远视性屈光参差时双焦镜的棱镜效应。

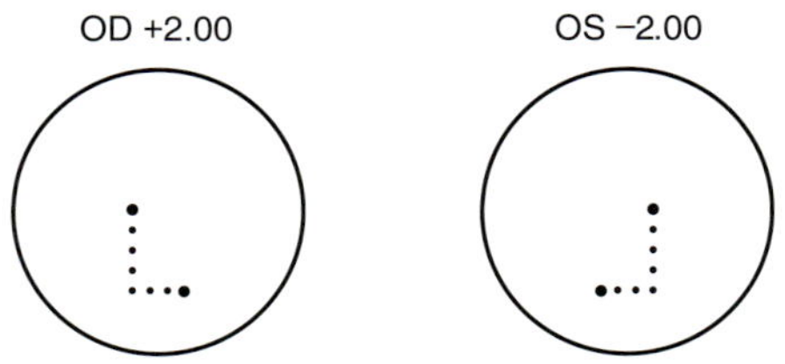

Vertical: OD 0.8 × +2 = 1.6Δ BU
Horizontal: OD 0.2 × +2 = 0.4Δ BO
Induced phoria: OD 1.6Δ + 1.6Δ = 3.2Δ BU
OD 0.4Δ BO – OS 0.4Δ BI = 0
(no horizontal induced phoria)

OS 0.8 × −2 = 1.6Δ BD
OS 0.2 × −2 = 0.4Δ BI

Figure 4-30 Prismatic effect of bifocal lenses in antimetropia.

For determination of the induced *horizontal phoria*, the induced prisms are added if both eyes are hyperopic or if both eyes are myopic. If 1 eye is hyperopic and the other is myopic, the smaller amount of prismatic displacement is subtracted from the larger (see Fig 4-30). Image displacement is minimized when round-top segment bifocal lenses are used with plus lenses and flat-top segment bifocal lenses are used with minus lenses (Fig 4-31).

Image jump

The usual position of the top of a bifocal segment is 5 mm below the optical center of the distance lens. As the eyes are directed downward through a lens, the prismatic displacement of the image increases (downward in plus lenses, upward in minus lenses). When the eyes encounter the top of a bifocal segment, they meet a new plus lens with a different optical center, and the object appears to jump upward unless the optical center of the add is at the very top of the segment (Fig 4-32). Executive-style segments have their optical centers at the top of the segment. The optical center of a typical flat-top segment is located 3 mm below the top of the segment. The closer the optical center of the segment approaches the top edge of the segment, the less the image jump. Thus, flat-top segments produce less image jump than do round-top segments because the latter have much lower optical centers. Patients with myopia who wear round-top bifocal lenses would be more bothered by image jump than would patients with hyperopia because the jump occurs in the direction of image displacement.

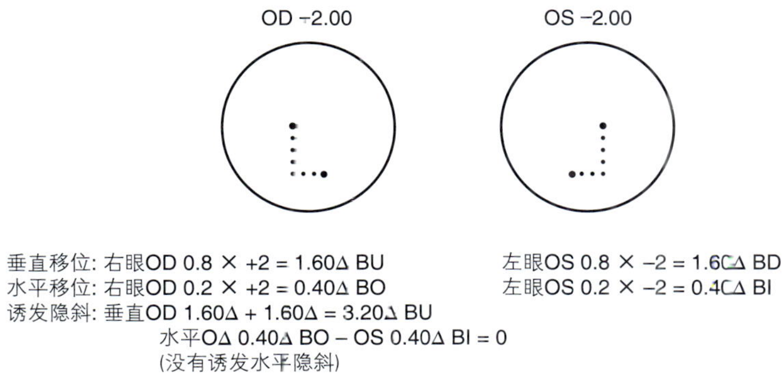

图 4–30　混合型屈光参差（即一只眼远视、一只眼近视）时双焦镜的棱镜效应。

在计算诱发的*水平隐斜*时，如果两眼都是远视或都是近视，则会增加棱镜效应。如果一只眼是远视而另一只眼近视，那么就用较大的棱镜位移量减去较小的棱镜位移量计算（见图 4–30）。当圆顶双焦镜用于正镜时，像移最小；而平顶双焦镜用于负镜时，像移最小（图 4–31）。

像跳跃

双焦镜子片顶通常位于视远镜片光学中心下方 5 mm 处。当眼竖直向下通过镜片时，像的棱镜移位增加（正镜朝下，负镜朝上）。当眼经过双焦子片顶时，会遇到一个具有不同光学中心的新正镜片，物体显现出上跳，除非附加子片的光学中心位于该子片的最顶部（图 4–32）。一线型双焦镜子片的光学中在它的顶部。典型的平顶子片的光学中心位于子片顶下方 3 mm 处。子片的光学中心越接近子片顶部边缘，像跳越少。因此，平顶子片产生的像跳比圆顶子片小，因为后者具有较低的光学中心。配戴圆顶双焦镜片的近视患者比远视患者更容易受到像跳的困扰，因为跳跃发生在像移的方向。

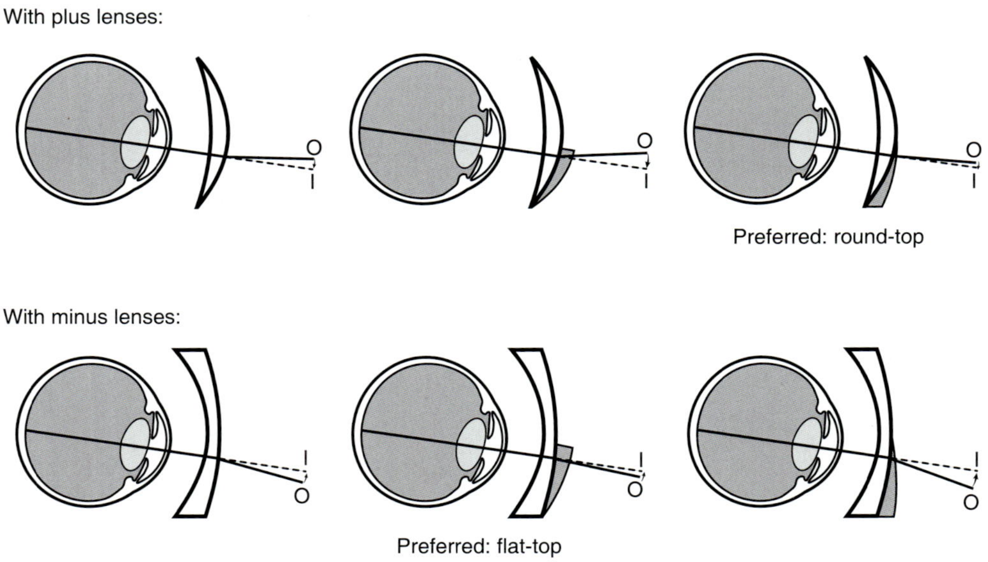

Figure 4-31 Image displacement through bifocal segments. *(From Wisnicki HJ. Bifocals, trifocals, and progressive-addition lenses. Focal Points: Clinical Modules for Ophthalmologists. San Francisco: American Academy of Ophthalmology; 1999, module 6. Reprinted with permission from Guyton DL. Ophthalmic Optics and Clinical Refraction. Baltimore: Prism Press; 1998. Redrawn by C. H. Wooley.)*

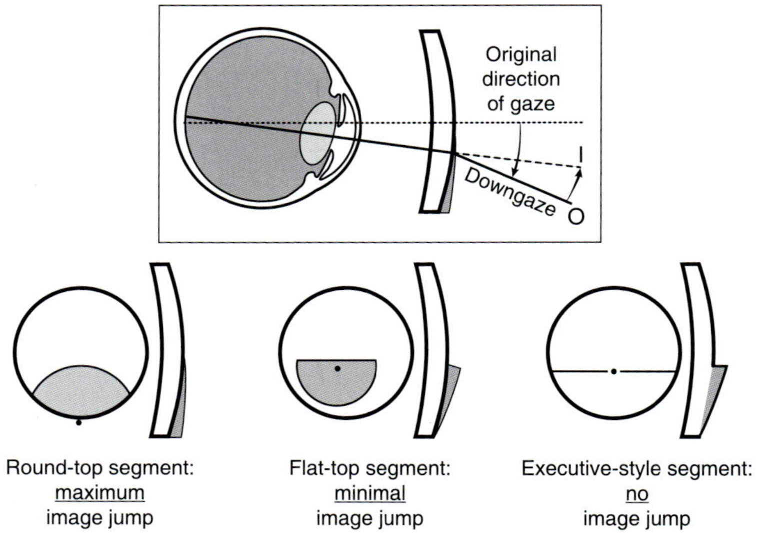

Figure 4-32 Image jump through bifocal segments. If the optical center of a segment is at its top, no image jump occurs. *(From Wisnicki HJ. Bifocals, trifocals, and progressive-addition lenses. Focal Points: Clinical Modules for Ophthalmologists. San Francisco: American Academy of Ophthalmology; 1999, module 6. Reprinted with permission from Guyton DL. Ophthalmic Optics and Clinical Refraction. Baltimore: Prism Press; 1998. Redrawn by H. Wooley.)*

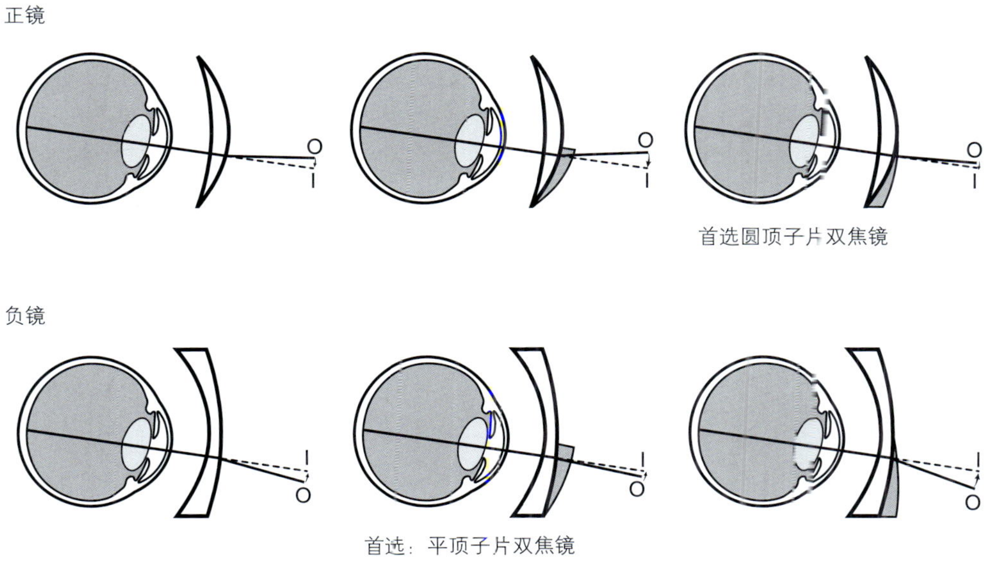

图 4-31　双焦镜的像移。*（译者注：资料来源见前页原文。）*

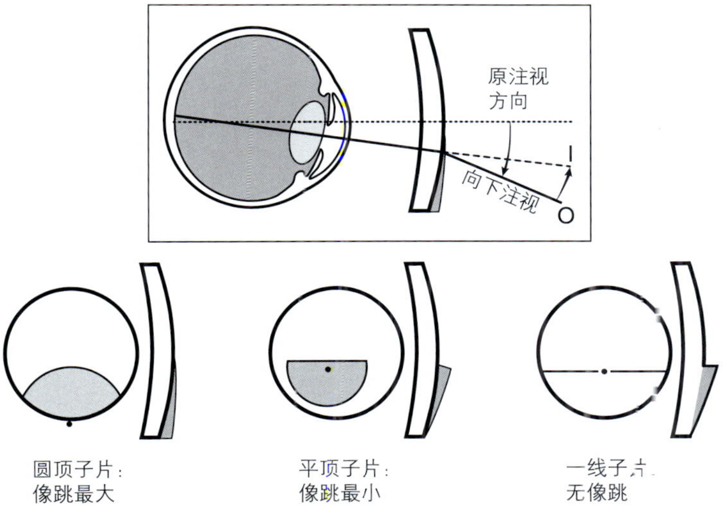

图 4-32　通过双焦镜的像跳。如果子片光学中心位于顶部，则不会发生像跳。*（译者注：资料来源见前页原文。）*

Compensating for induced anisophoria

When anisometropia is corrected with spectacle lenses, unequal prism is introduced in all secondary positions of gaze. This prism may be the source of symptoms, even diplopia. *Symptomatic anisophoria* occurs especially when a patient with early presbyopia uses his or her first pair of bifocal lenses or when the anisometropia is of recent and/or sudden origin, as occurs after retinal detachment surgery, with gradual asymmetric progression of cataracts, or after unilateral intraocular lens implantation. The patient usually adapts to horizontal imbalance by increasing head rotation but may have symptoms when looking down, in the reading position. Recall that horizontal vergence amplitudes are large compared with vertical fusional amplitudes, which are typically less than 2Δ. We can calculate the amount of induced phoria by using the Prentice rule (Fig 4-33; Clinical Example 4-5).

Rx: OD +4.00 sphere
OS +1.00 sphere
Add +2.50 OU

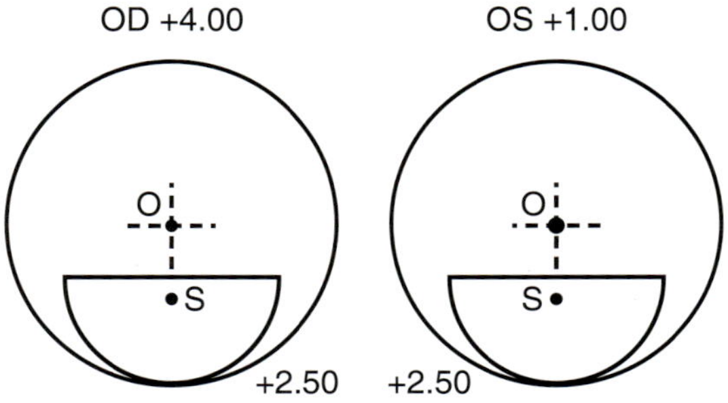

O = optical center, distance
S = optical center of segment
R (= S): Reading position 8 mm below distance optical center

Figure 4-33 Calculation of induced anisophoria.

CLINICAL EXAMPLE 4-5

This example demonstrates the Prentice rule. Consider a patient with the following reading point, 8 mm below distance optical center:

OD 4.00 D × 0.80 cm	=	3.20Δ base up (BU)
OS 1.00 D × 0.80 cm	=	0.80Δ BU
Net difference		2.40Δ BU

In this example, there is an induced right hyperdeviation of 2.40Δ. Conforming to the usual practice in the management of heterophorias, approximately two-thirds to three-fourths of the vertical phoria should be corrected—in this case, 1.75 D.

The correction of induced vertical prism may be accomplished in several ways:

Press-on (Fresnel) prisms With press-on prisms, 2.00Δ of base down (BD) prism may be added to the right segment in the preceding example or 2.00Δ of base up (BU) prism to the left segment.

诱发的不等隐斜的补偿

使用框镜矫正屈光参差时，在固视的所有第二眼位时会产生不等的棱镜效应。这是不适症状，甚至会是复视的原因。*有症状的不等隐斜*发生在戴第一副双焦镜的早期老视患者，或突然发病，如视网膜脱离手术后、白内障不对称进展或单眼人工晶体植入术后的患者。患者通常通过增加头部旋转来适应水平隐斜，但在阅读位置为向下看时出现症状。因为水平聚散幅度大于幅度小于 2Δ 的垂直融合幅度，我们可以用 Prentice 法则计算诱发隐斜量（图 4–33，临床案例 4–5）。

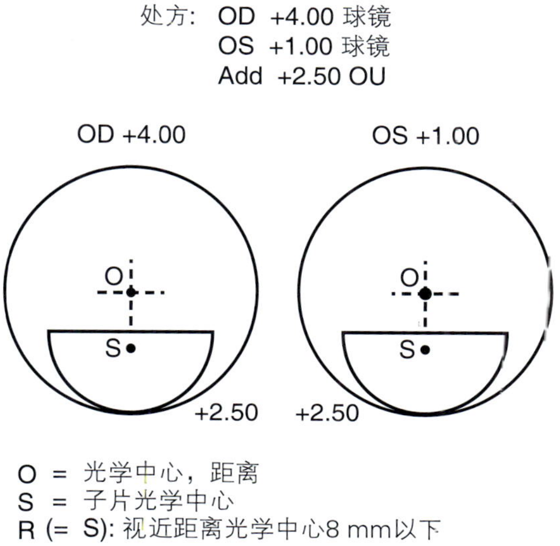

图 4–33　诱导的不等隐斜的计算。

临床案例 4–5

此例演示了 Prentice 法则。以光学中心下 8 mm 处为阅读点的患者为例:

OD 4.00 D × 0.80 cm	=	3.20Δ **底向上**(BU)
OS 1.00 D × 0.80 cm	=	0.80Δ BU
净差值		2.40Δ BU

在本例中，患者存在 2.40Δ 诱导的右眼上偏斜。按照常规隐斜的处理方法，应该矫正垂直隐斜的 2/3~3/4，在本例中，约为 1.75 D。

诱导垂直棱镜的矫正方法有以下几种：

压贴（Fresnel）三棱镜　利用压贴式棱镜，将 2.00Δ 底向下（BD）的棱镜贴在右眼子片前，或将 2.00Δ 底向上（BU）的棱镜贴在左眼子片前。

Slab-off The most satisfactory method of compensating for the induced vertical phoria in anisometropia is the technique of bicentric grinding, known as *slab-off* (Fig 4-34). In this method, 2 optical centers are created in the lens that has the greater minus (or less plus) power, thereby counteracting the base-down effect of the greater minus lens in the reading position. It is convenient to think of the slab-off process as creating *base-up prism* (or removing base-down prism—slab-off) over the reading area of the lens.

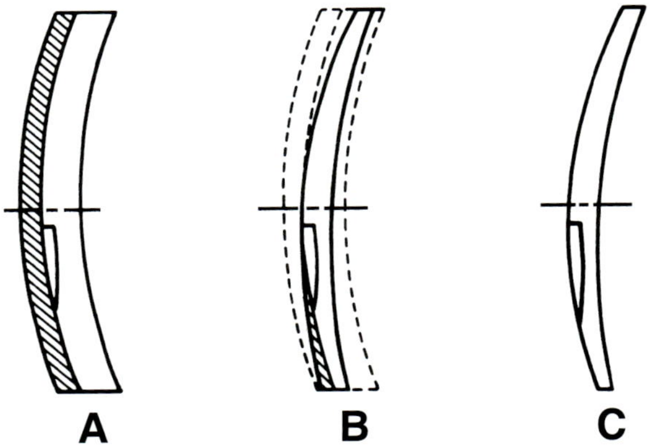

Figure 4-34 Bicentric grinding (slab–off). **A**, Lens form with a dummy lens cemented to the front surface. **B**, Both surfaces of the lens are reground with the same curvatures but removing base–up prism from the top segment of the front surface and removing base–down prism from the entire rear surface. **C**, The effect is a lens from which base–down prism has been removed from the lower segment only.

Bicentric grinding is used for single-vision lenses as well as for multifocal lenses. By increasing the distance between the 2 optical centers, this method achieves as much as 4.00Δ of prism compensation at the reading position.

Reverse slab-off Prism correction in the reading position is achieved not only by removing *base-down* prism from the lower part of the more minus lens (slabbing off) but also by adding base-down prism to the lower half of the more plus lens. This technique is known as reverse *slab-off.*

Historically, it was easy to remove material from a standard lens. Currently, because plastic lenses are fabricated by molding, it is more convenient to add material to create a base-down prism in the lower half of what will be the more plus lens. Because plastic lenses account for most lenses dispensed, reverse slab-off is the most common method of correcting anisometropically induced anisophoria. In theory, a minus powered spectacle lens will have less edge thickness with slab-off than with reverse slab-off.

When the clinician is ordering a lens that requires prism correction for an anisophoria in downgaze, it is often appropriate to leave the choice of slab-off versus reverse slab-off to the optician by including a statement in the prescription, such as, "Slab-off right lens 3.00Δ (or reverse slab-off left lens)." In either case, the prescribed prism should be measured in the reading position, not calculated, because the patient may have partially adapted to the anisophoria.

Dissimilar segments In anisometropic bifocal lens prescriptions, vertical prism compensation can also be achieved by using dissimilar bifocal segments with their optical centers at 2 different heights. The segment with the lower optical center should be placed in front of the more hyperopic (or less myopic) eye to provide base-down prism. (This method contrasts with the bicentric grinding method, which produces base-up prism and is therefore employed on the lesser plus or greater minus lens.)

In the example in Figure 4-35, a 22-mm round segment is used for the right eye, and the top of its segment is at the usual 5 mm below the distance optical center. For the left eye, a 22-mm flat-top segment is used, again with the top of the segment 5 mm below the optical center.

削薄镜 补偿屈光参差引起的垂直隐斜的最令人满意的方法是双中心磨削技术，又称为*削薄镜*（图 4–34）。在该方法中，镜片中有 2 个光学中心，会具有更大的负焦度（或更小的正焦度），从而可以抵消在视近时较大负镜的底向下效应。将削薄过程视为在镜片的视近区形成*底向上棱镜*（或移除底向下棱镜——削薄）。

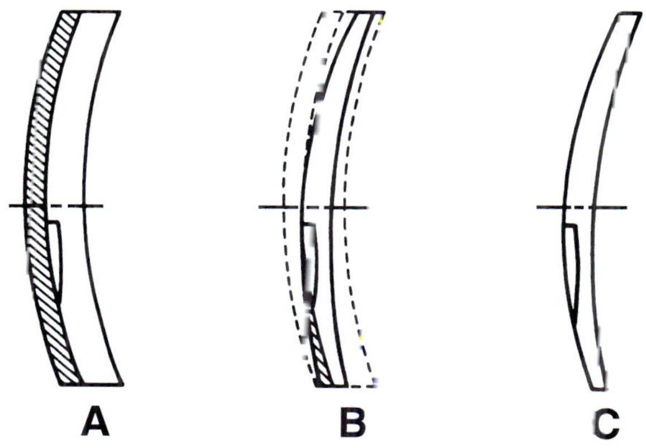

图 4–34 双向磨削（削薄）。**A**. 镜片形成，临时镜片粘合在前表面上。**B**. 透片的 2 个表面以相同的曲率重新研磨，但是从前表面的顶部区段移除底向上棱镜，并从整个后表面移除底向下棱镜。**C**. 效果是仅从下段移除底向下棱镜。

双中心磨削用于单焦镜及多焦镜。通过增加 2 个光学中心的距离的方法，最大可补偿的视近距离相当于 4.00 Δ 的棱镜。

反向削薄镜 视近区域的棱镜矫正不仅可以通过从负透镜的下部移心形成*底部向下*棱镜（削薄），而且还可以通过向正镜的下半部分添加底向下棱镜来实现。这种技术称为*反向削薄*。

过去，从标准镜片上移除材料很容易。目前常用的树脂镜片是模塑制造而成的，因此更方便添加材料，如在下半部分附加正镜，从而形成底向下棱镜。由于树脂镜片是目前镜片主流，因此反向削薄是矫正屈光参差产生的不等隐斜最常见的方法。理论上，削薄技术会使负镜片的边缘厚度减少。

当临床医生订购棱镜，并要求向下注视来消除不等隐斜时，通常会在处方中说明镜片是选择削薄还是反向削薄。“削薄右镜片 3.00 Δ（或反向削薄左镜片）。”这时，应在视近的状态下测量棱镜焦度，而不是计算，因为患者可能已经适应了一些不等隐斜。

不同的子片 在屈光参差双焦镜处方中，垂直棱镜补偿也可以通过使用不同的双焦子片获得，并使它们的光学中心在不同的高度。具有较低光学中心的子片应放置在远视较高（或近视较低）眼中，并提供底向下棱镜。（这种方法与双中心研磨方法形成对比，后者产生底向上棱镜，并且用于较小正镜或较大负镜。）

在图 4–35 的示例中，右眼使用 22 mm 的圆顶子片，子片顶部在光学中心下方 5 mm 处。左眼使用 22 mm 的平顶子片，子片顶同样在光学中心下方 5 mm 处。

Because the optical center of the flat-top segment is 3 mm below the top of the segment, it is at the patient's reading position and that segment will introduce no prismatic effect. However, for the right eye, the optical center of the round segment is 8 mm below the patient's reading position; according to the Prentice rule, this 2.50 D segment will pro- duce 2.50 × 0.8 = 2.00Δ base-down prism.

Single-vision reading glasses with lowered optical centers Partial compensation for the induced vertical phoria at the reading position can be obtained with single-vision reading glasses when the optical centers are placed 3–4 mm below the pupillary centers in primary gaze. The patient's gaze will be directed much closer to the optical centers of the lenses when reading.

OD	+4.00
OS	+1.00
Add	+2.50

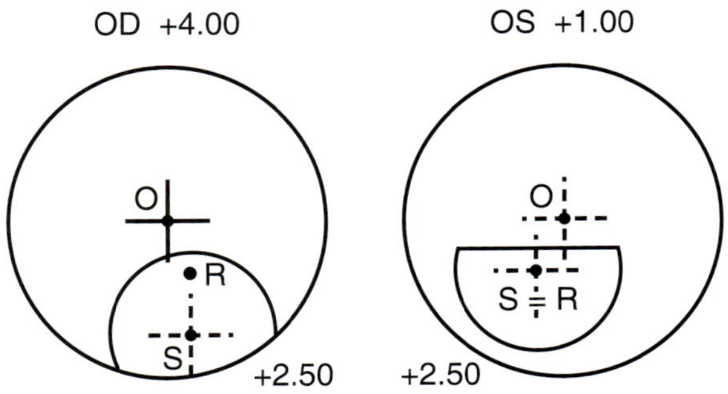

Figure 4-35 Dissimilar segments used to compensate for anisophoria in anisometropic bifocal prescriptions.

O = optical center, distance
S = optical center of segment
R (= S): Reading position 8 mm below distance optical center

Contact lenses Contact lenses can be prescribed for patients with significant anisometropia that causes a symptomatic anisophoria in downgaze. Reading glasses can be worn over the contacts if the patient's vision is presbyopic.

Refractive surgery Corneal refractive surgery may be an option for some patients with symptomatic anisometropia or anisophoria.

Occupation and Bifocal Segment

The *dioptric power* of a segment depends on the patient's accommodative reserve and the working distance required for a specific job. Such focal length determinations are a characteristic not of the job but of the individual patient's adaptation to that job. If the patient is allowed to use half of his or her available accommodation (which must be measured), the remainder of the dioptric requirement will be met by the bifocal add. For example, if the job entails proofreading at 40 cm, the dioptric requirement for that focal length is 2.50 D. If the patient's accommodative amplitude is 2.00 D, and half of that (1.00 D) is used for the job, the balance of 1.50 D becomes the necessary bifocal add. It is essential that the accommodative range (near point to far point) be measured and that it be adequate for the job tasks.

由于平顶子片的光学中心位于子片顶部下方 3 mm 处，因此它位于患者的阅读位置，并且该部分不会产生棱镜效应。而右眼圆顶子片的光学中心比患者的阅读位置低 8 mm，根据 Prentice 规则，若子片为 2.50D，将产生 2.50 × 0.8=2.00 Δ 底向下棱镜。

单焦阅读镜联合降低光学中心　当光学中心放置在第一眼位中瞳孔中心下方 3~4 mm 处时，可以补偿部分使用单焦镜在阅读时诱发的垂直隐斜。在阅读时，患者的注视将更加靠近镜片的光学中心。

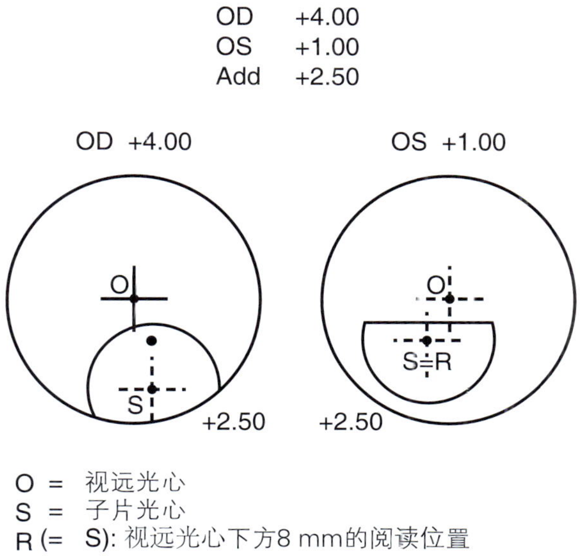

图 4-35　补偿不等双焦镜中不等隐斜的不同子片

接触镜　接触镜可以用于屈光参差的患者，这些患者向下固视时会出现不等隐斜的症状。如果患者是老花眼，可在接触镜上配戴阅读镜。

屈光手术　对于有症状的屈光参差或隐斜的患者，可以选择角膜屈光手术。

职业和双焦子片

子片*焦度*取决于患者的调节储备和所需的工作距离。这个焦距不是工作的特征，而是患者个人对该工作的适宜。如果患者使用可用调节储备的一半（必须测量），则剩余部分可用双焦镜子片来满足。例如，如果工作需要在 40 cm 处，对应焦距的屈光需求为 2.50 D。如果患者的调节幅度为 2.00 D，并且其中一半（1.00 D）用于该工作，则尚留有 1.50 D 需要双焦镜附加度。调节范围（近点至远点）需根据工作需求测量。

Lens design

The most important characteristic of the bifocal segment is the *segment height* in relation to the patient's pupillary center. The lenses will be unsuitable if the segment is placed too high or too low for the specific occupational need.

Segment width is substantially less important. The popular impression that very large bifocal lenses mean better reading capability is not supported by projection measurements. At a 40-cm reading distance, a 25-mm flat-top segment provides a horizontal reading field of 50–55 cm.

At a 40-cm distance, an individual habitually uses face rotation to increase his or her fixation field when it exceeds 45 cm (30° of arc); therefore, a 25-mm-wide segment is more than adequate for all but a few special occupations, such as a graphic artist or an architectural drafter using a drawing board. Furthermore, with a 35-mm segment producing a horizontal field 75 cm wide, the focal length at the extremes of the fixation field would be 55 cm, not 40 cm! Therefore, the split bifocal is useful not because it is a wider bifocal lens but because of its monocentric construction.

The *shape* of the segment must also be considered. For example, round-top segments require the user to look far enough down in the segment to employ his or her maximum horizontal dimension. In addition, these segments exaggerate image jump, especially in myopic corrections.

Segment decentration To avoid inducing a base-out prism effect when the bifocal lens–wearing patient converges for near-vision tasks, the reading segment is generally decentered inward. This design is especially important in aphakic spectacles. Consider the following points for proper decentration:

- *Working distance.* Because the convergence requirement increases as the focal length decreases, additional inward decentration of the bifocal segment is required.
- *Interpupillary distance.* The wider the interpupillary distance, the greater the convergence requirement and, correspondingly, the need for inward decentration ofthe segments.
- *Lens power.* If the distance lens is a high-plus lens, it will create a greater base-out prism effect (ie, induced exophoria) as the viewer converges. Additional inward decentration of the segments may be helpful. The reverse is true for high-minus lenses.
- *Existing heterophoria.* As with lens-induced phorias, the presence of an existing exophoria suggests that increasing the inward decentration would be effective. An esophoria calls for the opposite approach.

Prescribing Special Lenses

Aphakic Lenses

The problems of correcting aphakia with high-plus spectacle lenses include:

- magnification of approximately 20%–35%
- altered depth perception resulting from the magnification
- pincushion distortion; for example, doors appear to bow inward
- difficulty with hand–eye coordination
- ring scotoma generated by prismatic effects at the edge of the lens (causing the "jack-in-the-box" phenomenon)
- extreme sensitivity of the lenses to minor misadjustment in vertex distance, pantoscopic tilt, and height

镜片设计

双焦镜子片最重要的特征是确定患者瞳孔中心相对应的*子片高度*。如果针对特定的职业需求，镜片位置会偏高或偏低，则镜片就不合适。

*子片宽度*不太重要。一般认为宽大的子片意味着更好的阅读视野，但却无法进行专业检测。在 40cm 阅读距离处，25 mm 的平顶子片光可提供 50~55 cm 的水平阅读区域。

在 40 cm 的距离，当超过 45 cm（30° 弧度）的范围时，人会习惯性地转头来增加视野范围。因此，除了一些特殊职业，如图形艺术家或绘图板的建筑师等，一般人有 25 mm 宽的水平阅读视野就足够了。此外，35 mm 的子片产生 75 cm 宽的水平视野，固定视野极端的焦距是 55 cm，而不是 40 cm！ 因此，分离型双焦镜是有用的，不是由于它是较宽的双焦点镜片，而是因为它具有单中心结构。

还须考虑子片的*形状*。如圆顶子片要求尽量向下看，使用最大的水平空间。此外，这些子片，特别是在近视矫正中，还有像跳。

子片偏心 为了避免双焦镜配戴患者近距离工作集合时引起底向外棱镜效应，阅读子片时一般应向内偏位。这种设计在无晶状体眼配镜中尤其重要。如何合适地偏心应考虑到下列几点：

- *工作距离*。因为焦距减小时需要更多的集合，双焦子片也需要增加向内偏。
- *瞳距*。瞳距越宽，需要更多的集合。相应的，子片也需要更多的向内偏。
- *镜片度数*。如果远用镜是高度正镜片，集合时，将产生更大的底向外棱镜效应（即会诱发外隐斜），增加的子片会对向内偏位有帮助。对于高度负镜片则相反。
- 因为镜片诱导隐斜，存在外隐斜时建议增加向内偏是有效的。内隐斜相反。

特殊镜片处方

无晶体眼

用高度正镜片矫正无晶状体眼存在以下问题：

- 大约放大 20%~35%。
- 因放大作用，深度知觉的改变。
- 枕形畸变，如同大门向内弓形弯曲。
- 手眼协调困难。
- 镜片边缘的棱镜效应会产生暗环（产生“玩偶盒”现象）。
- 对顶点距、前倾角及高度的微调极为敏感。

- in monocular aphakia, loss of useful binocular vision because of differential magnification

In addition, aphakic spectacles create cosmetic problems. The patient's eyes appear magnified and, if viewed obliquely, may seem displaced because of prismatic effects. The high-power lenticular lens is itself unattractive, given its "fried-egg"appearance (Fig 4-36).

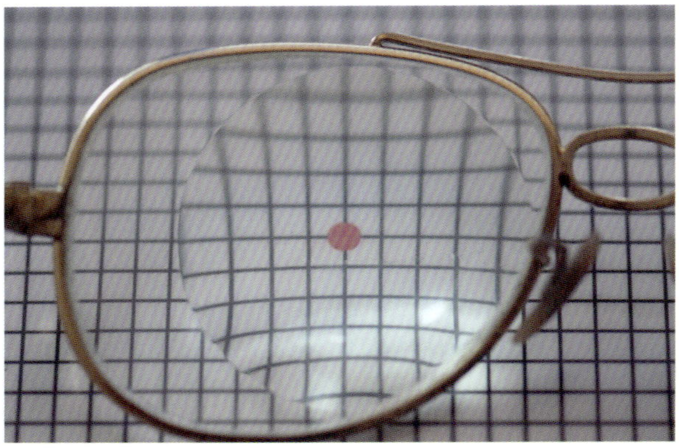

Figure 4-36 Aphakic lens with magnification and pincushion distortion. *(Courtesy of Tommy Korn, MD.)*

For these reasons, intraocular lenses and aphakic contact lenses now account for nearly all aphakic corrections. Nevertheless, spectacle correction of aphakia is sometimes appropriate, as in bilateral infantile pediatric aphakia.

Refracting technique

Because of the sensitivity of aphakic glasses to vertex distance and pantoscopic tilt, it is difficult to refract an aphakic eye reliably by using a phoropter. The vertex distance and the pantoscopic tilt are not well controlled, nor are they necessarily close to the values for the final spectacles. Rather than a phoropter, trial frames or lens clips are used.

The trial frame allows the refractionist to control vertex distance and pantoscopic tilt. It should be adjusted for minimal vertex distance and for the same pantoscopic tilt planned for the actual spectacles (approximately 5°–7°, not the larger values that are appropriate for conventional glasses). Pantoscopic tilt is desirable in spectacle lenses to maintain the vertex distance in downgaze. Excess tilt will induce oblique (marginal) astigmatism in the axis of rotation.

Refracting with clip-on trial lens holders placed over the patient's existing aphakic glasses (overrefraction) keeps vertex distance and lens tilt constant. Take care that the center of the clip coincides with the optical center of the existing lens. Even if the present lens contains a cylinder at an axis different from what is needed, it is possible to calculate the resultant spherocylindrical correction with an electronic calculator, by hand, or with measurement of the combination in a lensmeter.

Guyton DL. *Retinoscopy: Minus Cylinder Technique, 1986; Retinoscopy: Plus Cylinder Technique, 1986; Subjective Refraction: Cross-Cylinder Technique, 1987.* Reviewed for currency, 2007. Clinical Skills DVD Series [DVD]. San Francisco: American Academy of Ophthalmology.

Absorptive Lenses

In certain high-illumination situations, sunglasses allow for better visual function in a number of ways.

• 单眼无晶体眼时，因为不同的视网膜放大率，会使双眼视觉丧失。

另外，无晶体眼的框架镜还会产生美容问题。由于棱镜效应，患者的眼睛被放大了，如果侧目注视时，眼睛位置还会偏移。高度凸透镜片本身不美观，呈“煎蛋”样外观（图 4–36）。

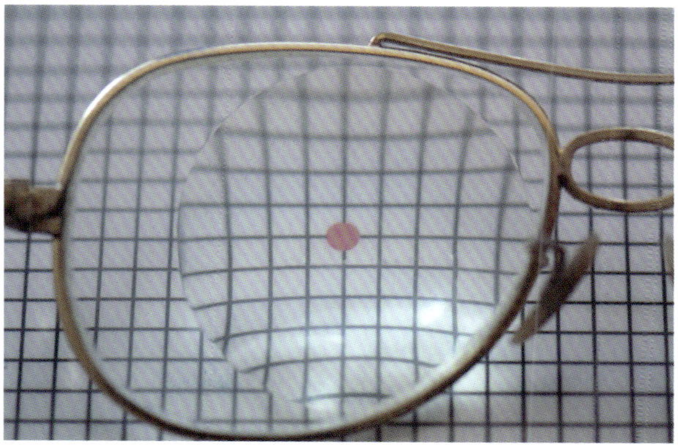

图 4–36　无晶体眼镜片的放大和枕样扭曲现象。*（译者注：资料来源见前页原文。）*

综上原因，大多数无晶体眼采用人工晶体和接触镜来进行屈光矫正。有时，无晶体眼更适合配戴框镜，如小儿双眼无晶体眼。

验光技术

因为无晶体眼镜片对顶点距及前倾角的敏感性，用综合验光仪很难可靠地对无晶体眼验光。因为用综合验光仪很难控制顶点距和前倾角大小，也就很难接近最终的镜片度数，所以常使用试镜架及镜片验光。

试镜架可以控制顶点距及前倾角，应根据实际眼镜的最小顶点距离和同样的前倾角（大约在 5° ~7° 之间，不适合常规眼镜的最大值）进行调整。在眼镜镜片中，前倾角是可以调整的，以保持俯视的顶点距离。过度倾斜会导致旋转轴上的斜（边缘）像散。

在患者的无晶体眼镜上，用夹持式试镜片进行验光（镜上验光），保持顶点距和镜片前倾不变。注意夹片中心与现有透镜的光学中心重合。即使目前镜片包含的柱镜轴位与验光检测的轴位不一样，也可以用电子计算器，或手动，或通过焦度计测量，合成的球柱矫正结果。

Guyton DL. *Retinoscopy: Minus Cylinder Technique, 1986; Retinoscopy: Plus Cylinder Technique, 1986; Subjective Refraction: Cross-Cylinder Technique, 1987.* Reviewed for currency, 2007. Clinical Skills DVD Series [DVD]. San Francisco: American Academy of Ophthalmology.

吸收镜片

在强光照的情况下，太阳镜可以通过一些路径获得更好的视觉功能。

Improvement of contrast sensitivity

On a bright, sunny day, irradiance from the sun ranges from 10,000–30,000 foot-lamberts. These high light levels tend to saturate the retina and therefore decrease finer levels of contrast sensitivity. The major function of dark (gray, green, or brown) sunglasses is to allow the retina to remain at its normal level of contrast sensitivity. Most dark sunglasses absorb 70%–80% of the incident light of all wavelengths.

Improvement of dark adaptation

A full day at the beach or on the ski slopes on a sunny day (without dark sunglasses) can impair dark adaptation for more than 2 days. Thus, dark sunglasses are recommended for prolonged periods in bright sun.

Reduction of glare sensitivity

Various types of sunglasses can reduce glare sensitivity. Because light reflected off a horizontal surface is polarized in the horizontal plane, properly oriented *polarized lenses* reduce the intensity of glare from road surfaces, glass windows, metal surfaces, and lake and river surfaces. *Graded-density sunglasses* are deeply tinted at the top and gradually become lighter toward the lens center. They are effective in removing glare from sources above the line of sight, such as the sun. Wide-temple sunglasses work by reducing glare from temporal light sources.

Use of photochromic lenses

When short-wavelength light (300–400nm) interacts with photochromic lenses, the lenses darken by means of a chemical reaction that converts silver ions to elemental silver. This process is similar to the reaction that occurs when photographic film is exposed to light. Unlike that in photographic film, however, the chemical reaction in photochromic lenses is reversible. Current photochromic lenses incorporate complex organic compounds in which UV light changes the molecules into different configuration states *(ie, cis to trans)*; this process darkens the lenses (Fig 4-37). Photochromic lenses can darken enough to absorb approximately 80% of the incident light; when the amount of illumination falls, they can lighten to absorb only a small part of the incident light. Note that these lenses take some time to darken and, in particular, take longer to lighten than to darken. This discrepancy can be problematic in patients who move frequently between outdoor and indoor environments. Because automobile glass and the window glass in many residences and commercial buildings absorb light in the UV spectrum, most photochromics do not darken inside cars or buildings. In colder weather, patients should also be warned that these lenses darken more than usual, especially during a cloudy day. Nevertheless, photochromic lenses are excellent UV absorbers.

对比敏感度的提高

在阳光明媚的日子，太阳辐照度为 10000~30000 ft·L（1 ft·L=3.426 26cd/m^2）。这些高光水平使视网膜光照度水平饱和，从而使对比敏感度水平降低。深色（灰色、绿色或棕色）太阳镜的主要功能是使视网膜保持正常的对比度敏感度水平。大多数深色太阳镜吸收了所有波长的入射光的 70%~80%。

暗适应的提高

在阳光明媚的日子里，在海滩或滑雪场待一整天（不戴墨镜），损害的暗适应能力需要 2d 才能恢复。当长时间处在强阳光下时，建议使用深色太阳镜。

炫光敏感性的降低

多种太阳镜可以降低眩光敏感度。因为从水平表面反射的光在水平平面上发生偏振，所以选择适当方向的*偏振镜*可降低来自路面、玻璃窗、金属表面、湖泊和河流表面的眩光强度。*分级密度太阳镜*在顶部着色深，向中心逐渐变浅，这样可以有效地去除视线上方的炫光，如阳光。侧边宽的太阳镜可以有效减少来自侧方光源的眩光。

变色镜片使用

当短波长光（300~400 nm）与变色镜相互作用时，通过将银离子转化为元素银的化学反应使镜片变暗。这个过程类似于照相感光胶片曝光时发生的反应。然而，与照相感光胶片不同的是，变色镜片中的化学反应是可逆的。目前的变色镜片加入了复杂的有机化合物，紫外光将其分子转化为不同的构型状态（*即顺式变成反式*），这个过程使镜片变暗（图 4-37）。变色镜片可以变暗到足以吸收大约 80% 的入射光；当光照量下降时，它们只吸收入射光的一小部分，从而可以使镜片变亮。使镜片发生变化是需要一些时间的，特别是变亮比变暗需要更长时间。对于频繁出入室外和室内的患者，这种延迟可能还会出现问题。由于汽车玻璃与许多住宅和商业建筑的窗户玻璃会吸收短波长的紫外光谱，大多数变色镜片不会在汽车或建筑物内变暗。在较冷的天气下，应该告知患者这些镜片会比平常更暗，尤其是在多云的阴天。毋庸置疑，变色镜片可以很好地吸收紫外线。

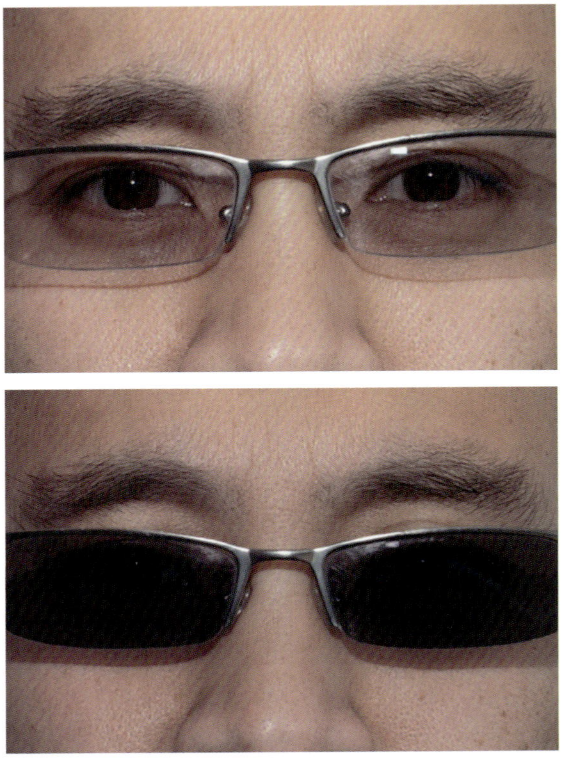

Figure 4-37 Photochromic lenses. *(Courtesy of Tommy Korn, MD.)*

Ultraviolet-absorbing lenses

The spectrum of ultraviolet (UV) light is divided into 3 types: UVA contains wavelengths of 400–320 nm, UVB contains wavelengths of 320–290 nm, and UVC contains wavelengths below 290 nm. The ozone layer of the atmosphere absorbs almost all UVC coming from the sun. Most exposure to UVC is from manufactured sources, including welding arcs, germicidal lamps, and excimer lasers. Of the total solar radiation falling on the earth, approximately 5% is UV light, of which 90% is UVA and 10% UVB.

The amount of UV light striking the earth varies with season (greatest in the summer), latitude (greatest near the equator), time of day (greatest at noon), and elevation (greatest at high elevation). UV light can also strike the eye by reflection. Fresh snow reflects between 60% and 80% of incident light; sand (beach, desert) reflects approximately 15% of incident light; and water reflects approximately 5% of incident light.

Laboratory experiments have shown that UV light damages living tissue in 2 ways. First, chemicals such as proteins, enzymes, nucleic acids, and cell-membrane components absorb UV light. When they do so, their molecular bonds (primarily the double bonds) may become disrupted. Second, these essential biochemicals may become disrupted by the action of free radicals (such as the superoxide radical). Free radicals can often be produced by UV light in the presence of oxygen and a photosensitizing pigment. For a fuller discussion of free radicals, see BCSC Section 2, *Fundamentals and Principles of Ophthalmology.*

Because it may take many years for UV light to damage eye tissue, a tight linkage between cause and effect is difficult to prove. Therefore, proof that UV light damages the eye comes primarily from acute animal experiments and epidemiologic studies covering large numbers of patients.

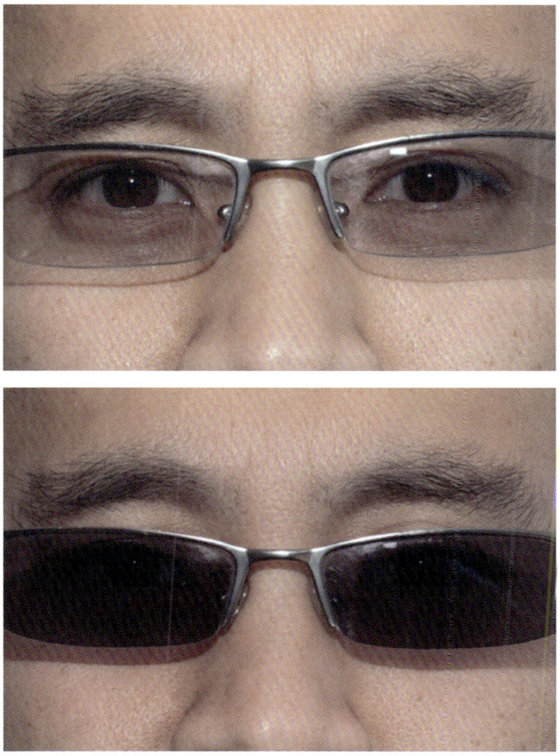

图 4–37　变色镜。*（译者注：资料来源见前页原文。）*

紫外线吸收镜片

紫外线（UV）光谱可分为 3 类：UV–A 包含 400~320 nm 波长，UV–B 包含 320~290 nm 波长，UV–C 包含 290 nm 以下波长。大气中的臭氧层吸收了几乎所有来自太阳的 UV–C。大多数暴露于空气中的 UV–C 来自人造光源，这些人造光源包括焊接电弧、杀菌灯和准分子激光。地球上的太阳总辐射中，大约 5% 是紫外光，其中 90% 是 UV–A，10% 是 UV–B。

地球上的紫外光总量随季节（夏季最大）、纬度（赤道附近最大）、日间时段（中午最大）和海拔（高海拔处最高）的变化而变化。紫外线也可以通过反射进入眼睛。雪地反射 60%~80% 的入射光；沙粒（海滩、沙漠）反射约 15% 的入射光；水反射约 5% 的入射光。

实验表明，紫外线通过 2 种途径损伤活体组织。第一，化学物质如蛋白质、酶、核酸和细胞膜成分吸收紫外光，使其分子键（主要是双键）断裂。第二，这些基本的生物化学物质被自由基（如超氧自由基）破坏。在氧和光敏色素存在条件下，紫外光会产生自由基。有关自由基更多的讨论，见 BCSC 第 2 册《*眼科基础与原理*》。

因为紫外线对眼组织造成损伤需要历经很多年，所以很难证明两者的相关因果关系。因此，紫外光的眼损伤结论主要来自急性动物实验和大样本患者的流行病学的研究结果。

Some surgeons routinely prescribe UV-absorbing glasses after surgery. Intraocular lenses incorporating UV-absorbing chromophores are now the norm. For further information regarding the effects of UV radiation on various ocular structures, see BCSC Section 8, *External Disease and Cornea*, and Section 12, *Retina and Vitreous*.

Almost all dark sunglasses absorb most incident UV light. The same is true for certain coated clear-glass lenses and clear plastic lenses made of CR-39 or polycarbonate. One suggestion has been that certain sunglasses (primarily light blue ones) may cause light damage to the eye. Proponents of this theory contended that the pupil dilates behind dark glasses and that if the sunglasses do not then absorb significant amounts of UV light, they will actually allow more UV light to enter the eye than if no sunglasses were worn. In fact, dark sunglasses reduce light levels striking the eye on a bright, sunny day to the range of 2000–6000 foot-lamberts. Such levels are approximately 10 times higher than those of an average lighted room. At such light levels, the pupil is significantly constricted. Thus, contrary to the preceding argument, dark sunglasses used on a bright day allow pupillary dilation of only a fraction of a millimeter and do not lead to light injury of the eye.

Special Lens Materials

It is important for the ophthalmologist to be aware of the variety of spectacle lens materials available. Four major properties are commonly discussed in relation to lens materials:

1. *Index of refraction.* As the refractive index increases, the thickness of the lens can be decreased to obtain the same optical power.
2. *Specific gravity.* As the specific gravity of a material decreases, the lens weight can be reduced.
3. *Abbe number (value).* This value indicates the degree of chromatic aberration or distortion that occurs because of the dispersion of light, primarily with off-axis viewing. Materials with a higher Abbe number exhibit less chromatic aberration and thus allow for higher optical quality.
4. *Impact resistance.* All lenses dispensed in the United States must meet impact-resistance requirements defined by the FDA (in 21CFR801.410), except in special cases wherein the physician or optometrist communicates in writing that such lenses would not fulfill the visual requirements of the particular patient. Lenses used for occupational and educational personal eye protection must also meet the impact-resistance requirements defined in the American National Standards Institute (ANSI) high-velocity impact standard (Z87.1). Lenses prescribed for children and active adults should also meet the ANSI Z87.1 standard, unless the patient is duly warned that he or she is not getting the most impact-resistant lenses available.

医生通常在手术后会开出吸收紫外线的眼镜处方，常规使用的是含有吸收紫外线成分的人工晶体。关于紫外线辐射对各眼部结构的影响，见 BCSC 第 8 册《*外眼疾病与角膜*》，以及第 12 册《*视网膜与玻璃体*》。

几乎所有的深色太阳镜都可以吸收大部分入射紫外光。某些镀膜镜片和 CR-39 或聚碳酸酯透明塑料镜片也是如此。某些建议提出一些特定的太阳镜（主要是浅蓝色的）可能会对眼睛造成轻微伤害。此理论支持者认为，在深色眼镜后面瞳孔会扩大，如果太阳镜不吸收紫外线，那么实际上会比不戴太阳镜时进入的紫外线更多。事实上，在明亮日光下，深色太阳镜会使进眼亮度降到 2 000~6 000ft · L。这种水平是房间平均照明水平的 10 倍。在这样的光照下，瞳孔明显收缩。因此，与前面的论点相反，在晴天使用的深色太阳镜，瞳孔开张不足 1mm，不会导致眼睛的光损伤。

特殊镜片材料

对于眼科医生来说，了解眼镜镜片材料的多样性是很重要的。与镜片材料有关的 4 个主要特性如下：

1. *折射率*。随着折射率的增加，透镜的厚度减小可以增加镜片的折射率，最终获得相同的屈光力。

2. *比重*。减少镜片材料的比重，可以减轻镜片重量。

3.*Abbe 数（值）*。这个值表示由于光的色散（主要是在离轴观看下）而发生的色差或失真的程度。Abbe 数较高的镜片材料表现出较少的色差，从而有更高的光学质量。

4.*抗冲击性*。在美国配制的所有镜片都必须符合 FDA（21CFR801.410）规定的抗冲击要求，除非由医生或验光师书面告知这种镜片不履行特殊患者视觉需求的职责。用于职业和教育要求的个人眼睛防护镜片也必须满足美国国家标准协会（ANSI）高速冲击标准（Z87.1）中规定的抗冲击要求。儿童和活动较多的成年人的镜片也应符合 ANSI Z87.1 标准，除非已提醒患者他们没有得到最有效的抗冲击镜片。

Standard glass

Glass lenses provide superior optics and are scratch resistant but also have several limitations, including low impact resistance, increased thickness, and heavy weight. Once the standard in the industry, glass lenses are less frequently used in current practice; many patients select plastic lenses. Without special treatment, glass lenses may be easily shattered. Chemical or thermal *tempering* increases the shatter resistance of glass, but if it is scratched or worked on with any tool after tempering, the shatter resistance is lost. Farmers appreciate photoreactive glass for its scratch resistance and easy care.Welders and grinders are better off with plastic, as small hot particles can become embedded in glass. Persons with myopia who desire thin glasses may choose high-index glass. The highest-index versions cannot be tempered and require that waivers be signed by patients who accept the danger of their breakage. High-index glass does not block UV light unless a coating is applied. (Characteristics of standard glass lenses are as follows: index of refraction, 1.52; Abbe number, 59; specific gravity, 2.54; impact resistance, pass FDA 21CFR801.410 if thick enough and chemically or heat treated.)

Standard plastic

Due to its high optical quality and light weight, standard plastic (also known as hard resin or CR-39) is the most commonly used lens material and is inexpensive. Standard plastic lenses are almost 50% lighter than glass lenses owing to the lower specific gravity of their material. They block 80% of UV light without treatment, can be tinted easily if desired, and can be coated to resist scratching and to provide further UV-light blocking. The index of refraction is not high, so the lenses are not thin. CR-39 lenses do not have the shatter resistance of polycarbonate or Trivex. (Characteristics of standard plastic lenses are as follows: index of refraction, 1.49; Abbe number, 58; specific gravity, 1.32; impact resistance, pass FDA 21CFR801.410.)

Polycarbonate

Introduced in the 1970s for ophthalmic lens use, the high-index plastic material polycarbonate has a low specific gravity and a higher refractive index, which allow for a light, thin lens. Polycarbonate is also durable and meets the high-velocity impact standard (ANSI Z87.1). One disadvantage of this material is the high degree of chromatic aberration, as indicated by its low Abbe number (30). Thus, color fringing can be an annoyance, particularly in strong prescriptions. Another disadvantage is that polycarbonate is the most easily scratched plastic, so a scratch-resistant coating is required. Also, if polycarbonate is cut too thin, it can flex on impact and pop out of the frame. (Characteristics of polycarbonate lenses are as follows: index of refraction, 1.58; Abbe number, 30; specific gravity, 1.20; impact resistance, pass FDA 21CFR801.410 and ANSI Z87.1.)

Trivex

Introduced in 2001, Trivex is a highly impact-resistant, low-density material that delivers strong optical performance and provides clear vision because of its high Abbe number. Its impact resistance is close to that of polycarbonate, and it blocks all UV light. Its index of refraction is not high, however, so the lenses are not thin. Trivex is the lightest lens material currently available and meets the high-velocity impact standard (ANSI Z87.1). Trivex material allows a comparably thin lens for the ±3.00D prescription range. A scratch-resistant coating is required. (Characteristics of Trivex lenses are as follows: index of refraction, 1.53; Abbe number, 45; specific gravity, 1.11; impact resistance, pass FDA 21CFR801.410 and ANSI Z87.1.)

标准玻璃镜片

玻璃镜片提供优越的光学性能和耐划伤性，但也有一些局限性，包括抗冲击性低、较厚和较重。一旦工业标准化，玻璃镜片则在实际中较少使用；许多患者会选择塑料镜片。如果没有特殊处理，玻璃镜片很容易破碎。化学或热*钢化*提高了玻璃的抗碎性，但如果在热钢化后用任何工具刮伤或加工，则会失去抗碎性。农场主多用光敏玻璃，因为其耐磨和易于护理；焊工和磨床工用塑料更好，因为小的热颗粒会嵌入玻璃中。近视眼可选择高折射率玻璃，但最高折射率型不能钢化，要求患者签署免责书，了解其破碎的危险。高折射率玻璃不阻挡紫外光，可以镀膜。（标准玻璃镜片的特性是：折射率 1.52；Abbe 数 59；比重 2.54；耐冲击性，如果足够厚并且经过化学或热处理，需达到 FDA 21CFR801.410 标准。）

标准塑料镜片

由于其光学质量高、重量轻，标准塑料（也被称为硬树脂或 CR–39）是最常用的镜片材料，并且价格便宜。标准塑料镜片比玻璃镜片轻近 50%，因为其材料的比重较低。它们不经过任何处理就可以阻挡 80% 的紫外光，如果需要很容易染色，还可以通过涂层抵抗划伤并阻挡紫外光。因折射率低，镜片较厚。CR–39 透镜不具有聚碳酸酯或 TrVeX 的抗碎性。（标准塑料镜片的特点是：折射率为 1.49；Abbe 数为 58；比重为 1.32；耐冲击性，达到 FDA 21CFR801.410 标准。）

聚碳酸酯镜片

20 世纪 70 年代聚碳酸酯镜片被引入眼用眼镜，塑料材料的聚碳酸酯具有高折射率、低比重和高折光率特性，所以制成的镜片更轻薄，很耐用，可以达到高速冲击标准（ANSI Z87.1）。这种材料的缺点是色差大，如其 Abbe 数（30）低。因此会产生干扰视觉的彩色条纹，特别是在高屈光度处方中。聚碳酸酯的另一个缺点是最容易被刮伤，需要一层耐刮擦涂层。此外，如果聚碳酸酯被切割得太薄，受冲击时会产生弯曲，并从镜框中被挤出。（聚碳酸酯透镜的特征是：折射率为 1.58；Abbe 数为 30；比重为 1.20；耐冲击性通过 FDA 21CFR801.410 和 ANSI Z87.1 标准。）

高氨基甲酸乙酯聚合物

Trivex 于 2001 年推出，是一种高抗冲击性、低密度材料，具有良好的光学性能，并因为阿贝数高，可提供清晰的视觉。它的抗冲击性接近聚碳酸酯，阻挡了所有的紫外光。然而，它的折射率并不高，所以镜片不薄。Trivex 是目前最轻的镜片材料，满足高速撞击标准（ANSI Z87.1）。Trivex 材料在 ±3.00 D 范围内时镜片较薄。需要一层耐刮擦涂层。（Trivex 透镜的特征是：折射率为 1.53；Abbe 数为 45；比重为 1.11；抗冲击性，达到 FDA 21CFR801.410 和 ANSI Z87.1 标准。）

High-index materials

A lens with a refractive index of 1.60 or higher is referred to as a high-index lens. High-index materials can be either glass or plastic and are most often used for higher-power prescriptions to create thin, cosmetically attractive lenses. The weight, optical clarity, and impact resistance of high-index lenses vary depending on the specific material used and the refractive index; in general, as the index of refraction increases, the weight of the material increases and the optical clarity (Abbe number) decreases. None of the high-index materials passes the ANSI Z87.1 standard for impact resistance. Plastic high-index materials require a scratch-resistant coating.

Strauss L. Spectacle lens materials, coatings, tints, and designs. *Focal Points: Clinical Modules for Ophthalmologists.* San Francisco: American Academy of Ophthalmology; 2005, module 11.

Therapeutic Use of Prisms

Small horizontal and vertical deviations can be corrected conveniently in spectacle lenses by the addition of prisms.

Horizontal heterophorias

Asthenopic symptoms may develop in patients (usually adults) if fusion is disrupted by inadequate vergence amplitudes; if fusion cannot be maintained, diplopia results. Thus, in patients with an exophoria at near, symptoms develop when the convergence reserve is inadequate for the task. Some patients can compensate for this fusional inadequacy through the improvement of fusional amplitudes. Younger patients may be able to do so through orthoptic exercises, which are sometimes used in conjunction with prisms that further stimulate their fusional capability (base-out prisms to enhance convergence reserve).

Symptoms may arise in some patients because of abnormally high accommodative convergence. Thus, an esophoria at near may be improved by full hyperopic correction for distance and/or by the use of bifocal lenses to decrease accommodative demand. In adult patients, orthoptic training and maximum refractive correction may be inadequate, and prisms or surgery may be necessary to restore binocularity.

Prisms are especially useful if a patient experiences an abrupt onset of symptoms secondary to a basic heterophoria or heterotropia. The prisms may be needed only temporarily, and the minimum amount of prism correction necessary to reestablish and maintain binocularity should be used.

Vertical heterophorias

Vertical fusional amplitudes are small ($<2.00\Delta D$). Thus, if a vertical muscle imbalance is sufficient to cause asthenopic symptoms or diplopia, it should be compensated for by the incorporation of prisms into the refractive correction. Once again, the minimum amount of prism needed to eliminate symptoms should be prescribed. In a noncomitant vertical heterophoria, the prism should be sufficient to correct the imbalance in primary gaze. With combined vertical and horizontal muscle imbalance, correcting only the vertical deviation may help improve control of the horizontal deviation as well. If the horizontal deviation is not adequately corrected, an oblique Fresnel prism may be helpful. A brief period of clinical heterophoria testing may be insufficient to unmask a latent muscle imbalance. Often, after prisms have been worn for a time, the phoria appears to increase, and the prism correction must be correspondingly increased.

高折射率材料

折射率为 1.60 或更高的镜片称为高折射率镜片。高折射率材料可以是玻璃或塑料，最常用于较高度数的处方，以便加工出较薄、美观的镜片。高折射率镜片的重量、光学清晰度和抗冲击性取决于所用的特定材料和折射率。一般来说，随着折射率的增加，材料的重量增加，光学清晰度（Abbe 数）降低。所有高折射率的材料都未达到 ANSI Z87.1 的耐冲击性标准。高折射率塑料材料则需要耐划伤涂层。

Strauss L. Spectacle lens materials, coatings, tints, and designs. *Focal Points: Clinical Modules for Ophthalmologists.* San Francisco: American Academy of Ophthalmology; 2005, module 11.

三棱镜的治疗作用

可以在眼镜镜片中附加棱镜有效地矫正小的水平和垂直斜视。

水平隐斜

如果聚散幅度不足导致的融合紊乱，患者（通常是成人）的视疲劳症状会发展；如果融合不能持久，就会出现复视。这样，有近距离外隐斜的患者，视近集合储备不足会加重症状。一些患者可以通过改善融合幅度来补偿融合不足。年轻患者可以通过视觉训练来达到目的，这些训练有时与棱镜结合使用，从而进一步刺激融合能力（底朝外棱镜加强集合储备）

一些患者可能会出现异常的高调调节性集合。因此，近距离内隐斜可以通过远距离远视全矫和（或）使用双焦镜减少调节需求来改善。在成人患者中，视觉训练和屈光全矫可能是不够的，还可能需要棱镜或手术恢复重建双眼视功能。如果患者突然出现继发于基本型隐斜或斜视的症状，棱镜尤其有用。棱镜可能只是暂时的需要，还需要使用最小量棱镜重新建立和维持双眼视。

垂直隐斜

垂直融合范围很小（＜ 2.00 ΔD），因此，如果一条垂直肌肉的不平衡就足以引起视疲劳症状或复视，应通过棱镜屈光矫正补偿。再次强调，应该用最小棱镜量来消除症状。在非共同的垂直隐斜，棱镜应纠正第一眼位的不平衡。同时有垂直和水平肌肉的不平衡时，只矫正垂直斜视也有助于改善水平斜视。如果水平斜视未被充分矫正，可使用斜向 Fresnel 棱镜。非功能性隐斜检查可能不足以发现潜在的肌肉不平衡。通常，在棱镜配戴一段时间后，隐斜可能增加，这时必须相应地增加矫正棱镜的数量。

Methods of prism correction

The potential effect of prisms should be evaluated by having the patient test the indicated prism in trial frames or trial lens clips over the current refractive correction. Temporary prisms in the form of clip-on lenses or Fresnel press-on prisms can be used to evaluate and alter the final prism requirement. The Fresnel prisms have several advantages: (1) they are lighter in weight (1 mm thick) and more acceptable cosmetically because they are affixed to the concave surface of the spectacle lens, and (2) they allow much larger prism corrections (up to 40.0Δ). With higher prism powers, however, it is not uncommon to observe a decrease in the visual acuity of the corrected eye. Patients may also observe chromatic fringes.

Prisms can be incorporated into spectacle lenses within the limits of cost, appearance, weight, and the technical skill of the optician. Prisms should be incorporated into the spectacle lens prescription only after an adequate trial of temporary prisms has established that the correction is appropriate and the deviation is stable.

Prism correction may also be achieved by decentering the optical center of the lens relative to the visual axis, although a substantial prism effect by means of this method is possible only with higher-power lenses. Aspheric lens designs are not suitable for decentration. (See earlier discussion of lens decentration and the Prentice rule.) Bifocal segments may be decentered in more than the customary amount to give a modest additional base-in effect to help patients with convergence insufficiency.

Management of Anisometropia

Table 4-4 highlights approaches to the management of anisometropia. These include full correction with adaptation, undercorrection of 1 eye to reduce anisometropia, contact lens wear (1 or both eyes), refractive surgery, reducing aniseikonia, and reducing induced vertical prismatic effect.

Table 4-4 Approaches to Anisometropia

- Full correction with adaptation: If the full correction of the more hyperopic eye is not tolerated, correct as much of the hyperopia as the patient can tolerate, and preserve the accurate difference between the 2 eyes. In children with refractive amblyopia, full correction of both eyes is frequently well tolerated, and may be sufficient to correct the amblyopia even without patching or atropine penalization.
- Under-correction of one eye to reduce anisometropia: In children under treatment for amblyopia, fully correct the amblyopic eye; in adults, fully correct the better-seeing (or dominant) eye.
- Contact lens wear (one or both eyes)
- Refractive surgery
- Reducing aniseikonia: Adjust lens base curve and center thickness of lenses to minimize effect on image size. Consider high refractive index lenses. Maintain the base curve and center thickness of current spectacles if they are well-tolerated.
- Reducing induced vertical prismatic effects: Separate single-vision distance and near glasses: Slab-off prism or dissimilar segment styles for bifocal corrections

棱镜矫正的方法

棱镜的潜在效果，应当通过让患者用插片法在屈光矫正的基础上来进行评估。可以临时用夹片或 Fresnel 压贴棱镜来评估和调整最终的棱镜需求。Fresnel 压贴棱镜有几个优点：①重量轻（1mm 厚），因为固定在镜片凹面上，所以更加美观；②棱镜矫正范围大（高达 40.0Δ）。然而，随着棱镜焦度的增高，有的患者矫正视力会下降，也会看到彩色条纹。

棱镜可以在成本、外观、重量和配镜师的技术等限制下被结合到眼镜的镜片中。只有充分地对临时棱镜进行矫正准确、眼位稳定之后，棱镜才能写入眼镜处方。

棱镜矫正也可以通过移心来实现，尽管这种方法只有在高度数镜片上才能产生显著的棱镜效果。非球面透镜设计不适合于移心。（见“镜片移心和 Prentice 规则”一节。）双焦点子片可超常移心，产生适度的底朝内效应，以补偿集合不足。

屈光参差处理

表 4–4 强调屈光参差的治疗方法。这些包括适应性全矫、单眼低矫以减少屈光参差、配戴接触镜（单眼或双眼）、屈光手术、减少双眼不等像，以及减少诱发的垂直棱镜效应。

表4–4　屈光参差的治疗

适应性全矫：如果高度远视眼不能够耐受全矫，则在患者可耐受范围内尽量多矫正远视，并保持两眼之间的准确差异。在屈光性弱视的患儿中，双眼全矫有很好的适应性，并且即使没有遮盖或使用阿托品压抑，弱视也可以被充分地矫治。

单眼低矫以减少屈光参差：在儿童弱视治疗中，应完全矫正弱视眼；在成人中，应完全矫正视力更好（或优势）的眼。

配戴膜接触镜（单眼或双眼）。
屈光手术。

减少双眼不等像：调整镜片基弧和中心厚度，以减小对像大小的影响。考虑高折射率镜片。如果它们被很好地耐受，就保持目前镜片的基弧和中心厚度。

减少诱发的垂直棱镜效应：分别用单焦的视远和视近眼镜；削薄棱镜或不同类型子片的双焦镜矫正。

Troubleshooting of Dissatisfied Spectacle Wearers

The management of dissatisfied spectacle wearers is both an art and a science. As in many areas of medicine, the management of expectations is critical. Demonstrations with trial frames and overrefracting with the patient's existing spectacles may be helpful tools. Major changes (such as cylinder axis changes) should be carefully evaluated and discussed with the patient prior to prescribing. Many potential problems can be prevented with appropriate attention during the prescribing and fitting process. A good working relationship with the optometrist and dispensing optician is critical. The written prescription is helpful in preventing problems. The interpupillary distance (monocular for PALs) should be included. Vertex distance should be specified for high prescriptions. The exact type of bifocal, trifocal, or PAL should be specified or noted if it should remain the same as in the current glasses. Any prismatic correction should be carefully noted, mentioning whether it is the same as the current glasses so that the dispensing optician can verify this. The dispensing optician has extensive latitude in the actual materials and coatings of the lens as well as the type and style of the bifocal and the vertex distance unless it is written on the prescription. For instance, if the prescriber wishes to keep the same base curve as the current spectacles (to decrease changes in image size in the case of anisometropia) this should be specified on the prescription. The lens material should be indicated, especially if it is a high-index or impact-resistant material. Any photochromic or lens tint or other coatings that the prescriber wants the spectacles to have should be specified.

A "balance lens" may be specified for a completely blind eye. This allows the dispensing optician to place a lens that is cosmetically similar to the fellow eye. In some cases, this may lessen the cost of the lens for the patient. Care must be taken in prescribing this for an eye with limited but usable vision (amblyopia, macular degeneration). Leaving the power of this lens at the discretion of the optician with only cosmetic concerns may cause functional problems.

Once the patient presents with dissatisfaction with a new spectacle correction, a detailed history of the problem must be performed. The nature of the complaint should be isolated, if possible, to its source: distance or near vision, static or dynamic, and blurring, distortion, and/or diplopia. The spectacle power and optic center should be determined and confirmed with that ordered. The refraction should be rechecked, especially in the case of a significant difference from the previous spectacle correction.

In the case where the previous spectacle correction is not different from the new one, then a comparison of other properties of the spectacles is helpful. In addition to the verification of the optical centers (induced prism), prismatic correction, or slab-off in the previous correction should also be present in the new prescription. Changes in base curve and center thickness (from old to new) may cause aniseikonia symptoms. If the previous prescription is very old, it should be checked with a Geneva lens clock for plus (front) cylinder design. Differences in bifocal type and position should be noted. Positioning and alignment of PALs should be noted. A change in model of PAL may cause significant problems. A change from traditional bifocals or trifocals to PALs may also be a source of problems. Vertex distance changes and pantoscopic tilt may lead to effective lens power differences. Finally, lens material changes may cause chromatic aberrations.

Milder B, Rubin M. *The Fine Art of Prescribing Glasses: Without Making a Spectacle of Yourself.* 3rd ed. Gainesville, FL: Triad Publishing Company; 2004.

处理戴镜不适的投诉

对眼镜配戴者不满意配戴效果的管理既是一门艺术，也是一门科学。和许多医学领域一样，对患者期望值的管理至关重要。用试镜架演示和在患者现有眼镜上验光都是有用的手段。根据患者先前的处方，主要变化（如柱镜轴的变化）应被仔细评估和探讨。只要在处方和装配中给予适当的注意，许多潜在的问题是可以避免的。视光师和配镜师良好的工作关系是至关重要的。书面处方有助于预防问题。瞳距（渐进多焦镜需单眼瞳距）也应包括在内。对于高度数处方，应指定顶点距离。如果瞳距保持与当前眼镜相同，则应该指定或注意双焦镜、三焦镜或渐进多焦镜的精确类型。任何棱镜矫正都应被仔细标注，提及是否与当前眼镜相同，以便配镜师能够核实到这点。配镜师在镜片的实际材料、涂层、双焦镜的类型和样式，以及顶点距离方面具有较大的自由度，但处方上没有注明的除外。例如，如果处方医师希望保持与现有眼镜相同的基弧（在屈光参差的病例减少像大小的变化），则应在处方上说明。应该指定镜片材料，特别是高折射率或抗冲击材料。处方医师希望镜片具有的变色或染色或镀膜明确指定。

一个“平衡镜片”可以被认定为完全盲眼。这允许配镜师放置一个外观与另外一只眼相似的眼镜。在一些病例中，这可以节约患者的镜片成本。开具处方时必须注意眼睛（弱视，黄斑变性）有限但可用的视力。配镜师仅考虑外观的处置而不管镜片的度数，可能会导致镜片的功能性问题。

一旦患者对新的眼镜矫正提出不满，就应该询问详细的病史。不应关注投诉的性质，应尽可能地了解投诉的根源：远视力或近视力、静态或动态、模糊、变形和（或）复视。眼镜的度数和光学中心应被确定。屈光度应该被重新检查，尤其是在与先前的眼镜矫正有显著差异的病例中。

在以前眼镜矫正和新的眼镜矫正没有差别的病例中，比较眼镜的其他特性是有帮助的。除了对光学中心（诱导棱镜）的验证外，在新处方中还应出现棱镜矫正或之前屈光矫正中的削薄。基弧和中心厚度的变化（从旧到新）可能引起双眼不等像症状。如果以前的处方很久了，应该用 Geneva 镜度表检查正（前表面）柱面设计。应注意双焦点类型和位置的差异。应注意渐进多焦点的定位和对准。渐进多焦镜样式的改变可能会引起明显问题。从传统的双焦镜或三焦镜到渐进多焦镜的改变也可能是问题的根源。顶点距离变化和前倾角可能导致有效的镜片度数的改变。最后，透镜材料的变化可能引起色差。

Milder B, Rubin M. *The Fine Art of Prescribing Glasses: Without Making a Spectacle of Yourself.* 3rd ed. Gainesville, FL: Triad Publishing Company; 2004.

Chapter Exercises

Questions

4.1. Which prescription represents a Jackson cross cylinder?

a. −2.00 +4.00 × 180

b. −1.00 +3.00 × 90

c. +2.00 +3.00 × 180

d. +1.00 −1.00 × 90

4.2. When performing cycloplegic retinoscopy on an anxious 7-year-old boy, you notice that the central reflex shows *with* movement while the peripheral reflex shows *against* movement. What is the most likely cause?

a. keratoconus

b. congenital cataract

c. spherical aberration

d. insufficient time for maximum cycloplegia

4.3. What type of distortion is shown in Figure 4-38 (page 394)?

a. pincushion distortion

b. barrel distortion

c. image jump

d. image displacement

4.4. A patient with +9.00 D spectacle lenses (vertex distance is 12 mm) requires a new spectacle frame because of recent nasal surgery. The vertex distance of the new frame is required to be 22 mm to avoid any nasal discomfort. What power is required for the new spectacles?

a. +7.25 D

b. +8.25 D

c. +9.25 D

d. +10.25 D

4.5. Based on the type of spectacle lenses shown in Figure 4-39, what is the patient's probable occupation?

a. retired investment banker or stockbroker

b. professional senior golfer

c. airline p ilot

d. jewelry or watch-repair technician

4.6. The Abbe number is a measure of what characteristic?

a. spherical aberration

b. chromatic aberration

c. image displacement in plus lenses

d. curvature of spectacle lenses

章节练习

问题

4.1　下面哪个处方代表 Jackson 交叉柱镜？

a.–2.00 +4.00 × 180

b.–1.00 +3.00 × 90

c.+2.00 +3.00 × 180

d.+1.00 –1.00 × 90

4.2　当对一个焦虑的 7 岁男孩做睫状肌麻痹检影时，你注意到中央反光*顺动*，而周边反光*逆动*。最可能的原因是什么？

a. 圆锥角膜

b. 先天性白内障

c. 球差

d. 最大化睫状肌麻痹时间不足

4.3　图 4–38（第 395 页）显示哪种类型的变形？

a. 枕形畸变

b. 桶形畸变

c. 像跳

d. 像移

4.4　一个戴 +9.00 D 眼镜的患者（顶点距离是 12 mm）最近做了鼻部手术，因而要求一个新的眼镜框。新镜框的顶点距离要求 22 mm，以避免鼻部不适。新眼镜的度数要求是多少？

a. +7.25 D

b. +8.25 D

c. +9.25 D

d. +10.25 D

4.5　根据图 4–39 所示的眼镜类型，患者可能的职业是什么？

a. 退休的投资银行家或股票经纪人

b. 职业年长的高尔夫球手

c. 航空飞行员

d. 珠宝或手表修理技师

4.6　Abbe 数是衡量什么特征的指标？

a. 球面像差

b. 色差

c. 正镜像移

d. 眼镜镜片曲率

4.7. Your refraction determines that a –8.00 D lens in a trial frame with a vertex distance of 10 mm from the patient's cornea provides 20/15 visual acuity. What is the minus power lens needed if the patient requires a vertex distance of 14 mm to use her favorite existing spectacle frame?
   a. –7.25 D
   b. –8.25 D
   c. –9.25 D
   d. –10.25 D

4.8. What is the primary reason that patients with presbyopia cannot tolerate significant anisometropia in bifocal lenses?
   a. asthenopia
   b. inability of the lens to accommodate and correct any hyperopic error
   c. reduced vertical fusion amplitude
   d. spherical aberration

4.9. In bifocal lens design, image jump may be minimized by which step?
   a. placing the optical center of the segment as close as possible to the top of the segment
   b. placing the top of the segment as close as possible to the distance optical center
   c. using a smaller bifocal segment
   d. using a blended bifocal segment that has no visible line of separation
   e. lowering the bifocal segment by 3 mm

4.10. An angle of 45° corresponds to how many prism diopters (Δ)?
   a. 45.0 Δ
   b. 22.5 Δ
   c. 90.0 Δ
   d. 100.0 Δ

4.11. Which statement applies to bifocal lenses that are prescribed for a patient with myopia?
   a. The practitioner should leave the choice of the segment type to the optician.
   b. A round-top segment is preferred because of its thin upper edge, which causes less prismatic effect.
   c. A flat-top segment is preferred because it lessens image jump.
   d. The 1-piece shape is indicated for adds greater than +2.00 D.
   e. A split bifocal should be used because patients with myopia do not accept bifocal lenses easily.

4.12. An aphakic contact lens wearer (+13.00 soft contact lens in each eye) needs to switch to spectacles but finds that she experiences diplopia at near. What prismatic correction would you expect to correct her diplopia?
   a. base-up prism
   b. base-in prism
   c. oblique prism
   d. base-out prism

4.7　你的验光决定了试镜架上 –8.00 D 镜片距患者角膜 10 mm 的顶点距离可以提供 20/15 的视力。如果患者要使用顶点距离为 14 mm 的最喜欢的镜架，那么需要多少负镜度数？

a. –7.25 D
b. –8.25 D
c. –9.25 D
d. –10.25 D

4.8　戴双焦镜片老视患者不能耐受显著屈光参差的主要原因是什么？

a. 眼疲劳
b. 镜片的调节和矫正远视的不适应
c. 减少垂直融合像的幅度
d. 球面像差

4.9　在双焦点镜片设计中，像跳可以通过哪一步来最小化？

a. 将子片的光学中心尽量靠近子片顶部
b. 将子片顶部尽可能靠近远用区光心
c. 使用较小的双焦子片
d. 使用没有可见分离线的双焦子片
e. 双焦子片下降 3 mm

4.10　45° 角对应多少棱镜度（Δ）？

a. 45.0 Δ
b. 22.5 Δ
c. 90.0 Δ
d. 100.0 Δ

4.11　哪种说法适用于近视患者的双焦镜？

a. 执业者应当把子片类型的选择给验光师。
b. 推荐圆顶子片，因为其更薄的边缘使得棱镜效应不明显。
c. 推荐平顶子片，因为其减少像跳。
d. 附加度超过 +2.00 D，使用整体形状。
e. 由于近视患者很难接受双焦点镜片，应当使用分离双焦镜。

4.12　一个无晶体隐形眼镜的配带者（双眼均为 +13.00 软性隐形眼镜）需要更换眼镜，但发现近距离复视。用什么样的棱镜矫正可以纠正她的复视？

a. 底向上三棱镜
b. 底向内三棱镜
c. 斜向三棱镜
d. 底向外三棱镜

4.13. A patient who has just been prescribed new progressive addition lenses returns with the complaint that he needs to tilt his chin up in order to see clearly at distance. What is the most likely source of the problem?
a. add power that is too strong
b. add power that is positioned too high
c. undercorrected hyperopia or overcorrected myopia
d. incorrect optical centers

4.14. Following cataract surgery in the left eye, the patient has a refraction of right, −3.50 D; left, −0.50 D. You prescribe this with a +2.50 flat-top bifocal set 3 mm below the optical center of the lens. How much induced prism will there be when the patient is looking 4 mm below the top of the bifocal?
a. 1.2Δ base down in the right eye
b. no induced prism
c. 0.9Δ base down in the right eye
d. 2.1Δ base down in the right eye

Answers

4.1. **a.** The Jackson cross cylinder is a lens made of 2 cylinders of equal but opposite magnitude placed at 90° relative to each other; the spherical equivalent of the resulting lens is zero (see Fig 4-17). High-power Jackson cross cylinders are especially useful in refining the refraction in low vision patients.

4.2. **c.** Spherical aberration occurs in patients with large or dilated pupils. This aberration is caused when light rays are refracted as they travel through a widely dilated pupil and strike the peripheral crystalline lens. The periphery of the human lens is more curved than the center, so the incoming light rays show increased refraction compared with the light rays that strike the central lens. In retinoscopy, this can result in the appearance of different central and peripheral reflexes. Thus, it is always important to concentrate on the central light reflex when performing retinoscopy.

4.3. **b.** Figure 4-38 depicts a high-minus spectacle lens where there is minification of the image. Note the barrel-shaped distortion of the Amsler grid as viewed through the lens.

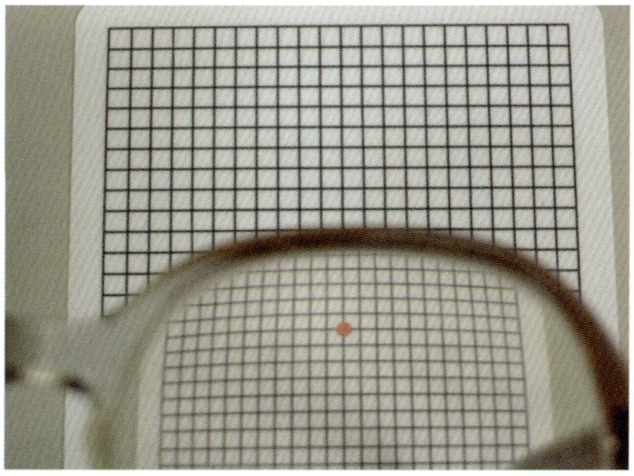

Figure 4-38 *(Courtesy of Tommy Korn, MD.)*

4.13 一位刚配了新型渐进多焦点镜片的患者回来时抱怨说，他需要抬起下巴才能看清远处。这个问题最有可能的原因是什么？

a. 附加度数过多
b. 附加度数位置过高
c. 欠矫远视或过矫近视
d. 光学中心不正确

4.14 在左眼白内障手术后，患者验光为右眼 –3.50D，左眼 –0.50D。你的配镜处方里使用 +2.50 平顶双焦镜设置在镜片光学中心下方 3mm 处。当患者看双焦镜顶部下方 4mm 时，会有多少诱导棱镜？

a. 右眼 1.2Δ 底向下
b. 无诱导棱镜
c. 右眼 0.9Δ 底向下
d. 右眼 2.1Δ 底向下

答案

4.1 **a**。Jackson 交叉柱镜是由 2 个大小相等、符号相反、相互垂直轴的柱镜构成的镜片，联合镜片的球镜等效为零（参见图 4–17）。高度数 Jackson 交叉柱镜特别适用于改善低视力患者的验光。

4.2 **c**。瞳孔较大或散瞳者出现球面像差。这种像差是由于光线在通过扩大的瞳孔并穿过晶状体周边形成的。人晶状体的周边比中心更弯曲，所以入射的光线与入射到晶体中央的光线相比折射作用增加。在检影中，这会导致中央和周边反光出现不同。因此，在进行检影时，注意力始终集中于中央光反光是非常重要的。

4.3 **b**。图 4–38 描述了高度数负镜缩小的像。注意透过镜片看到 Amsler 方格的桶形畸变。

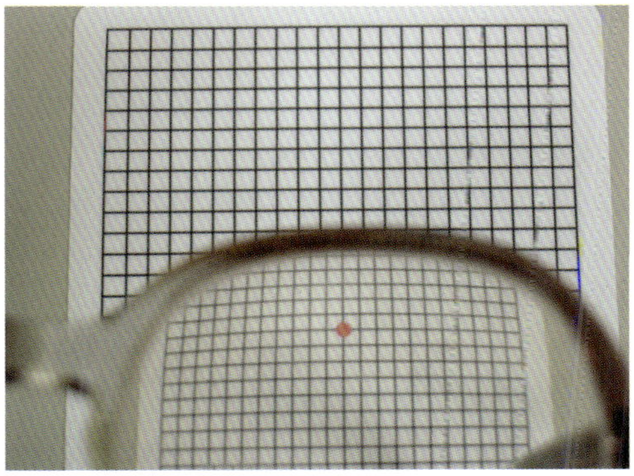

图 4–38　高度数负镜缩小的像。*（译者注：资料来源见前页原文。）*

4.4. **b.** The far point of a +9.00 D lens is 111 mm (1/9 m) behind the lens. However, for the old lens to focus the image on the retina, it must be held by the frame 12 mm in front of the cornea. Thus, the far point of the patient's hyperopia is located 99 mm (111 mm –2 mm) behind the cornea. If the new frame is to be located 22 mm in front of the cornea, it should be placed 121 mm (99 mm + 22 mm) in front of the far point of the patient's hyperopia. The power required for this new lens, therefore, is 1/0.121 m = +8.26 D. Because spectacle lenses come in 0.25 D steps, the answer is +8.25 D + 9.00 D.

4.5. **c.** Figure 4-39 depicts an occupational multifocal lens known as a double D. This type of lens has the additive near power at the top and bottom of the spectacle lens; the distance power is in the middle. This design is especially useful for airline pilots, who must frequently look up at cockpit instrument panels that are in close proximity to one another and look down at printed flight material.

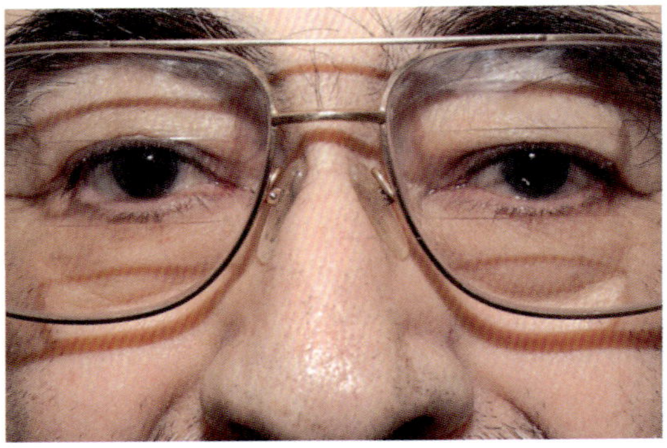

Figure 4-39 *(Courtesy of Tommy Korn, MD.)*

4.6. **b.** The Abbe number is a measure of chromatic aberration. The lower the Abbe number, the higher the amount of chromatic aberration present in the lens material. Spectacle lenses with a low Abbe number often require antireflective coating to minimize chromatic aberration that arises particularly when bright indoor light reflects off the lenses.

4.7. **b.** The far point of a –8.00 D lens is 125 mm (1/8 m) and is located in front of the lens. A patient's myopic refractive error is corrected with a –8.00 D trial lens when the lens is placed 10 mm in front of the cornea (Fig 4-40). If the lens is moved to 14 mm in front of the cornea with her existing frame, the far point remains the same distance from the original –8.00 D lens. The location of the existing frame from the far point is 135 mm –14 mm = 121 mm. The power of the lens must then be 1/0.121 m = –8.26 D. Because spectacle lenses come in 0.25 D increments, the answer is –8.25 D.

4.8. **c.** When a patient has anisometropia, which may arise after cataract surgery, for example, a large vertical prismatic effect is induced in the bifocal add. When the patient suddenly looks through the top of the bifocal segment, image jump occurs because of vertical prismatic effects through the spectacle lenses. Image jump is a problem because the human brain has a very limited capacity to fuse 2 images that are separated vertically, as in the case of a bifocal lens with anisometropia.

4.9. **a.** As the eyes look down to read through the add segment, there is an abrupt upward image jump at the top edge of the segment. This jump is due to the prismatic effect of the plus lens (the add segment). On the basis of the Prentice rule, the amount of jump depends on the power of the segment and on the distance from the top of the segment to the optical center of the segment.

4.4　**b**。透镜的远点在透镜后面 111mm（1/9m）。然而，为了用旧镜将像聚焦在视网膜上，框架镜必须保持在角膜前 12mm。因此，远视患者的远点立于角膜后 99mm（111mm–12mm）。如果新框架镜位于角膜前面 22mm，它应该放置在患者远视远点前面 121mm（99mm+22mm）。因此，这个新镜片所需的度数为 1 / 0.121m = 8.25 D。因为眼镜片 0.25D 的间隔，所以答案是 8.25 D。

4.5　**c**。图 4–39 描述了一种被称为双 D 的职业多焦点透镜。这种镜片具有在眼镜镜片的顶部和底部有增加的近度数，远距离度数在中间。这种设计尤其对航空飞行员有用，他们必须经常抬头看身边的驾驶舱仪表板，并向下看打印的飞行材料。

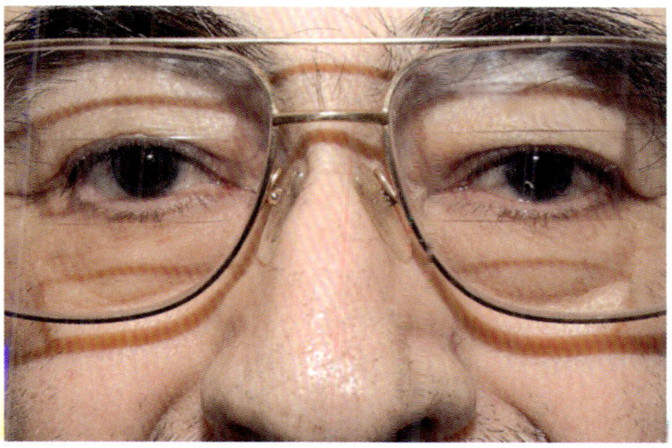

图 4–39　双 D 职业多焦点透镜。

（译者注：资料来源见前页原文。）

4.6　**b**。阿贝数是评估色差的。阿贝数越低，镜片材料中的色差量越高。低阿贝数的镜片通常需要抗反射涂层，以最小化色差，尤其是当明亮的室内光从镜片上反射的时候。

4.7　**b**。–8.00 D 镜片的远点立于镜片前 125 mm（1/8 m）处。当镜片放置在角膜前 10mm 时，–8.00 D 试验镜片矫正患者的近视屈光不正（图 4–40）。如果用现有的框架将镜片移动到角膜前面 14 mm，则远点与原来的 –8.00 D 镜片保持相同的距离。现有镜框的位置远点是 135 mm–14 mm = 121 mm。镜片的屈光力现在是 1/0.121 m = –8.26 D。因为眼镜镜片以 0.25 D 递增，所以答案是 8.25 D。

4.8　**c**。当患者有屈光参差，在白内障手术后可能会加重。例如，在双焦镜附加诱发一个大的垂直棱镜效应。当患者突然从双焦镜子片的顶部看时，由于通过眼镜的垂直棱镜效应，发生像跳。像跳是一个重要问题，因为人脑融合垂直分离的 2 个像的能力非常有限，就像戴双光镜具有屈光参差一样。

4.9　**a**。当眼睛通过附加子片向下看时，在子片的顶端边缘出现突然向上的像跳。这种跳跃是由于正镜片的棱镜效应（附加子片）。根据 Prentice 原则，跳跃量是由子片焦度及从子片顶部到子片光学中心的距离决定的。

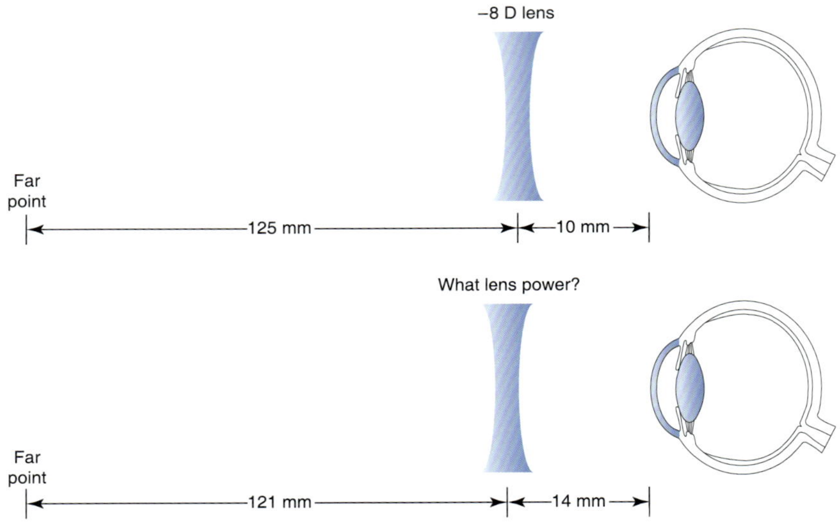

Figure 4-40 *(Illustration developed by Tommy Korn, MD.)*

4.10. **d.** As a general rule, the number of prism diopters is approximately twice the angle in degrees. However, this equation works only for small angles (<20°). An angle of 45° means that at 1 m, a beam is deviated by 1 m (100 cm). Thus, 45° corresponds to 100.0Δ. An angle of 90° corresponds to infinity in prism diopters.

4.11. **c.** In general, patients perceive image jump as a greater problem than image displacement. Flat-top segments minimize image jump because the optical center is near the top. In patients with myopia, flat-top segments also reduce prism displacement because the base-down effect of the distance portion is reduced by the base-up effect of the segment.

4.12. **d.** Aphakic spectacles will generate base-in prism with convergence when compared to contact lens correction. Adjustment of the optical centers, addition of base-out prism, or single-vision reading glasses may improve this problem.

4.13 **c.** In the chin-up position, the patient is effectively adding plus power to the distance prescription by viewing through the upper portion of the add. The patient has either undercorrected hyperopia or overcorrected myopia.

4.14 **d.** The induced prism is a result of the anisometropia of the distance correction. The bifocal add is equal, and there should be no induced prism contribution from that. If the top of the bifocal is 3 mm below the optical center of the lens and the patient is looking 4 mm below that, then the distance for the Prentice rule is 7 mm and the power difference is 3 D; therefore, 2.1Δ with the induced prism base in the more myopic correction (right side).

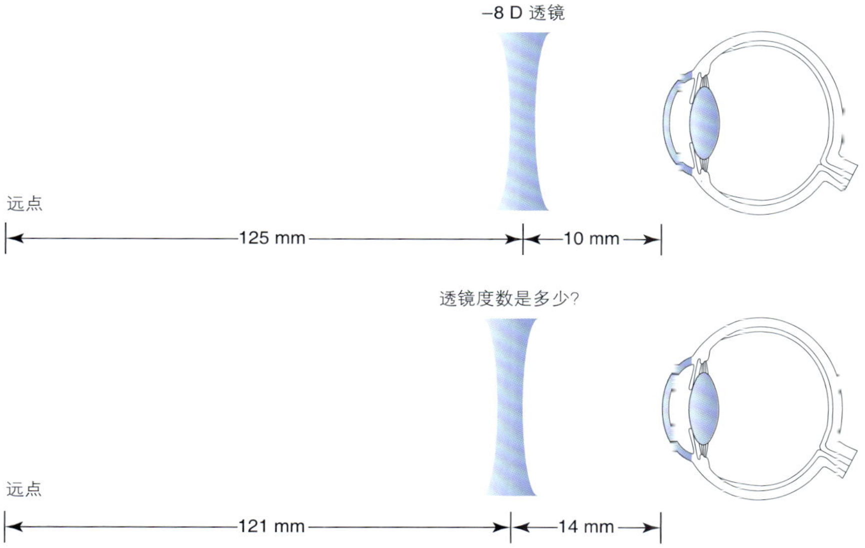

图 4–40　近视屈光不正的矫正。*（译者注：资料来源见前页原文。）*

4.10　**d**。一般来说，棱镜度的数量大约是圆周度的 2 倍。然而，这个方程只适用于小角度（< 20°）。45° 角意味着在 1 m 处，光束偏离 1m（100 cm）。因此，45° 对应于 100.0 Δ。90° 角对应于无穷大棱镜度。

4.11　**c**。一般来说，患者感觉像跳比像移问题更大。因为光学中心接近顶部，顶部平坦子片可使像跳最小化。在近视患者，平顶子片还减少棱镜位移，因为子片的底向上效应可降低远距离部分的底向下效应。

4.12　**d**。与接触镜矫正相比，无晶状体眼集合时，眼镜将产生底向内棱镜作用。调整光学中心，添加底向外棱镜，或者单焦点阅读眼镜可以改善这个问题。

4.13　**c**。在下颌上抬位，患者通过从下加镜上部分观看，有效地给远距离处方增加了正度数。患者要么有欠矫远视，要么有过矫近视。

4.14　**d**。诱导棱镜是远距矫正屈光参差的结果。双焦镜附加度是相等的，不应该有诱导棱镜的作用。如果双焦镜的顶部比镜片光学中心低 3 mm，并且患者通过子片顶下方 4 mm 看，那么 Prentice 规则的距离是 7mm，并且焦度差是 3.00 D。因此，在近视度更高的眼（右眼），底向下 2.1Δ 诱导棱镜。

（翻译　石蕊　杨乐　谭薇　王涛　张乐　肖勇 // 审校　肖勇　石一宁）

CHAPTER 5

Contact Lenses

Highlights

- optical differences between spectacles and contact lenses.
- contact lens types: soft and rigid, gas permeability, surface characteristics.
- contact lens correction of astigmatism.
- contact lenses for abnormal corneas.
- care of contact lenses, roles of the practitioner and patient.
- contact lens complications.

Glossary

Apical zone of the cornea, corneal apex The steepest part of the cornea, normally including its geometric center, usually 3–4 mm in diameter.

Base curve The curvature of the central posterior surface of the lens, which is adjacent to the cornea, described by its radius of curvature (mm). Base curves and peripheral curvatures of contact lenses are chosen to achieve a good fit of the lens to the cornea.

Diameter (chord diameter) The width of the contact lens, from edge to edge. The diameter of soft contact lenses, for example, ranges from 13 mm to 15 mm, whereas that of rigid gas-permeable (RGP) lenses ranges from 9 mm to 10 mm.

Optical zone The central area of the contact lens. The curvature of its anterior surface is designed to yield the desired refractive power of the lens.

Peripheral curves Secondary curves of the posterior lens surface away from the center, nearer the lens edge. These curves are flatter than the central posterior "base" curve to approximate the normal flattening of the peripheral cornea and achieve a desired fit. Junctions between central and more peripheral curvatures are smoothed or "blended" or maybe continuously graduated.

Sagittal depth or vault The distance between the center of the posterior surface to the plane of the edges of the lens. If the diameter of the lens is held constant, the sagittal depth decreases as the base curve radius increases.

Tear lens The lens formed by the tears that fill in the space between a contact lens and the cornea.

第 5 章

接触镜

重点

- 框架眼镜与接触镜的光学差异。
- 接触镜种类：软镜和硬镜、透氧率、表面特性。
- 接触镜矫正散光。
- 异常角膜的接触镜验配。
- 接触镜的护理，验配师和患者的角色。
- 接触镜并发症。

术语

角膜顶点区域，角膜顶点 包括角膜几何中心，3~4 mm 直径内最陡峭的区域。

基弧 与角膜相邻的接触镜中央后表面的曲率，用曲率半径（mm）来记录。接触镜的基弧和边弧选择应和角膜相匹配。

直径（弦长） 接触镜边到边的距离。软镜的直径为 13~15 mm，硬性透气性接触镜（RGP）的直径为 9~10 mm。

光学区 接触镜的中央区域。前表面曲率决定了镜片的焦度。

边弧 接触镜后表面远离中央区、靠近边缘部分的第二弧区。边弧曲率较基弧平坦，这是为了配合这一区域角膜的曲率变平、达到理想适配而设计的。中央区与多个边弧区的连接部变得平滑、协调、逐渐接续。

矢深或拱高 后表面中心到镜片边缘平面的垂直距离。如果镜片直径不变，矢高减小，表示镜片的基弧半径变大。

泪液镜 由充满在接触镜与角膜表面间的泪液形成。

Wetting angle The wettability of a lens surface. A low wetting angle means water will spread over the surface, increasing surface wettability, whereas a high wetting angle means that waterwill bead up, decreasing surface wettability. A lower wetting angle (greater wettability) generally translates into better lens comfort and vision.

Introduction

About 50% of adults in the United States (US) use glasses or contact lenses. A quarter of those use contact lenses; 90%, soft lenses; and 10%, rigid gas-permeable (RGP) lenses. There is increasing use of scleral RGP lenses. These preferences vary around the world; for example, half the lenses fit in Germany are RGP material. Table 5-1 summarizes optical considerations of contact lenses

Morgan PB, Woods CA, Tranoudis IG, et al. International contact lens prescribing in 2016.*Contact Lens Spectrum.* 2017(1):30–35.

Nichols JJ. Contact lenses 2016. *Contact Lens Spectrum.* 2017;32(1):22–25, 27, 29, 55.

Contact Lens Optics

When a contact lens is in placed on the cornea, most of the refraction occurs at the interface between air and the tear film on the anterior surface of the contact lens. Corneal contact lenses are only about 3 mm in front of the eye's first principal plane, where refraction may be considered to occur. The lenses turn with the eye, so that compared to a spectacle lens 12 mm in front of a rotating eye, there is less aberrational blur, distortion, and magnification/minification. Spectacle lenses have complementary optical advantages, offering stable vision and the ability to design more useful bifocals and to apply prism when needed.

Anisometropia and Image Size

When one eye is much more myopic or hyperopic than the other, spectacle correction creates retinal images of unequal size, unless the difference is caused primarily by unequal axial lengths (Clinical Example 5-1). Also, as the eyes look off-axis, through parts of the spectacle lenses farther from their optical centers, the eyes encounter unequal prism, following the Prentice rule (see Chapter 4). This is particularly disturbing, looking down to view through bifocal segments, as it does not take much unequal vertical prism to cause discomfort or diplopia. To deal with this, it may be necessary to "slab-off" prism on one of the bifocal segments (see Chapter 4).

On the other hand, contact lenses of unequal powers yield retinal images that are of almost equal size, if the eyes are of similar length. The lenses move with the eyes, so there is little induced prismatic effect. Unilateral aphakia is an extreme example of anisometropia, with the aphakic eye usually much more hyperopic than its fellow eye. Typically, the aphakic spectacle lens magnifies the retinal image about 25% larger than it would be in an emmetropic eye of the same length, whereas a contact lens magnifies it about 7%. To understand this "relative spectacle magnification," imagine starting with emmetropic eyes and instead of removing the natural lens of one eye, neutralize the lens's power with a minus lens just in front of the natural lens, and place a correcting plus-powered spectacle lens 12 mm in front of the eye. Those 2 lenses create a magnifying Galilean telescope effect, which enlarges the retinal image.

湿润角　描述接触镜表面的湿润性。湿润角小意味着水将扩散到镜片表面上，表面润湿性增加。而湿润角大，意味着镜片表面形成水珠，表面润湿性降低。较小的湿润角（更大的湿润性）通常意味着更好的戴镜舒适度和视觉效果。

引言

美国约有 50% 的成人使用框架镜或接触镜。戴镜人群中 1/4 配戴接触镜，其中 90% 配戴软性接触镜，另外 10% 配戴硬性透气性接触镜（RGP）。现在配戴巩膜 RGP 镜的人也在增加。各国人群的偏好不同，例如在德国，一半的人配戴 RGP。表 5-1 总结了接触镜的光学特性与选择。

Morgan PB, Woods CA, Tranoudis IG, et al. International contact lens prescribing in 2016.*Contact Lens Spectrum*. 2017(1):30–35.

Nichols JJ. Contact lenses 2016. *Contact Lens Spectrum*. 2017;32(1):22–25, 27, 29, 55.

接触镜光学

当接触镜放置到角膜上，大部分的折射发生在镜片前表面由泪液与空气形成的界面上。接触镜在眼的第一主平面前约 3 mm 处，主平面被认为发生折射。接触镜随眼球一起转动，框架镜距离眼表 12 mm。与框架镜相比，接触镜有更小的像差性模糊，畸变和放大 / 缩小。框架镜也有一些互补的光学优势，可以提供稳定的视觉，可以有更有效的双焦点设计，还能按需提供棱镜。

屈光参差与成像大小

当一只眼的近视或远视较对侧眼严重时，除了眼轴差异这一因素造成视网膜成像大小有差异（临床案例 5-1）外，框架镜的矫正也会造成视网膜成像大小的差异。而且，依据 Prentice 法则（见第 4 章），当眼睛离轴注视，即从框架镜远离光学中心处看出去时，产生双眼的不等棱镜效果。当向下通过双焦点镜片看时，不适症状会加重，因为少量的不等量垂直棱镜就会带来不适或复视。为解决这一问题，需要“去除”一边双焦点镜片上的棱镜来补尝（见第 4 章）。

另外，双眼眼轴相同而接触镜度数不一致时，视网膜成像大小也基本一致。接触镜随眼球一起运动，所以很少带来棱镜效应。单眼无晶体眼是屈光参差的一个特例，无晶体眼远视度数较对侧眼高很多。与同等眼轴的正视眼视网膜像相比，无晶体眼的框架镜视网膜像放大了 25%，而接触镜仅放大 7%。为了理解这种“相对眼镜放大率”的效果，我们可以设想成用正视眼代替无晶体眼，并在晶状体前用 1 个负透镜中和晶状体的屈光力，再在眼前 12mm 处放置 1 个矫正性的正度数框架镜。这 2 个镜片产生了 Galileo 望远镜的放大效果，从而使视网膜成像变大。

Table 5-1 Optical Considerations of Contact Lenses

Type of Lens	Indications	Optical Characteristics
Soft spherical	Myopia or hyperopia with little or no astigmatism	May "mask" mild astigmatism.
Soft toric	Myopia, hyperopia, mild to moderate amount of regular astigmatism	Lens must maintain toric axis position through ballast, thin areas, or edge shape. May be used to correct corneal and lenticular astigmatism.
Soft bifocal alternating vision	Presbyopia, regular refractive errors	The lens translates up on the cornea during downgaze by the lower lid. The inferior periphery of the lens contains the near prescription.
Soft bifocal simultaneous vision	Presbyopia, regular refractive errors	Concentric rings or aspheric design gives simultaneous focus of distance and near objects.
Rigid gas-permeable (RGP) spherical	Myopia, hyperopia, regular and irregular astigmatism	Corrects corneal but not lenticular astigmatism.
RGP posterior toric	Has a posterior toric surface to match the cornea; especially effective to treat against-the-rule astigmatism	The toric surface matching that of the cornea helps position the lens.
RGP bitoric	Useful for higher amounts of astigmatism, has toric shape on both sides	The anterior toric shape can be used to correct whatever "residual" refractive error is not corrected by the posterior surface.
RGP bifocal alternating or simultaneous	May be used with regular and irregular corneas	Similar to soft bifocal lenses.
Hybrid	Keratoconus, postkeratoplasty; other irregular corneas	Combines the comfort and fitting properties of soft contact lenses with the ability of rigid lenses to correct irregular corneas.
Scleral	Keratoconus, postkeratoplasty; other irregular corneas. Also useful in creating a therapeutic environment in ocular surface disease such as Stevens–Johnson syndrome and graft-vs-host disease	

Accommodation

When an eye is corrected for distance, how much accommodation is required to focus the image of a near object? Compared with spectacles, contact lenses increase the accommodative demand for myopic eyes and decrease it for hyperopic eyes in proportion to the size of the refractive error.

表5–1　接触镜的光学特性与选择

类型	适应症	光学特性
软性球镜	伴有少量散光或无散光的近视或远视	可矫正少量散光
软性复曲面镜	近视、远视、轻度/中度规则散光	镜片轴位维持需通过镜片的垂重、薄型区域、边缘形状设计等方法，可用于矫正角膜及晶状体散光
软性双焦点镜 交替视	老视，规则的屈光不正	向下注视时，下眼睑将镜片上移到角膜上。镜片下方区域包含了近用度数
软性双焦点镜 同时视	老视，规则的屈光不正	同心环或非球面设计，同时视远和视近
球面硬性透气性接触镜（RGP）	近视、远视、规则和不规则散光	矫正角膜散光，但不矫正晶状体散光
后复曲面RGP	后表面为复曲面设计,用来契合角膜形态，尤其适用于矫正逆规散光	后表面的复曲面设计与角膜形态契合，有助于镜片位置的稳定
双复曲面镜RGP	前后表面均为复曲面设计，适用于高散光	前复曲面设计可用于矫正无法被后复曲面矫正的“残余”散光度数
RGP双焦点镜 交替视或同时视	可用于规则或不规则角膜	同软性双焦点镜
混合镜片	圆锥角膜，角膜移植术后及其他不规则角膜	软镜的舒适性和适应性与硬镜对不规则角膜的矫正功能相结合
巩膜镜	用于圆锥角膜，角膜移植术后及其他不规则角膜。也用于诸如Stevens－Johnson综合征和移植排斥反应等眼表疾病，有助建立眼表治疗环境	

调节

当一只眼视远已矫正，即视近时需要多少调节？与框架镜相比较，接触镜增加了近视眼的调节需求，减少了远视眼的调节需求，并且依屈光不正的程度不同或比例改变。

Clinical Example 5-2 and Figure 5-1 illustrate accommodative demand. For an emmetropic eye to read print that is one-third meter away, it needs to accommodate 3 diopters. Suppose that the eye is myopic, instead of emmetropic, and has a –7.00 D spectacle lens 15 mm in front of it, which exactly corrects its myopia for distance viewing. Parallel rays passing through the lens have divergence of –6.3 D when they reach the cornea, and the eye effortlessly focuses those rays on the retina. A pencil of rays coming from an object one-third meter in front of that eye has about –3 D divergence when it reaches the –7.00D lens, and therefore –10 D leaving the lens. After traversing the 15 mm from the lens to the cornea, it has –8.7 D divergence. In order to focus the pencil on the retina, which requires the pencil to have –6.3 D divergence at the cornea, the required accommodation is the difference, which is 2.4 D. This is the "near effectivity" of the myopic spectacles, reducing accommodative demand, in this case, from 3 D to 2.4 D. If we correct the same eye with a contact lens, a –6.30 D contact lens is required to replace the –7.00 D spectacle lens for distance viewing, and the full 3 D of accommodation is required to read the print at one-third meter. Thus, contact lenses eliminate the *accommodative advantage* enjoyed by those with spectacle-corrected myopia and the *disadvantage* experienced by those with spectacle-corrected hyperopia. A 42-year-old person with myopia who is getting along well enough with –5.00 D glasses may find reading with contact lenses difficult, even though both the glasses and contacts are correct for distance. Conversely, a 38-year-old person with hyperopia, beginning to have symptoms of presbyopia with glasses, will have easier near vision with contact lenses fitted to correct distance vision, than with the glasses.

CLINICAL EXAMPLE 5-1

Fitting a unilateral aphakic eye causes diplopia that persists in the presence of prisms that superimpose the 2 images. The refractive error of the fellow eye is –5.00 D, and the image of the aphakic eye is described as larger than that of the fellow myopic eye. How can the diplopia be resolved?

The goal is to reduce the aniseikonia of the 2 eyes by magnifying the image size of the phakic eye and/or reducing the image size of the contact lens–corrected aphakic eye. To achieve the former, correct the myopic phakic eye with a contact lens to increase its image size. If this is inadequate, overcorrect the contact lens for the aphakic eye by +5.00 D and prescribe a spectacle lens of –5.25 D for that eye, in effect introducing a reverse Galilean telescope. If, however, the phakic eye were hyperopic, its image size would be increased by correcting its refractive error with a spectacle lens rather than a contact lens.

CLINICAL EXAMPLE 5-2

What is the accommodative demand of a –7 D myopic eye corrected with a spectacle lens compared with a contact lens? A +7 D hyperopic eye? Assume a vertex distance of 15 mm and a near-object distance of 33.3 cm.

The myopic refractive error of the first eye is –7 D at a vertex distance of 15 mm, and the object distance is 33.3 cm. The vergence of rays originating at infinity and exiting the spectacle lens is –7 D. Due to the vertex distance, the vergence of these rays at the front surface of the cornea (which is approximately the location of the first principal point) is –6.3 D. Use the focal point of the –7 D spectacle lens, 1/7 = 0.143 m, plus the vertex distance of 0.015 m (0.158 m) to find the vergence at the corneal surface: 1/0.158 m = –6.3 D (see Fig 5-1A).

临床案例 5-2 和图 5-1 阐述了调节需求。正视眼需要在 1/3 m 处阅读，需要 3.00 D 调节。如果是近视，在眼前 15 mm 处戴 -7.00 D 框架眼镜（完全矫正），平行光线通过镜片，到达角膜的发散度为 -6.30 D，不需要眼调节即可聚焦在视网膜。位于眼前 1/3 m 处的物体发出的光线产生了 -3.00 D 的发散度，通过 -7.00 D 的镜片后发散度达到 -10.00 D。再经过从镜片到角膜的 15 mm 距离，变为 -8.70D 的发散度。为使物体清晰成像于视网膜上，需要在角膜上产生 -6.30 D 的发散度，这就产生了调节需求的差异 2.40 D。这称作近视性框架镜的“近效应”，调节需求从 3.00 D 减少为 2.40 D。如果用接触镜来矫正同一只眼，看远时可用 -6.30 D 的接触镜替代 -7.00D 的框镜，在 1/3 m 处阅读时调节的需求是 3.00 D。因此，配戴接触镜后，近视患者失去了近用减少*调节的优势*，以及远视患者增加*调节的缺点*。一位 42 岁近视患者配戴 -5.00 D 框架镜，无不适；尽管框架镜和接触镜的矫正视力都很好，但配戴接触镜可能阅读困难。相反地，一位 38 岁远视患者开始出现老视症状，使用远用接触镜视近时，较框架镜更舒适。

临床案例 5-1

一单眼无晶体眼验配接触镜时产生了复视，即使用棱镜使 2 个像叠加，复像仍持续存在。此眼的屈光不正度数为 -5.00 D，患者感觉无晶体眼的像比另一个近视眼的像更大。如何解决复视的问题？

通过放大有晶体眼的像像或减小接触镜矫正的无晶体眼的像，实现减少双眼不等像的目的。对于有晶体眼，用接触镜矫正近视可使成像变大。如果仍不能消除不等像，用 +5.00D 的接触镜过矫无晶体眼，并在眼前加用一个 -5.25 D 的框架镜，引入反向的 Galileo 望远镜。如果有晶体眼是远视，用框架眼镜而不是接触镜来矫正屈光不正，像大小将会增大。

临床案例 5-2

与接触镜相比，用框架镜矫正一个 -7.00 D 的近视眼，调节需求是多少？如果是一个 +7.00 D 远视眼呢？假设顶点距离为 15mm，物体距离为 33.3cm。

对于 -7.00 D 的近视屈光不正眼，顶点距离为 15 mm，视标距离为 33.3 cm。来自无穷远处的光线经由框架镜片后聚散度为 -7.00 D。因顶点距离的存在，这些光线在角膜前表面（位置大约等同于第一主点）形成的聚散度为 -6.30 D。用 -7.00 D 框架镜片的焦点 1/7 = 0.143 m，加上顶点距离 0.015 m（总长度为 0.158 m），计算出相对角膜面的聚散度为：1/0.158 m =-6.30 D（见图 5-1A）。

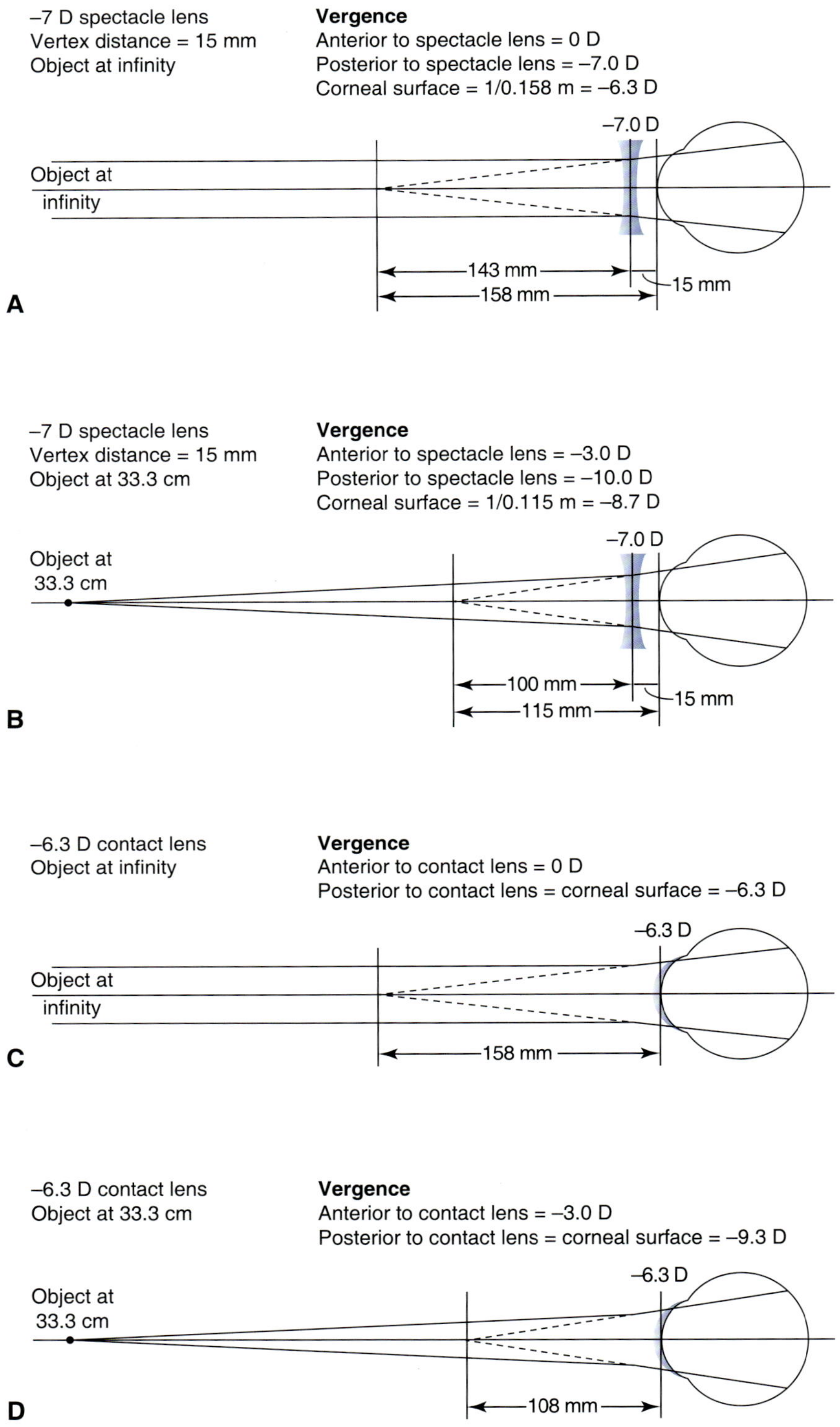

Figure 5-1 Accommodative demand. **A**, Effective spectacle lens power at the corneal surface. **B**, Accommodative demand with a –7.0D spectacle lens. **C**, Correction with a –6.3 D contact lens. **D**, Accommodative demand with a –6.3 D contact lens. *(Illustrations developed by Thomas F. Mauger, MD.)*

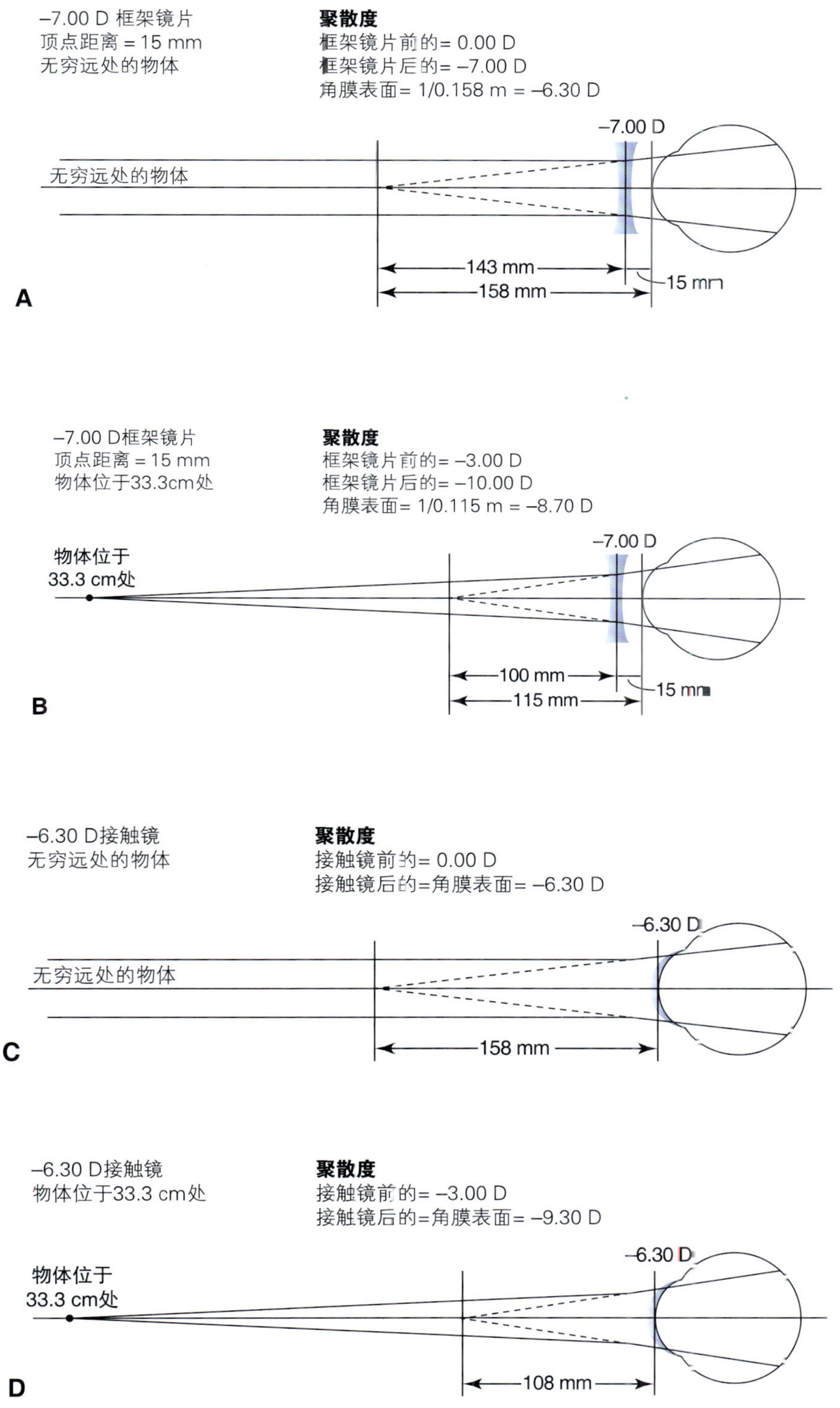

图 5–1 调节需求 **A**. 角膜面的有效眼镜焦度。**B**. 使用 –7.00D 框架镜矫正时的调节需求。**C**. 用 –6.30 D 接触镜矫正。**D**. 用 –6.30 D 接触镜矫正时的调节需求。*（译者注：资料来源见前页原文。）*

The vergence of rays originating at 33.3 cm after exiting the spectacle lens is −10 D (see Fig 5-1B). The vergence is calculated by using the vergence of the light after it leaves the spectacle lens: −3 + (−7) = −10. Due to the vertex distance, the vergence of these rays at the front surface of the cornea (which is approximately the location of the first principal point) is −8.7 D. Use the focal point of the rays after the light travels through the lens, −10 D, 1/10 = 0.1 m, plus the vertex distance of 0.015 m (0.115 m) to find the vergence at the corneal surface: 1/0.115 m = −8.7 D).

Accommodative demand is the difference between the vergence at the first principal point between rays originating at infinity and the vergence of rays originating at 33.3 cm. In this case, the accommodation is 2.4 D: −6.3 − (−8.7) = 2.4. In contrast, the accommodation required with a contact lens correction is approximately 3 D (see Figs 5-1C, D). Therefore, this myopic eye would need 0.6 D more accommodation to focus an object at 33.3 cm when wearing a contact lens compared with correction with a spectacle lens. Similarly, the accommodative demand of an eye corrected with a +7.00 D spectacle lens would be 3.5 D compared with approximately 3 D for a contact lens (Table 5-2).

Table 5-2 Accommodative Demand Through Spectacles and Contact Lenses

	−7.0 D Spectacle Lens		**−6.3 D Contact Lens[a]**	
Object at:	Infinity	33.3 cm	Infinity	33.3 cm
Vergence *(D)* at anterior spectacle lens surface	0	−3.0		
Power of lens	−7.0	−7.0	−6.3	−6.3
Vergence at posterior spectacle lens surface	−7.0	−10.0		
Vergence at corneal surface with 15 mm vertex distance	−6.3	−8.7	−6.3	−9.3
Accommodative demand	−6.3 − (−8.7) = **2.4 D**		−6.3 − (−9.3) = **3.0 D**	
	+7.0 D Spectacle Lens		**+7.8 D Contact Lens[b]**	
Vergence *(D)* at anterior spectacle lens surface	0	−3.0		
Power of lens	+7.0	+7.0	+7.8	+7.8
Vergence at posterior spectacle lens surface	+7.0	+4.0		
Vergence at corneal surface with 15-mm vertex distance	+7.8	+4.3	+7.8	+4.8
Accommodative demand	+7.8 − (+4.3) = **3.5 D**		+7.8 − (+4.8) = **3.0 D**	

[a] The equivalent power at the cornea of a −7.0 D spectacle lens with a vertex distance of 15 mm is −6.3 D.

[b] The equivalent power at the cornea of a +7.0 D spectacle lens with a vertex distance of 15 mm is +7.8 D.

来自 33.3 cm 处的光线，通过框架镜后聚散度为 –10.00D（见图 5–1 B）。聚散度是经由光线通过框镜镜片之后的聚散计算得出的：–3 + (–7) = –10。由于顶点距离的存在，角膜前表面光线的聚散度（大致相当于眼的第一主点位置）是 –8.70D。用光线通过 –10.00D 镜片的焦点为 1/10 = 0.1 m, 加上顶点距离 0.015 m（总共 0.115 m)，由此得出角膜表面的聚散度为 1/0.115 m = –8.70D。

来自无穷远处的光线与来自 33.3 cm 处的光线，在第一主点位置的聚散度不同，因此调节需求也不同。在这个案例中，调节是 2.40D：–6.3 – (–8.7) = 2.4。相反，使用接触镜矫正的调节大约是 3.00D（见图 5–1C、D）。所以，近视眼用接触镜矫正比配戴框架镜，需要多付出 0.6 D 的调节才能看清 33.3 cm 处的物体。同样，远视眼用 +7.00D 框架镜矫正所需的调节是 3.50D，若换为接触镜矫正，则所需的调节大约是 3.00D（表 5–2）。

表5–2　框架镜与接触镜的调节需求比较

	–7.00 D框架镜		–6.30 D接触镜[a]	
物体位置	无穷远	33.3 cm	无穷远	33.3 cm
框架镜前表面的调节 (D)	0	–3.0		
镜片的焦度	–7.0	–7.0	–6.3	–6.3
框架镜平面后的光束聚散度	–7.0	–10.0		
顶点距离为15 mm时的角膜面的光束聚散度	–6.3	–8.7	–6.3	–9.3
调节需求	–6.3 – (–8.7) = 2.40 D		–6.3 – (–9.3) = 3.00 D	
	+7.00 D框架镜		**+7.80 D接触镜[b]**	
框架镜平面前的光束聚散度 (D)	0	–3.0		
镜片的焦度	+7.0	+7.0	+7.8	+7.8
框架镜平面后的光束聚散度	+7.0	+4.0		
顶点距离为15 mm时的角膜面的光束聚散度	+7.8	+4.3	–7.8	+4.8
调节需求	+7.8 – (+4.3) = 3.50 D		+7.8 – (+4.8) = 3.00 D	

[a] 顶点距离为15 mm时，–7.00 D框架镜在角膜处的等效焦度为–6.30 D。

[b] 顶点距离为15 mm时，+7.00 D框架镜在角膜处的等效焦度为+7.80 D。

Depending on their power, spectacle lenses, whose optical centers are positioned for distance viewing, and contact lenses require different amounts of convergence to achieve fusion, looking at a near object. Contact lenses turn with the eyes; therefore, no prism is encountered, looking through the contact lenses, when the eyes converge. Myopic spectacle lenses induce *base-in prisms* for near objects, following the Prentice rule, so that the eyes do not have to turn in as much to look at the near object. Hyperopic spectacles increase the convergence needed for fusion by inducing *base-out prisms*.

In summary, correction of myopia with contact lenses, as opposed to spectacle lenses, increases both accommodative and convergence demands of focusing and fusion for near objects, proportional to the size of the refractive error, and decreases both demands in hyperopia (Fig 5-2). These effects may be welcome, unwelcome, or of no consequence, depending on the patient's muscle balance and ability to accommodate.

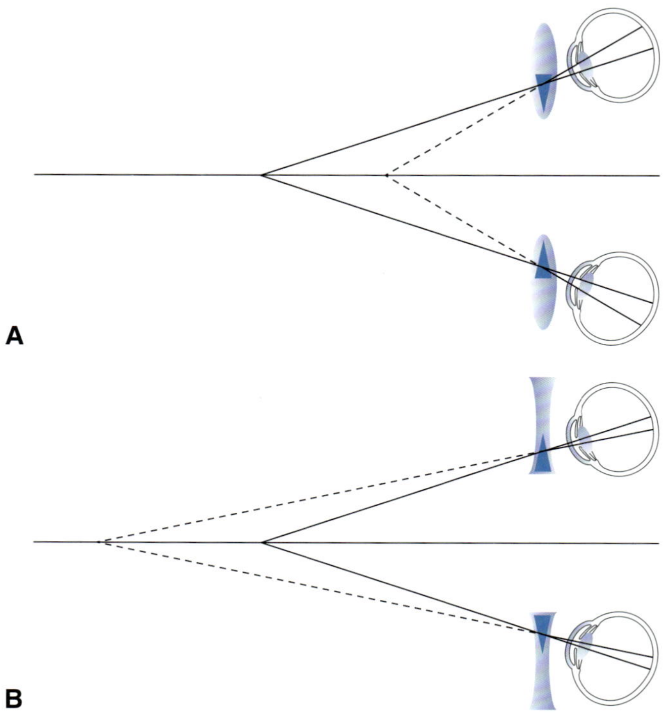

Figure 5-2 Effect of spectacle lenses on convergence demands. **A**, Lenses for correction of hyperopia create induced base-out prism with convergence, which increases the convergence demand. **B**, Lenses for correction of myopia create induced base-in prism, which decreases the convergence demand. *(Illustrations developed by Thomas F. Mauger, MD.)*

框架镜与接触镜需要不同的集合来看清近物，框镜的光学中心是在视远的位置，所以不同焦度的框架镜看近时产生的棱镜效果不同。接触镜随眼球运动，眼睛会聚看近物时，不产生棱镜效应。依据 Prentice 法则，近视框架镜视近时，会产生*底向内的棱镜效果*，所以眼睛不必内转太多；远视框架镜看近时，会产生*底向外的棱镜效果*，所以需要增加双眼的集合需求。

总之，与框架镜相比，使用接触镜矫正近视，会增加视近时的调节和集合。增加的量与屈光不正的大小成比例。而在远视眼则相反（图 5–2）。患者对产生的这些效果的感受是好是坏，或有无影响，取决于眼外肌平衡和调节能力。

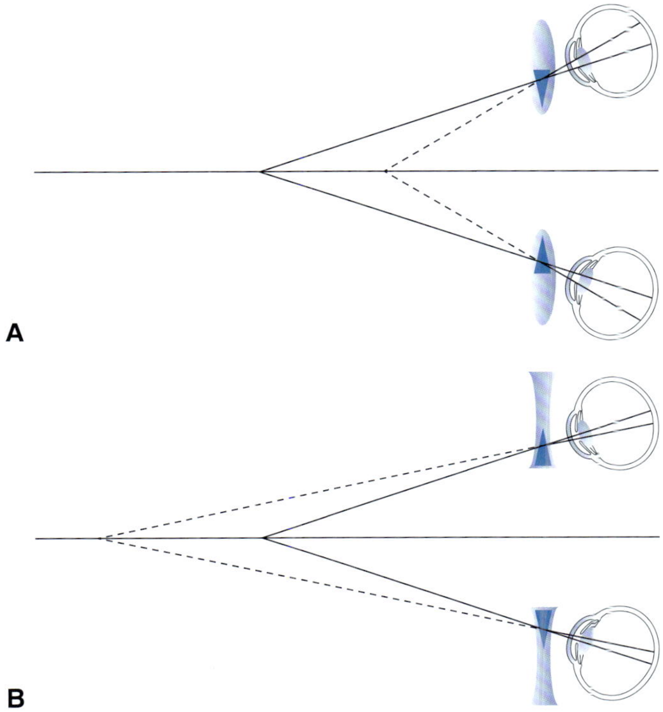

图 5–2　框架镜对集合需求的影响。**A**. 远视框架眼镜产生底朝外的棱镜效应，导致集合需求增加。**B**. 近视框架眼镜产生底朝内的棱镜效应，使集合需求减少。*（译者注：资料来源见前页原文。*

Correcting Astigmatism

Rigid lenses with a spherical rear surface form a *tear lens* in the space between the lens and the cornea. When rigid (and toric soft) contact lenses neutralize astigmatism at the corneal surface, the meridional aniseikonia created with toric-surfaced spectacle lenses is avoided. For this reason, people whose astigmatism has been corrected with contact lenses often experience an annoying change in spatial orientation when they switch to spectacles. However, refractive astigmatism is the sum of *corneal* and *lenticular astigmatism.* Lenticular astigmatism, if present, is not corrected by spherical contact lenses, so it persists as "residual" astigmatism when the corneal astigmatism component is neutralized by spherical rigid contact lenses. This finding is more common among older patients and often explains why their hard contact lenses fail to provide full correction. These cases can be identified by refracting while the contact lenses are in place. If it happens that the eye has lenticular astigmatism against the rule and a similar amount of corneal astigmatism with the rule, a soft contact lens may be used, so that the astigmatism of the cornea and of the lens continue to compensate for each other.

For example, consider a patient whose refraction is -3.50 -0.50×180 and keratometry measurements of the affected eye are 42.50 D (7.94 mm) horizontal and 44.00 D (7.67 mm) vertical. Would a soft or rigid contact lens provide better vision (ie, less residual astigmatism)? The disparity between the corneal astigmatism of 1.50 D and the refractive astigmatism of 0.50 D reveals 1.00 D of against-the- rule lenticular astigmatism that neutralizes a similar amount of with-the-rule corneal astigmatism. Neutralizing the corneal component of the refractive astigmatism with a rigid contact lens exposes the 1.00 D of lenticular residual astigmatism. Therefore, a spherical soft contact lens would, in this case, provide better vision than a spherical RGP lens.

Contact Lens Materials

What would we ask of a material to make a contact lens? The material would fit a variety of corneal shapes, be durable, easy to handle, comfortable, and transparent. Its surface would be "wettable" and stay wet between blinks, but we do not want deposits to stick to it, or for pseudomonas to find it a congenial home. We would want the lens to transmit oxygen and carbon dioxide and flush new tears under it with each blink, to maintain corneal metabolism. We would not want the lens to contribute to dry eye problems by soaking up water from the cornea.

Dk, Dk/t, and *wetting angle* are some terms used to describe oxygen permeability andwettability: *Dk* refers to the oxygen permeability of a lens material, where *D* is the diffusion coefficient for oxygen movement in the material, and k is the solubility constant of oxygen in the material. *Dk/t* refers to the oxygen transmissibility of a lens, depending on its material and central thickness *(t)*. *Wetting angle* refers to the wettability of a lens surface (Fig 5-3). A low wetting angle means water will spread over the surface, increasing surface wettability. Both a high Dk/t and a low wetting angle are desirable.

"Hard" contact lenses were introduced in the 1940s and were made of *polymethylmethacrylate (PMMA)*, the same plastic used subsequently for the first intraocular lenses. These lenses were very durable, but oxygen passed only around them, not through them.

散光矫正

硬性接触镜在镜片后表面和角膜间形成一个*泪液镜*。当硬性（和复曲面软性）接触镜在角膜界面中和散光时，可以避免复曲面框架镜的子午线不等像。所以，配戴接触镜的散光患者，更换戴框架镜时，对空间方向感到不适。验光的散光是指*角膜*和*晶状体散光*的总和。球面接触镜不能矫正晶状体散光，当角膜散光被矫正后，晶状体散光就表现为“残余”散光。这一现象在老年患者中常见，这也解释了为什么接触镜很难全部矫正这些患者的散光。可以通过配戴接触镜后的屈光状态来判别有无残余散光。如果发现一只眼有逆规性晶状体散光，同时还有散光度相同的顺规性角膜散光，角膜和晶状体的散光相互抵消，可以使用软性接触镜来矫正。

例如，一位患者的验光度数是 −3.50 −0.50 × 180，角膜曲率水平方向为 42.50 D (7.94 mm)，垂直方向为 44.00 D (7.57 mm)。选用接触镜矫正，软性和硬性哪种效果更好（即残留的散光少）？ 1.50 D 角膜散光和 0.50 D 总散光之间的差异提示，存在有 1.00 D 的晶状体逆规性散光，中和了等量的角膜顺规散光度数。如果用硬镜矫正了角膜散光，就会暴露出晶状体散光。因此，在这个案例中，使用球面软镜较球面 RGP 效果更好。

接触镜材料

制作接触镜需要什么材料？材料必须适应不同的角膜形态、经久耐用、易于操作、舒适、透明。表面可“湿润”，在不眨眼时也保持湿润，但不能有沉淀物黏附，也不希望假单胞菌在镜片上繁殖。镜片能透过氧气和二氧化碳，在每次瞬目时能交换镜片下泪液，保持角膜的新陈代谢。镜片不吸收角膜的水分而造成干眼。

Dk、*Dk/t* 和*润湿角*是描述透氧性和湿润性的常用术语：*Dk* 指的是镜片材料的透氧性，其中 *D* 是氧在材质中的扩散系数，*k* 是氧在材料中的溶解度系数。*Dk/t* 是指镜片的透氧率，取决于材料和中心厚度（*t*）。湿润角描述透镜表面的湿润性（图 5–3）。湿润角小意味着泪液将会扩散覆盖于镜片表面，增加表面的湿润性。高 Dk/t 和湿润角小都是理想的镜片参数。

“硬性”接触镜在 20 世纪 40 年代出现，是由*聚甲基丙烯酸甲酯*制成（*PMMA*），同样的材质用于第一枚人工晶体。这种镜片非常耐用，但氧气只能“绕过”镜片传递到角膜，而不是透过镜片。

Soft contact lenses are made of a hydrogel polymer, *hydroxyethylmethacrylate* or, more often now, a silicone hydrogel. Hydrogels have more oxygen permeability when they have higher water content, but the higher-water-content lenses tend to cause dryness of the cornea if they are made thin, and they may form deposits and require frequent replacement. Modifying the hydrogels yielded "silicone hydrogels," used for daily and extended wear. These lenses achieve their oxygen permeability with less water content, using pores induced by the presence of silicon atoms, rather than high water content. Some patients are more comfortable with the hydrogels than the silicone hydrogels. Available lenses differ in chemistry throughout the lens or at its surfaces with differing wettability, flexibility, clarity, resistance to deposit retention, and suitability for those with dry eye. They also differ in their longevity and should be replaced at recommended intervals.

RGP lenses were developed in the latter 20th century, using the architecture of large-polymer plastics to allow passage of oxygen. RGP lenses allow oxygen to pass through and allow more tear exchange around the lens with each blink than soft lenses allow, so that oxygen-depleted tears are not trapped between the lens and the cornea. The addition of fluorine to the silicone/acrylate material increases oxygen permeability and encourages the coating of the lens with mucin, which improves wettability. There are various chemistries, with differing advantages.

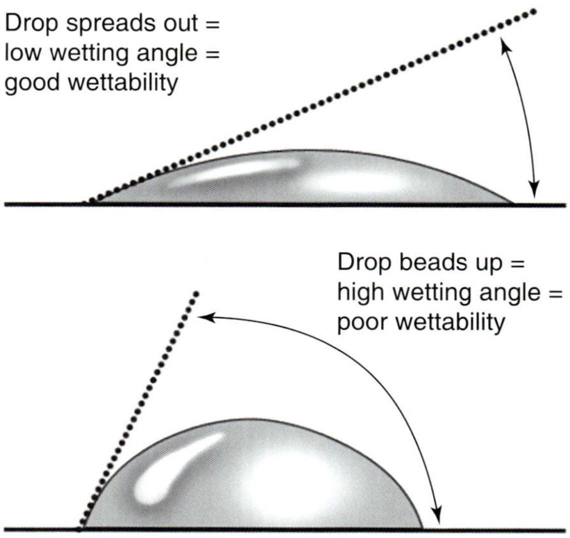

Figure 5-3 The wettability of a lens surface determines whether a wetting angle will be low (greater wettability, greater comfort) or high (less wettability, less comfort). *(Modified with permission from Stein HA, Freeman MI, Stein RM.CLAO Residents Contact Lens Curriculum Manual. New Orleans: Contact Lens Association of Ophthalmologists; 1996. Redrawn by Christine Gralapp.)*

Table 5-3 Comparative Advantages of Soft and Rigid Gas-Permeable Contact Lenses

Soft Contact Lenses	RGP Contact Lenses
Shorter adaptation period	Clear vision
More comfortable for occasional wear than rigid gas-permeable lenses	Correction of regular and irregular corneal astigmatism
Variety of lens types (eg, disposable lenses, lenses replaced frequently)	Ease of handling
Ability to change eye color	Stability and durability
Easier to fit, inexpensive to replace	Ease of care

Table 5-3 summarizes the comparative advantages of soft and RGP contact lenses.

软性接触镜由水凝胶聚合物、*甲基丙烯酸羟乙酯*制作而成　现在通常用的是硅水凝胶材质。水凝胶因为含水量高，所以具有更高的透氧性，但如果镜片较薄，高含水会导致角膜干燥；易于沉淀物附着，需要频繁更换。将水凝胶改良为“硅水凝胶”，适用于日戴和超长时配戴。这些镜片利用硅原子形成的孔隙，以较少的含水量来达到透氧性，而非高含水。一些患者配戴水凝胶镜片舒适感较硅水凝胶更好。不同镜片的化学性质不同，镜片表面的湿润性、柔韧性、透明度、抗沉积物性和是否对干眼患者适用等都不同，它们的寿命也不同，应按推荐的时间进行更换。

RGP 是 20 世纪末发展起来的，利用大聚合物树脂材料的结构实现透氧性。和软镜相比，RGP 能在每次眨眼时透过氧气，泪液交换更多，所以，缺氧的泪液不会滞留在镜片和角膜间。在硅 / 丙烯酸酯材料中添加氟可增加透氧性，最好再用黏液涂覆镜片处理，从而提高湿润性。不同的化学物质具有不同的优点。

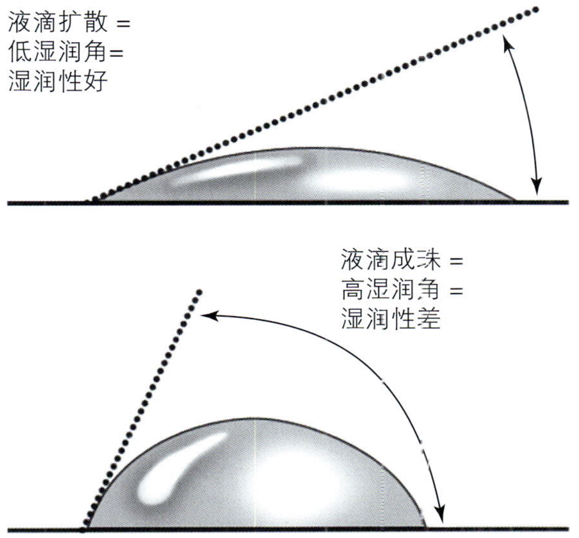

图 5–3　镜片表面的湿润性决定了湿润角是小（湿润性好，舒适感好）还是大（湿润性差，舒适感差）。（译者注：资料来源见前页原文。）

表5–3　软镜与RGP比较

软性接触镜	RGP镜
更短适应期	视觉质量清晰
偶尔配戴舒适感比RGP镜好	矫正规则和不规则散光
种类多（如每日抛弃型镜片，可频繁更换）	操作简单
可改变眼睛颜色	稳定和耐久
容易验配，更换便宜	容易护理

表 5–3 比较了软镜与 RGP 的优点。

Patient History and Examination

Factors that increase the risk of complications with contact lens use include diabetes mellitus, especially if poorly controlled; immunosuppression; long-term use of topical ocular medications, such as corticosteroids; and occupational chemical or foreign body exposure. Other relative contraindications to contact lens use include an inability or history of failure to care for contact lenses, monocularity, abnormal eyelid function such as Bell palsy, severe dry eye, and corneal neovascularization.

The eyes and adnexa are examined for abnormalities of eyelid and lash position, tear film, and ocular surface. Eyelid movement should be observed. The cornea and conjunctiva should be evaluated carefully for signs of allergy, scarring, symblepharon, or other signs of conjunctival scarring diseases, such as ocular cicatricial pemphigoid and giant papillary conjunctivitis or abnormal vascularization resulting from previous lens wear. Through refraction and keratometry, the ophthalmologist can determine whether there is significant corneal, lenticular, or irregular astigmatism. The identification of irregular astigmatism may suggest other pathologies, such as keratoconus.

Contact Lens Selection

The main advantages of soft contact lenses are their comfort and shorter period of adaptation (see Table 5-3). They are available with a wide range of shapes and materials and are usually easier to fit than rigid lenses. A lost or damaged lens is readily replaced without much cost.

Soft lenses are designed for monthly, daily, and 1–2-week replacement. Very few soft lenses dispensed now are intended for longer-duration duty cycles.

Daily-wear lenses have been favored in the United States ever since reports in the 1980s showed increased incidence of keratitis with extended-wear lenses. Improved materials that have greater oxygen permeability (Dk = 60–140) have been approved for extended wear. Use of these materials may decrease the risk of infection compared with the risk associated with earlier materials, but patients who want extended-wear lenses should understand the increased risk of bacterial keratitis and the signs and symptoms that require the attention of a physician. Additional risk factors for extended-wear complications include previous eye infections, lens use while swimming, exposure to smoke, dry eye, eyelid margin disease, and allergy. Daily-wear users are exposed to the same risks, only less so.

About 10% of contact lenses fit in the United States are RGP lenses. Some with high-oxygen permeability are approved for extended wear. They are typically replaced yearly. The main advantages of RGP lenses are the high quality of vision they offer, including the correction of corneal astigmatism (see Table 5-3), durability, and simplicity of lens care. The main disadvantages of RGP contact lenses are initial discomfort, longer period of adaptation, greater knowledge and effort required for fitting, and the greater cost of replacing a lost or damaged lens. People who use contacts only sporadically are generally more comfortable with a soft lens.

病史和检查

接触镜并发症的风险因素包括糖尿病，尤其是血糖控制欠佳者；使用免疫抑制剂；长期使用眼药，如糖皮质激素类；职业性化学或异物暴露。接触镜使用的相对禁忌症包括不能护理或曾经护理不当、独眼、眼睑功能异常如 Bell 麻痹、严重干眼和角膜新生血管。

眼及附属器检查，注意有无眼睑和睫毛位置异常，有无泪膜和眼表异常。观察眼睑运动。仔细评估角膜和结膜是否有过敏、瘢痕、睑球粘连或其他结膜瘢痕疾病的征象，如眼部瘢痕性天疱疮、巨乳头状结膜炎或以前戴镜导致的异常血管化。通过屈光检查和角膜曲率测量，确定是否有明显的角膜、晶状体散光或不规则散光。发现不规则散光提示有其他病理性疾病，如圆锥角膜。

接触镜选择

软镜最主要的优点在于舒适性和适应期短（见表 5-3）。它们有多种形态设计和材质可供选择，通常比硬镜更容易验配。丢失或损坏时容易更换，成本也不高。

软镜的设计是每月、每天和 1~2 周更换。没有更长使用周期的软镜。

自从 20 世纪 80 年代有报道显示，长时间配戴接触镜会增加角膜炎的发病率以来，日抛型接触镜一直在美国受到青睐。具有更大透氧性 (*Dk* = 60~140) 的改良镜片已用于超长时间配戴。与早期材料相比，使用这些材料可降低感染风险。但是这类患者应该了解，超长时间戴镜也会增加细菌性角膜炎的风险，需要医生注意相关体征和症状。超长时间配戴并发症的其他危险因素包括以前的眼部感染、游泳时使用接触镜、吸烟、干眼、睑缘疾病和过敏。日抛型用户也面临着同样的风险，只是要小一些。

美国约 10% 的患者配戴 RGP。一些高透氧性的 RGP 是批准用于超长时间配戴的，只需每年更换一次镜片。RGP 的最主要优点在于提供清晰的视觉，包括矫正角膜散光（见表 5-3）、耐用、护理简单；主要缺点是初始戴镜不适、适应期长、需有验配知识和技能，如果镜片破损或丢失后，更换成本高。偶尔使用接触镜的人通常觉得软镜更舒服。

Contact Lens Fitting

The goals of lens fitting are good vision that does not fluctuate with blinking or eye movement, comfort for the entire day, and low risk of complications. Terms used to describe lens geometry, illustrated in Figure 5-4, include the following: The *apical zone of the cornea (corneal apex)* is the steepest part of the cornea, normally including its geometric center. The *base curve* is the curvature of the central posterior surface of the lens, which is adjacent to the cornea, described by its radius of curvature. The *diameter (chord diameter)* is the width of the contact lens from edge to edge. The *optical zone* is the central area of the lens; curvature of its front surface is chosen to achieve the desired power of the lens. *Peripheral* or secondary curves of the posterior lens surface farther from its center are designed to follow the shape of the cornea, which is normally flatter toward its periphery. *Sagittal depth or vault* is the distance between the center of the posterior surface to the plane of the edges of the lens.

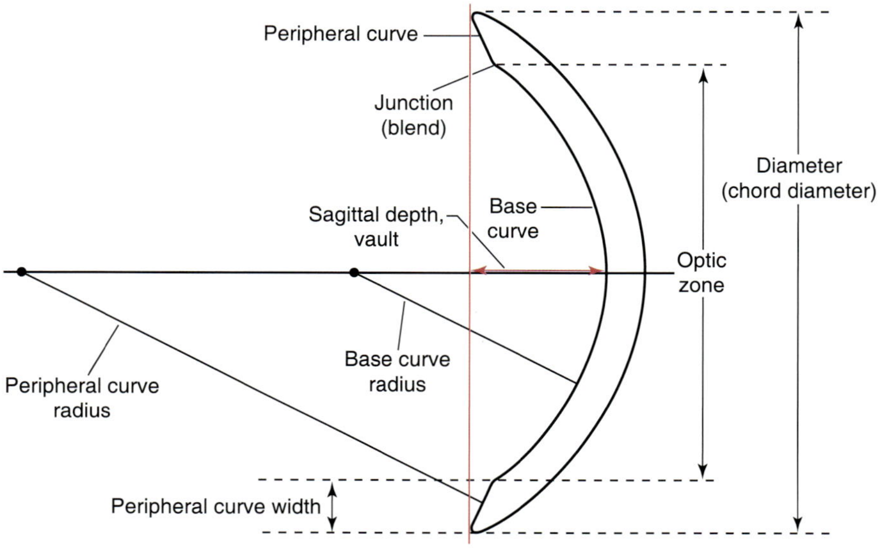

Figure 5-4 Contact lens. Note the relationship among the parts. *(Modified with permission from Stein HA, Freeman MI, Stein RM. CLAO Residents Contact Lens Curriculum Manual. New Orleans: Contact Lens Association of Ophthalmologists; 1996. Redrawn by Christine Gralapp.)*

Contact lenses are described by their rear vertex power, which can be checked for rigid lenses by placing the back of the lens on the nose cone of a lensmeter (done less frequently for soft lenses, similarly or in a liquid chamber, correcting for index of refraction). The required contact lens power may differ slightly from the power of the appropriate spectacle correction, to adjust for the difference in position of the correcting lens. This disparity is known as the correction for the effectivity of lenses, and is discussed in Chapter 1. The magnitude of the correction depends on the strength of the lenses, and can be readily obtained from standard tables (Table 5-4).

接触镜的适配

适配的目标是获得良好的视觉效果、视力不会因眨眼或眼球运动而波动、全天配戴舒适、并发症少。用于描述镜片几何形态的术语如图 5–4 所示，包括*角膜顶点区域*（*角膜顶点*），这是角膜最陡峭的部分，通常包括其几何中心。*基弧*是镜片中央后表面与角膜相邻部分的曲率，以其曲率半径来描述。*直径*(*弦长*)是指接触镜从边缘到边缘的宽度。*光学区*是镜片的中央区域，其前表面曲率由镜片焦度决定。*边弧*或第二弧是在远离中央部分的后表面、依据角膜形态变化进行的设计，通常角膜从中心到周边部分逐渐平坦。*矢高*（*拱高*）是镜片后表面中心到镜片边缘平面的距离。

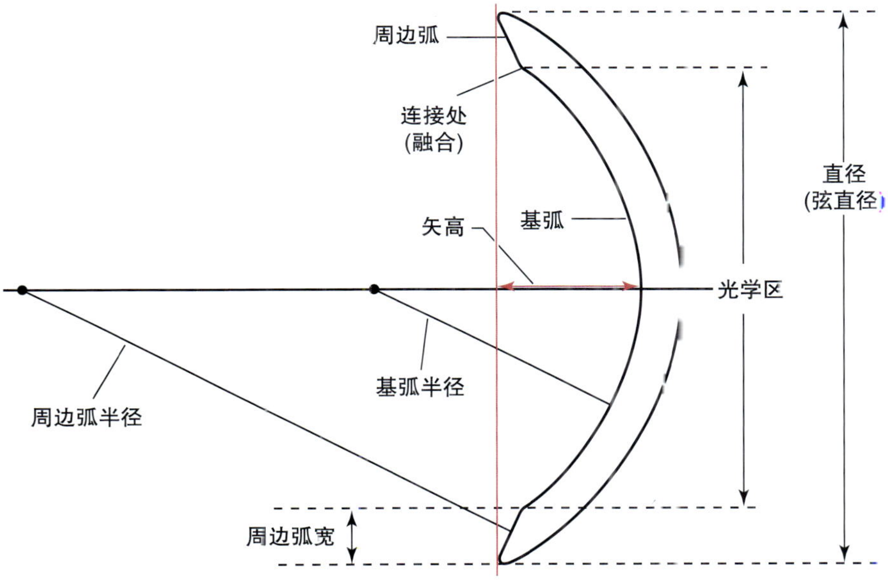

图 5–4　接触镜的各参数及关系。*（译者注：资料来源见前页原文。）*

接触镜的焦度是指它的后顶点焦度，可以将硬性接触镜镜片的后面置于焦度计的测量鼻锥上测量(对软镜少用此方法测量，可放入液体室内用相似的方法测量，但须修正折射率)。接触镜的焦度与框架镜略有不同，要根据矫正眼镜的位置进行调整。这被称为透镜的有效矫正，已在第 1 章讨论过相关的内容。矫正值的大小取决于镜片的焦度值，可以从对照表(表 5–4)中得到换算值。

Table 5-4 "Vertexing" Chart for Converting From Spectacle Prescription to Expected Contact Lens Prescription

Spectacle Lens Power[a]	Range of Normal Values
−5.00	−4.75
−6.00	−5.50
−8.00	−7.25
−10.00	−9.00
−14.00	−12.00
+5.00	+5.25
+6.00	+6.50
+8.00	+9.00
+10.00	+11.25
+14.00	+17

[a] Rear vertex at 12 mm

Soft Contact Lenses

Soft contact lenses are comfortable, thanks to the thin edges encountered by the eyelids. The lenses extend beyond the cornea to the conjunctiva overlying the sclera. A good soft contact lens fit is often described as having a "light 3-point touch," the lens touching the surface of the eye at the corneal apex and at the limbus on either side of the cornea. A soft or rigid lens can be made to fit tighter by either choosing a smaller radius to steepen the base curve or by increasing the lens chord diameter without changing the radius. Either way, we are increasing the "sagittal depth," the height of the lens's rear surface, if it were placed edge-down on a table (Table 5-5 and Fig 5-5).

Evaluating the soft lens fit, the clinician should observe the lens movement and centration after the lens has been in the eye for a while, until the fit has stabilized. In a good fit, the lens will move about 1 mm with upward gaze or blink, or with gentle pressure on the lower eyelid. A tight lens resists movement, and a loose lens will move too much. By evaluating a patient's vision and comfort, slit-lamp findings (eg, lens movement, lens edge, limbal injection), and keratometry mires, the clinician can determine whether the lens fits well (see Table 5-5).

Once a fit is deemed adequate, an overrefraction is performed to check whether the power needs to be adjusted.

When the initial fitting process is complete, the final lens parameters should be clearly identified (Table 5-6). The clinician should teach the patient how to insert and remove the contact lenses, how to care for them, and how to recognize the signs and symptoms of eye emergencies. Follow-up appointments are scheduled depending on the lens and patient.

表 5-4　镜眼距转换表（将框架镜焦度换算为等效的接触镜焦度）

框架镜焦度[a]	接触镜焦度换算值
−5.00	−4.75
−6.00	−5.50
−8.00	−7.25
−10.00	−9.00
−14.00	−12.00
+5.00	+5.25
+6.00	+6.50
+8.00	+9.00
+10.00	+11.25
+14.00	+17

[a] 镜眼距离为12 mm。

软性接触镜

软性接触镜与睑缘接触的边缘很薄，所以配戴很舒服。镜片从角膜延伸到巩膜上的球结膜表面。理想的软性接触镜适配经常被描述为“轻 3 点接触”，镜片在角膜顶点和两侧角膜缘处接触。软镜或硬镜都可以通过选择较小的曲率半径使基弧变陡峭，或通过增加镜片弦长（而不改变基弧）的 2 种方法使其适配更紧。无论哪种方式都是在增加‘矢高”（即把镜片边向下放置于一水平面时镜片后表面的高度）(表 5-5 和图 5-5)。

软性接触镜的适配评估，应在镜片置入一段时间、待适配稳定后，再观察镜片的运动和中心定位。良好适配的特征包括：眼睛向上方注视、瞬目或轻推下睑时，镜片移动约 1mm。适配过紧，会阻碍镜片的移动度；适配过松，会使移动度过大。通过评估患者的视力和舒适度、裂隙灯检查(如镜片活动度、镜片边缘适配、角膜缘是否充血)和角膜曲率计检查的曲面，来确定镜片配戴是否适合(见表 5-5)。

一旦确认镜片适配合适，还需要进行片上验光，核查接触镜的焦度是否需要调整。

初步的适配流程完成后，确认最终定片参数(表 5-6)。医生需要教会患者如何戴镜和摘镜，指导如何护理操作，讲解如何识别眼部紧急情况的先兆和症状。按接触镜验配的类型和患者的具体情况做随访和预约。

Table 5-5 Basic Soft Contact Lens Fitting

Initial Lens Selection	
Parameter	**Description**
Diameter	Approximately 2 mm larger than the horizontal corneal diameter
Base curve	0.2–0.6 mm greater (flatter) than the radius of the flattest *K* reading
Power	Close to the patient's refraction corrected for the vertex distance; refined after fit is achieved

Evaluating Soft Contact Lens Fit	
Loose Fit	**Tight Fit**
Excessive movement	No lens movement
Poor centration; lens easily dislocates off the cornea	Centered lens
Lens-edge standoff	"Digging in" of lens edge
Blurred mires after a blink	Clear mires with blink
Fluctuating vision	Good vision initially
Continuing lens awareness	Initial comfort, but increasing lens awareness with continued use
Air bubbles under the lens	Limbal–scleral injection at lens edge

Adjusting Soft Contact Lens Fit	
Create a Looser Fit	**Create a Tighter Fit**
Decrease the sagittal depth	Increase the sagittal depth
Choose a flatter base curve (increase the radius of curvature)	Choose a steeper base curve (decrease the radius of curvature)
Choose a smaller diameter	Choose a larger diameter

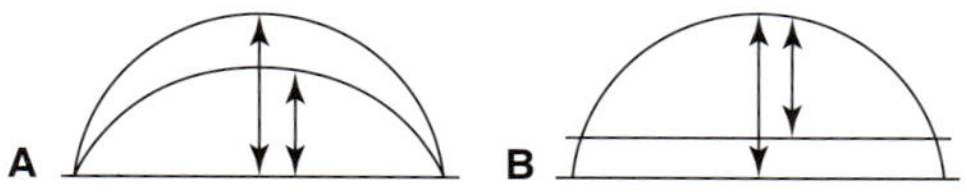

Figure 5-5 Changing the sagittal depth. **A**, Changing the base curve of a contact lens changes the sagittal depth. **B**, Changing the diameter with equal base curve also changes sagittal depth.

Table 5-6 Soft Contact Lens Parameters

Parameter	Common Abbreviation (in the United States)	Typical Range of Values
Overall diameter	OAD	12.5–16.0 mm, extended ranges available for therapeutic purposes
Base curve	BC	8.0–9.5 mm
Center thickness	CT	0.04–0.20 mm (varies with the power of the lens and is set by the manufacturer)
Prescription	RX	Sphere and astigmatism, if any, in diopters
Manufacturer	Varies	Company name and lens style

Rigid Gas-Permeable Contact Lenses

Rigid gas-permeable lenses have smaller chord diameters than soft lenses, and allow more circulation of fresh tears under the lens with each blink. Central and peripheral curves, edge shape, and central thickness can be tailored for stable vision, comfort, and tear exchange.

表 5-5　软性接触镜验配基础

初始镜片选择	
参数	描述
直径	镜片直径比水平角膜直径大2mm
基弧	基弧比角膜曲率平坦 *K* 读数大（平 0.2~0.6 mm
焦度	患者的屈光被有一定顶点距离的眼镜矫正后，要换算成接触镜焦度
软性接触镜适配的评估	
适配松	适配紧
活动度太大 定位偏中心，镜片容易脱出 镜片边缘翘离角膜表面 瞬目后视标模糊一段时间 视力波动 一直感觉到镜片存在 镜片下气泡	镜片不活动 镜片中心定位 镜片边缘紧触角膜 瞬目时视标清晰 初始视力清晰 初始舒适，但随着持续戴镜，镜片感逐渐增加 镜片边缘角巩缘充血
调整软镜适配	
放松适配	收紧适配
减少矢高 选择更平的基弧（增大基弧） 选择更小的直径	增加矢高 选择更陡的基弧（减少基弧） 选择更大的直径

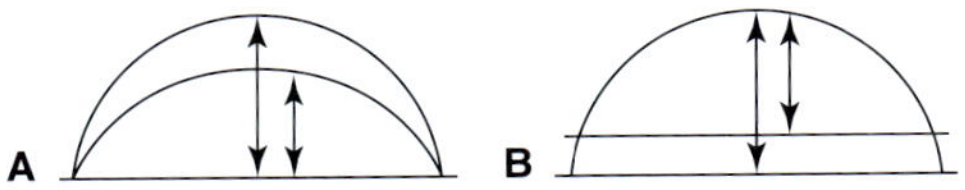

图5-5　改变矢高。**A**. 改变基弧，改变矢高。**B**. 基弧不变，但直径变化最终改变了矢高。

表5-6　软镜参数

参数	常规缩写（美国）	常规值范围
总直径	OAD	12.5 ~ 16.0mm（治疗性接触镜直径更大）
基弧	BC	8.0 ~ 9.5mm
中心厚度	CT	0.04 ~ 0.20mm（随镜片焦度和制造商而不同）
处方	RX	球镜和散光（如果有），以D为单位
制造商	不统一	制造商名称和镜片类型

硬性透气性接触镜

硬性透气性接触镜直径较软镜小，每次瞬目时有较多新鲜泪液循环。通过定制镜片的基弧、边弧，边缘形状和中央厚度，可获得稳定的视觉质量、舒适的配戴，以及泪液交换。

Unlike a soft contact lens, an RGP lens maintains its shape when placed on the cornea, and a tear lens fills the space between the lens and the cornea. The power of the tear lens is determined by the difference between the curvature of the cornea (K) and that of the base curve of the contact lens (Fig 5-6). The fit is described as *apical alignment* (*on K*), when the base curve matches that of the cornea; *apical clearance* (*steeper than K*), when the base curve has a steeper fit, with radius shorter than that of the cornea; and *apical bearing* (*flatter than K*), when the base curve is flatter than the cornea.

To fit an RGP lens of a particular design and material, one can consult the laboratory fashioning the lens, a fitting guide for the lens, or use trial lenses. In designing the lens, consideration is given to pupil size and lid tension, as well as refractive error, keratometry, and possibly topography.

The most common type of RGP lens fit is an *apical alignment fit* with the upper edge of the lens under the upper eyelid (Fig 5-7). This "lid attachment" fit allows the lens to move with each blink, enhances tear exchange, and decreases lens sensation, because the upper eyelid does not strike the lens edge with each blink.

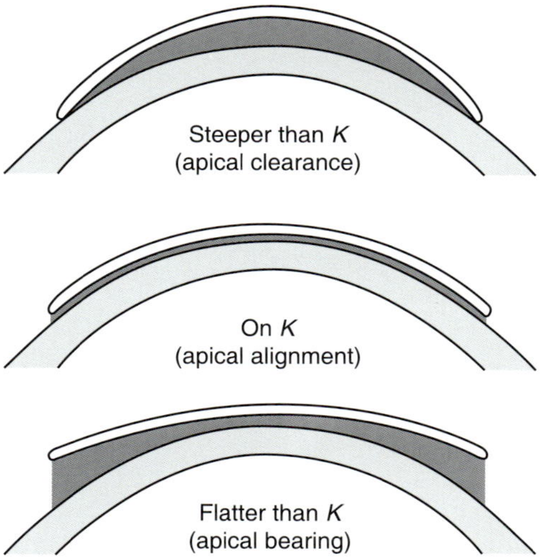

Figure 5-6 A rigid contact lens creates a tear (or fluid) lens whose power is determined by the difference between the curvature of the cornea (*K*) and that of the base curve of the contact lens. *(Courtesy of Perry Rosenthal, MD. Redrawn by Christine Gralapp.)*

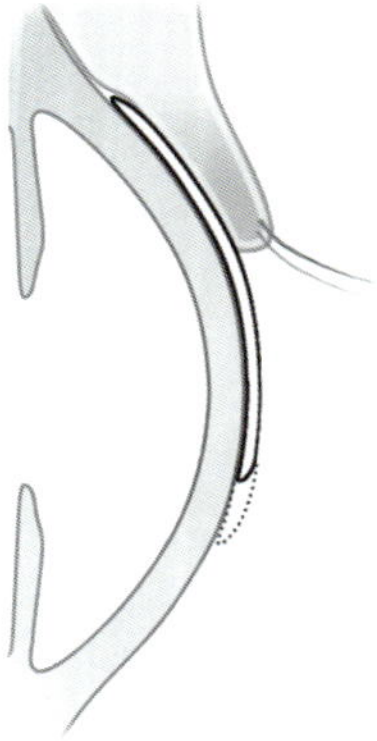

Figure 5-7 The most common and most comfortable type of rigid gas permeable lens fit is apical alignment, in which the upper edge of the lens fits under the upper eyelid. *(Modified with permission from Albert DM, Jakobiec FA, eds. Principles and Practice of Ophthalmology. Philadelphia: Saunders; 1994;5:3630. Redrawn by Christine Gralapp.)*

Alternatively, *a central* or *interpalpebral fit* is achieved when the lens rests between the upper and lower eyelids. The diameter of the lens is smaller than with a lid-attachment fit. There may be greater lens sensation, because the eyelid strikes the lens edge with each blink. This type of fit may be preferable for patients who have high upper eyelids, hyperopia, or Asian eyes.

与软性接触镜不同，RGP 置于角膜表面时，镜片形状保持不变，并在角膜和 RGP 之间形成泪液镜。角膜曲率（K 值）和接触镜的基弧决定了泪液镜的焦度（图 5–6）。基弧与角膜匹配时描述为*顶点平行适配*（*等于 K*）；当基弧比角膜曲率半径小、适配陡峭时描述为*顶点间隙*（*陡于 K*）；当基弧比角膜曲率半径大、适配平坦时描述为*顶点接触*（*平于 K*）。

适配特殊设计或材料的 RGP 镜片，可以咨询生产镜片的厂商，索要适配指南或试戴镜组。镜片设计需要考虑瞳孔大小、眼睑张力、屈光不正、角膜曲率，甚至是角膜地形图的测量结果。

RGP 最常见的适配类型是*顶点平行适配*，镜片的上缘适配在上眼睑的下面（图 5–7）。这种“睑裂后接触”的适配方式允许镜片随着每次瞬目移动，增加泪液交换，减少对镜片的感知，因为每次眨眼时眼睑不会碰到镜片的边缘。

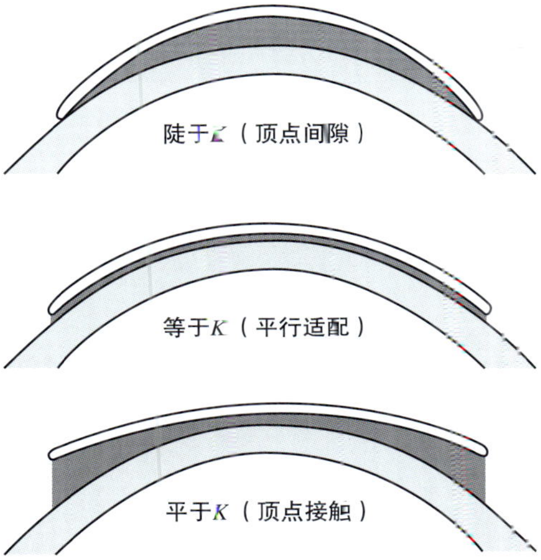

图 5–6 硬性接触镜会产生泪液镜，角膜曲率（*K* 值）和接触镜的基弧决定了泪液镜的焦度（*译者注：资料来源见前页原文。*）

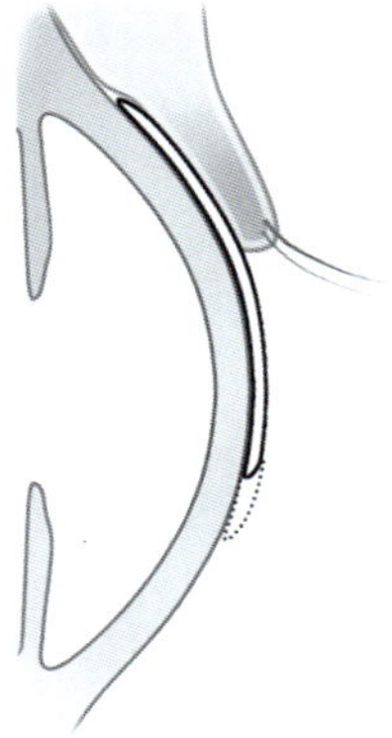

图 5–7 RGP 最常见、最舒适的适配类型是顶点平行适配，镜片的上缘适配在上眼睑的下面。（*译者注：资料来源见前页原文。*）

另一种适配称为*中央*或*睑裂间适配*，是指镜片定位于上下眼睑之间。这种适配要求镜片直径比睑裂后适配的镜片小，因为每次瞬目时眼睑都碰触镜片，对镜片的感知也会更明显。这种适适配用于上眼睑位置高，远视眼或亚洲人的面型。

To evaluate the fit of a contact lens, the clinician looks for stability of vision and appropriate lens movement. The fluorescein pattern is evaluated at the slit lamp (Fig 5-8). If there is apical clearing of the cornea, pooling or a bright green area will be observed centrally; if the RGP lens is touching the cornea, this area will appear dark. Over-refraction determines whether a power change is needed, when the fit is satisfactory. Table 5-7 summarizes RGP lens parameters and the range of normal values.

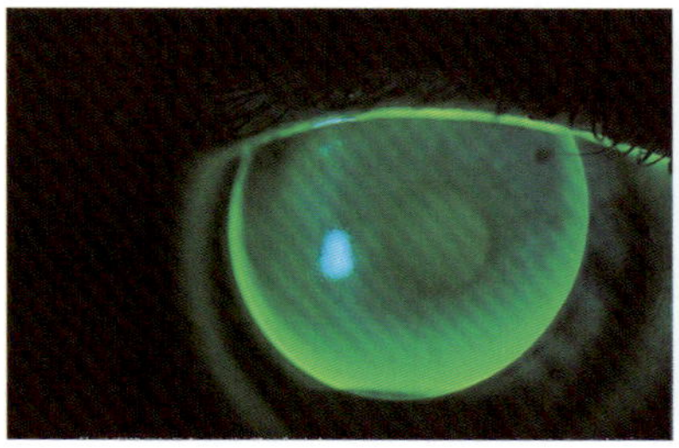

Fluorescein pattern of a good fit with minimal apical clearance.

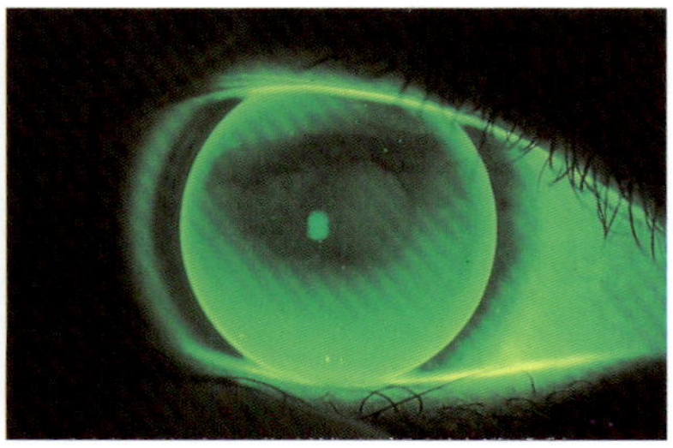

Fluorescein pattern demonstrating a flat fit.

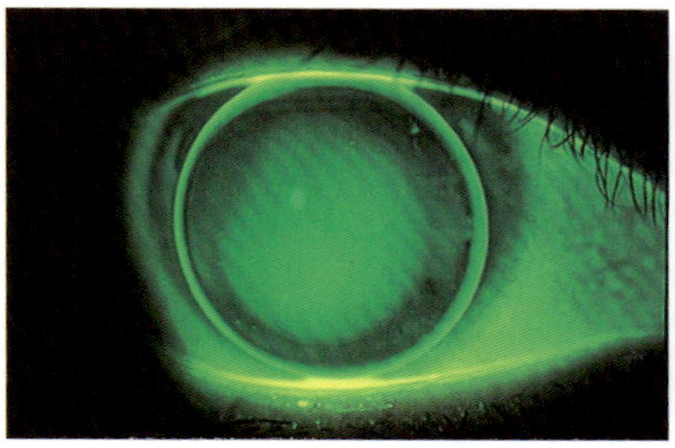

Fluorescein pattern showing a steep fit.

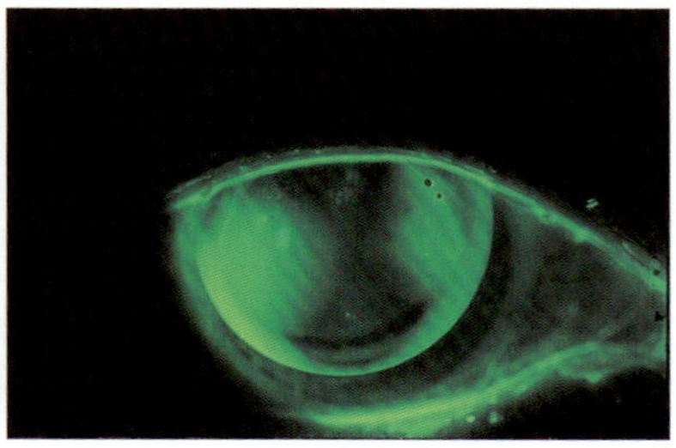

Against-the-rule astigmatic band.

Figure 5-8 Examples of fluorescein patterns in contact lens fitting. *(Courtesy of Perry Rosenthal, MD.)*

Bennett ES, Henry VA. *Clinical Manual of Contact Lenses.* 4th ed. Philadelphia: Lippincott Williams & Wilkins; 2014:133.

Table 5-7 Rigid Gas-Permeable Lens Parameters

Parameter	Common Abbreviation (in the United States)	Range of Normal Values
Overall diameter	OAD	8.0–11.5 mm
Optic zone diameter	OZD	7.0–8.5 mm
Peripheral curve width	PCW	0.1–1.0 mm
Base curve	BC	7.0–8.5 mm
Center thickness	CT	0.08–0.30 mm
Prescription	RX	Any power required

医生通过评估视觉的稳定性和镜片的活动度来判断接触镜的适配是否合适。裂隙灯荧光素染色评估(图 5-8)，观察镜片和角膜的适配状态，如果是顶点间隙适配，镜片下有荧光淤积，观察到亮绿色的区域；如果是顶点接触适配，镜片与角膜接触则表现为暗黑色区域。当获得满意的适配后，还需要做片上验光以确定是否需要修正屈光度。表 5-7 总结了 RGP 镜的参数及其常规范围。

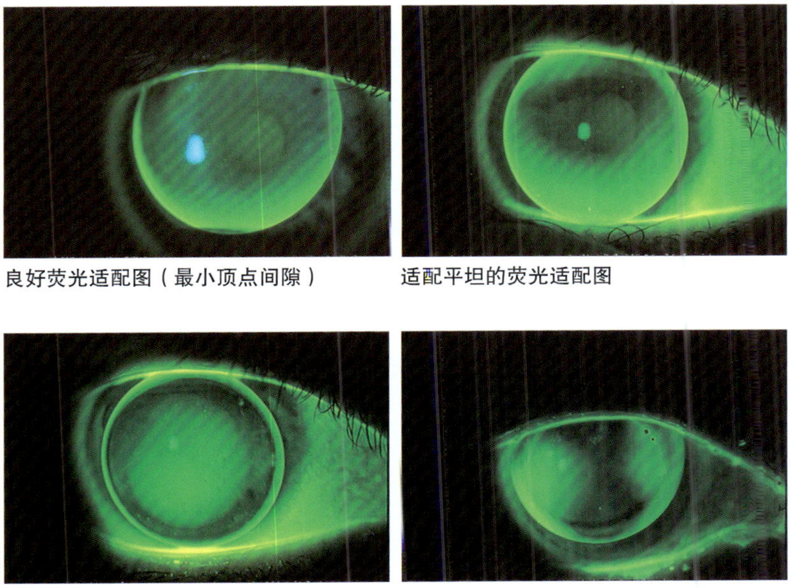

良好荧光适配图（最小顶点间隙）　适配平坦的荧光适配图

适配陡峭的荧光适配图　逆规散光的适配图

图 5-8　接触镜适配的荧光素评估图示（*译者注：资料来源见前页原文。*）

Bennett ES, Henry VA. *Clinical Manual of Contact Lenses.* 4th ed. Philadelphia: Lippincott Williams & Wilkins; 2014:133.

表5-7　硬性透气性接触镜参数

参数	常用缩写（美国）	常规范围
总直径	OAD	8.0~11.5 mm
光学区直径	OZD	7.0~8.5 mm
边弧宽度	PCW	0.1~1.0 mm
基弧	BC	7.0~8.5 mm
中央厚度	CT	0.08~0.30 mm
处方光度	RX	需要的焦度值

Power

The power of the tear lens is approximately 0.25 D for every 0.05-mm radius-of-curvature difference between the base curve of the contact lens and the central curvature of the cornea (*K*), and this power becomes somewhat greater for corneas steeper than 7.00 mm. Tear lenses created by rigid contact lenses with base curves that are steeper than *K* (smaller radius of curvature) have plus power, whereas tear lenses formed by base curves that are flatter than *K* (larger radius of curvature) have minus power (Figs 5-9, 5-10). Therefore, the power of a rigid contact lens must account for both the eye's refractive error and the power introduced by the tear lens. An easy way of remembering this is to use the rules SAM (*steeper add minus*) and FAP (*flatter add plus*). Clinical Example 5-3 illustrates these calculations.

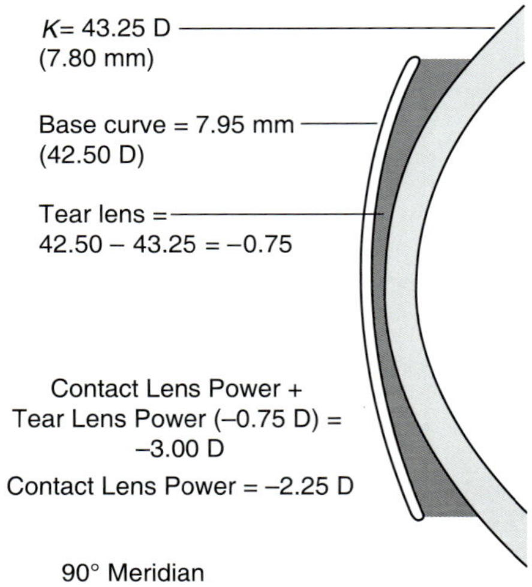

Figure 5-9 Determining the power of a contact lens using the FAP-SAM rules. *(Illustration developed by Thomas F. Mauger, MD.)*

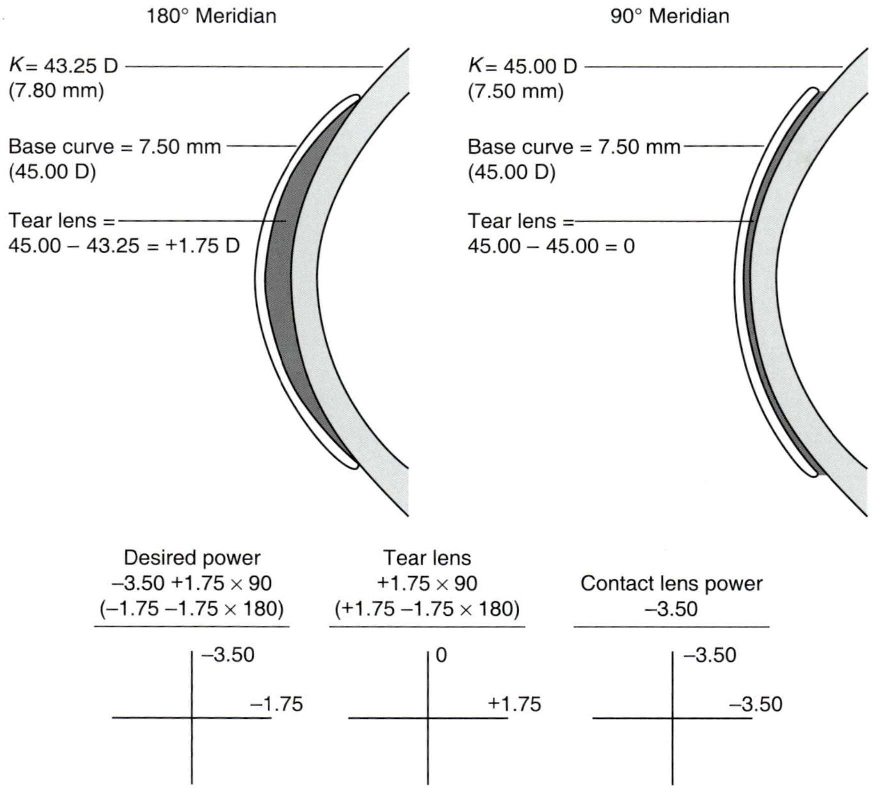

Figure 5-10 Determining the power of a contact lens using the FAP-SAM rules. *(Illustration developed by Thomas F. Mauger, MD.)*

屈光度

接触镜的基弧和中央角膜曲率（*K*）之间的差值是，每变化 0.05 mm，对应泪液镜 0.25D 变化，角膜曲率半径较 7.00 mm 陡峭时，这种对应的变化量更大。当基弧比角膜 *K* 值陡峭（即曲率半径更小）时，会产生正的泪液镜；反之，当基弧比角膜 *K* 值平坦（即曲率半径更大）时，会产生负的泪液镜（图 5-9、图 5-10）。所以，硬性接触镜的焦度必须要同时考虑眼的屈光度和泪液镜。有一个法则方便记忆这个规则：SAM（*陡峭增加负度数 / 陡加负*）和 FAP（*平坦增加正度数 / 平加正*）。临床案例 5-3 说明了计算的过程。

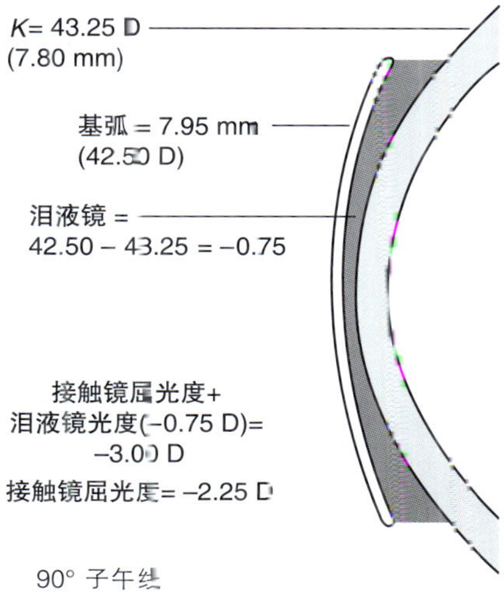

图 5-9　用 FAP-SAM 法则计算接触镜的屈光度。*（译者注：资料来源见前页原文。）*

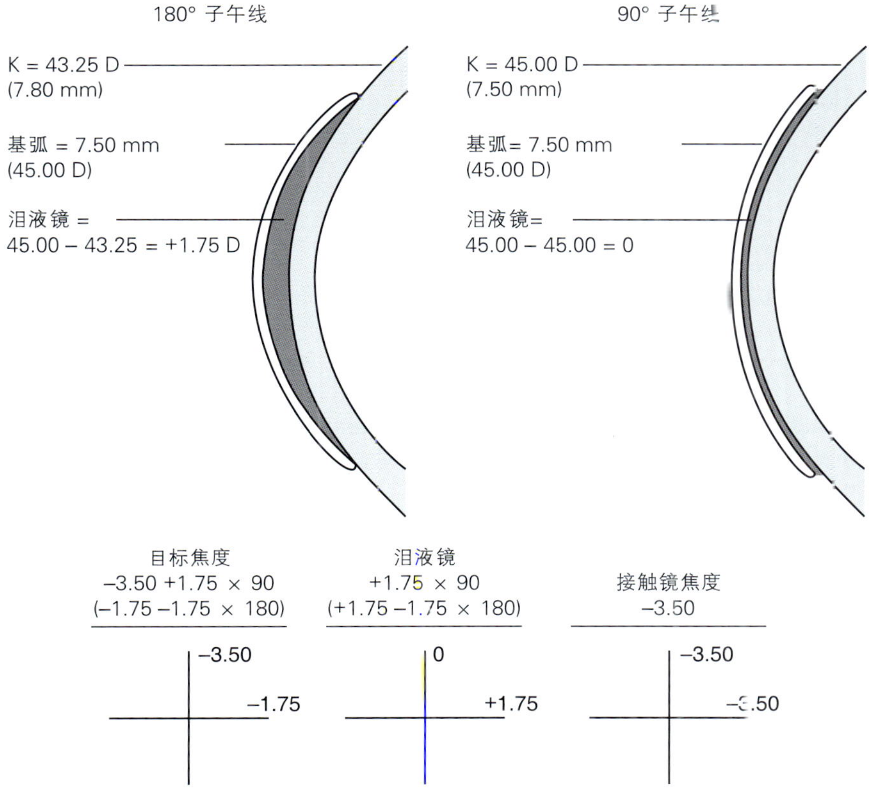

图 5-10　用 FAP-SAM 法则计算接触镜的光度。*（译者注：资料来源见前页原文。）*

CLINICAL EXAMPLE 5-3

The refractive error of an eye is –3.00D, the K measurement is 7.80 mm (43.25 D), and the base curve chosen for the rigid contact lens is 7.95 mm (42.50D). What is the anticipated power of the contact lens?

The power of the resulting tear lens is –0.75 D. This power would correct –0.75 D of the refractive error. Therefore, the remaining refractive error that the contact lens is required to correct is –2.25 D (recall the FAP rule: flatter add plus). Conversely, if the refractive error were +3.00D (hyperopia), then the necessary contact lens power would be +3.75 D to correct the refractive error and the –0.75 D tear lens (see Fig 5-5).

Because the refractive index of the tear lens (1.336) is almost identical to that of a cornea (1.3765), it masks the optical effect of the corneal surface. If the back surface of a contact lens is spherical, then the anterior surface of the tear lens is also spherical, regardless of the corneal topography. Thus, the tear layer created by a spherical rigid contact lens neutralizes more than 90% of regular and irregular corneal astigmatism. This principle simplifies the calculation of the tear lens power on astigmatic corneas: the powers of the steeper corneal meridians can be ignored, and only the flattest meridians need to be considered. The refractive error along the flattest meridian is represented by the spherical component of refractive errors expressed in *minus cylinder form*. For this reason, it is simpler to use the minus cylinder format when dealing with rigid contact lenses (Clinical Example 5-4). When a spherical contact lens is in place, there may still be "residual" astigmatism, which may be caused by the eye's natural lens and the shape of the posterior surface of the cornea. There are "back surface toric" gas permeable lenses with toric back surfaces, chosen to match the shape of the cornea, stabilizing the lens position, with a spherical front surface. There are also "bitoric" RGP lenses, whose back surface matches that of the cornea, while the front toric surface is chosen to correct the residual refractive error (Clinical Example 5-5).

CLINICAL EXAMPLE 5-4

The refractive correction is –3.50 +1.75 × 90, and the K measurements along the 2 principal meridians are 7.80 mm horizontal (43.25 D at 180°) and 7.50 mm vertical (45.00 D at 90°). The contact lens base curve is 7.50 mm. What is the anticipated power of the contact lens?

The refractive correction along the flattest corneal meridian (7.80 mm) is –1.75 D (convert the refractive error to minus cylinder form), and the lens has been fitted steeper than flat *K*, creating a tear lens of +1.75 D. Thus, a corresponding amount of minus power must be added (recall the SAM rule: *steeper* add *minus*), giving a corrective power of –3.50 D in that meridian.

The refractive correction along the steepest meridian (7.50 mm) is –3.50D. The lens is fitted "on K"; therefore, no tear lens power is created. The corrective power for this meridian is also –3.50 D.

Accordingly, the power of the contact lens should be –3.50 D (see Fig 5-6).

临床案例 5–3

–3.00 D 的屈光不正，K 值测量为 7.8 mm（43.25 D），为硬性接触镜选择的基弧是 7.95 mm（42.50 D）。那接触镜的焦度应该是多少呢?

泪液镜是 –0.75 D，这个焦度矫正了 –0.75 D 的屈光不正。所以，剩下的需要由接触镜来矫正的屈光不正度数为 –2.25 D（记住 FAP 平加正法则）。反之，如果屈光不正是 +3.00 D（远视），那么接触镜的焦度是 +3.75 D，泪液镜是 –0.75 D（见图 5–5）。

由于泪液镜的折射率（1.336）与角膜的折射率（1.3765）基本相同，泪液镜就能重建角膜表面的屈光效果。不论角膜地形图的形态如何，如果接触镜后表面的形态是球面的，那泪液镜前表面的形态也是球面的。所以，球面硬性接触镜产生的泪液镜可以中和 90% 以上的规则和不规则角膜散光。这个原理简化了散光角膜上的泪液镜焦度计算：不必考虑陡峭子午线上的焦度，只考虑平坦子午线上的焦度。平坦子午线上的焦度与转换为*负柱镜形式*的球镜。所以，硬性接触镜验配时，用负柱镜形式较简单（临床案例 5–4）。球面接触镜还可能“残余散光”，这是由于晶状体和角膜后表面的形态造成的。有一种“后复曲面”透气性接触镜，其设计是前表面为球面，而后表面是复曲面，后表面与角膜的形态一致，可以稳定镜片的定位。还有一种“双复曲面”设计的 RGP 镜，其后表面与角膜形态一致，而前表面设计为可以矫正残余散光的复曲面（临床案例 5–5）。

临床案例 5–4

验光为 –3.50+1.75 x 90，K 值测量两主子午线为水平 7.8mm（43.25D at 180°）和垂直 7.5 mm（45.00D at 90°）。接触镜的基弧为 7.5mm。接触镜的焦度应该是多少?

沿平坦子午线（7.80mm）的焦度是 –1.75D（转换为负柱镜形式），镜片比平坦 *K* 更陡峭，会产生 +1.75D 的泪液镜。所以需要增加相应负焦度（SAM 法则，平加负），在平坦子午线上的焦度就是 –3.50D。

沿陡峭子午线（7.50 mm）的焦度是 –3.50 D。镜片适配是“等于 K”的，所以不会产生泪液镜，在陡峭子午线上的焦度也是 –3.50 D。

综上所述，接触镜的焦度应该是 –3.50 D（图 5–6）。

CLINICAL EXAMPLE 5-5

A patient with a refraction of −2.00 −2.00 × 180 desires contact lens correction. The keratometry measurement is 44.00 sphere. What is the residual refractive error if this eye is fitted with a spherical RGP contact lens? A spherical soft contact lens? A toric soft contact lens?

This eye has lenticular but not corneal astigmatism. Correction with spherical soft or rigid contact lenses will result in residual astigmatism. A soft toric contact lens may be used to correct the lenticular astigmatism.

Toric Soft Contact Lenses

Perhaps one-third of contact lens wearers have at least 1.00 D of astigmatism. Up to 0.75 or 1.00 D of astigmatism will likely be "masked" by a spherical soft contact lens enough to offer best acuity (Table 5-8). Greater degrees of astigmatism will usually not be well-corrected by spherical soft contact lenses.

Table 5-8 Astigmatism and Lens Fitting

Degree of Astigmatism	First Choice of Lens
Less than 1 D	Spherical soft or rigid gas permeable (RGP) lens
1–2 D	Toric soft contact or spherical RGP lens
2–3 D	Custom soft toric or spherical RGP lens
More than 3 D	Toric RGP or custom soft toric lens

Soft toric contact lenses are available in several designs. To prevent lens rotation, various techniques are used:

- adding prism ballast, placing extra lens material on the bottom edge of the lens, whose weight aligns the lens—commonly used
- creating thin zones; that is, making lenses with a thin zone on the top and bottom, so that eyelid pressure tends to keep the lens in the appropriate position
- truncating or removing the bottom of the lens to form a straight edge that aligns with the lower eyelid—not as commonly used

Fitting soft toric lenses is similar to fitting other soft lenses, except that lens rotation must also be evaluated. Toric lenses typically have a mark to note their 6-o'clock position. If a slit-lamp examination shows that the lens mark is consistently rotated to one side of the 6-o'clock axis, the amount of rotation should be noted, in degrees (1 clock-hour equals 30°). To adjust the prescription for lens rotation, follow the *LARS rule (left add; right subtract)*. This is illustrated in Clinical Example 5-6 and Figure 5-11.

Contact Lenses for Presbyopia

Presbyopia affects virtually everyone older than 40 years. Thus, as contact lens wearers age, their accommodation needs must be considered. Three options are available for these patients: (1) use of reading glasses with contact lenses, (2) monovision, and (3) bifocal contact lenses.

The first option, using reading glasses over contact lenses, has the advantages of being simple, inexpensive, and effective.

临床案例5-5

一个患者验光 -2.00-2.00×180，验配接触镜。角膜曲率计测量 K 值为 44.00 球面。如果这眼睛配的是球面的 RGP 接触镜，它的残余散光会是多少？如果配的是球面软镜呢？如果配的是复曲面软镜呢？

眼睛有晶状体散光，而不是角膜散光。配戴球面的软镜或硬性接触镜会导致残余散光的暴露，可以使用软性复曲面接触镜来矫正晶状体散光。

复曲面软性接触镜

1/3 的接触镜配戴者有近 1.00D 的散光。球面软性接触镜最多能矫正 0.75D 或 1.00D 的散光，以获得最佳的视力（表 5-8）。球面软性接触镜难以矫正更大的散光。

表5-8　散光和镜片配适

散光量	首选镜片
＜ 1.00D	球面软镜或RGP
1~2.00D	复曲面软镜或球面RGP
2~3.00D	定制复曲面软镜或球面RGP
＞ 3.00D	复曲面RGP或定制复曲面软镜

软性复曲面接触镜有很多种设计，用于避免镜片旋转，使用了以下的技术：

- 比较常用的是棱镜垂重法。在镜片底部边缘增加额外的镜片材料，使其重力与镜片一致。
- 制作薄区。在镜片上、下方做薄，这样利用眼睑的压力就能使镜片保持在合适的位置。
- 还有一种不太常用的截边法。把镜片下方横截，使之与下眼睑平行。

复曲面软镜的适配与其他软镜适配类似，但复曲面软镜还要评估镜片的旋转。一般复曲面软镜会在 6 点钟的位置做一个标记。如果裂隙灯检查发现镜片标记偏离，需记录旋转角度（1 个钟点 =30°），用 *LARS 法则*（*左加右减*），调整处方中的柱镜轴向。临床案例 5-6 和图 5-11 做了说明。

老视眼的接触镜验配

年龄超过 40 岁几乎都会受到老视的影响。因此，对于这个年龄段的接触镜配戴者，需考虑调节问题。这些患者有 3 种选择：①戴接触镜的同时使用阅读镜；②单眼视；③双焦接触镜。

第 1 种选择，即在配戴接触镜的同时使用阅读镜，其操作简便、经济有效。

CLINICAL EXAMPLE 5-6

An eye with a refraction of −3.00 −1.00 × 180 is fitted with a toric contact lens with an astigmatic axis given as 180°. Slit-lamp examination shows that the lens is well centered, but lens markings show that the 6-o'clock mark is located at the 7-o'clock position. What axis should be ordered for this eye?

Because the trial contact lens rotated 1 clock-hour, or 30°, to the left, the contact lens ordered (recall the LARS rule: left add; right subtract) should be 180° + 30° = 210°, which is the same as 30°, so the lens to order is: −3.00 −1.00 × 30°.

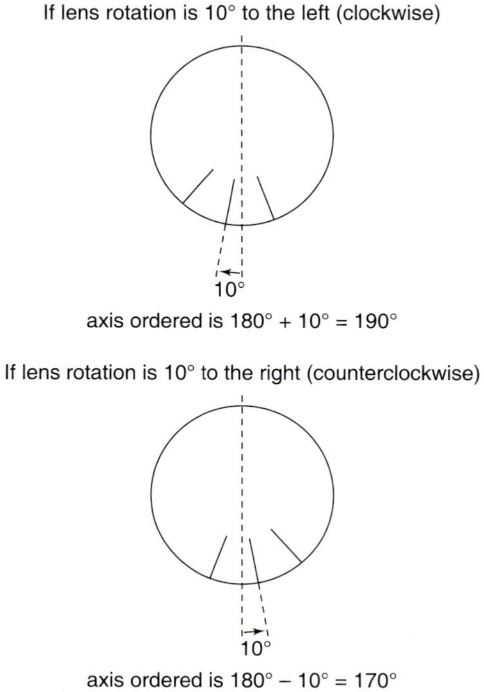

Figure 5-11 Evaluating lens rotation in fitting soft toric contact lenses using the LARS rule of thumb (left add; right subtract). The spectacle prescription in this example is −2.00 −1.00 ×180°. *(Modified with permission from Key JE II, ed. The CLAO Pocket Guide to Contact Lens Fitting. 2nd ed. Metairie, LA: Contact Lens Association of Ophthalmologists; 1998. Redrawn by Christine Gralapp.)*

The second option, monovision, involves correcting one eye, usually the dominant eye, for distance and the other eye for near (see BCSC Section 13, *Refractive Surgery*). Many patients are satisfied with this correction, tolerating the reduced binocular acuity and depth perception. Typically, the dominant eye is corrected for distance. For driving and other critical functions, overcorrection with glasses may be necessary. A temporary trial of monovision contact lenses is often useful when considering a permanent monovision option with laser refractive surgery or lens implant surgery.

The third option for patients with presbyopia is to use bifocal contact lenses, either soft or RGP. There are 2 types of bifocal lenses: alternating vision lenses and simultaneous vision lenses. *Alternating vision bifocal contact lenses* are similar in function to bifocal spectacles in that there are separate areas for distance and near, and the retina receives a focused image from only 1 object plane at a time (Fig 5-12). *Segmented contact* lenses have 2 areas, top and bottom, like bifocal spectacles, whereas concentric contact lenses have 2 rings, 1 for far and 1 for near. For alternating vision contact lenses, the position on the eye is critical and must change as the patient switches from distance to near viewing. The lower eyelid controls the lens position, so that as a person looks down, the lens stays up, and the eye's visual axis moves into the reading portion of the lens. The need for this "translation" of the lens in downgaze makes RGP lenses work well for these designs.

临床案例5-6

眼的屈光状态为 -3.00 -1.00 × 180°，验配散光轴在 180° 的散光接触镜。裂隙灯检查显示镜片居中性良好，但镜片 6 点位的标记位于角膜 7 点位。应该为此眼预订哪个轴位的镜片？

由于试戴片向左转动 1 个钟点位，即 30°，所以接触镜的轴位（LARS 规则：左加右减）为 180° +30° =210°，即 30°，所以应为此眼预订片为：-3.00 -1.00 × 30° 。

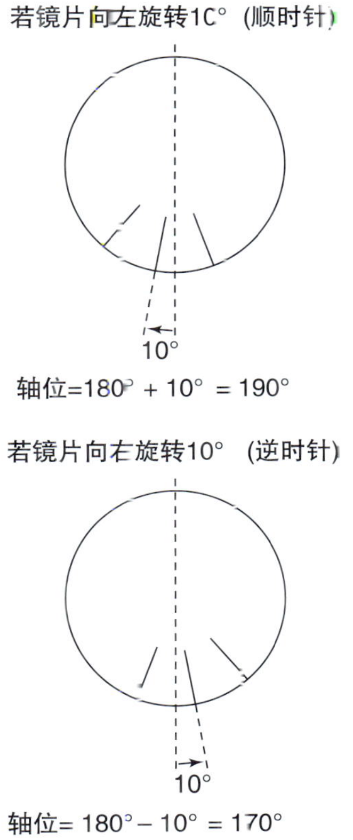

图 5-11　LARS 法则评估复曲面软镜的适配（左加右减）。眼镜处方是 -2.00 -1.00 ×180°。*（译者注 资料来源见前页原文。）*

第 2 种选择为单眼视，即一眼（通常主导眼）视远，另一眼视近（见 BCSC 第 13 册《*屈光手术*》）。虽然此矫正方法会使双眼视力和深度知觉下降，但可获得满意的效果。一般来讲，以主视眼视远。对于驾车和在其他重要场合，需要利用框架镜再次进行屈光矫正。若因激光屈光手术或人工晶体植入手术形成单眼视，可临时选择单眼视接触镜。

第 3 种选择是双焦点接触镜，即软性或硬性接触镜。有 2 种类型的双焦点接触镜：交替视接触镜和同时视接触镜。*交替视双焦点接触镜*在功能上与双焦点眼镜相似，分别有视远和视近的区域，视网膜 1 次只接收来自一个物平面的聚焦像（图 5-12）。与双焦眼镜一样，*分段式接触镜*有 2 个区域，即顶部和底部；而同心圆式接触镜有 2 个环，1 个为视远、1 个为视近。交替视接触镜在角膜上的位置至关重要，必须随着患者从视远到视近不断切换。下眼睑确定镜片的位置，以便向下看时，镜片向上移动、视轴移动到镜片的视近部分。这种镜片的“切换”使 RGP 镜在向下注视时发挥出作用。

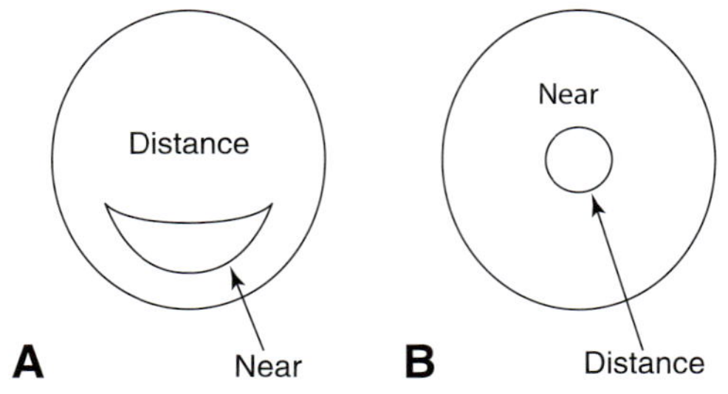

Figure 5-12 Alternating vision bifocal contact lenses. **A**, Segmented lens. **B**, Concentric (annular) lens.

Simultaneous vision bifocal contact lenses, in soft multifocal lenses and some RGP, provide the retina with focused images of near and far simultaneously. This requires the patient's brain to ignore one or the other and accept the reduction in contrast (Fig 5-13). These lenses have various optical designs, with rings of differing focal lengths to provide a bifocal or multifocal effect. The most central portion may be used for either near or distance. Another strategy is to have less add for the dominant eye, so that it has better distance vision, and more add in the nondominant eye.

Jain S, Arora I, Azar DT. Success of monovision in presbyopes: review of the literature and potential applications to refractive surgery. *Surv Ophthalmol.* 1996;40(6):491–499.

Infantile aphakia

Avoiding amblyopia is a major goal in the management of aphakia in infants and young children. When contact lens wear is not feasible, intraocular lens placement is considered for the initial surgery (see BCSC Volume 6, *Pediatric Ophthalmology and Strabismus).*

Infant Aphakia Treatment Group; Lambert SR, Buckley EG, et al. The infant aphakia treatment study: design and clinical mea sures at enrollment. *Arch Ophthalmol.* 2010;128(1):21–27.

Keratoconus and the Abnormal Cornea

Contact lenses can provide better vision than spectacles by *masking* irregular corneal astigmatism. For mild or moderate irregularities, soft spherical, soft toric, or custom soft toric contact lenses are used. Large irregularities typically require an RGP lens to mask the abnormal surface; the anterior surface of the contact lens creates a smooth, spherical air–tear interface, and the tear lens fills the corneal irregularities. As with nonastigmatic eyes, fitters first find the best alignment fit and then determine the optimal power. Three-point touch can be successfully used for larger keratoconus cones to ensure lens centration and stability with slight apical and paracentral touch or *bearing* (dark areas on the fluorescein evaluation; Fig 5-14). Alternatively, apical clearance fitting technique places a lens vault slightly over the cone, avoiding the risk of contributing to apical scarring.

图 5-12　交替视双焦点接触镜。**A**. 分段式接触镜。**B**. 同心圆式接触镜。

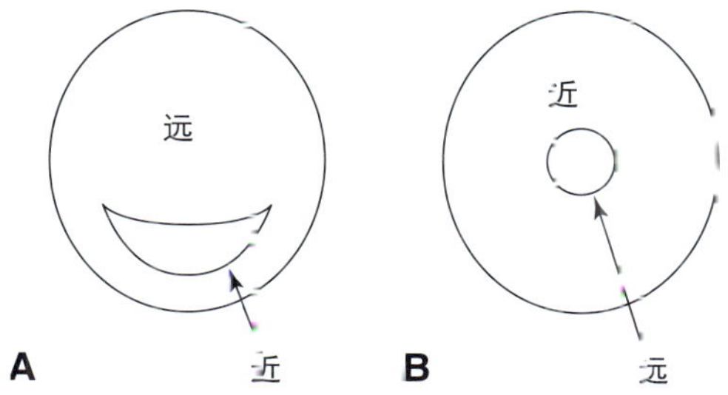

同时视双焦接触镜，软性多焦点镜片和部分 RGP 均有，在视网膜上同时投射近、远聚焦图像。这需要大脑忽略其中一个图像，并接受对比敏感度的降低（图 5-13）。这些镜片有多种光学设计，多个不同焦距环形成双焦点或多焦点。最中心部分可用于视近或视远。另一种策略是减少主导眼的近附加，使它具有更好的远视力，主要是在非主导眼近附加。另一种方法是在主视眼减少近附加，使其具有更好的视远功能，而在非主视眼增加近附加。

Jain S, Arora I, Azar DT. Success of monovision in presbyopes: review of the literature and potential applications to refractive surgery. Surv Ophthalmol. 1996;40(6):491–499.

无晶体眼的婴幼儿

婴幼儿无晶状体眼治疗的主要目标是避免弱视。当不能配戴接触镜时，首次手术时即需要考虑放置人工晶体（参见 BCSC 第 6 册《*小儿眼科与斜视*》）。

Infant Aphakia Treatment Group; Lambert SR, Buckley EG, et al. The infant aphakia treatment study: design and clinical mea sures at enrollment. *Arch Ophthalmol.* 2010;128(1):21–27.

圆锥角膜和异常角膜

接触镜可以通过*消除*不规则角膜散光来获得比框架眼镜更好的视力。对于轻度或中度的角膜不规则，软性球面、软性复曲面或定制的软性复曲面接触镜可以矫正。大的不规则角膜通常需要 RGP 镜覆盖异常的角膜表面，镜片的前表面形成光滑的球性空气 – 泪液交界面，泪液镜填充不规则的角膜表面。与非散光眼一样，首先找到最佳的适配，然后确定度数。三点接触可以成功地验配较大的圆锥角膜，以确保镜片的居中性和稳定性，顶点轻轻接触和旁中心接触或*托举*（荧光素评估上的暗区；图 5-14）。或者，使用顶点间隙技术使镜片稍陡于圆锥，避免角膜顶点瘢痕的形成。

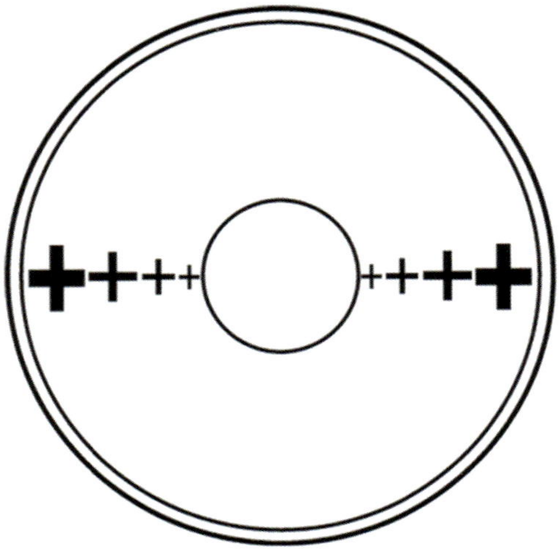

Figure 5-13 Simultaneous vision bifocal design. *(Modified with permission from Key JE II, ed. The CLAO Pocket Guide to Contact Lens Fitting. 2nd ed. Metairie, LA: Contact Lens Association of Ophthalmologists; 1998. Redrawn by Christine Gralapp.)*

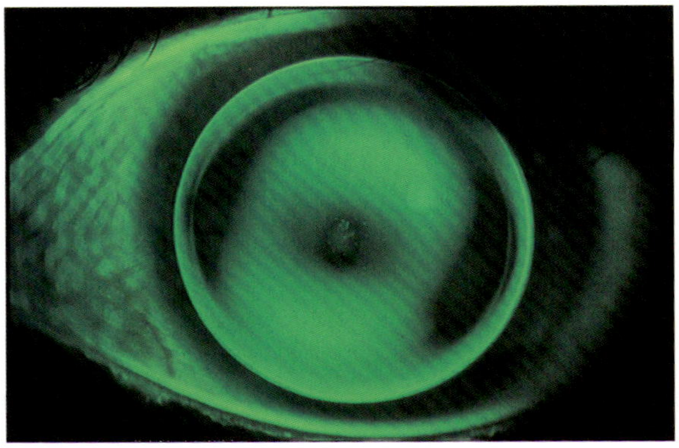

Figure 5-14 Three-point touch in keratoconus. *(Courtesy of Perry Rosenthal, MD.)*

Specialized RGP lenses have been developed for keratoconus. Most provide a steep central posterior curve to vault over the cone and flatter peripheral curves to approximate the more normal peripheral curvature. Larger RGP contact lenses with larger optical zones (diameters >11 mm) are available for keratoconus and post-transplant fitting; they are known as intralimbic contact lenses.

A hybrid contact lens has a rigid center and a soft skirt. The aim is to provide the good vision of an RGP lens and the comfort of a soft lens.

Piggyback lens systems involve the fitting of a soft contact lens with an RGP lens fitted over it. This system may allow comfort benefits like those offered by hybrid lenses, with a greater choice of contact lens parameters, if the combination of lenses allows sufficient gas permeability to avoid hypoxia.

Scleral lenses provide an increasingly popular alternative for corneas that cannot be fit with corneal gas-permeable lenses.

Finding a good fit for an abnormal cornea is well worth the determination and patience required of both fitter and patient. The lens will need refitting after any surgical intervention.

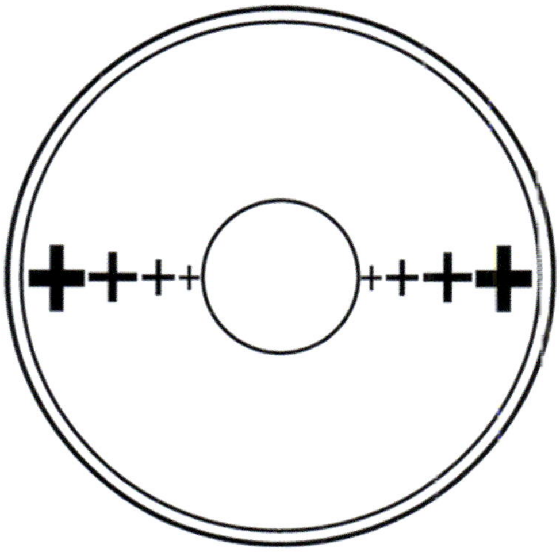

图 5-13 同时视双焦接触镜。*（译者注：资料来源见前页原文。）*

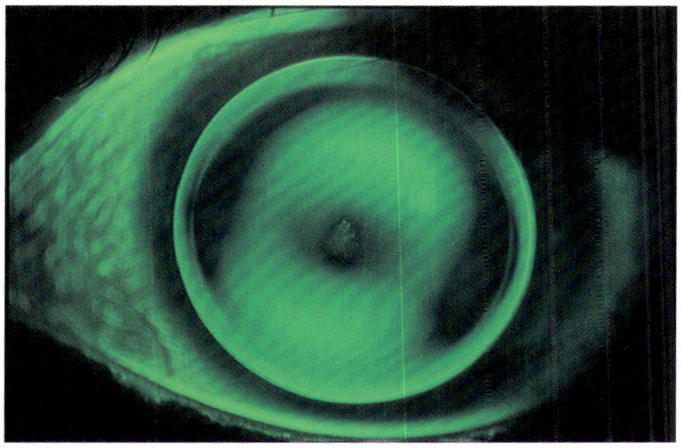

图 5-14 圆锥角膜的三点接触。*（译者注：资料来源见前页原文。）*

已有专门针对圆锥角膜的 RGP。大多数设计为圆锥区陡峭的中央弧和接近较平坦的正常的边弧。具有较大的光学区较大直径的 RGP（直径 >11mm）可用于圆锥角膜和角膜移植后的适配，称为角膜缘内接触镜。

混合性接触镜具有硬性的中央区和软性周边区，可以提供 RGP 镜片良好的视觉和软性接触镜良好的舒适性。

背驮镜系统由软性接触镜以及适配其上的 RGP 组成。若能够提供足够的透气性以避免缺氧，该系统可能像混合接触镜那样，提供良好的舒适性、有更多的镜片参数的选择。

对于不适宜 RGP 的角膜，巩膜镜为其提供了另一种选择。

对于异常形态的角膜，需要患者和医师共同努力和耐心寻找合适的适配。如果实施过手术，接触镜需要重新适配。

Gas-Permeable Scleral Contact Lenses

A scleral lens has a central optic that vaults over the cornea and a peripheral haptic that rests on the scleral surface (Fig 5-15). The shape of the posterior optic surface is chosen to minimize the volume of the fluid compartment while avoiding corneal contact. The posterior haptic surface is configured to minimize localized scleral compression; the transitional zone that joins the optic and haptic surfaces is designed to vault over the limbus.

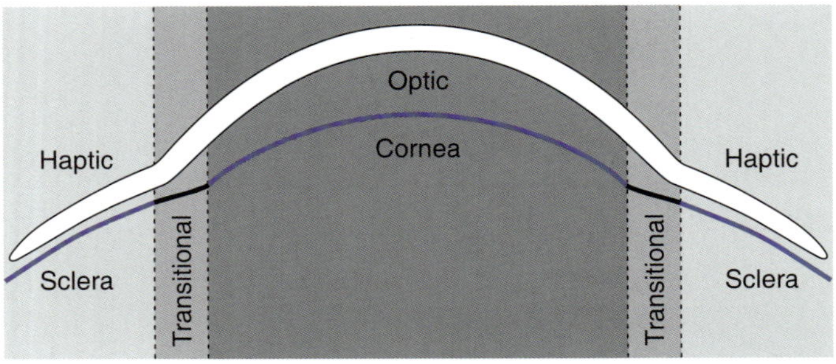

Figure 5-15 Scleral contact lens. *(Redrawn with permission from Albert DM, Jakobiec FA, eds. Principles and Practice of Ophthalmology. Philadelphia: Saunders; 1994;5:3643. Redrawn by Christine Gralapp and modification redeveloped by Leon Strauss, MD, PhD.)*

These RGP lenses, with or without channels, must vent tears in and out to prevent buildup of suction onto the cornea and allow ample circulation of fresh tears beneath the lens. Improved RGP chemistry has enabled these lenses to be well tolerated. They have 2 primary indications: (1) correcting abnormal regular and irregular astigmatism in eyes that cannot be fit with corneal contact lenses, and (2) managing ocular surface diseases that benefit from the constant presence of a protective, lubricating layer of oxygenated tears, such as pellucid degeneration, Terrien marginal degeneration, keratoconus, Ehlers–Danlos syndrome, elevated corneal scars, and astigmatism following penetrating keratoplasty.These lenses can be helpful with complications of Stevens–Johnson syndrome, graft-vs- host disease, tear layer disorders, and ocular cicatricial pemphigoid, protecting the fragile epithelium of these corneas from the abrasive effects of keratinized eyelid margins associated with distichiasis and trichiasis and from exposure to air. They have promoted the healing of some persistent epithelial defects, where other strategies have been unsuccessful. Semi-scleral lenses, extending not as far onto the sclera, have diameters 15–18 mm; scleral lenses have larger diameters, 18.1–24 mm.

Contact Lens Overrefraction

Sometimes we wish to determine the etiology of poor vision of an eye with an irregularly shaped cornea and other possible causes of decreased acuity, such as macular degeneration. Finding out whether refraction over a rigid contact lens achieves good acuity is then diagnostically useful, even when actual contact lens wear is not being considered.

透气性巩膜接触镜

巩膜镜的中央光学区呈拱形，凸出于角膜表面，周边接触区巩膜表面（图 5–15）。镜片后表面的形状设计旨在避免接触角膜，同时使泪液镜的体积最小。巩膜支撑的后表面设计应尽可能减小对局部巩膜的压迫；镜片的巩膜部分和角膜部分的交界处设计为拱形，越过角巩膜缘。

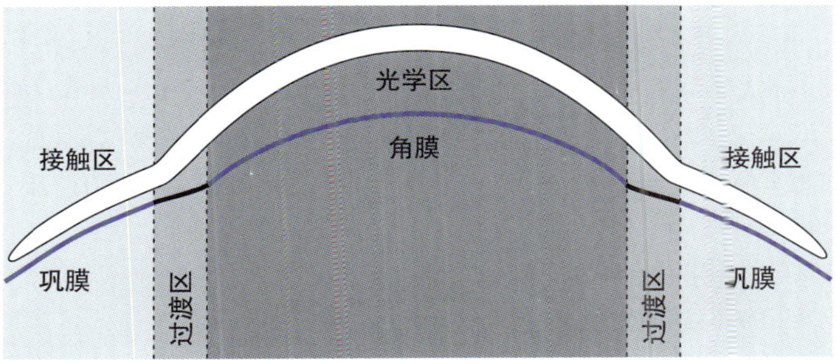

图 5–15　巩膜接触镜。*（译者注：资料来源见前页原文。）*

不论有无通道，这些 RGP 必须使泪液进出，以防止镜片吸附在角膜上，以及镜片下新鲜泪液的充分循环。改进的 RGP 能够很好地耐受。它们有 2 个主要适应症：①矫正不适合接触镜的规则和不规则散光；②治疗眼表疾病，其需要稳定的含氧泪液层的保护和润滑，如角膜透明变性、Terrien 边缘变性、圆锥角膜、Ehlers–Danlos 综合征、隆起的角膜瘢痕和穿透性角膜移植引起的散光。这些镜片还有助于 Stevens–Johnson 综合征、移植物抗宿主病、泪液层紊乱和眼瘢痕性天疱疮等的并发症，保护脆弱的角膜上皮免受角质化睑缘、倒睫、双行睑的磨损，并且避免暴露于空气中，促进持久性上皮缺损的愈合。半巩膜镜直径为 15~18 mm，巩膜镜片直径为 18.1~24 mm。

接触镜矫正后验光

为了确定形状不规则角膜眼视力不良的病因，和其他可能导致视力下降的原因，如黄斑变性，即使不考虑配戴接触镜，也可用硬性接触镜矫正后进行验光，发现是否提高视力，有助于诊断。

Therapeutic Use of Contact Lenses

Contact lenses may be used to enhance epithelial healing, prevent epithelial erosions, or control surface-generated pain. These lenses are sometimes referred to as *bandage contact lenses.* Typically, a disposable plano soft lens of high oxygen permeability is left on the eye for an extended period.Fitting principles are similar to those of other soft lenses, although for therapeutic use, a somewhat tighter fit maybe be preferable, as lens movement could further injure the healing epithelium. Some fitters prefer high-water- content lenses, but high oxygen permeability is usually the chief factor in lens selection.

Conditions and circumstances in which bandage contact lenses might be useful include

- bullous keratopathy
- recurrent erosions
- Bell palsy, exposure keratopathy
- keratitis, such as filamentary or post–chemical exposure
- corneal dystrophy with erosions
- post-surgery, such as corneal transplant, laser in situ keratomileusis (LASIK), or photorefractive keratectomy (PRK)
- nonhealing epithelial defect, such as geographic herpes keratitis, slow-healing ulcer, or abrasion
- eyelid abnormalities, such as entropion, eyelid lag, or trichiasis
- bleb leak after glaucoma filtration surgery

These patients need to be made especially aware of the signs and symptoms of infection, as the vulnerability to infection is increased by the abnormality of the cornea. Some practitioners prefer to use prophylactic topical antibiotics with these lenses.

Orthokeratology and Corneal Reshaping

Orthokeratology refers to the overnight use of RGP contact lenses to temporarily mechanically reshape the cornea. For myopia, lenses are designed to flatten the central cornea for a period after the lenses are removed. The objective is to wear the lenses only during sleep, and not need glasses or contacts during the day. For further information, see the section Orthokeratology in BCSC Section 13, *Refractive Surgery.*

To provide similar temporary correction for hyperopia, soft lenses are also used. There is interest recently in attempting to use contact lenses to reduce progression of myopia in children. This subject remains controversial.

Bennett ES, Henry VA. Orthokeratology. In: *Clinical Manual of Contact Lenses.* 4th ed. Phila-delphia: Lippincott Williams & Wilkins; 2014.

Van Meter WS, Musch DC, Jacobs DS, Kaufman SC, Reinhart WJ, Udell IJ; American Acad-emy of Ophthalmology. Safety of overnight orthokeratology for myopia: a report by the American Acad emy of Ophthalmology. 2008;115(12):2301–2313.e1.

接触镜的治疗应用

接触镜可用于促进角膜上皮愈合、防止上皮糜烂，或控制眼表的疼痛。这些镜片有时被称为*绷带镜*。一次性高氧透性平光软性接触镜可以配戴较长时间。配戴原则与其他软性镜相同，治疗镜的适配可以略紧，因为镜片移动可能进一步损伤愈合中的角膜上皮。尽管有人喜欢配戴高含水量镜片，但应该主要选择高透氧性。

应用绷带接触镜的疾病有：

- 大泡性角膜病变。
- 复发性糜烂。
- Bell 麻痹，暴露性角膜病变。
- 角膜炎，如丝状角膜炎或化学伤后的暴露。
- 角膜营养不良伴糜烂。
- 手术后，如角膜移植、准分子激光原位角膜磨镶术（LASIK）或 PRK 术后。
- 不愈合的上皮缺损，如地图样疱疹病毒性角膜炎、愈合迟缓性角膜溃疡、角膜上皮剥脱。
- 眼睑异常，如睑内翻、眼睑迟落或倒睫。
- 青光眼滤过术后滤泡漏。

这些患者需要特别注意感染的体征和症状，因为角膜病变增加了感染的可能性。一些医师在使用接触镜的同时联合应用预防性眼局部抗生素。

角膜塑形术与角膜形态重塑

角膜塑形术是指夜间使用的 RGP 接触镜，暂时机械地重塑角膜。近视镜片的设计是，在取出镜片后的一段时间内，中央角膜变平。目的是只在睡眠期间配戴镜片，而白天不需要眼镜或接触镜。有关进一步的信息，请参阅 BCSC 第 13 册《*屈光手术*》。

也有使用软性镜片来临时矫正远视的方法。最近也尝试用接触镜减缓儿童近视的进展。这种方法目前仍然存在争议。

Bennett ES, Henry VA. Orthokeratology. In: *Clinical Manual of Contact Lenses*. 4th ed. Phila-delphia: Lippincott Williams & Wilkins; 2014.

Van Meter WS, Musch DC, Jacobs DS, Kaufman SC, Reinhart WJ, Udell IJ; American Academy of Ophthalmology. Safety of overnight orthokeratology for myopia: a report by the American Academy of Ophthalmology. Ophthalmology. 2008;115(12):2301–2313.e1.

Custom Contact Lenses

A normal cornea is generally steepest near its geometric center; beyond the center, the surface flattens. The steep area is known as the *apical zone*, and its center is the *corneal apex*. Outside the apical zone, which is approximately 3–4 mm in diameter, the rate of peripheral flattening may vary significantly in the different corneal meridians. This variation is important, because peripheral corneal topography significantly affects the position, blink-induced excursion patterns, and, therefore, wearing comfort of corneal contact lenses, especially gas-permeable lenses.

The availability of corneal topography and wavefront aberrometers, together with desktop graphics programs and computerized lathes, enables the preparation of individually tailored contact lenses that assist with otherwise difficult fits, such as keratoconus, trauma, and transplant. There is interest in the attempt to design lenses in this way to optimize wavefront correction for normal corneas, with the caveat that contact lenses constantly change their position on the cornea. Specially painted lenses, another custom service, are provided to reduce glare in aniridia and albinism by providing a pupil.

Contact Lens Care and Solutions

Contact lenses are cleaned and disinfected after use, unless they are 1-day disposable lenses. Lens-care systems have been developed to remove deposits and microorganisms from lenses, enhance comfort, and decrease the risk of eye infection and irritation. They include, in 1 or more bottles, cleaning, disinfection, and storage functions (Table 5-9). Enzymatic cleaners, which remove protein deposits from the lens surface, provide additional cleaning for lenses that are not replaced frequently. Alternatively, patients whose eyes form deposits can be switched to lenses that are more frequently replaced. Serious eye infections may occur with any disinfection system, and there is more risk when patients do not follow instructions (eg, to discard and replace solutions). Lens cases must be replaced, unless they are treated with boiling water. Rinsing the lens or case with tap water risks contamination. If a practitioner uses trial lenses, one of the peroxide systems can be used for disinfection of soft and RGP lenses. Peroxide, however, does not kill *Acanthamoeba* species.

Several methods have been developed for disinfecting lenses, including the use of

- chemicals
- hydrogen peroxide
- ultraviolet light exposure

Table 5-9 Contact Lens–Care Systems

Type	Purpose	Lens Use	Comments
Saline	Rinsing	All types	May be used with, but not instead of, disinfecting systems
Daily cleaner	Cleaning	All types	Used with some disinfecting systems
Multipurpose solution	Cleaning, disinfecting, rinsing, and storing	All types	Rubbing with a daily cleaner is usually preferred for RGP lenses
Hydrogen peroxide solution	Cleaning, disinfecting, rinsing, and storing	All types	Risk of chemical burn, if instructions are not followed
Enzymatic cleaner	Removal of deposits	All types	Used to remove deposits from lenses that are not replaced frequently

定制的接触镜

正常的角膜通常在其中央附近最为陡峭；在中央之外，前表面变平。陡峭的区域称为*顶区*，其中心是*角膜顶点*，顶区直径为 3~4 mm。顶区之外的周边角膜变平，不同子午线上的改变比较大。这种变化很重要，因为周边角膜的形态会显著影响接触镜的位置、眨眼引起的偏移，会影响接触镜配戴的舒适性，尤其是透气性接触镜。

角膜地形图和波前像差仪，以及图形处理程序和计算机车床的应用，使我们能够个性化定制接触镜，这些接触镜有助于复杂眼部情况的适配，如圆锥角膜、外伤和角膜移植术后。这种设计可实施正常角膜的优化波前相差矫正，同时预测镜片在角膜上变化的位置。另一种特殊着色的定制镜片，可通过人工瞳孔减少无虹膜症和白化病患者的眩光。

接触镜的护理和护理液

除了一次性镜片，接触镜在使用后都需要清洗和消毒。镜片护理系统用于去除镜片的沉积物和微生物，提高舒适度，并降低眼部感染的风险和刺激。其包括 1 个或多个瓶子，具有清洁、消毒和储存的功能（表 5–9）。酶清洗剂可以去除镜片表面的蛋白质沉积物，为不经常更换的镜片提供额外的清洗。另外，对于镜片经常有沉积物的患者，需选经常更换的镜片。任何消毒系统都不能避免严重眼部感染的发生，当患者不遵医嘱时风险更大（如丢弃和更换护理液）。镜片盒须更换，或用沸水处理。用自来水冲洗镜片或镜片盒有污染的危险。医生使用的试戴片，需要用过氧化物消毒剂消毒软镜和 RGP，但过氧化物不能杀死*棘阿米巴*。

几种消毒镜片的方法包括：

- 化学方法。
- 使用过氧化氢。
- 紫外线照射。

表5–9　接触镜护理系统

类型	目的	可使用的镜片类型	备注
盐溶液	冲洗	所有类型	可和消毒液一同使用，但不可替代消毒液
日常清洗液	清洁	所有类型	与消毒液一同使用
多用途溶液	清洁、消毒、冲洗和保存	所有类型	护理RGP和日常清洗液一同使用效果更佳
过氧化氢溶液	清洁、消毒、冲洗和保存	所有类型	如果未按照操作规程可能造成镜片化学损害
含酶清洗液	去除沉淀	所有类型	用于去除镜片上不易清除的沉淀

Heat disinfection is not commonly used now. The care system selected depends on the personal preference of the fitter and patient, the simplicity and convenience of use, cost, and possible allergies to solution components. Currently, multipurpose solutions are the most popular care systems in the United States.

The fitter should instruct the patient in the care and use of contact lenses:

- Clean and disinfect a lens whenever it is removed. Rubbing cleans the lens more thoroughly.
- Follow the instructions included with the lens-care system.
- Do not use tap water, saliva, home-made solutions, and so on.
- Do not reuse contact lens–care solutions.
- Note that swimming with contact lenses increases the risk of infection.
- Do not allow the dropper tip or bottle to be contaminated.
- Clean the contact lens case daily; disinfect with boiling water and/or replace it every 2–3 months.
- Follow the recommended lens replacement schedule.
- Seek medical assistance promptly, when indicated.

In addition to teaching appropriate contact lens and case care, the fitter should instruct the patient in proper lens insertion and removal techniques, determine a wear schedule, and decide when the lens should be replaced. Insertion and handling techniques vary significantly among various lenses; manufacturers provide written information and videos to instruct staff and patients in appropriate insertion and removal techniques.

Recommendations for preventing possible transmission of human T-lymphotropic virus Type Ⅲ / lymphadenopathy-associated virus from tears. *MMWR.* 1985;34(34):533-534. Available at www .cdc .gov / mmwr /preview /mmwrhtml /00033677 .htm. A ccessed O ctober 8, 2017.

Contact Lens–Related Problems and Complications

Contact lens problems can be categorized as follows: infectious, hypoxic/metabolic, toxic, mechanical, inflammatory, and dry eye (Table5-10).

Infections

With the increased use of disposable lenses, better patient education, more convenient care systems, and the availability of more oxygen-permeable lens materials, serious eye infections from lens use have become less common. However, practitioners should be aware of unusual infections that can occur, such as *Acanthamoeba*, fungal keratitis, and Pseudomonas (Fig 5-16A). Diagnosis and treatment of corneal infections are covered in BCSC Section 8, *External Disease and Cornea.*

Hypoxic/Metabolic Problems

Contact lens overwear syndromes can take several forms. Hypoxia, lactate accumulation, and impaired carbon dioxide efflux are responsible for these complications.

高温消毒已不使用。根据验配者和患者的个人偏好、简便性和易用性、成本，以及对消毒液成分是否过敏，选择护理方法。目前，多功能护理液是美国最流行的护理方法。

验配者应指导患者护理和使用接触镜：

- 每次取出镜片时都要清洗消毒。揉搓能更彻底地清洁镜片。
- 按照镜片护理方法所包括的指导。
- 不要使用自来水、唾液、自制溶液等。
- 不要重复使用接触镜护理液。
- 注意配戴接触镜游泳会增加感染的风险。
- 不要让滴管口或瓶子受到污染。
- 每天清洁镜盒；用沸水消毒或每 2~3 个月更换 1 次。

- 按照建议的镜片更换时间表更换镜片。
- 如有需要，立即寻求医师的帮助。

除了指导患者正确地护理接触镜和镜盒外，验配人员还应指导患者正常地配戴和取出镜片，交代清楚配戴时间，并告知应何时更换镜片。各种镜片的配戴和护理差别很大；制造商提供书面信息和视频，以指导工作人员和患者使用正确的配戴和取出方法。

Recommendations for preventing possible transmission of human T-lymphotropic virus Type Ⅲ/lymphadenopathy-associated virus from tears. *MMWR*. 1985;34(34):533-534. Available at www.cdc.gov/mmwr/preview/mmwrhtml/00033677.htm. Accessed October 8, 2017.

接触镜相关问题与并发症

接触镜问题可按以下情况分类：感染性、缺氧性/代谢性、中毒性、机械性、炎症性和干眼性（表 5-10）。

感染

随着一次性接触镜使用的增加、更完善的患者宣教、更方便的护理程序和更好透氧性材料的应用，镜片使用引起的眼部严重感染已非常少见。然而，医生应当注意仍可能发生罕见感染，例如*棘阿米巴性*、真菌性角膜炎和假单胞菌感染（图 5-16A）。角膜感染的诊断与治疗见 BCSC 第 8 册《*外眼疾病与角膜*》。

缺氧与代谢问题

接触镜的过度磨损综合征可以表现为多种形式。组织缺氧，乳酸堆积和二氧化碳释放造成损害是这些并发症的原因。

Table 5-10 Contact Lens–Related Problems and Complications

Category	Problem or Complication
Infectious	Conjunctivitis
	Keratitis
	Bacterial
	Fungal
	Acanthamoebal
Hypoxic/metabolic	Metabolic epithelial damage
	Corneal neovascularization
Toxic	Punctate keratitis
	Toxic conjunctivitis
Mechanical	Corneal warpage
	Spectacle blur
	Ptosis
	Corneal abrasions
	3-o'clock and 9-o'clock staining
Inflammatory	Contact lens–induced keratoconjunctivitis (CLIK)
	Allergic reactions
	Giant papillary conjunctivitis (GPC)
	Sterile infiltrates
Dry eye	Punctate keratitis
	Keratitis sicca

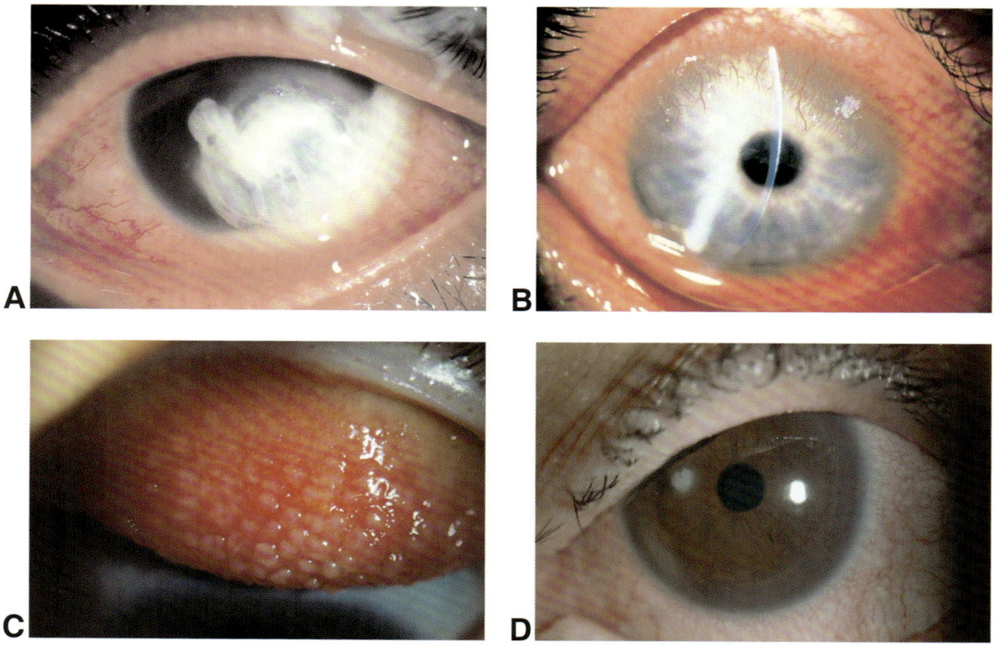

Figure5-16 Contact lens complications. A, Pseudomonas corneal ulcer. B, Corneal neovascularization (vascular pannus). C, Giant papillary conjunctivitis. D, Sterile corneal infiltrates. *(Parts Cand D courtesy of Deborah S. Jacobs, MD.)*

Central epithelial edema (Sattler veil) may present after many hours of wear, more commonly with hard contact lenses. This epithelial edema causes blurred vision that may persist for many hours or, in rare instances, progress to acute epithelial necrosis.

表 5－10　接触镜相关问题和并发症

分类	问题或并发症
感染性	结膜炎
	角膜炎
	细菌性
	真菌性
	棘阿米巴性
缺氧/代谢性	代谢性上皮损伤
	角膜新生血管
中毒性	点状角膜炎
	中毒性结膜炎
机械性	角膜翘曲
	眼镜片模糊
	上睑下垂
	角膜擦伤
	3点和9点着色
炎症性	接触镜诱发的结膜角膜炎 (CLIK)
	过敏反应
	巨乳头结膜炎 (GPC)
	无菌浸润
干眼	点状角膜炎
	干燥性角膜炎

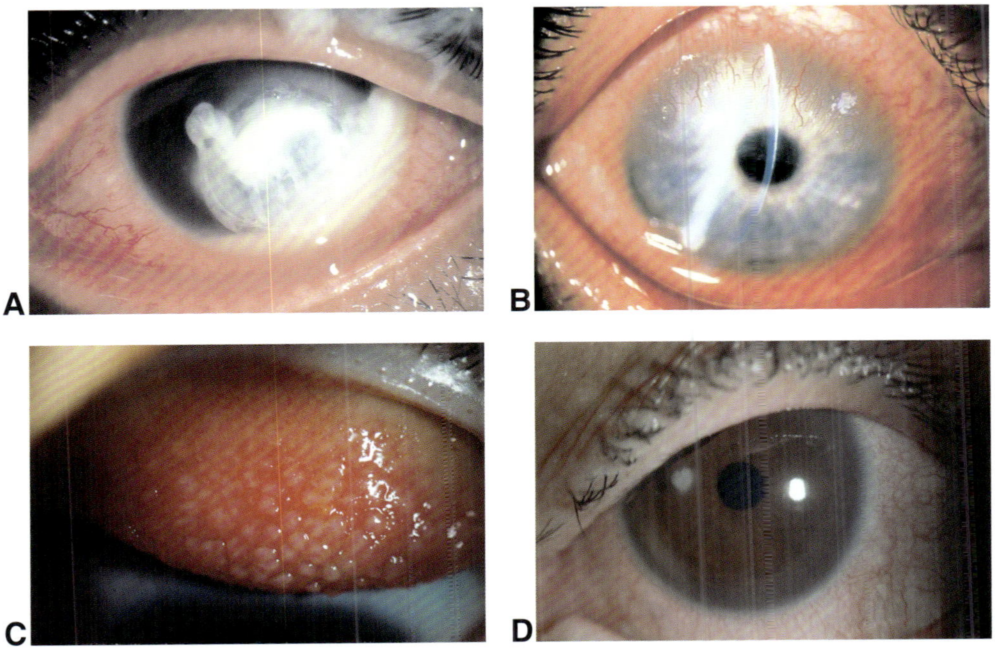

图 5–16　接触镜并发症。**A**. 假单胞菌角膜溃疡。**B**. 角膜新生血管形成（血管翳）。**C**. 巨乳头结膜炎。**D**. 无菌性角膜浸润。*（译者注：资料来源见前页原文。）*

角膜上皮水肿（Sattler 薄雾症）见于配戴接触镜数小时后，更常见于硬性接触镜。这种上皮水肿中央造成持续数小时的视觉模糊，或者偶然发展成急性上皮坏死。

Microcystic epitheliopathy, another condition caused by impaired metabolism in the corneal epithelium, shows fine epithelial cysts, which are most easily observed with retroillumination. This condition is more common with extended wear. The cysts may either be asymptomatic or cause recurrent brief episodes of pain and epiphora. It takes up to 6 weeks following discontinuation of contact lens wear for the cysts to resolve. In some cases, this epitheliopathy may have a dendritic appearance.

Corneal neovascularization (Fig 5-16B) is usually a sign of hypoxia. Refitting with lenses of higher-oxygen-permeability material or with a looser fit, requiring fewer hours of lens wear per day, or switching to disposable lenses can prevent further progression. If neovascularization is extensive, it can lead to corneal scarring and lipid deposition or intracorneal hemorrhage. Superficial pannus is rarely associated with RGP contact lens wear, but is encountered more frequently in patients who use soft lenses either as extended wear or daily wear with less frequent replacement. This type of neovascularization is probably caused by hypoxia and chronic trauma to the limbus. Other causes of pannus, such as staphylococcal and chlamydial keratoconjunctivitis, should be considered in the presence of accompanying signs that suggest them.

Deep stromal neovascularization has been associated with extended-wear contact lenses, especially in aphakia. This condition is not usually symptomatic unless there is secondary lipid deposition. Deep neovascularization of the cornea is often irreversible and is best managed by discontinuing contact lens wear.

Toxicity

Punctate keratitis

Punctate keratitis may be related to poor contact lens fit, toxic reaction to contact lens solutions, or dry eye.

Toxic conjunctivitis

Conjunctival injection, epithelial staining, punctate epithelial keratopathy, erosions, microcysts, and limbal stem cell deficiency are all potential findings of conjunctival or corneal toxicity arising from contact lens solutions. Any of the proteolytic enzymes or chemicals used for cleaning contact lenses, or the preservative-containing soaking solution, may be the culprit. Cleaning and disinfecting agents can cause an immediate, painful epitheliopathy.

Mechanical Problems

Corneal warpage

Change in corneal shape from contact lens use occurs with both soft and RGP lenses, but it is more commonly associated with hard lenses. Most warpage resolves after the patient discontinues wearing the lens. To evaluate corneal shape on an ongoing basis, the clinician can follow keratometry or corneal topography and manifest refraction as part of the contact lens follow-up examination. The common term *spectacle blur* misleadingly suggests that these changes are somehow due to a problem with the spectacle correction. If there is more than a little fluctuation of refractive error, the contact lens fit should be reevaluated.

微囊性上皮病变，是另一种由于代谢引起的角膜上皮损伤，用后照法可观察到上皮微囊。这种情况常见于超时配戴，可能无症状，也可引起反复发作的短暂的疼痛和流泪。需要停戴 6 周。有些病例可能表现为树枝状。

角膜新生血管 (图 5–16B) 是缺氧的表现。改用高透氧材料的镜片或略松的适配、每天减少戴镜时间，或者改用一次性镜片，可以阻止新生血管进一步进展。如果新生血管范围比较大，会导致角膜瘢痕和脂类沉积或者角膜内出血。RGP 镜片少有浅层血管翳，软性接触镜的患者，无论是长时间配戴或日戴，都常见，可能是缺氧和角膜缘慢性损伤造成的。其他引起血管翳的原因有金黄色葡萄性和衣原体性角结膜炎的伴随症状。

*基质层新生血管*常见于长戴型接触镜，尤其是无晶体眼。一般没有症状，除非伴有中度脂质沉积。角膜深层新生血管常是不可逆的，停戴接触镜可以控制发展。

毒性反应

点状角膜炎

点状角膜炎与接触镜不良适配、接触镜护理液毒性反应或者干眼有关。

中毒性结膜炎

结膜充血、上皮点染、点状角膜上皮病变、糜烂、微囊肿和角膜缘干细胞缺失等，都可能是接触镜护理液引起的角膜结膜毒性反应，包括所有用于清洁镜片的蛋白水解酶和化学性制剂，或者含有防腐剂的浸泡液。清洁剂和消毒剂都可以引起剧痛的急性上皮性病变。

机械性问题

角膜翘曲

软镜和 RGP 镜都可以引起角膜形状的改变，但更常见于硬镜，停戴后可以恢复。为了对角膜形状持续地进行评估，医生复查时应该进行角膜曲率计、角膜地形图和显然验光等检查。常见的“*眼镜模糊*”一词误导我们认为这些变化在某种程度上是由于眼镜矫正的问题。如果屈光不正度数波动较大，接触镜的适配需要重新评估。

Ptosis

Ptosis related to dehiscence of the levator aponeurosis has been associated with long-term use of RGP lenses.

Corneal abrasions

Corneal abrasions can result from foreign bodies under a lens, poor insertion or removal technique, or a damaged contact lens. Most clinicians treat abrasions with topical antibiotics and try to avoid patching, particularly in the context of contact lens wear, to reduce the likelihood of infection.

3-o'clock and 9-o'clock staining

This specific superficial punctate keratitis staining pattern may be observed in RGP contact lens users, especially with interpalpebral fit, and is probably related to poor wetting (Fig 5-17). Paralimbal staining is characteristic of lowriding lenses and is associated with an abortive reflex blink pattern, insufficient lens movement, inadequate tear meniscus, and a thick peripheral lens profile. Refitting the lens or regular use of rewetting drops may help.

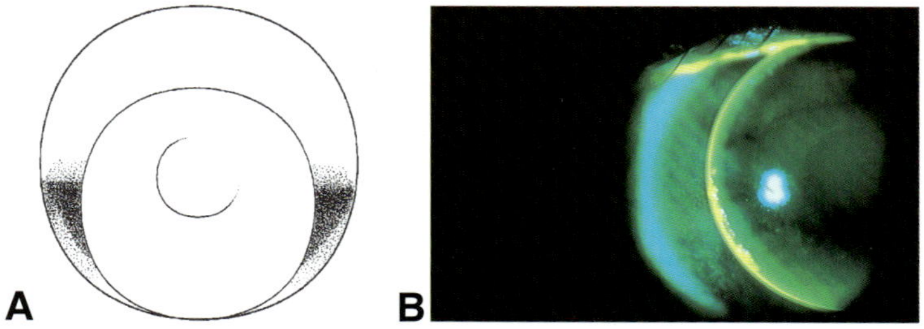

Figure 5-17 Three-o'clock and 9-o'clock corneal staining. **A**, Inferior corneal desiccation of the tear film. **B**, Peripheral corneal desiccation. *(Part B courtesy of Perry Rosenthal, MD.)*

Inflammation

Contact lens–induced keratoconjunctivitis

Contact lens–induced keratoconjunctivitis (CLIK) can be ascribed to allergy, dry eye, infection, and deposits on lenses. Patients with ocular prostheses and exposed monofilament sutures have similar reactions. Findings suggest a combined mechanical and immune-mediated pathophysiology.

Allergic reactions

Preservative chemicals can produce a type IV delayed hypersensitivity response, resulting in conjunctivitis, keratitis, coarse epithelial and subepithelial opacities, and superior limbic keratoconjunctivitis. This condition has become less common, probably because of the replacement of thimerosal by other preservatives in contact lens solutions and the introduction of disposable contact lenses.

Giant papillary conjunctivitis

Giant papillary conjunctivitis (GPC) (Fig 5-16C) tends to develop more frequently with extended-wear soft contact lenses, dry eye, and meibomian gland dysfunction. It may also be induced by other irritants, such as loose sutures or prosthetics. Symptoms include contact lens intolerance, itching, excessive mucus discharge, and blurred vision with mucus coating the contact lens, contact lens decentration, and conjunctival redness. Sometimes, there may be bloody tears and ptosis secondary to inflammation of the superior tarsal conjunctiva.

上睑下垂

上睑下垂与长期配戴 RGP 镜片引起的提上睑肌腱膜撕裂有关。

角膜擦伤

角膜擦伤可能是镜片下异物、不良配戴或摘取，或者镜片损坏造成的。多数医生使用抗生素以降低感染风险，避免包扎，特别是在接触镜配戴时。

3 点和 9 点着色

特殊的表层点状角膜染色见于 RGP，特别是睑裂间适配型、湿润性差的情况（图 5–17）。角膜缘染色提示低骑适配，还与不完全的眨眼反应、镜片移动度不足、泪湖高度不足以及镜缘厚有关。镜片重新适配或者常规使用湿润滴眼液有助于改善。

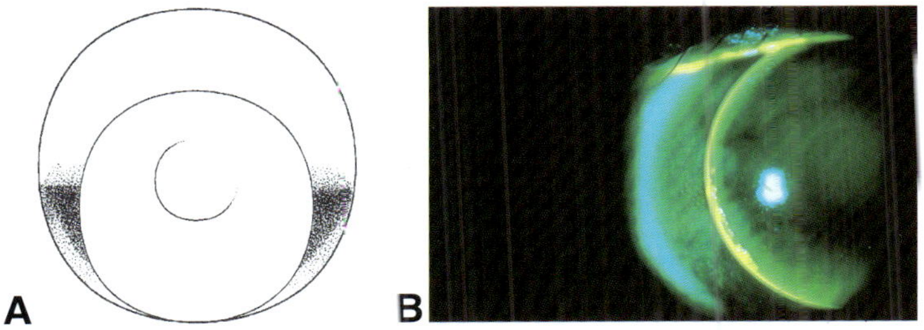

图 5–17　3 点和 9 点角膜着色。**A**. 下方角膜的泪膜干燥。**B**. 周边角膜干燥。*（译者注：资料来源见前页原文。）*

炎症

接触镜引发的结角膜炎

接触镜性角结膜炎（CLIK）由过敏、干眼、感染和镜片沉积物引发。义眼和暴露的单丝缝线也有类似反应，提示是一种机械与免疫联合介导的病理生理反应。

过敏反应

防腐剂可以引起 IV 型迟发型变态反应，导致结膜炎、角膜炎、上皮粗糙和上皮下混浊，以及上方角膜缘的角结膜炎。由于取代了护理液中防腐剂的硫柳汞，以及一次性接触镜，已经较少见。

巨乳头结膜炎

巨乳头结膜炎（GPC）（图 5–16C）常见于长戴型软性接触镜、干眼和睑板腺功能障碍。也可能是其他的刺激物，如松动的手术缝线或义眼。症状包括不能耐受接触镜、眼痒、黏性分泌物增加和黏性分泌物覆盖在镜片上引起的视物模糊、接触镜偏心和结膜充血。可有血性泪水、上睑结膜炎症导致的继发性上睑下垂。

The signs of GPC consist of hyperemia, thickening, and abnormally large papillae (diameter >0.3 mm) of the superior tarsal conjunctiva due to disruption of the anchoring septae. In some cases, the giant papillae cover the entire central tarsus from the posterior eyelid margin to the upper border of the tarsal plate; involvement in other cases may be less extensive. Long-standing or involuted giant papillae on the superior tarsus may resemble follicles. The symptoms of GPC generally resolve when contact lens wear is discontinued. The tarsal conjunctival hyperemia and thickening may resolve in several weeks, but papillae or dome-shaped scars on the superior tarsus can persist for years.

If GPC persists, the clinician should consider changing the lens to a different polymer or to daily-wear disposable lenses. Some patients prefer low-water-content lenses. In persistent cases, consider fitting the patient with RGP contact lenses, which are associated with a lower incidence of GPC, or discontinuing contact lens wear.

Many practitioners recommend discontinuing lens wear for 2–3 weeks while treatment is initiated. Mast-cell stabilizer/antihistamine topical medications are used for mild GPC. Topical corticosteroids may be used for several weeks for these or more advanced cases, with appropriate monitoring of the increased long-term risks of infection, elevated intraocular pressure, and cataract formation. Topical cyclosporine and tacrolimus may be helpful in some cases. In the most severe cases, it may be necessary to discontinue contact lens wear.

Sterile infiltrates

Typically, sterile infiltrates are observed in the peripheral cornea. They occur more often in younger patients. Often there is more than one spot, the epithelium over the spots is intact, and they are relatively small (Fig 5-16D). Discontinuing lens use can usually solve the problem quickly, but clinicians often prescribe an antibiotic, even though cultures tend to show no growth. Increased bacterial bioburden has been found on these lenses.

Dry Eye

Patients with severe dry eye probably are not good candidates for contact lens use. However, patients with moderate to mild dry eye may do well with contact lenses. Some soft lenses are marketed for dry eye patients; these lenses often have lower water content, more thickness, and/or better wettability. They may be made of material that is less prone to lens deposit formation.

Some patients may succeed in contact lens wear with the placement of punctal plugs. Occasionally, the signs and symptoms of dry eye result from incomplete or infrequent blinking (fewer than 12 times per minute). Scleral lenses are being used for some cases of severe dry eye.

Over-the-Counter Contact Lenses

Of course, contact lenses should not be sold over-the-counter without being fitted by someone qualified to do so. Unfortunately, this has occurred. Colored contacts, circle lenses, sclera contacts, and other costume contact lenses may be advertised like toys.

Colored contact lenses. Available at www.aao.org/eye-health/glasses-contacts/colored-lenses. Accessed October 8, 2017.

巨乳头结膜炎的体征有上睑结膜充血、增厚和异常的巨大乳头 (直径 >0.3 mm)，这是睑板隔破坏而引起的。有时巨大乳头覆盖整个上睑板。上睑板长期存在的或者非典型的巨乳头可类似滤泡。接触镜停戴后巨乳头结膜炎消失。睑结膜充血和增厚可在几周后恢复，但上睑的乳头状突起和圆顶状瘢痕可能会持续数年。

如果巨乳头结膜炎持续存在，应当考虑改用不同聚合物的镜片或者日抛镜片。有些患者喜爱低含水量镜片。在顽固病例中，考虑为患者适配 RGP，或者停戴接触镜。

建议在治疗初始阶段，停戴镜片 2~3 周。肥大细胞稳定剂或抗组胺药物局部治疗用于轻度巨乳头结膜炎。局部类固醇皮质激素用于严重的病例，并应密切监测可能产生的感染、升高眼压和白内障的风险。还可以使用局部环孢霉素和他克莫司（免疫抑制药）。严重的病例应该停戴接触镜。

无菌浸润

典型的无菌浸润出现在周边角膜，常见于年纪较小的患者。常常多个较小的点状浸润，且浸润处上皮完整 (图 5–16D)。停戴后快速消失。即使微生物培养阴性，也会使用抗生素，因为在这些镜片上会有微生物污染。

干眼

严重干眼不适合配带接触镜，但是中、轻度干眼可能适应接触镜。市场上有干眼专用接触镜，其含水量低、较厚、具有较好的湿润性，所用材料不易形成沉积物。

有些干眼通过放置泪点塞，再配带接触镜。有时干眼是由于不完全眨眼，或眨眼较少造成的（＜ 12 次 /s）。严重干眼可以使用巩膜镜。

非处方接触镜

当然，接触镜不应未经有资质的人员验配在柜台销售。令人感到遗憾的是，这样的事情常有发生。彩色接触镜、环形接触镜、巩膜镜和其他美容接触镜与玩具一起在广告中出现。

Colored contact lenses. Available at www.aao.org/eye-health/glasses-contacts/colored-lenses. Accessed October 8, 2017.

Federal Law and Contact Lenses

The Federal Fairness to Contact Lens Consumers Act (PL 108-164) "increases consumers' ability to shop around when buying contact lenses." The patient must be given, without having to ask, a copy of the prescription. If the patient calls in contact lens parameters to a seller, and the seller leaves a message for the prescriber, it is considered "verified" if the prescriber doesn't reply within 8 business hours, Monday – Friday, except federal holidays. Although the fit of a rigid lens may depend on the laboratory's machinery, and modifications the practitioner may have made, these lenses are not excluded from this law, which also forbids the prescriber from asking the patient to sign a waiver of responsibility for the prescription. State laws may also address these issues.

Contact lens law is clarified by EU court. Available at www.eubusiness.com/topics/eulaw /lens.01. Accessed July 31, 2017.

Federal Trade Commission. The contact lens rule: a guide for prescribers and sellers. Available at www.ftc.gov/tips-advice/business-center/guidance/contact-lens-rule-guide -prescribers-sellers. Accessed October 8, 2017.

Chapter Exercises

Questions

5.1 A 40-year-old patient is prescribed single-vision glasses –6.00 D OU and also fitted with contact lenses –5.50 D OU. He calls to complain that he has trouble reading when wearing the contacts. What is the most likely explanation?
  a. The contact lenses are "over-minused."
  b. With the contacts, he is losing near effectivity, which the glasses give him.
  c. Looking through the contacts causes base-in prism, making it difficult for the eyes to converge.
  d. The contacts have plus-powered tear lenses, which increase accommodative demand.

5.2 A patient tore her soft contact lens, and it has caused a corneal abrasion. What is the next step?
  a. Put in a fresh lens, which will have a bandage effect, while the abrasion heals.
  b. Put in a fresh lens and use topical antibiotics for several days.
  c. Pressure-patch the eye with antibiotic and see the patient the next day.
  d. Do not use a contact lens; use lubrication and perhaps antibiotic drops.

5.3 A trial soft contact lens moves excessively with eyelid blinks. Which of the following would decrease lens movement?
  a. flattening the base curve while maintaining the diameter
  b. decreasing the diameter while maintaining the base curve
  c. increasing the power of the contact lens
  d. steepening the base curve while maintaining the diameter
  e. flattening the base curve and decreasing the diameter

联邦法律和接触镜

接触镜消费者的联邦公平法案 (PL 108–164) “增加了接触镜的购买者货比三家的消费权益”。在不提供接触镜处方复印件的情况下，必须付货给患者。当患者向医生电话询问接触镜参数、同时卖家记录这些信息时，如果医生没有在 8 个工作小时（除外法定假日的周一至周五）回复，视为医生“认可”这个电话记录。尽管硬镜的适配要依靠诊室的设备，以及医师做出相应的参数调整，这些镜片依然受法律限制，即法律禁止开具处方者要求患者签署处方免责声明。国家法律也关注这些问题。

Contact lens law is clarified by EU court. Available at www.eubusiness.com/topics/eulaw /lens.01. Accessed July 31, 2017.

Federal Trade Commission. The contact lens rule: a guide for prescribers and sellers. Available at www.ftc.gov/tips-advice/business-center/guidance/contact-lens-rule-guide -prescribers-sellers. Accessed October 8, 2017.

章节练习

问题

5.1　一个 40 岁的患者的处方是：单焦框架眼镜，双眼 –6.00 D；接触镜双眼 –5.50 D。他抱怨戴接触镜时阅读出现问题。最可能的解释是什么？
a. 接触镜负镜过大
b. 戴接触镜时丧失了戴框镜所带来的视近效率
c. 接触镜引起了底向内的棱镜效应使眼睛会聚困难
d. 接触镜增加了泪液镜的焦度，这增大了调节需求

5.2　患者的接触镜破损，引起角膜擦伤。下一步如何处理？
a. 戴新镜片，可以在擦伤愈合的过程中起绷带镜的作用
b. 戴新镜片，同时局部使用数日抗生素
c. 使用抗生素并加压包扎患眼，第 2 天复诊
d. 停用接触镜，给予舒润液或抗生素滴液

5.3　接软性接触镜试戴片随着眼睑眨动过度移动。以下哪项可以减少镜片移动？
a. 保持直径不变，基弧变平
b. 保持基弧不变，减小直径
c. 增加接触焦度
d. 保持直径不变，基弧变陡
e. 基弧变平，同时减小直径

5.4 You fit a patient who has −3.50 D of myopia with an RGP contact lens that is flatter than *K*. If the patient's average *K* reading is 7.80 mm and you fit a lens with a base curve of 8.00 mm, what is the shape of the tear lens?

a. plano
b. teardrop
c. concave
d. convex

5.5 For the patient in question 5.4, what power RGP lens should you order?

a. −3.50D
b. −4.00D
c. −2.00D
d. −2.50D

5.6 You fit a toric soft contact lens on a patient with a refractive error of −2.50 D −1.50 × 175. The trial lens centers well, but the lens mark at the 6-o'clock position appears to rest at the 5-o'clock position when the lens is placed on the patient's eye. What power contact lens should you order?

a. −2.50D −1.50 × 175
b. −2.50D −1.50 × 145
c. −2.50D −1.50 × 55
d. −2.50D −1.00 × 175

Answers

5.1.**b.** The near effectivity of the glasses decreases accommodative demand, making it easier to read than when the myopia is corrected at the cornea by the contact lenses. The glasses have their optical centers placed for distance viewing. Converging to read induces base-in prism, so that less convergence is required to look at near objects, when wearing the glasses. If the contacts are rigid, and form a plus-powered tear lens, they would blur distance vision and aid reading vision, unless the power of the lenses is properly adjusted by over-refracting with the lenses in place. The contact lens has slightly less power than the spectacle lens, because of the difference in vertex distance (see Table 5-4).

5.2 **d.** With contact lens involvement, we are more concerned than otherwise about infection. Use no lens or patch, consider lubrication and topical antibiotic, and see the patient soon for follow-up.

5.3 **d.** Increasing the sagittal depth of the contact lens tightens the fit and decreases lens movement, which may be achieved through steepening (decreasing) the base curve or increasing the diameter of the contact lens. Flattening (increasing) the base curve or decreasing the diameter of the lens decreases sagittal depth and increases the movement of the lens on the cornea. The power of the contact lens should not affect the fitting relationships.

5.4 **c.** The tear lens is formed by the posterior surface of the contact lens and the anterior surface of the cornea. If these 2 curvatures are the same, as with a soft lens, the tear lens is plano. If they are different (as is typical of RGP lenses), a plus or minus tear lens forms. In this case, the contact lens is flatter than *K*, so the tear lens is negative, or concave, in shape.

5.4　近视患者 –3.50 D 适配 RGP，镜片比 *K* 值平坦。如果这个患者的平均 *K* 值读数为 7.80mm，而试戴镜片的基弧是 8.00 mm，泪液镜的形状是什么样的？
a. 平光
b. 泪滴状
c. 凹透镜
d. 凸透镜

5.5　对于问题 5.4 的患者，订制 RGP 镜片的焦度是多少？
a.–3.50D
b.–4.00D
c.–2.00D
d.–2.50D

5.6　屈光不正 –2.50 D –1.50 × 175，适配复曲面软镜。试片中心定位良好，但是，在患者戴镜后，镜片 6 点钟标记位于 5 点钟。应该订制多少焦度的接触镜？
a.–2.50 D –1.50 × 175
b.–2.50 D –1.50 × 145
c.–2.50 D –1.50 × 55
d.–2.50 D –1.00 × 175

答案

5.1　**b**。由于框架眼镜的视近效率减少了调节需求，使近视眼戴框架眼镜看近时，比戴接触镜更容易。框镜的光学中心是视远的，当视近时产生底向内的棱镜，这样减少了视近所需集合。硬性接触镜形成一个正焦度泪液镜，使视远视力模糊而有助于近阅读。还可调整戴镜时的焦度。由于顶点距离的原因，接触镜的焦度稍小于框架眼镜的焦度 (见表 5–4)。

5.2　**d**。涉及接触镜时，应该关注感染问题。不用镜片或眼罩，使用局部润眼液和抗生素，并且密切随访。

5.3　**d**。增加镜片矢高，收紧适配来减少镜片移动，可以通过变陡（减小）镜片基弧，或加大直径来实现。镜片基弧变平（增加），或减小镜片直径，使镜片矢高降低，增加镜片在角膜上的移动。镜片焦度不影响与角膜的适配关系。

5.4　**c**。泪液镜是由接触镜的后表面和角膜的前表面形成的。如果这 2 个曲面是相同的，如软镜，则泪液镜是平光；如果是不同的（如 RGP），将形成一个正的或负的泪液镜。在本例中，接触镜比 *K* 值平坦，所以，泪液镜是负的或者说是凹透镜形状。

5.5 **d.** For every 0.05mm radius -of- curvature difference between the base curve and *K*, the induced power of the tear film is 0.25 D. The power of the concave tear lens in this case is −1.00D. The power of the RGP contact lens you should order is −3.50D−(−1.00D)= −2.50D. An easy way to remember this formula is to use the following rule: SAM = steeper add minus and FAP = flatter add plus.

5.6 **b.** The amount and direction of rotation should be observed. In this case, they are, respectively, 1 clock-hour and rotation to the right. Each clock-hour represents 30° (360°/12 = 30°), so the adjustment should be 30°. Because the rotation is to the right, you should order a contact lens with axis 145° instead of 175°— that is, −2.50D −1.50 × 145. An easy rule to remember is LARS = left add, right subtract.

5.5　**d**。由于在基弧和 K 值之间，曲率半径变化为 0.05mm，产生 0.25D 的泪液镜。本例中的凹透镜泪液镜的焦度为 –1.00D。需要订制的这片 RGP 镜片的屈光力是 –3.50D–（–1.00D）=–2.50D。容易记住的规则：SAM= 陡加负和 FAP 平加正。

5.6　**b**。注意观察旋转的方向和量。本例向右方旋转了 1 个点钟。每个点钟 =30°(360°/12 = 30°)，所以需要调整 30°。因为向右旋转，需要订制轴向是 145°，而不是 175°，即 –2.50D–1.50 × 145。容易记住的规则是：LARS= 左加右减。

（翻译　唐志萍　梅颖　杨嘉嵩　姚春艳　郑玲 // 审校　石一宁　吴捷 // 章节审校　郑玲）

CHAPTER 6

Intraocular Lenses

This chater includes related videos, which can be accessed by scanning the QR codes provided in the text or going to www.aao.org/bcscvideo_section03.

Highlights

- IOL design influences the development of posterior capsular opacity, and intraocular lens (IOL) presence influences the likelihood of retinal detachment.
- Different axial lengths require different IOL power calculation formulae.
- Postrefractive eyes require different calculation methods from surgically naïve eyes.
- The presence of silicone oil in the eye necessitates adjustments to biometry. If silicone oil is to remain in the eye, adjustment to refractive target is necessary.
- Small angular misalignments of toric lenses can produce substantial reductions in net astigmatic correction.
- Modulation transfer function (MTF) curves are a good tool for distinguishing different sorts of multifocal IOLs.

Glossary

Apodization The gradual tapering of the diffractive steps from the center to the outside edge of a lens to create a smooth transition of light between the distance, intermediate, and near vision focal points.

Dysphotopsias Various light-related vision disturbances encountered by pseudophakic (and phakic) patients. Positive dysphotopsias are characterized by brightness, streaks, and rays emanating from a central point source of light, sometimes with a diffuse, hazy glare. Negative dysphotopsias are characterized by subjective darkness or shadowing.

Estimated lens position An estimation of the distance at which the principal plane of the IOL will be situated behind the cornea. Derived from biometric measurement of the eye used in IOL power calculation.

Modulation transfer function A measure of optical performance that describes contrast degradation of a sinusoidal pattern as it passes through the optical system as well as the cutoff special frequency beyond which fine detail will not be resolved. Often used when discussion wavefront aberrations.

第 6 章

人工晶体

本章的相关录像可通过扫描文中二维码或登录 www.aao.org /bcscvideo_section03 获取。

重点

- 人工晶体的设计影响后囊膜混浊的发展，同时人工晶体的存在影响视网膜脱离发生的可能性。
- 不同的眼轴长度，需要不同的 IOL 度数计算公式。
- 屈光术后的眼需用与未行屈光手术的眼不同的计算方法。
- 眼内硅油的存在需要调整生物测量方法。如眼内有硅油填充，对屈光目标的调整是必要的。
- 复曲面晶体位置的小角度偏转可显著降低散光矫正效果。
- 调制传递函数（MTF）曲线是一种很好的工具，可区分不同类别的多焦点人工晶体。

术语

衍射控像法　人工晶体衍射环从中央到周边逐渐变窄造成远、中和近视觉焦点之间光的平稳过渡。

不良闪光　人工晶体（或有晶体）的患者会遇到各种光相关的视觉干扰。正不良闪光特征表现为明亮、条纹和从点光源发散的光线，有时伴有弥漫的眩光。负不良闪光特征表现为主观的阴暗或暗影。

预测晶体位置　预估的从角膜后到 IOL 主平面的距离，源于 IOL 度数计算时的生物测量。

调制传递函数　一种光学表现的衡量方法。它描述了光线穿过光学系统时，正弦模式的对比度衰减以及截止频率（超过截止频率时，细节将无法分辨）。经常被用于波前像差的讨论中。

Monovision A refractive strategy for the selection of contact lens or IOL powers such that one eye has better distance vision and the other eye has better near vision.

Piggyback intraocuar lens A second IOL inserted in an eye that already has an IOL in place. A piggyback lens may be used when the postoperative IOL power is incorrect or when the needed IOL power is higher than what is commercially available.

Introduction

Progress in the accuracy of intraocular lens (IOL) biometry, new IOL designs, and the concomitant rise in patients' refractive expectations has brought emphasis to the optics of intraocular lenses. This chapter focuses on the optical considerations relevant to IOLs. For information on the history and development of IOLs, and more surgical information with respect to IOLs, see BCSC Section 11, *Lens and Cataract.*

In the 1970s, surgeons implanting IOLs included those who used *intracapsular cataract extraction (ICCE)* and those who used *small-incision phacoemulsification (phaco)*. The IOL optic was made from polymethylmethacrylate (PMMA), with supporting haptics of metal, polypropylene, or PMMA. The rigidity of these materials required that a small phaco incision be enlarged for IOL insertion. However, following the introduction of a foldable optic (made from silicone) in the late 1980s, enlargement was no longer required, and the combination of phaco and IOL implantation became the standard of care.

The basic lens designs currently in use are differentiated by the plane in which the lens is placed (posterior chamber or anterior chamber) and by the tissue supporting the lens (capsule/ciliary sulcus or chamber angle). Figure 6-1 illustrates the major types of IOLs and optics.

The effect of lens material on factors such as *posterior capsular opacification (PCO)* has been investigated. Earlier studies suggested that IOLs made from acrylic are associated with lower rates of PCO than are those made from silicone or PMMA. However, more recent studies suggest that lens edge design is a more important factor in PCO than is lens material, as Hoffer proposed in 1979 in the lens edge barrier theory. An IOL with an annular, ridged edge or a square, truncated edge creates a barrier effect at the optic edge, exerting a 69% increase in pressure of the IOL edge against the posterior capsule. This reduces cell migration behind the optic and thus reduces PCO (Figs 6-2, 6-3, 6-4). The ridge concept led to the development of partial-ridge and meniscus IOLs, which were used for a time, and the sharp-edge designs now in use.

Plano and even negative-power IOLs are available for patients with very high myopia. The presence of even a plano IOL helps maintain the structural integrity of the anterior segment and decreases the incidence of posterior capsular opacity over simply leaving the eye aphakic. Moreover, yttrium-aluminum-garnet (YAG) capsulotomy in aphakic eyes is associated with a higher incidence of retinal detachment than in eyes with IOLs.

"Piggyback" lenses (ie, 2 IOLs in 1 eye; biphakia), implanted either simultaneously or sequentially, may be used when the postoperative IOL power is incorrect or when the needed IOL power is higher than what is commercially available. Minus-power IOLs can be used to correct extreme myopia and (as piggybacks) to correct IOL power errors. Intralenticular fibrosis may occur after placement of a piggyback lens arrangement. To the extent that this fibrosis may displace or tilt the piggyback IOL, it will change the refractive effect of the IOL and result in ametropia.

单眼视　一种接触镜或 IOL 度数的屈光选择策略，设计一眼的远视力较好，对侧眼的近视力较好。

背驮 IOL　对已经植入一片 IOL 的眼内，再植入一枚。这种方法多用于白内障术后 IOL 度数不准确或所需 IOL 度数高于市面上提供的单片 IOL 的度数。

引言

IOL 生物测量准确性和 IOL 的新型设计的进展，以及伴随着的患者屈光期望值的升高，让人工晶体的光学性能受到了重视。本章着重于与 IOL 相关的光学问题。有关人工晶体的历史与发展，以及其他更多的相关手术内容见 BCSC 第 11 册《*晶状体与白内障*》。

20 世纪 70 年代，IOL 植入的手术医生包括实施*白内障囊内摘除*（*ICCE*）和*小切口超声乳化*（*phaco*）的医生。那时 IOL 的光学部分由聚甲基丙烯酸甲酯（PMMA）制成，金属、聚丙烯或 PMMA 材料制成的襻作支撑。材料的硬度决定了小切口超乳手术时必须扩大切口，才可将晶体植入眼内。而随着 80 年代后期可折叠光学部的出现（由硅胶制成），切口不再扩大，Phaco 联合 IOL 植入成为标准的白内障治疗方法。

目前使用的人工晶体根据植入的位置（后房或前房），以及晶体的支持组织（囊袋 / 睫状沟或房角）的不同而区分。图 6-1 描述了主要的人工晶体种类和光学部。

晶体材料对其他因素的影响，比如*后囊混浊*（PCO），已得到研究。早期的研究提示，与硅胶或 PMMA 制成的 IOL 相比，丙烯酸酯 IOL 的后囊混浊发生率较低。而近期更多的研究表明，晶体的边缘设计在后囊混浊的发生中是比材料更重要的影响因素，如 1979 年 Hoffer 提出了晶体边缘阻碍理论。人工晶体环状、脊状或方形、钝边缘设计在晶体光学部边缘产生阻碍效应，晶体边缘对后囊的压力增加了 69%，从而减少细胞向光学部的迁移，降低了后囊混浊的发生（图 6-2、图 6-3、图 6-4）。根据脊状边缘理论，还曾设计了部分脊状 IOL 和弯月状 IOL，目前多用直角方边设计 IOL。

高度近视眼可以使用无度数或负度数的人工晶体。无度数人工晶体的使用可维持眼前节结构的稳定，与无晶状体眼相比，减少了 PCO 的发生。此外，与植入 IOL 的眼相比，对无晶状体眼施行钇铝石榴石（YAG）激光囊膜切开术，可视网膜脱离发生率增高。

当白内障手术植入 IOL 度数不准确或所需晶体度数高于市面可用人工晶体度数时，可术中或二次植入“背驮”晶体（1 眼植入 2 枚人工晶体，即双人工晶体眼）。对于超高度近视可植入负度数 IOL，或背驮晶体以矫正人工晶体屈光误差。背驮晶体植入后可能会发生人工晶体间纤维化。严重的纤维化可能导致 IOL 异位或倾斜，改变 IOL 的屈光效果，导致屈光不正。

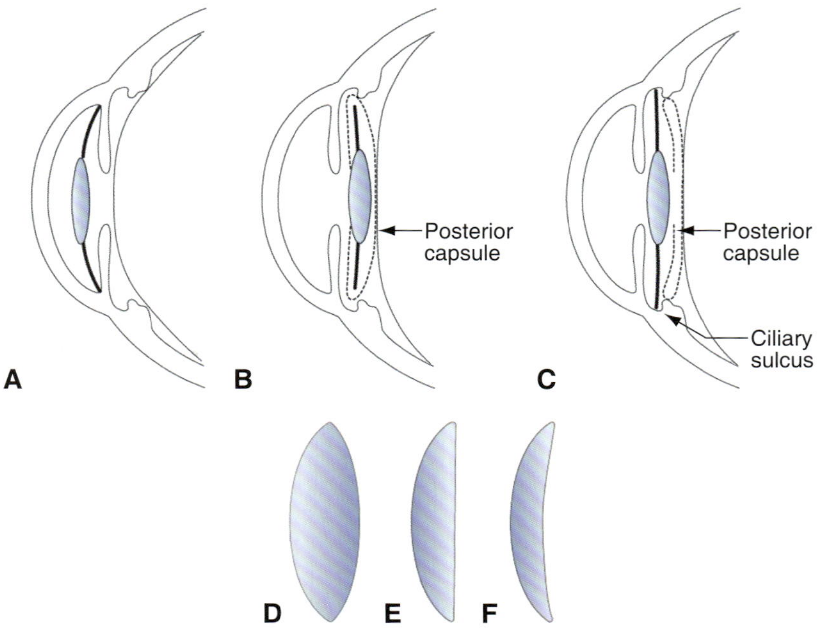

Figure 6-1 The major types of intraocular lenses (IOLs) and optics. **A**, Anterior chamber lens. **B**, Posterior chamber lens in the capsular bag. **C**, Posterior chamber lens in the ciliary sulcus. **D**, Biconvex optic. **E**, Planoconvex optic. **F**, Meniscus optic. *(Redrawn by C. H. Wooley.)*

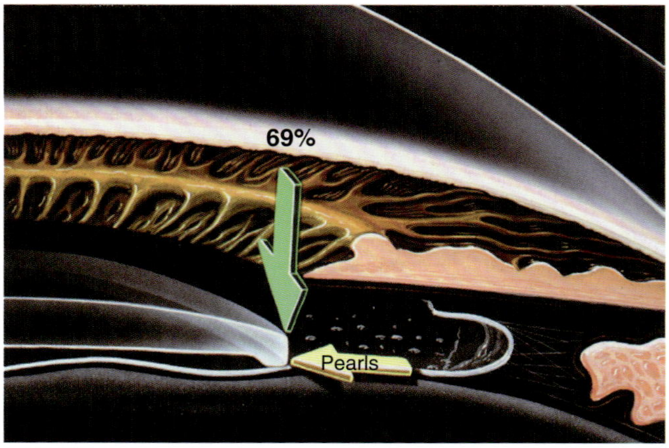

Figure 6-2 Schematic illustrating the concept of a 69% increase in pressure *(green arrow)* at the edge of an intraocular lens. *(Courtesy of Kenneth J. Hoffer, MD.)*

Current IOLs are foldable, injectable, aspheric, sharp edged, and single piece (or 3 piece), and they have higher refractive indices; together, these features allow for implantation through smaller incisions than used for the earlier designs.

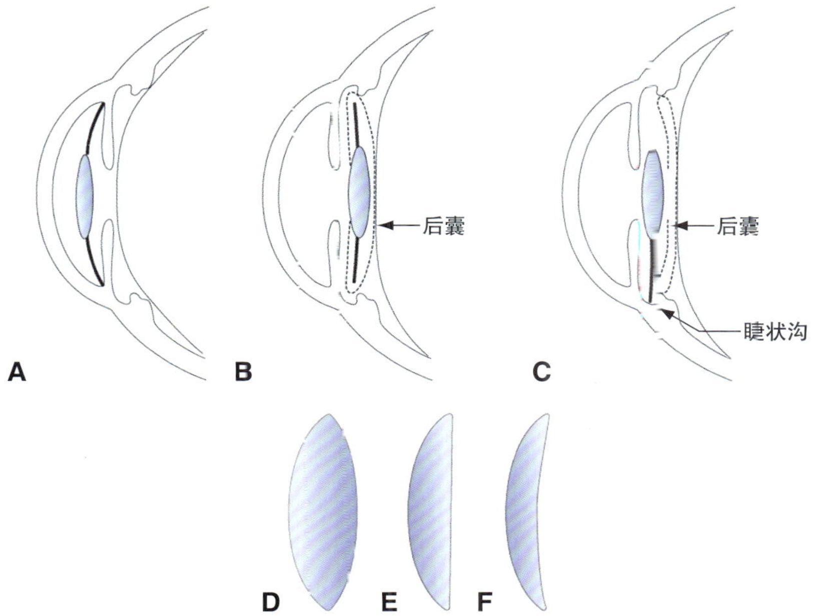

图 6–1　人工晶体和光学部的主要类型。**A**. 前房型人工晶体。**B**. 后房型人工晶体植入囊袋。**C**. 后房型人工晶体植入睫状沟。**D**. 双凸型光学部。E. 平凸型光学部。F. 凹凸型光学部。*（译者注：资料来源见前页原文。）*

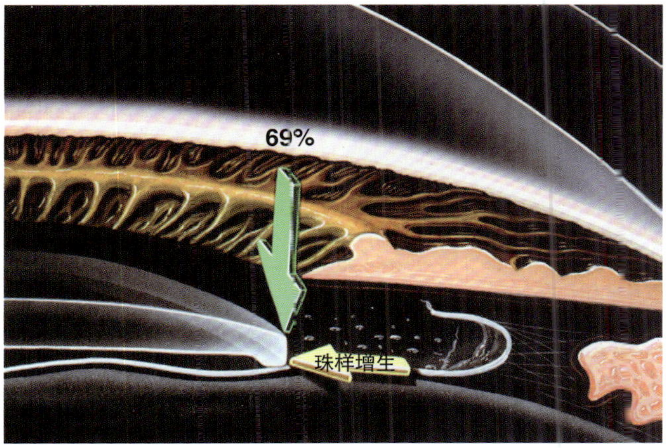

图 6–2　示意图说明了人工晶体边缘压力（*绿箭头*）增加了 69%。*（译者注：资料来源见前页原文。）*

目前的人工晶体有可折叠式、注入式、非球面、锐利边缘的；有 1 片（或 3 片）式设计；晶体材料折射率较高。这些因素使其可以通过更小的切口植入眼内。

A B

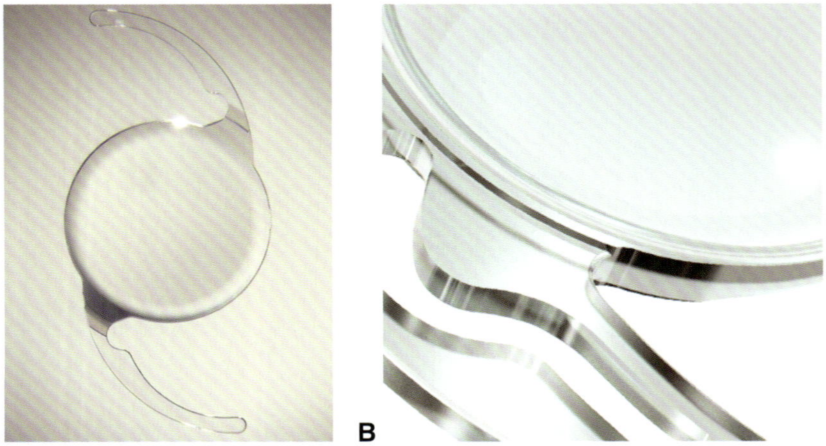

Figure 6-3 Square edge intraocular lens (IOL) design. **A**, TECNIS 1-piece IOL with the square edge design extending to the haptics. **B**, Detail of Rayner Superflex aspheric IOL demonstrating a square edge design. *(Courtesy of Baye Vision.)*

A B

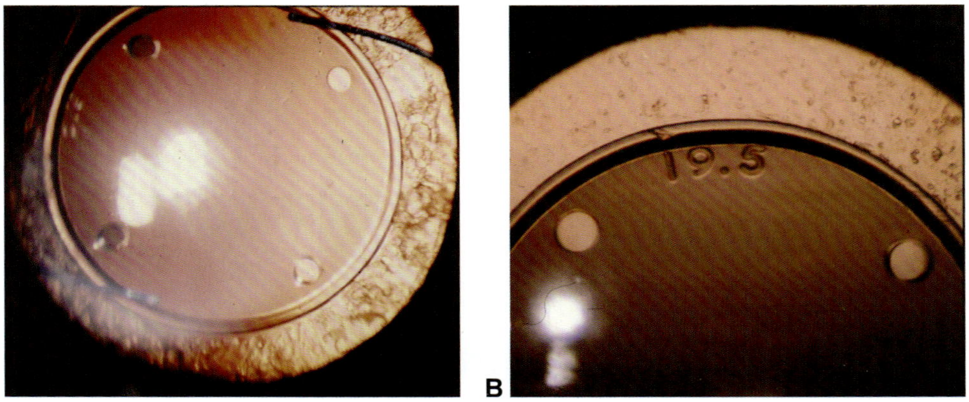

Figure 6-4 Increasing the pressure at the edge of an intraocular lens leads to a blockage of cells to the central posterior capsule (**A**, **B**). *(Courtesy of Kenneth J. Hoffer, MD.)*

Apple DJ. Influence of intraocular lens material and design on postoperative intracapsular cellular reactivity. *Trans Am Ophthalmol Soc.* 2000;98:257–283.

Badr IA, Hussain HM, Jabak M, Wagoner MD. Extracapsular cataract extraction with or without posterior chamber intraocular lenses in eyes with cataract and high myopia. *Ophthalmology.* 1995;102(8):1139–1143.

Behrendt S, Giess L, Duncker G. Incidence of retinal detachment after treatment with the Nd:YAG laser, *Fortschr Ophthalmol.* 1991;88(6):809–811.

Boyce JF, Bhermi GS, Spalton DJ, El-Osta AR. Mathematical modeling of the forces between an intraocular lens and the capsule. *J Cataract Refract Surg.* 2002;28(10): 1853–1859.

Hoffer KJ. Hoffer barrier ridge concept [letter]. *J Cataract Refract Surg.* 2007;33(7):1142–1143; author reply 1143.

Nagamoto T, Fujiwara T. Inhibition of lens epithelial cell migration at the intraocular lens optic edge: role of capsule bending and contact pressure. *J Cataract Refract Surg.* 2003; 29(8):1605–1612.

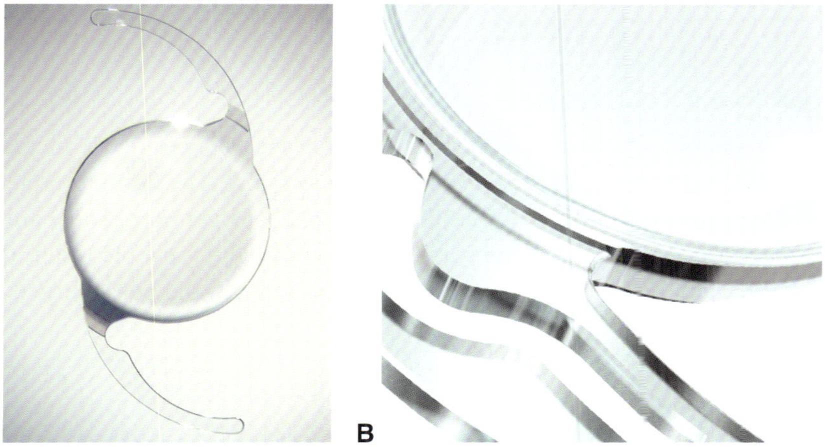

图 6-3　IOL 的方边设计。A. TECNIS 一片式方边设计的 IOL，可见舒展的襻。B. Rayner 的 Superflex 非球面晶体方边设计的细节。（译者注：资料来源见前页原文。）

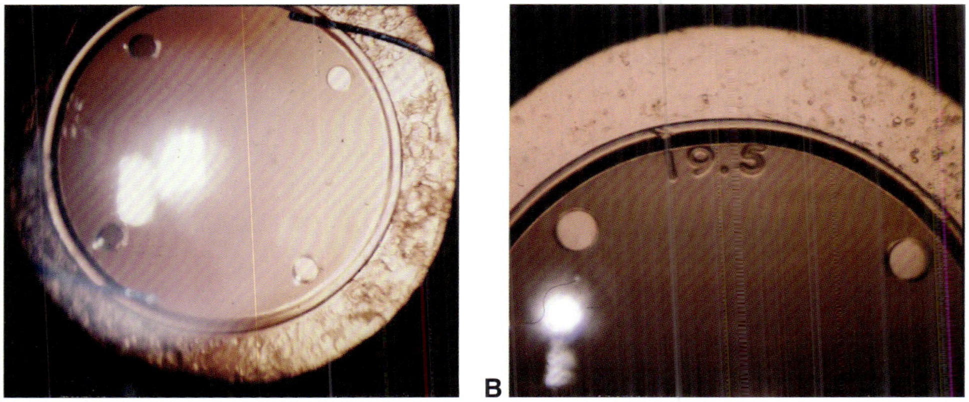

图 6-4　IOL 边缘压力的增加阻止了细胞到达中央区后囊膜（A, B）。（译者注：资料来源见前页原文。）

Apple DJ. Influence of intraocular lens material and design on postoperative intracapsular cellular reactivity. *Trans Am Ophthalmol Soc.* 2000;98:257–283.

Badr IA, Hussain HM, Jabak M, Wagoner MD. Extracapsular cataract extraction with or without posterior chamber intraocular lenses in eyes with cataract and high myopia. *Ophthalmology.* 1995;102(8):1139–1143.

Behrendt S, Giess L, Duncker G. Incidence of retinal detachment after treatment with the Nd:YAG laser, *Fortschr Ophthalmol.* 1991;88(6):809–811.

Boyce JF, Bhermi GS, Spalton DJ, El-Osta AR. Mathematical modeling of the forces between an intraocular lens and the capsule. *J Cataract Refract Surg.* 2002;28(10): 1853–1859.

Hoffer KJ. Hoffer barrier ridge concept [letter]. *J Cataract Refract Surg.* 2007;33(7):1142–1143; author reply 1143.

Nagamoto T, Fujiwara T. Inhibition of lens epithelial cell migration at the intraocular lens optic edge: role of capsule bending and contact pressure. *J Cataract Refract Surg.* 2003; 29(8):1605–1612.

Optical Considerations for Intraocular Lenses

Intraocular Lens Power Calculation

In IOL power calculation, a formula is used that requires accurate biometric measurements of the eye, the visual *axial length* (*AL*), and the *central corneal power* (*K*). The desired "target" postoperative refraction and the estimated position of the IOL *(estimated lens position [ELP])* are added to these factors for use in power calculation. Some surgeons target a slightly myopic result, the advantage of which is that it allows for some degree of near vision and reduces the possibility of a postoperative hyperopic refractive surprise.

Power prediction formulas

IOL power prediction formulas are termed *theoretical* because they are based on theoretical optics, the basis of which is the Gullstrand eye (see Chapter 3). In the 1980s, regression formulas (eg, Sanders, Retzlaff, Kraff [SRK] formulas I and II) were popular because they were simple to use. However, the use of these formulas often led to power errors that subsequently became the major reason IOLs were explanted or exchanged. In the 1990s, regression formulas were largely replaced by more accurate, newer theoretical or ray tracing formulas.

Geometric optics was used to generate basic theoretical formulas for IOL power calculation, an example of which is shown below. The pseudophakic eye can be modeled as a 2-element optical system (Fig 6-5). Using Gaussian reduction equations (see Chapter 1), the IOL power that produces emmetropia may be given by

$$P=\frac{n_V}{AL-C}-\frac{K}{1-K\times\frac{C}{n_A}}$$

where

P=power of the target IOL (in diopters [D])

n_V=index of refraction of the vitreous

AL=visual axial length (in meters)

C=ELP (in meters), the distance from the anterior corneal surface to the principal plane of the IOL

K=average dioptric power of the central cornea

n_A=index of refraction of the aqueous

Most of the advances in newer theoretical formulas (such as the Haigis, Hoffer Q, Hoffer H5, Holladay 1 and 2, Olsen, and SRK/T formulas) concerned improved methods of predicting the *ELP*, as described later in this chapter. These formulas are complex and cannot be used easily for calculation by hand. However, programmable calculators and applicable computer programs are widely available. These formulas are also programmed into automated optical biometers like the IOLMaster (Carl Zeiss Meditec, Jena, Germany) and the Lenstar (Haag-Streit, Köniz, Switzerland) and most modern ultrasonographic instruments.

人工晶体的光学问题

人工晶体度数的计算

使用计算公式计算 IOL 度数时，需要精确的眼部生物测量数据、*眼轴*（*AL*）和*中央角膜曲率*（*K*）。此外，还需考虑预期的术后“目标”屈光状态和预测的人工晶体位置（*ELP*）。有些术者会预留轻度的近视，这样处理的好处是，既可以保留一定的近视力，又减少了术后远视的发生。

焦度预测公式

基于 Gullstrand 模型眼的理论光学原理推导出的 IOL 度数预测公式被称为*理论型公式*（见第 3 章）。20 世纪 80 年代，回归型公式（比如，Sanders, Retzlaff, Kraff [即 SRK]–I 和 II 公式）因其使用方便而广受欢迎。然而，这些公式也常常导致屈光误差，这些误差成为 IOL 取出或置换的主要原因。到了 90 年代，回归型公式被更准确的新理论公式，即光线追踪公式所取代。

几何光学是理论型 IOL 计算公式的基础，如下所示。人工晶体眼可视为二元光学系统（图 6–5）。使用 Gaussian 简化方程（见第 1 章），术后正视的 IOL 度数计算方法如下：

$$P=\frac{n_{\mathrm{V}}}{AL-C}-\frac{K}{1-K\times\frac{C}{n_{\mathrm{A}}}}$$

其中：

P 代表目标焦度（单位：D）；

n_v 代表玻璃体的折射率；

AL 代表视轴长度（单位：m）；

C 代表*预测人工晶体位置*，即角膜前表面到 *IOL* 主平面的距离（单位：m）；

K 代表中央角膜平均屈光力；

n_A 代表房水的折射率。

更新的理论型计算公式（如 Haigis、HofferQ、Hoffer H5、Holladay 1 和 Holladay 2、Olsen 以及 SRK/T 公式）的进步在于改进了 *ELP* 的预测方法，具体内容见本章后一部分。这些公式比较复杂，手工计算困难，可通过编程的计算器和计算机程序计算。这些公式也被编入自动光学生物测量仪，如 IOLMaster（Carl Zeiss Meditec, Jena, 德国）和 Lenstar（Haag–Streit, Könitz, 瑞士）和大多数现代超声测量仪。

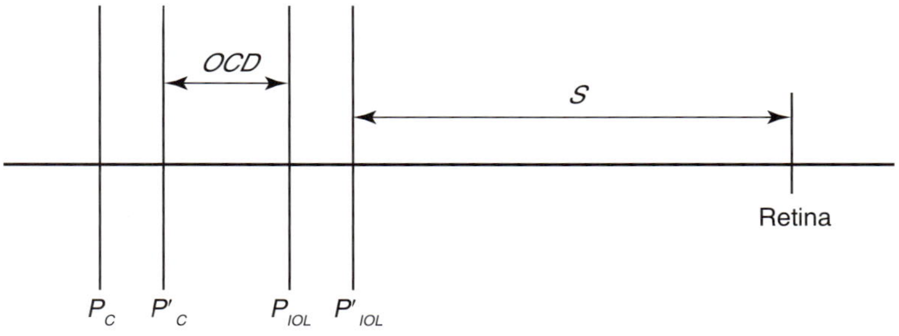

Figure 6-5 Schematic eye. P_C and P'_C are the front and back principal planes of the cornea, respectively. Similarly, P_{IOL} and P'_{IOL} are the front and back principal planes of the intraocular lens (IOL). *OCD* = optical chapter depth and represents a mathematical construct of this simplified model and is not identical to the anatomical anterior chamber depth; *S* = distance between back principal plane of the IOL and retina. (The drawing is not to scale.) *(Redrawn by C. H. Wooley.)*

Biometric formula requirements

Axial length The *AL* is the most important factor in these formulas. A 1-mm error in *AL* measurement results in a refractive error of approximately 2.35 D in a 23.5-mm eye. The refractive error declines to only 1.75 D/mm in a 30-mm eye but rises to 3.75 D/mm in a 20-mm eye. Therefore, accuracy in *AL* measurement is more important in short eyes than in long eyes.

ULTRASONIC MEASUREMENT OF AXIAL LENGTH When *A-scan ultrasonography* is used to measure *AL*, we either assume a constant ultrasound velocity through the entire eye or measure each of the various ocular structures at its individual velocity. A-scans measure not distance but rather the time required for a sound pulse to travel from the cornea to the retina and back again. Sound travels faster through the crystalline lens and the cornea (1641 m/s) than it does through aqueous and vitreous (1532 m/s). Even within the lens itself, the speed of sound can vary in different layers and is altered by nuclear sclerosis.

The average velocity through a phakic eye of normal length is 1555 m/s; however, it rises to 1560 m/s for a short (20-mm) eye and drops to 1550 m/s for a long (30-mm) eye. This variation is due to the presence of the crystalline lens; 1554 m/s is an accurate value for an aphakic eye of any length.

The following formula can be used to easily correct any *AL* measured with an incorrect average velocity:

$$AL_C = AL_M \times \frac{V_C}{V_M}$$

where AL_C is the *AL* value at the correct velocity, AL_M is the resultant *AL* value at the incorrect velocity, V_C is the correct velocity, and V_M is the incorrect velocity.

In eyes with *AL* values greater than 25 mm, *staphyloma* should be suspected, especially when numerous disparate readings are obtained. Such errors occur because the macula is located either at the deepest part of the staphyloma or on the "side of the hill." To measure such eyes and obtain the true measurement to the fovea, the patient must fixate on the light in the center of the A-scan probe. If such a lighted probe is unavailable or if the patient is unable to fixate upon it, the clinician must use a *B-scan technique*. Optical methods (eg, IOLMaster, Lenstar) are very useful in such cases (see the following section).

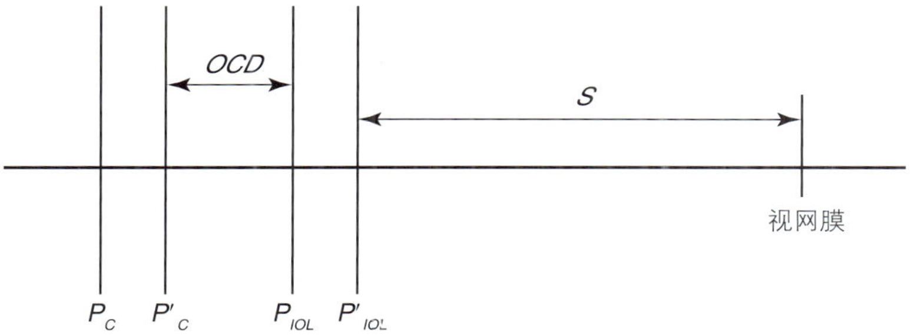

图 6–5　模型眼。P_C 和 P'_C 分别代表角膜的前、后主平面。而 P_{IOL} 和 P'_{IOL} 分别是人工晶体（IOL）的前、后主平面。*OCD*= 光学深度，代表这个简单模型的数学结构，但不等于解剖学上的前房深度；*S*=IOL 后主平面到视网膜的距离。（此图未按比例绘制）*（译者注：资料来源见前页原文。）*

生物测量参数的要求

眼轴长度　*AL* 是 IOL 计算公式中最重要的因素。在 23.5 mm 的眼球中，*眼轴*测量时 1 mm 的误差导致大约 2.35 D 的屈光度；在 30 mm 的眼球中，屈光度下降到仅 1.75 D/mm；在 20 mm 的眼球中，则上升至 3.75 D/mm。因此，*眼轴*测量的准确性，在短眼轴眼球比长眼轴眼球更重要。

眼轴长度的超声测量　当使用*超声*测量 *AL* 时，我们通常假定超声以一个恒定的速度通过整个眼球，或在测量不同部分的眼组织时采用相应的声速。A 超测量的并非距离，而是声波从角膜到视网膜往返所需的时间。声波在晶状体和角膜中的传播速度（1641 m/s）高于房水和玻璃体中的传播速度（1532 m/s）。即使在晶状体内部，声波在不同层面内的速度也是不一样的，会受到核硬化的影响而改变。

声波在正常眼轴的有晶体眼内的平均传播速度是 1555 m/s；而在短眼轴（20 mm）眼球中，速度可达 1560 m/s；在长眼轴（30 mm）眼球中，可降至 1550 m/s。这种变化是因为晶状体的存在。在任何长度眼轴的无晶体眼中，1554 m/s 是准确的声波速度。

下面的公式用于校正任何用未校正平均声速测得的眼轴 *AL*：

$$AL_C = AL_M \times \frac{V_C}{V_M}$$

AL_C 代表校正声速下的 *AL*；AL_M 是未校正声速测得的 *AL*；V_C 是校正的声速；V_M 是测量所用的未校正的声速。

当眼轴长大于 25 mm 时，尤其是当获得完全不同的多个测量值时，需怀疑*葡萄肿*的存在。这种误差的发生是因为黄斑或置于葡萄肿的最深处，或置于葡萄肿的侧壁上。测量这种类型的眼球时，为了获得真实的对准中心凹的测量，患者必须注视 A 超探头中心的光点。如果没有这种带注视点的探头或患者无法注视，医师必须使用 *B 超扫描*。在这类患者中，光学生物测量（如 IOLMaster、Lenstar）是很有帮助的（见下文）。

When ultrasonography is used to measure the *AL* in *biphakic* eyes (ie, a phakic IOL in a phakic eye), it is difficult to eliminate the effect of the sound velocity through the implanted phakic lens. To correct for this potential error, one can use the following published formula:

$$AL_{corrected}=AL_{1555}+C \times T$$

where

AL_{1555} = the measured *AL* of the eye at a sound velocity of 1555 m/s

C = the material-specific correction factor, which is +0.42 for PMMA, –0.59 for silicone, +0.11 for collamer, and +0.23 for acrylic

T = the central thickness of the implanted phakic IOL

Published tables list the central thickness of phakic IOLs available on the market (for each dioptric power). The least degree of error (in terms of *AL* error) is associated with use of a very thin myopic collamer lens, and the greatest amount of error is associated with use of a thick hyperopic silicone lens.

The primary A-scan techniques—*applanation* (contact) and *immersion* (noncontact)—often give different results (Figs 6-6, 6-7). Although the immersion method is accepted as the more accurate of the 2 techniques, it is more difficult to perform and less widely employed than the applanation method. The applanation method is susceptible to artificially shortened *AL* measurement because of inadvertent corneal indentation.

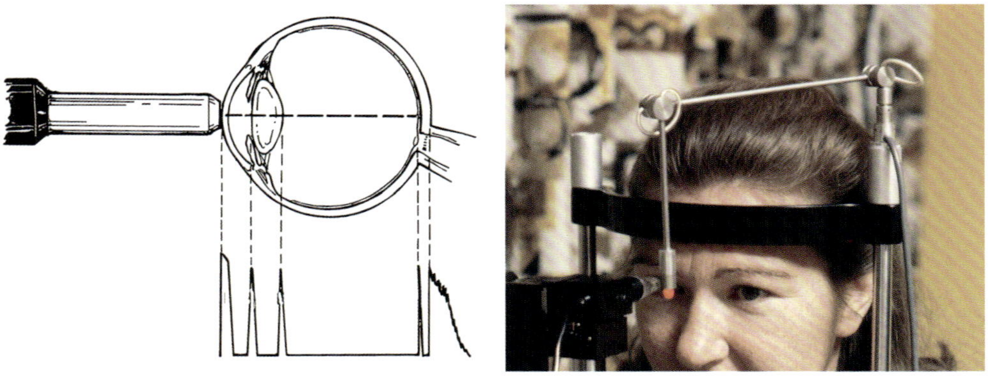

Figure 6-6 In applanation ultrasonography, the probe must contact the cornea, which causes corneal depression and shortening of the axial length reading. *(Courtesy of Kenneth J. Hoffer, MD.)*

当使用超声技术测量*双晶体*眼（比如，植入了 IOL 的有晶体眼）的 *AL* 时，很难消除声波穿过不同晶体时声速不同产生的影响。为了矫正这种潜在的误差，可使用如下公式：

$$AL_{矫正}=AL_{1555}+C\times T$$

其中：

AL_{1555}= 以 1555m/s 声速测得的眼轴长度；

C= 材料特异性矫正因子，PMMA 时 +0.42，硅油时 −0.59，胶原多聚物时 +0.11，丙烯酸酯时 +0.23；

T= 植入 IOL 的中心厚度

可查找到市面上不同 IOL 的中心厚度（每个屈光度）。很薄的矫正近视的胶原多聚物材质的 IOL 的误差最小（*AL* 误差），较厚的远视硅胶材质的 IOL 的误差最大。

A 超主要的技术——*压平式*（接触式）和*浸润式*（非接触式）——常常给出不同的结果（图 6-6、图 6-7）。尽管浸润式 A 超更为准确，但因其操作难度较大，导致其没有压平式 A 超应用得多。由于压平法测量时可能人为压平角膜，*眼轴*可能人为变短。

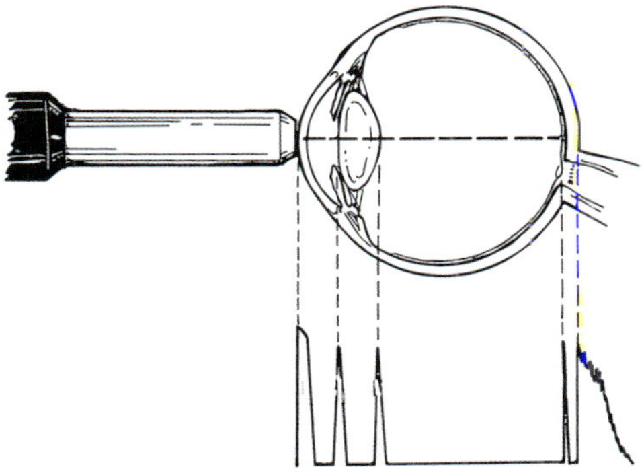

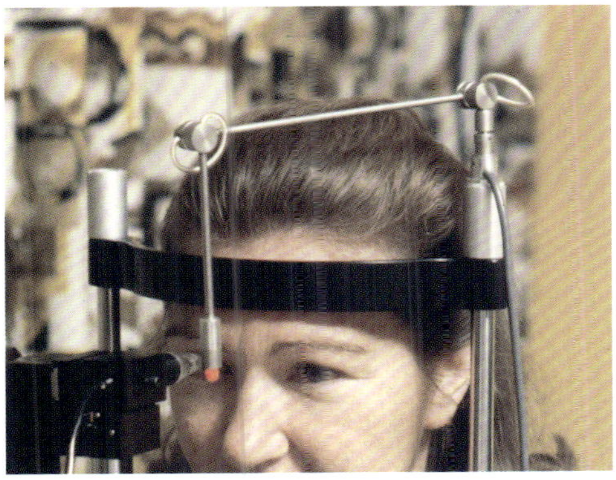

图 6-6　压平式超声测量，探头必须接触角膜，可导致角膜压平、测量结果眼轴变短。*（译者注：资料来源见前页原文。）*

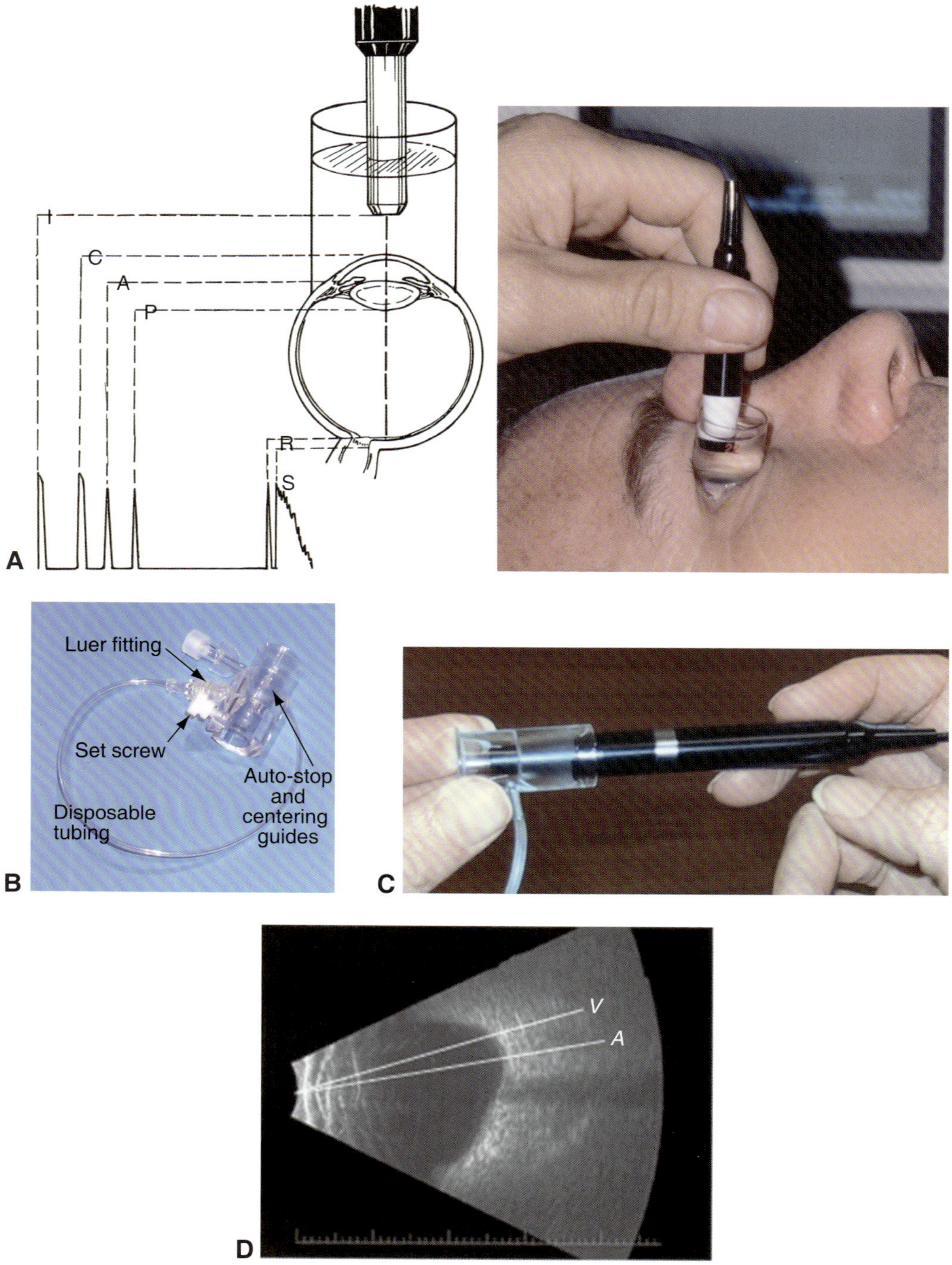

Figure 6-7 Ultrasonography techniques. **A**, In immersion ultrasonography, the probe is immersed in the solution, placing it away from the cornea. **B**, Prager shell for immersion A-scan. **C**, Ultrasound probe and Kohn shell. **D**, B–scan of an eye with staphyloma, showing the difference between the anatomical length *(A)* and the visual length *(V)*. *(Courtesy of Kenneth J. Hoffer, MD.)*

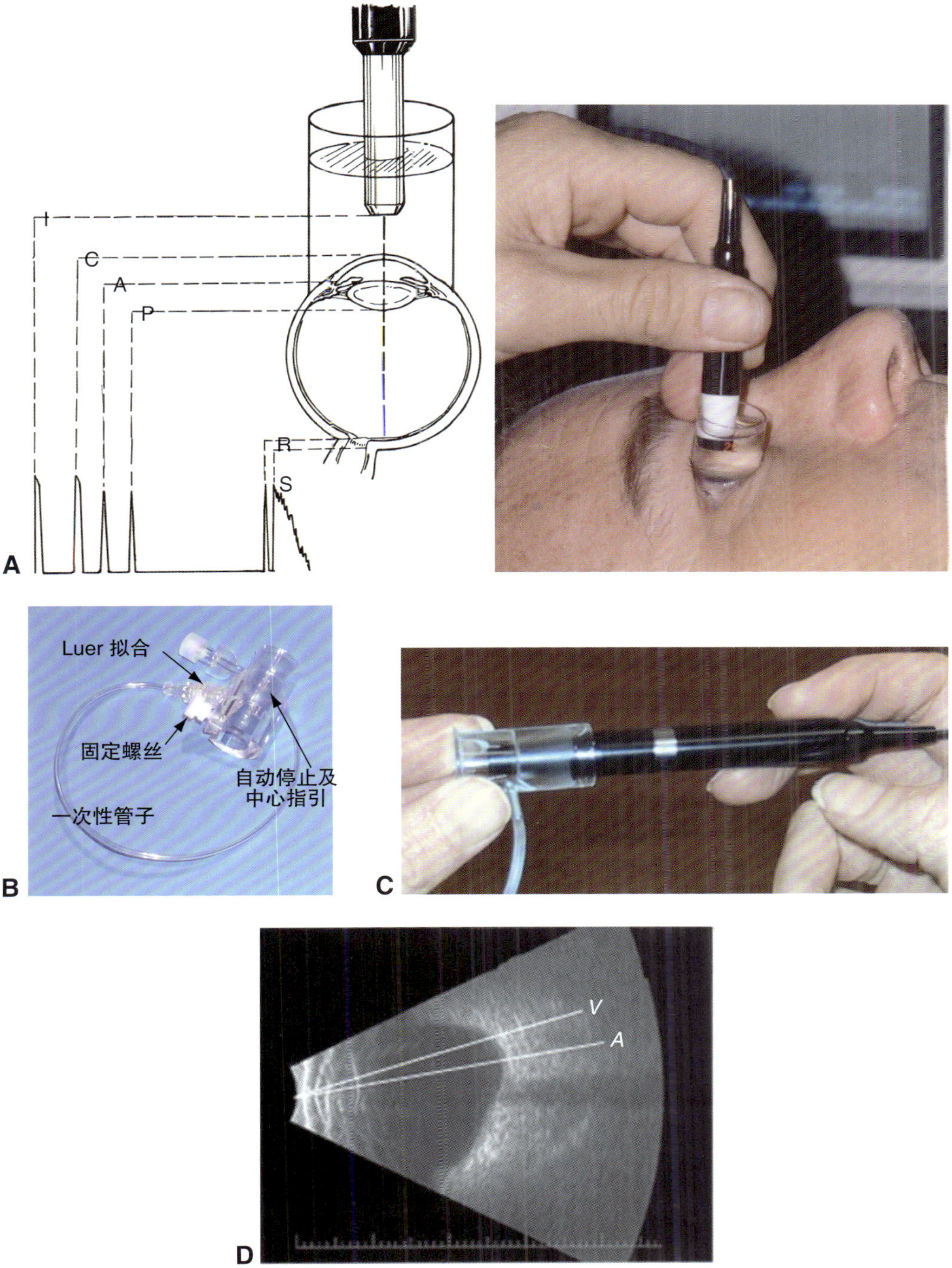

图 6–7　超声成像技术。**A.** 浸润式超声检查时，探头浸没于溶液中，放置于远离角膜的位置。**B.** 浸润式 *A* 超的 Prager 杯。**C.** 超声探头和 Kohn 杯。**D.** 巩膜葡萄肿的眼部 B 超图像，显示了解剖学眼轴长度（*A*）和视轴长度（*V*）。*（译者注：资料来源见前页原文。）*

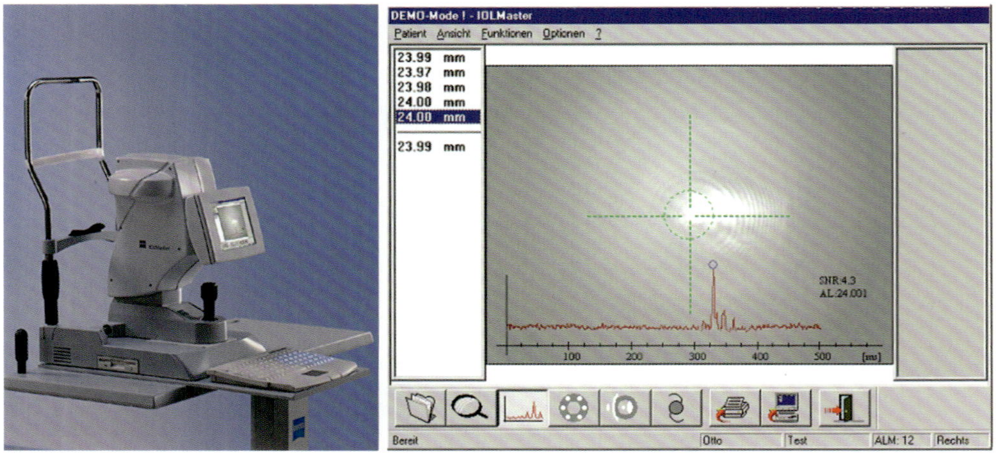

Figure 6-8 An optical biometer *(left)* and view of the instrument's axial length screen *(right)*. *(Courtesy of Kenneth J. Hoffer, MD.)*

OPTICAL MEASUREMENT OF AXIAL LENGTH Optical biometry uses a partial coherence laser for *AL* measurement (Fig 6-8). In a manner analogous to ultrasonography, this device indirectly measures the time required for infrared light to travel to the retina. Because light travels at too high a speed to be measured directly, light interference methodology (interferometry) is used to determine the transit time and thus the *AL*. This technique does not require contact with the globe, so corneal compression artifacts are eliminated. This instrument was developed such that its readings would be equivalent to those of the immersion ultrasound technique. Because this device requires the patient to fixate on a target, the length measured is the path the light takes to the fovea: the "visual" *AL*. The ocular media must be clear enough to allow voluntary fixation and light transmission. Thus, in dense cataracts (especially posterior subcapsular cataracts), ultrasound biometry is still necessary (in 5%–8% of cataract patients). Compared with ultrasonography, this technique provides more accurate, reproducible *AL* measurements. In addition, optical measurement is ideal in 2 clinical situations that are difficult to achieve using ultrasonography: eyes with staphyloma and eyes filled with silicone oil, although such measurements require adjustment.

If removal of the silicone oil is not intended, additional optical accommodations must be made. Because of the element of reduced vergence (see Chapter 1) introduced by a medium with a difference refractive index, IOL power must be increased to achieve the intended refractive target. This problem is further compounded by the decreased refractive power achieved at the interface between the posterior surface of the IOL and the silicone oil. When these elements are not considered, Grinbaum and colleagues demonstrated that patients exhibit a mean postoperative hyperopic surprise of close to 4 diopters (D). This hyperopic shift may be minimized by avoiding the use of IOLs with convex posterior surfaces.

Dong J, Tang M, Zhang Y, et al. Comparison of Anterior Segment Biometric Measurements between Pentacam HR and IOLMaster in Normal and High Myopic Eyes. *PLoS One.* 2015; 10(11): e0143110.

Freeman G, Pesudovs K. The impact of cataract severity on measurement acquisition with the IOLMaster. *Acta Ophthalmol TablScand.* 2005;83(4):439–442.

Grinbaum A, Treister G, Moisseiev J. Predicted and actual refraction after intraocular lens implantation in eyes with silicone oil. *J Cataract Refract Surg.* 1996;22(6): 726–729.

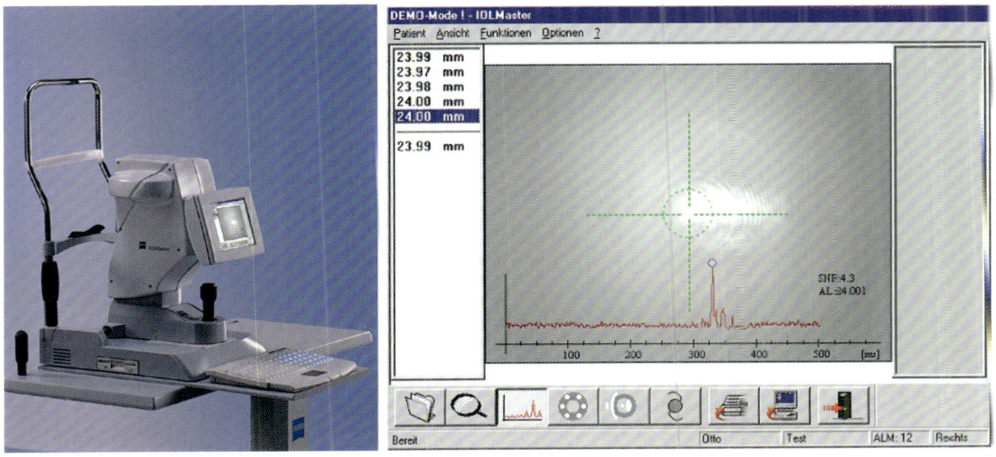

图 6-8 光学生物测量仪（左）和眼轴测量的界面（右）。*（译者注：资料来源见首页原文。）*

眼轴长度的光学测量 光学生物测量仪使用部分相干激光测量眼轴（图 6-8）。光学生物测量仪与超声成像技术类似，间接地测量红外光到达视网膜所用的时间。由于光的传播速度太快，无法直接测量，所以使用光干涉法（干涉仪）获得传播所需的时间，进而得到眼轴。这种技术不需要接触眼球，因此没有压迫角膜产生的人工误差。光学生物测量仪的测量结果可等同于浸润式超声技术的结果。由于测量时需要患者注视目标，因此所测得的长度是光线到达中心凹的距离，即视轴的长度。眼部的屈光介质必须足够透明，以便实现固视和使测量的光线穿过。因此，硬核白内障（尤其是后极性后囊下白内障）超声生物测量仍是必要的（占白内障患者的 5%~8%）。与超声生物测量相比，光学生物测量的眼轴更准确、重复性更好。此外，超声测量对以下 2 种情况的测量有困难，即伴葡萄肿的眼球以及硅油填充眼，光学生物测量是理想的选择，但需要一些修正。

如果不打算取出眼内的硅油，必须附加光学调节。由于不同折射率的屈光介质导致了会聚的减少（见第 1 章），必须提高 IOL 的度数以实现预期的屈光目标。在 IOL 后表面与硅油接触面之间，屈光力的下降会使这一问题更为复杂。如果不考虑这一因素的影响，Grinbaum 见到，患者术后可出现近 4.00D 的远视。通过避免使用后凸面人工晶体，可使这种远视漂移最小化。

Dong J, Tang M, Zhang Y, et al. Comparison of Anterior Segment Biometric Measurements between Pentacam HR and IOLMaster in Normal and High Myopic Eyes. *PLoS One*. 2015; 10(11): e0143110.

Freeman G, Pesudovs K. The impact of cataract severity on measurement acquisition with the IOLMaster. *Acta Ophthalmol TablScand*. 2005;83(4):439–442.

Grinbaum A, Treister G, Moisseiev J. Predicted and actual refraction after intraocular lens implantation in eyes with silicone oil. *J Cataract Refract Surg*. 1996;22(6): 726–729.

Corneal power The central corneal power, *K*, is the second most important factor in the calculation formula; a 1.0 D error in corneal power causes a 1.0 D postoperative refractive error. Corneal power can be estimated by keratometry or corneal topography, neither of which measures corneal power directly. The standard manual keratometer (Fig 6-9A) measures only a small central portion (3.2-mm diameter) of the cornea and views the cornea as a convex mirror. The corneal radius of curvature can be calculated from the size of the reflected image. Both front and back corneal surfaces contribute to corneal power, but the keratometer power "reading" is based on measurement of the radius of curvature of only the front surface and assumptions about the posterior surface.

Two imaging systems are commonly used in measuring corneal power. The Pentacam (Oculus Optikgeräte GmbH, Wetzlar, Germany, Fig 6-9B) system uses a single Scheimpflug camera to measure the radius of curvature of the anterior and posterior corneal surfaces, as well as the corneal thickness, for the calculation of corneal power. Early studies questioned the accuracy of the Pentacam in eyes that had undergone laser corneal refractive procedures. Newer software has made dramatic improvements. The Galilei (Ziemer Ophthalmic Systems AG, Port, Switzerland) system measures corneal power by use of a dual Scheimpflug camera integrated with a Placido disk.

Estimated lens position All formulas require an estimation of the distance at which the principal plane of the IOL will be situated behind the cornea—a factor now known as the *ELP*. Initially, most IOLs were either anterior chamber or prepupillary IOLs. Thus, in the original theoretical formulas, this factor was called the *anterior chamber depth* (*ACD*), and it was a constant value (usually 2.8 or 3.5 mm). This value became incorporated in the A constant of the regression formulas of the 1980s.

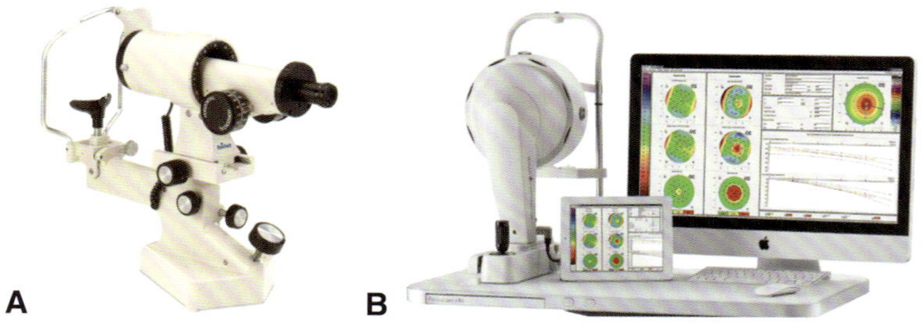

Figure 6-9 Instruments for measuring corneal power. **A**, Manual keratometer. **B**, Oculus Pentacam. *(Part A courtesy of Reichert Technologies; part B courtesy of Oculus Optikgeräte GmbH.)*

In 1983, using pachymetry studies of posterior chamber IOLs as a basis, Hoffer introduced an *ACD* prediction formula for posterior chamber lenses that was based on the eye's *AL*:

$$ACD = 0.293 \times AL - 2.92$$

Other adjustments (second-generation formulas) were also based on the *AL*. The Holladay 1 formula used the *K* reading and *AL* value as factors (in a corneal height formula by Fyodorov), as did the later SRK/T formula, whereas the Hoffer Q formula used the *AL* value and a tangent factor of *K* (all these formulas are third generation). Olsen added other measurements of the anterior segment, such as the preoperative *ACD*, lens thickness, and corneal diameter (this formula is fourth generation). Subsequently, Holladay used these factors, as well as patient age and preoperative refraction, in his Holladay 2 formula. Haigis eliminated *K* as a prediction factor and replaced it with the preoperative *ACD* measurement. These newer formulas are more accurate than those of the first and second generations, and all are currently in use (Fig 6-10).

角膜屈光力　中央角膜屈光力，*K*，是 IOL 计算公式中第二重要因素；中央角膜 1.0 D 的误差引起 1.0 D 的术后屈光不正。角膜屈光力可通过角膜曲率计或角膜地形图估算，这 2 种方法都不能直接测量角膜屈光力。标准的手动曲率计（图 6–9A）仅测量角膜小的中央区域（3.2 mm 直径），并把角膜视为凸面镜。角膜的曲率半径可通过反射像的大小计算得出。尽管角膜的前后表面都对角膜屈光力有贡献，但角膜曲率计的读数结果是基于前表面的测量值和后表面的推测值。

2 种成像系统常用于角膜屈光力的测量。Pentacam 系统（Oculus Optikgeräte GmbH, Wetzlar, Germany, 图 6–9B）利用单个 Scheimpflug 摄像头测量角膜前、后表面的曲率半径，以及角膜厚度，来计算角膜屈光力。早期的研究曾质疑 Pentacam 对角膜屈光术后眼球测量的准确性，新软件的应用改进了该项技术。Galilei 系统（Ziemer Ophthalmic Systems AG, Port, Switzerland）则使用了双 Scheimpflug 摄像头和 Placido 盘联合测量角膜屈光力。

预测晶体位置　所用的公式都需要一个距离的预估值，即放置于角膜后的 IOL 的主平面位置，这一因子即预测晶体位置 *ELP*。起初，大多数人工晶体置于前房或瞳孔前，因此在原始的理论计算公式中，这一因子被称为*前房深度*（*ACD*），它是一个固定值（通常是 2.8 mm 或 3.5 mm）。在 80 年代的回归公式中，这一值被纳入 *A* 常数。

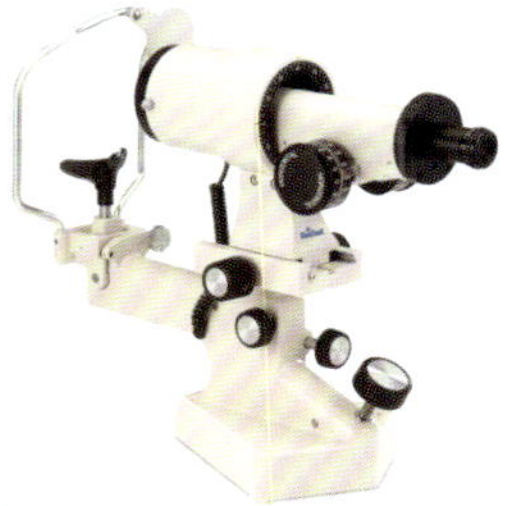
A

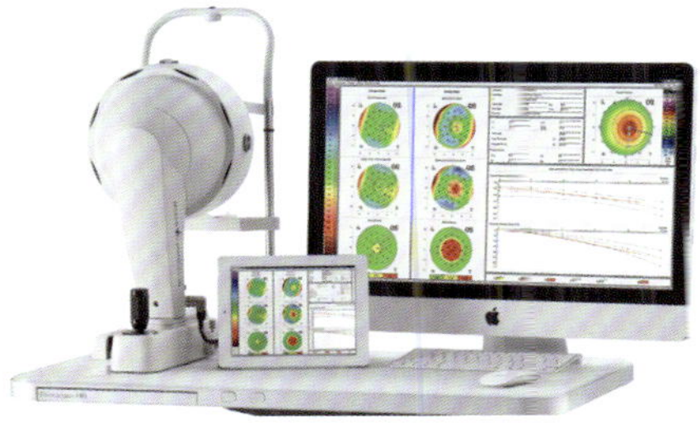
B

图 6–9　角膜屈光力的测量设备。**A.** 手动曲率计。**B.** Oculus Pentacam。*（译者注：资料来源见前页原文。）*

1983 年，应用角膜厚度计研究后房型 IOL，Hoffer 引入了基于眼轴长度 *AL* 的后房型晶体的 *ACD* 预测公式：

$$ACD=0.293 \times AL-2.92$$

其他调整（第二代公式）也是基于眼轴长度。Holladay 1 公式与后来的 SRK/T 公式一样，使用 *K* 值和 *AL* 进行计算；而 Hoffer Q 公式使用 *AL* 和切线方向的 *K* 值进行计算（这些公式为第三代）。Olsen 则增加了眼前节其他测量值，比如术前前房深度 *ACD*、晶状体厚度和角膜直径（第四代公式）。之后，Holladay 在 Holladay 2 公式中也考虑了这些因素，同时还考虑了患者年龄和术前屈光状态。Haigis 用术前 *ACD* 值取代 *K* 作为预测因素。这些更新的公式比第一、第二代公式更准确，目前均在用（图 6–10）。

The most accurate way to measure the preoperative *ACD* or the postoperative *ELP* is by optical means, using scanning slit topography, Scheimpflug imaging, or optical interferometry. Ultrasonography is usually less precise and provides a shorter reading.

Most formulas use only one constant, such as the *ACD*, the A constant, or the *surgeon Factor (SF)*. One exception is the Haigis formula, which uses 3 constants (a_0, a_1, a_2). The *A* constant, developed as a result of regression formulas, was widely used in the 1980s, so much so that manufacturers assigned each lens design a specific *A* constant, as well as an *ACD* value. Even though regression formulas (eg, SRK formula) are no longer recommended and rarely used for IOL calculation, the *A* constant still exists for the SRK/T formula.

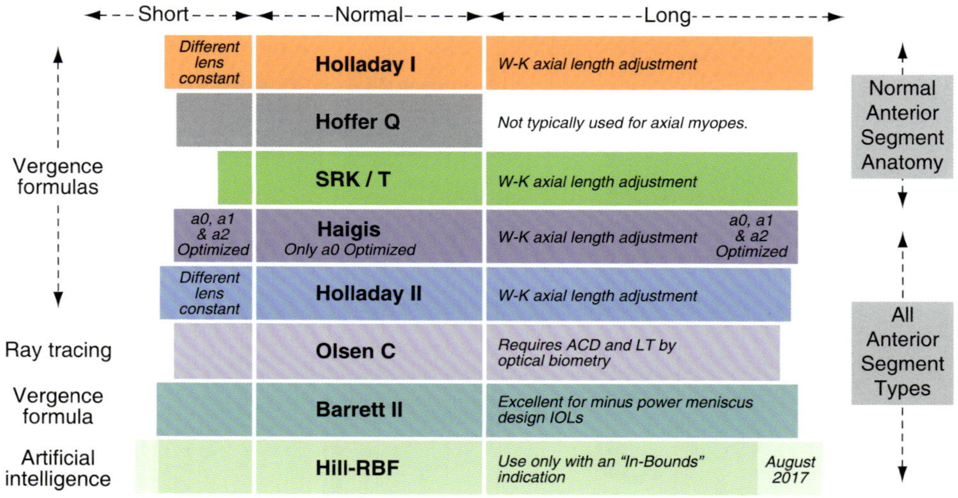

Figure 6-10 Accuracy range of commonly used formulas by axial length. *(Courtesy of Warren Hill, MD.)*

Holladay developed 2 formulas that convert a lens's *A* constant to another factor. The first converts the *A* constant to an *SF* for the Holladay formula:

$$SF = (0.5663 \times A) - 65.6$$

where *A* is the IOL-specific *A* constant and SF is the Holladay surgeon factor. The second formula converts a lens's *A* constant to a personalized *ACD* (p*ACD*) for the Hoffer Q formula:

$$\text{p}ACD = \frac{(0.5663 \times A) - 62.005}{0.9704}$$

where *A* is the IOL-specific *A* constant and p*ACD* is the Hoffer p*ACD (ELP)*. So, for example, an *A* constant of 113.78, 116.35, or 118.92 converts to a p*ACD* of 2.50 mm, 4.00 mm, or 5.50 mm, respectively.

It is prudent to calculate the power of an alternate IOL before surgery. If not calculated in advance, the power of an IOL intended for bag placement can be decreased for sulcus placement with subtraction of 0.75–1.50 D, depending on the *AL* value (Table 6-1). This need to reduce IOL power is not necessary if posterior optic capture is performed. If the haptics are in the sulcus but the optic is "buttonholed" through the anterior capsulorrhexis into the capsular bag, no IOL power adjustment need be made.

测量术前的前房深度 *ACD* 或术后的预测晶体位置 *ELP* 最准确的方法是光学测量法，包括扫描裂隙角膜地形图、Scheimpflug 成像技术以及光学干涉测量仪。超声检测精确性低，且测量值较短。

大多数公式只使用一个常数，比如 *ACD*，*A* 常数或*医生因子*（SF）。Haigis 是一个例外，使用了 3 个常数（a0, a1,a2）。*A* 常数，作为回归公式的成熟结果，在 20 世纪 80 年代被广泛使用，以至于厂商为每一个晶体设计了一个特定的 *A* 常数以及 *ACD* 值。即使已不推荐使用回归公式（如 SRK 公式）计算 IOL，SRK/T 公式中依然有 *A* 常数。

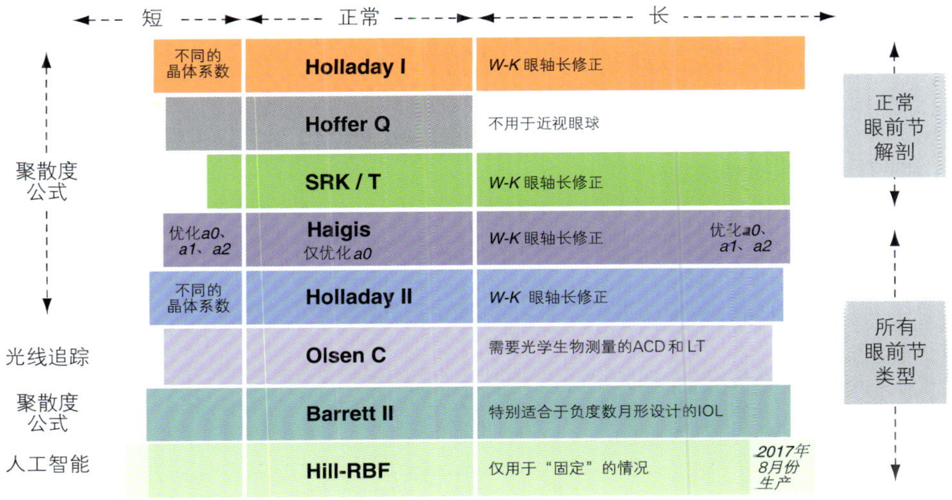

图 6-10　常用公式按不同眼轴长度的精确范围（*译者注：资料来源见前页原文。*）

Holladay 研发的 2 个公式，都将晶体的 *A* 常数转化为另一个因子。第一个 Holladay 公式是将 *A* 常数转化成 *SF*：

$$SF=(0.5663\times A)-65.6$$

A 是 IOL 特殊 *A* 常数，SF 是 Holladay 医生因子。在第二个公式，即 Hoffer Q 公式中，晶体的 *A* 常数转化为个性化 *ACD*(p*ACD*)：

$$pACD=\frac{(0.5663\times A)-62.005}{0.9704}$$

A 代表 IOL 特异的 *A* 常数，p*ACD* 即 Hoffer p*ACD*（预测晶体位置 *ELP*)。例如，分别为 113.78、115.35 或 118.92 的 *A* 常数转化成别为 2.50 mm、4.00 mm 或 5.50 mm 的 p*ACD*。

白内障手术前应该认真计算替换的 IOL 度数。如果没有提前计算，原计划放置于囊袋内的 IOL 如放在了睫状沟，IOL 的度数需根据眼轴长度不同，减少 0.75~1.50 D（表 6-1）。若进行了光学部向后夹持，则无须减少 IOL 度数。如果晶体的襻置于睫状沟而光学部向后，通过前囊膜撕囊口改置于囊袋内，也无须调整 IOL 的度数。

Careful attention to avoiding IOL tilt is important, especially in cases of sutured-in IOLs. Such tilt will induce astigmatism of oblique incidence. For plus-power IOLs, the induced astigmatism will be of with-the-rule orientation in the case of a lens tilted about the horizontal axis and against-the-rule astigmatism in the case of an IOL tilted about the vertical axis. The opposite holds true for the much less common minus-powered IOLs.

Douthwaite WA, Spence D. Slit-lamp measurement of the anterior chamber depth. *Br J Ophthalmol.* 1986;70(3):205–208.

Millar ER, Allen D, Steel DH. Effect of anterior capsulorhexis optic capture of a sulcus-fixated intraocular lens on refractive outcomes. *J Cataract Refract Surg.* 2013;39(6):841–844.

Savini G, Hoffer KJ, Lombardo M, Serrao S, Schiano-Lomoriello D, Ducoli P. Influence of the effective lens position, as predicted by axial length and keratometry, on the near add power of multifocal intraocular lenses. *J Cataract Refract Surg.* 2016;42(1):44–49.

Formula choice

Several studies have indicated that the Hoffer Q formula is more accurate for eyes shorter than 24.5 mm; the Holladay 1, for eyes ranging from 24.5 to 26.0 mm; and the SRK/T, for eyes longer than 26.0 mm (very long eyes). A 2011 study conducted in the United Kingdom proved the statistical significance of these recommendations in more than 8000 eyes by use of optical *AL* values. For long eyes, the Haigis formula may achieve equivalent results.

Table 6-1 IOL Power Adjustment for Sulcus Placement

IOL Power Calculated for In-the-Bag Placement	Power Adjustment for Sulcus Placement
+28.50 D to +30.00 D	Subtract 1.50 D
+17.50 D to +28.00 D	Subtract 1.00 D
+9.50 D to +17.00 D	Subtract 0.50 D
+5.00 D to +9.00 D	No change

The choice of formula is, of course, up to the surgeon, but whatever the method, every effort should be made to ensure that the biometry is as accurate as possible. The operating surgeon should review preoperative *AL* values and *K* readings. If a reading is suspect because it lies outside normal limits, biometry should be repeated during or immediately after the initial reading. Similarly, it is prudent to measure both eyes and recheck the readings if there is a large discrepancy between the 2 eyes. Great care should be taken in the measurement of eyes that have undergone previous refractive surgery (corneal procedures or placement of a phakic IOL), as well as those that have undergone an encircling band treatment of a retinal detachment.

Abulafia A, Barrett GD, Rotenberg M, et al. Intraocular lens power calculation for eyes with an axial length greater than 26.0 mm: comparison of formulas and methods. *J Cataract Refract Surg.* 2015;41(3):548–556.

Aristodemou P, Knox Cartwright NE, Sparrow JM, Johnston RL. Formula choice: Hoffer Q, Holladay 1, or SRK/T and refractive outcomes in 8108 eyes after cataract surgery with biometry by partial coherence interferometry. *J Cataract Refract Surg.* 2011;37(1):63–71.

Cooke DL, Cooke TL. Comparison of 9 intraocular lens power calculation formulas. *J Cataract Refract Surg.* 2016;42(8):1157–1164.

避免人工晶体倾斜很重要，尤其在 IOL 缝合固定的病例中。这种倾斜可导致斜向散光的发生。对于正度数的人工晶体，水平轴上的倾斜会导致顺规散光；而垂直轴向上的倾斜则导致逆规散光。对于较更少用的负度数人工晶体，结果则相反。

Douthwaite WA, Spence D. Slit-lamp measurement of the anterior chamber depth. *Br J Ophthalmol.* 1986;70(3):205–208.

Millar ER, Allen D, Steel DH. Effect of anterior capsulorhexis optic capture of a sulcus-fixated intraocular lens on refractive outcomes. *J Cataract Refract Surg.* 2013;39(6):841–844.

Savini G, Hoffer KJ, Lombardo M, Serrao S, Schiano-Lomoriello D, Ducoli P. Influence of the effective lens position, as predicted by axial length and keratometry, on the near add power of multifocal intraocular lenses. *J Cataract Refract Surg.* 2016;42(1):44–49.

公式的选择

多项研究表明，Hoffer Q 公式对短于 24.5 mm 的眼球更准确；Holladay 1 公式更适用于 24.5~26.0 mm 的眼轴；SRK/T 公式对长于 26.0 mm 的眼球更准确。2011 年英国的研究证实，在 8000 多只眼的光学生物测量中，以上推荐公式具有统计学意义。Haigis 公式对于长眼轴眼球也同样准确。

表6–1　IOL睫状沟植入的度数调整

植入囊袋内的IOL度数	植入睫状沟的度数调整
+28.50 D 至+30.00 D	减去1.50 D
+17.50 D 至+28.00 D	减去1.00 D
+9.50 D 至+17.00 D	减去 0.50 D
+5.00 D 至+9.00 D	不变

当然，公式的选择应当由手术医生决定，但不管用哪种方法，应努力确保生物学测量尽可能准确。手术医生应检查术前 *AL* 和 *K* 值结果。如果超出正常范围，应该尽快重复检查。谨慎地测量双眼；如果双眼差异太大，应重复检查。有屈光手术史（角膜屈光手术或 ICL 植入术）以及视网膜脱离扣带术的眼球，应特别注意。

Abulafia A, Barrett GD, Rotenberg M, et al. Intraocular lens power calculation for eyes with an axial length greater than 26.0 mm: comparison of formulas and methods. *J Cataract Refract Surg.* 2015;41(3):548–556.

Aristodemou P, Knox Cartwright NE, Sparrow JM, Johnston RL. Formula choice: Hoffer Q, Holladay 1, or SRK/T and refractive outcomes in 8108 eyes after cataract surgery with biometry by partial coherence interferometry. *J Cataract Refract Surg.* 2011;37(1):63–71.

Cooke DL, Cooke TL. Comparison of 9 intraocular lens power calculation formulas. *J Cataract Refract Surg.* 2016;42(8):1157–1164.

Piggyback and Supplemental Intraocular Lenses

When an IOL is inserted into an eye that already has an IOL in place, the second IOL is called a *piggyback IOL*. The piggyback IOL can be inserted at the time the first IOL is implanted to produce a high power that is commercially unavailable. It can also be inserted secondarily to correct a postoperative refractive error. Computer programs can be used to calculate the power of the second IOL and to make adjustments, which may be needed if the posterior IOL is displaced posteriorly. However, these adjustments are minor, and using one of the following formulas is the easiest way to calculate them:

Myopic correction: $P = 1.0 \times \text{error}$
Hyperopic correction: $P = 1.5 \times \text{error}$

where P is the needed power in the piggyback lens, and *error* refers to the residual refractive error that needs to be corrected.

Intraocular Lens Power Calculation After Corneal Refractive Surgery

Intraocular lens power calculation is a problem in eyes that have undergone *radial keratotomy (RK)* or laser corneal refractive procedures. The difficulty stems from 3 sources of errors: (1) instrument error, (2) index of refraction error, and (3) formula error.

Instrument Error

Instrument error was first described by Koch in 1989. The instruments used by phthalmologists to measure corneal power (keratometers and corneal topographers) cannot obtain accurate measurements in eyes that have undergone corneal refractive surgery. These instruments often miss the central, flatter zone of effective corneal power. The flatter the cornea is, the larger the zone of measurement is, and the greater the error. Placido disk topography is susceptible to similar errors and usually overestimates the central corneal power, leading to a postoperative hyperopic refractive surprise in myopic eyes. Emerging technologies based on direct anatomical analysis of the cornea (Scheimpflug and computer modeling techniques) may offer a truer measure of corneal central power.

Index of Refraction Error

The assumed index of refraction (IR) of the normal cornea is based on the relationship between the anterior and posterior corneal curvatures. This relationship changes in eyes treated with ablative laser procedures. Ophthalmologists long believed that IR error did not occur in eyes that have undergone RK. This situation leads to an overestimation of the corneal power by approximately 1 D for every 7 D of correction obtained and results in hyperopic refractive surprise. A recent study showed that in eyes treated with RK, there is greater flattening of the posterior curvature than of the anterior curvature. Both manual keratometers and computerized corneal topographers that measure only the front surface curvature convert the radius of curvature (r) obtained to diopters (D), usually by using an *IR* value of 1.3375. The following formula can be used to convert diopters to radius:

背驮和附加 IOL

对已植入 IOL 的眼，在这个 IOL 处再植入一个 IOL，第二个 IOL 被称为*背驮 IOL*。如果需植入的 IOL 度数过高，超过了市场上现有的 IOL 度数范围，则需要植入背驮 IOL。它也可以用于矫正白内障术后残留的屈光度。可使用计算机程序计算第二片晶体的度数，如果后方的 IOL 植入位置后移，也可使用程序调整度数。然而，调整通常比较小，可通过下面最简单的方法进行计算：

近视屈光度矫正：$P=1.0\times$ 误差
远视屈光度矫正：$P=1.5\times$ 误差

P 是指所需的背驮晶体度数，*误差*是指需要被矫正的残余屈光度。

角膜屈光术后的 IOL 度数计算

行*放射状角膜切开*（*RK*）或激光角膜屈光手术的眼，*存在* IOL 度数的计算问题。有 3 个方面：① 设备的误差；② 折射率误差；③ 公式的误差。

设备的误差

设备的误差是 Koch 首次于 1989 年提出的。眼科医生所用的测量角膜曲率的设备（角膜曲率计和角膜地形图）无法对做过角膜屈光手术的眼球获得准确的测量结果。这些设备经常会漏掉中央较平坦的区域，其存在有效角膜屈光力。角膜越平坦，测量区域越大，误差就越大。基于 Placido 盘的角膜地形图易产生类似误差，高估中央角膜屈光力，导致近视眼术后的远视。基于直接角膜解剖分析的测量技术（Scheimpflug 和计算机建模技术）可能会提供更真实的中央角膜屈光力测量结果。

折射率的误差

正常角膜的折射率（IR）是基于前、后表面角膜曲率关系的推定值。激光消融术后的角膜这种关系发生了改变。长期以来，眼科医生认为做了 RK 手术的眼不存在角膜 IR 的误差。这种状况导致每矫正 7D，角膜屈光力约高估 1D，导致出现意外的远视。近期的一项研究表明，行 RK 手术的眼球，其后表面会比前表面更平坦。手动角膜曲率计和计算机角膜地形图都只测量了前表面的弯曲度，使用常用的*角膜折射率* 1.3375，将曲率半径（r）转化为屈光力（D）。转化公式如下：

$$r = \frac{337.5}{D}$$

To convert r to D, use

$$D = \frac{337.5}{r}$$

Formula Error

Except for the Haigis formula, all the modern IOL power formulas (eg, Hoffer Q, Holladay 1 and 2, and SRK/T) use the *AL* values and *K* readings to predict the postoperative position of the IOL *(ELP)*. The flatter-than-normal *K* value for eyes that have undergone myopic refractive surgery causes an error in this prediction because the anterior chamber dimensions do not actually change in these eyes commensurately with the much flatter *K* .These ELP errors also tend to result in hyperopic refractive surprise.

Power Calculation Methods for the Post–Keratorefractive Procedure Eye

The double-*K* method uses the pre-LASIK corneal power (or, if unknown, 43.50 D) to calculate the *ELP*, and the post-LASIK (much flatter) corneal power to calculate the IOL power. These calculations can be performed automatically with computer programs.

The double-*K* method is only one of more than 20 methods proposed over the years to either calculate the true corneal power or adjust the calculated IOL power to account for the errors discussed in the preceding sections. Some methods require knowledge of pre-refractive surgery values such as refractive error and *K* reading. Many of these methods have come in and out of favor based on studies investigating their accuracy. More recent theoretical or ray tracing formulas (Olsen, Barrett) may offer a more accurate alternative in abnormally sized eyes in which previous refractive procedures have been performed, especially corneal refractive surgery. It is up to the surgeon to keep abreast of the most accurate available methods.

It is not possible to describe all these methods in this chapter. Several excellent calculators are available online, including tools from Warren Hill and Graham Barrett at ASCRS.org, APACRS .org, and www .doctor-hill .com, as well as the Hoffer/Savini LASIK IOL Power Tool, which can be downloaded for free (see the Hoffer reference below).

Perhaps in the future there will be a more satisfactory method of measuring true corneal power by use of topography and advanced measuring techniques. At present, the ideal method for use with post-refractive surgery patients has yet to be determined.

Abulafia A, Hill WE, Koch DD, Wang L, Barrett GD. Accuracy of the Barrett True-K Formula for intraocular lens power prediction after laser in situ keratomileusis or photorefractive keratectomy for myopia. *J Cataract Refract Surg*. 2016;42(3):363–369.

Alió JL, Abdelghany AA, Abdou AA, Maldonado MJ. Cataract surgery on the previous corneal refractive surgery patient. *Surv Ophthalmol*. 2016;61(6):769–777.

Fernández-Buenaga R, Alió JL, Pérez Ardoy AL, Quesada AL, Pinilla-Cortés L, Barraquer RI. Resolving refractive error after cataract surgery: IOL exchange, piggyback lens, or LASIK. *J Refract Surg*. 2013;29(10):676–683.

Hill W, Wang L, Koch D.IOL Power Calculation in Eyes That Have Undergone LASIK/PRK/RK. Available at www.iolcalc.ascrs.org.

Hoffer KJ. The Hoffer/Savini LASIK IOL Power Tool. Available at www.iolpowerclub.org /post-surgical-iol-calc. Accessed June 3, 2013.

$$r=\frac{337.5}{D}$$

将 r 转化为 D，使用公式：

$$D=\frac{337.5}{r}$$

公式的误差

除了 Haigis 公式，其他所有的现代人工晶体计算公式（比如，Hoffer Q、Holladay 1 和 2 以及 SRK/T 公式）都使用 *AL* 和 *K* 值预测白内障术后 IOL 的位置（*ELP*）。对于做了近视性角膜屈光术的眼球，其角膜 *K* 值较正常变平坦，而前房深度实际上并没有随着变平的角膜发生匹配的改变，这导致了预测术后 IOL 位置时产生误差。ELP 的误差也会导致远视的出现。

角膜屈光术后眼球的 IOL 度数计算方法

双 *K* 法采用 LASIK 术前的角膜屈光力（如果未知，使用 43.50 D）计算 *ELP*，以计算 LASIK 术后（更平坦的）的角膜屈光力，算出 IOL 度数。计算过程通过计算机软件自动完成。

这些年前提出了许多计算法，双 K 法仅仅是 20 多个方法之一，用以计算真实的角膜屈光力，或调整前面讨论的 IOL 度数误差。有些方法需要屈光术前的资料，比如屈光不正和 *K* 值。有许多方法基于其准确性被应用或被淘汰。最近的理论公式或光路追踪公式（Olsen, Barrett）可作为更准确的选择用于曾接受了屈光手术的异常大小的眼球，特别是角膜屈光手术。这是目前医生了解到的最精确可用的方法。

在本章无法描述所有方法。可在线获取一些好的计算方法，包括从 ASCRS.org，APACRS.org 和 www.doctor-hill.com 获取的 Warren Hill 和 Graham Barrett 的工具，以及免费下载的 Hoffer/Savini LASIK IOL 度数计算工具（见参考文献）。

也许将来会有更为满意的方法使用角膜地形图和先进的测量技术测量真实的角膜屈光力，目前，供屈光术后患者使用的理想方法尚未确定。

Abulafia A, Hill WE, Koch DD, Wang L, Barrett GD. Accuracy of the Barrett True-K Formula for intraocular lens power prediction after laser in situ keratomileusis or photorefractive keratectomy for myopia. *J Cataract Refract Surg*. 2016;42(3):363–369.

Alió JL, Abdelghany AA, Abdou AA, Maldonado MJ. Cataract surgery on the previous corneal refractive surgery patient. *Surv Ophthalmol*. 2016;61(6):769–777.

Fernández-Buenaga R, Alió JL, Pérez Ardoy AL, Quesada AL, Pinilla-Cortés L, Barraquer RI. Resolving refractive error after cataract surgery: IOL exchange, piggyback lens, or LASIK. *J Refract Surg*. 2013;29(10):676–683.

Hill W, Wang L, Koch D.IOL Power Calculation in Eyes That Have Undergone LASIK/PRK/RK. Available at www.iolcalc.ascrs.org.

Hoffer KJ. The Hoffer/Savini LASIK IOL Power Tool. Available at www.iolpowerclub.org /post-surgical-iol-calc Accessed June 3, 2013.

Koch DD, Liu JF, Hyde LL, Rock RL, Emery JM. Refractive complications of cataract surgery after radial keratotomy. Am *J Ophthalmol*. 1989;108(6):676–682.

Special Consideration: Postoperative Refractive Surprise in Patients Who Have Undergone Myopic Keratorefractive Correction

- Keratometers fail to measure the flattest portion of the cornea. This overestimation of corneal power will result in a hyperopic refractive surprise.
- Keratometers and computerized corneal topographers underestimate the relative contribution of the posterior cornea and therefore overestimate the net corneal refractive index and overall corneal refractive power. This overestimation of corneal power will result in a hyperopic refractive surprise.
- Standard IOL formulas estimate the ELP to be too anterior and therefore overestimate the refractive contribution of the IOL. This overestimation of IOL refractive contribution will result in a hyperopic refractive surprise.

Intraocular Lens Power in Corneal Transplant Eyes

It is very difficult to predict the ultimate power of the cornea after the eye has undergone penetrating keratoplasty. Thus, in 1987 Hoffer recommended that the surgeon wait for the corneal transplant to heal completely before implanting an IOL. The current safety of intraocular surgery allows for such a double-procedure approach in all but the rarest cases. Geggel has proven the validity of this approach by showing that posttransplant eyes have better uncorrected visual acuity (68% with 20/40 or better) and that the range of IOL power error decreases from 10 D to 5 D (95% within±2.00 D).

If simultaneous IOL implantation and corneal transplant are necessary, surgeons may use either the *K* reading of the fellow eye or the average postoperative *K* value of a previous series of transplants, but these approaches are fraught with error. When there is corneal scarring in an eye but no need for a corneal graft, it might be best to use the corneal power of the other eye or even a power that is commensurate with the eye's *AL* and refractive error.

Flowers CW, McLeod SD, McDonnell PJ, Irvine JA, Smith RE. Evaluation of intraocular lens power calculation formulas in the triple procedure. *J Cataract Refract Surg*. 1996;22(1): 116–122.

De Bernardo M, Capasso L, Caliendo L, Paolercio F, Rosa N. IOL power calculation after corneal refractive surgery. *Biomed Res Int*. 2014;33(6):e2.

Geggel HS. Intraocular lens implantation after penetrating keratoplasty. Improved unaided visual acuity, astigmatism, and safety in patients with combined corneal disease and cataract. *Ophthalmology*. 1990;97(11):1460–1467.

Hoffer KJ. Triple procedure for intraocular lens exchange. *Arch Ophthalmol*. 1987;105(5): 609–610.

Koch DD, Liu JF, Hyde LL, Rock RL, Emery JM. Refractive complications of cataract surgery after radial keratotomy. *Am J Ophthalmol.* 1989;108(6):676–682.

特别注意：近视角膜屈光矫正术后行白内障手术的术后屈光变化

- 角膜曲率计无法测量最平坦部分的角膜导致的角膜屈光力高估将产生远视。
- 角膜曲率计和计算机角膜地形图低估了角膜后表面的相对作用，导致了高估净角膜折射率和全角膜屈光力而产生远视。
- 标准的 IOL 计算公式预估 ELP 偏前，而高估了 IOL 的屈光作用，产生远视。

角膜移植眼的 IOL 度数

很难预测穿透性角膜移植术后眼球最终的角膜屈光力。因此，1987 年 Hoffer 建议，推迟植入 IOL，直到角膜移植片完全愈合。目前，内眼手术的安全性允许在这种罕见病例中进行双步法。Geggel 已经证实了这种方法的有效性。角膜移植术后眼可以获得较好的裸眼视力（68% 视力 ≥ 20/40，或 0.5），IOL 度数的误差从 10.00D 下降到 5.00D（95% 在 ± 2.00D 以内）。

如果必须同时进行 IOL 植入和角膜移植，手术医生可以使用对侧眼的 *K* 值或前一批角膜医生患者术后平均的 *K* 值进行计算，但这些方法存在误差。当角膜存有瘢痕、但无须角膜移植时，最好用另一眼的角膜屈光力，或匹配眼球长度和屈光度的角膜屈光力进行计算。

Flowers CW, McLeod SD, McDonnell PJ, Irvine JA, Smith RE. Evaluation of intraocular lens power calculation formulas in the triple procedure. *J Cataract Refract Surg.* 1996;22(1): 116–122.

De Bernardo M, Capasso L, Caliendo L, Paolercio F, Rosa N. IOL power calculation after corneal refractive surgery. *Biomed Res Int.* 2014;33(6):e2.

Geggel HS. Intraocular lens implantation after penetrating keratoplasty. Improved unaided visual acuity, astigmatism, and safety in patients with combined corneal disease and cataract. *Ophthalmology.* 1990;97(11):1460–1467.

Hoffer KJ. Triple procedure for intraocular lens exchange. *Arch Ophthalmol.* 1987;105(5): 609–610.

Silicone Oil Eyes

Ophthalmologists considering IOL implantation in eyes filled with silicone oil encounter 2 major problems.The first is obtaining an accurate *AL* measurement with the ultrasonic biometer. Recall that this instrument measures the transit time of the ultrasound pulse and, using estimated ultrasound velocities through the various ocular media, calculates the distance. This concept must be taken into consideration when velocities differ from the norm, for example, when silicone oil fills the posterior segment (980 m/s for silicone oil vs 1532 m/s for vitreous). Use of optical biometry to measure *AL* solves this problem somewhat. It is recommended that retinal surgeons perform an optical or immersion *AL* measurement before silicone oil placement, but doing so is not common practice. The second problem is that, as the refractive index of silicone oil is greater than that of the vitreous humor, the oil filling the vitreous cavity reduces the optical power of the posterior surface of the IOL in the eye when a biconvex IOL is implanted. This problem must be counteracted by an increase in IOL power of 3–5 D.

Suk KK, Smiddy WE, Shi W. Refractive outcomes after silicone oil removal and intraocular lens implantation. *Retina*. 2013;33(3):634–641.

Symes RJ. Accurate biometry in silicone oil-filled eyes. *Eye (Lond)*. 2013;27(6):778–779.

Pediatric Eyes

Several issues make IOL power selection for children much more complex than that for adults. The first challenge is obtaining accurate *AL* and corneal measurements, which is usually performed when the child is under general anesthesia. The second issue is that, because shorter *AL* causes greater IOL power errors, the small size of a child's eye compounds power calculation errors, particularly if the child is very young. The third problem is selecting an appropriate target IOL power, one that will not only provide adequate visual acuity to prevent amblyopia but also allow adequate vision with the expected growth of the eye after the IOL implantation.

A possible solution to the third problem is to implant 2 (or more) IOLs simultaneously: one IOL with the predicted adult emmetropic power placed posteriorly and the other (or others) with the power that provides childhood emmetropia placed anterior to the first lens. When the patient reaches adulthood, the obsolete IOL(s) can be removed (sequentially). Alternatively, corneal refractive surgery may be used to treat myopia that develops in adulthood. Most recent studies have shown that the best modern formulas do not perform as accurately for children's eyes as they do for adults' eyes.

Hoffer KJ, Aramberri J, Haigis W, Norrby S, Olsen T, Shammas HJ; IOL Power Club Executive Committee. The final frontier: pediatric intraocular lens power. *Am J Ophthalmol*. 2012; 154(1):1–2.e1.

O'Hara MA. Pediatric intraocular lens power calculations. *Curr Opin Ophthalmol*. 2012;23(5): 388–393.

硅油眼

眼科医生在考虑用硅油填充眼的 IOL 植入时，面临 2 个主要问题。第一个问题是，使用超声生物测量仪获得准确的 AL。回顾一下，这种设备测量的是超声脉冲的传播时间，通过估计的声波穿过不同眼部介质时的速度，计算出距离。当声速改变时，这一概念必须要考虑，比如，硅油填充的眼后节（声波在硅油中的传播速度是 980 m/s，而在玻璃体内是 1532 m/s）。使用光学生物测量可解决这个问题。推荐视网膜手术医生在填充硅油前，用光学或浸润式超声测量 AL，但常规不做。第二个问题是，硅油的折射率高于玻璃体，当植入双凸 IOL 时，填充于玻璃体腔的硅油减少了 IOL 后表面的屈光力，需要调高 3.00~5.00 D IOL 度数。

Suk KK, Smiddy WE, Shi W. Refractive outcomes after silicone oil removal and intraocular lens implantation. *Retina*. 2013;33(3):634–641.

Symes RJ. Accurate biometry in silicone oil-filled eyes. *Eye (Lond)*. 2013;27(6):778–779.

小儿眼球

多个因素使儿童 IOL 度数的选择比成人更困难。首先，患儿是在全麻下测量准确的 *AL* 和角膜屈光力。第二个，由于较短的 *AL* 可产生较大的 IOL 度数误差，较小的儿童眼球增加 IOL 度数计算的误差，特别是患儿年龄很小。第三，选择合适的目标 IOL 度数，这个度数不仅能提供足够的视力预防弱视的发生，同样需要在 IOL 植入后为预期的眼球生长提供足够的视力。

对第三个问题，解决的方法是同时植入 2 片（或更多的）人工晶体：一片满足成人正视需求的 IOL 放在后面；另一片是提供儿童正视所需度数的晶体放在第一片前面。当患儿成年时，将不需要的晶体取出（按顺序），或使用角膜屈光手术矫正成人后发生的近视。大多数近期的研究表明，最现代的公式在儿童眼球中不如在成人眼中准确。

Hoffer KJ, Aramberri J, Haigis W, Norrby S, Olsen T, Shammas HJ; IOL Power Club Executive Committee. The final frontier: pediatric intraocular lens power. Am *J Ophthalmol*. 2012; 154(1):1–2.e1.

O'Hara MA. Pediatric intraocular lens power calculations. *Curr Opin Ophthalmol*. 2012;23(5): 388–393.

Image Magnification

Image magnification of as much as 20%–35% is the major disadvantage of aphakic spectacles. Contact lenses magnify images by only 7%–12%, whereas IOLs magnify images by 4% or less. An IOL implanted in the posterior chamber produces less image magnification than does an IOL in the anterior chamber. The issue of magnification is further complicated by the correction of residual postsurgical refractive errors. A Galilean telescope effect is created when spectacles are worn over pseudophakic eyes. Clinically, each diopter of spectacle overcorrection at a vertex of 12 mm causes a 2% magnification or minification (for plus or minus lenses, respectively). Thus, a pseudophakic patient with a posterior chamber IOL and a residual refractive error of −1 D would have 2% magnification from the IOL and 2% minification from the spectacle lens, resulting in little change in image size.

Aniseikonia is defined as a difference in image size between the 2 eyes and can cause disturbances in stereopsis. Generally, a person can tolerate spherical aniseikonia of 5%–8%. In clinical practice, aniseikonia is rarely a significant problem; however, it should be considered in patients with unexplained vision symptoms.

Gobin L, Rozema JJ, Tassignon MJ. Predicting refractive aniseikonia after cataract surgery in anisometropia. *J Cataract Refract Surg*. 2008;34(8):1353–1361.

Lens-Related Vision Disturbances

The presence of IOLs may cause numerous optical phenomena. Various light-related visual phenomena encountered by pseudophakic (and phakic) patients are termed *dysphotopsias*. These phenomena are divided into positive and negative dysphotopsias. Positive dysphotopsias are characterized by brightness, streaks, and rays emanating from a central point source of light, sometimes with a diffuse, hazy glare. Negative dysphotopsias are characterized by subjective darkness or shadowing. Such optical phenomena may be related to light reflection and refraction along the edges of the IOL. High-index acrylic lenses with square or truncated edges produce a more intense edge glare (Fig 6-11A).These phenomena may also be due to internal re-reflection within the IOL itself; such re-reflection is more likely to occur with materials that have a higher refractive index, such as acrylic (Fig 6-11B). With a less steeply curved anterior surface, the lens may be more likely to have internal reflections that are directed toward the fovea and are therefore more distracting (Fig 6-11C, D).

成像放大

无晶体眼配镜主要的缺点是成像放大 20%~35%。接触镜成像放大仅 7%~12%，而人工晶体放大仅 4% 或更少。后房型 IOL 植入较前房型时的成像放大更少。成像放大的问题，对屈光矫正术后的残留屈光不正会更为复杂。当人工晶体眼配戴框架眼镜时，会产生 Galileo 望远镜效应。临床上镜眼距离为 12 mm 时，每 1.00 D 的框架眼镜矫正可产生约 2% 的放大或缩小（分别是正镜片或负镜片）。因此，后房型 IOL 植入的患者残留 –1.00 D 的度数时，会产生来自 IOL 的 2% 的放大率和来自框架眼镜 2% 的缩小率，结果成像变化很小。

*物象不等症*是指双眼间的物象差异引起立体视的干扰。一般来说，人可以耐受 5%~8% 的球面物象不等。在临床中，物象不等症不会产生严重的问题，但当患者出现无法解释的视觉症状时，需要考虑物象不等。

Gobin L, Rozema JJ, Tassignon MJ. Predicting refractive aniseikonia after cataract surgery in anisometropia. J *Cataract Refract Surg*. 2008;34(8):1353–1361.

晶体相关视觉干扰

人工晶体可导致多种光学现象。人工晶体眼（和有晶状体眼）的患者出现各种与光学相关的视觉现象被称为*失能性炫光*。这些现象分为正失能性炫光和负失能性炫光。正失能性炫光的特征表现为明亮、条纹和从点光源发散的光线，有时伴有弥漫的眩光。负失能性炫光的特征表现为主观的阴暗或暗影。这些光学现象可能与 IOL 边缘的光线反射和折射有关。方边或钝边的高折射率丙烯酸酯人工晶体可产生更多的边缘眩光（图 6–11A）。这些现象也可能源于 IOL 内部的光线再反射。这些再反射多发生在较高折射率的物质，如丙烯酸酯（图 6–11B）。当晶体前表面不太陡峭弯曲时，更可能发生晶体内部反射，导致光线反射到中心凹，进而产生更多的干扰（图 6–11C、D）。

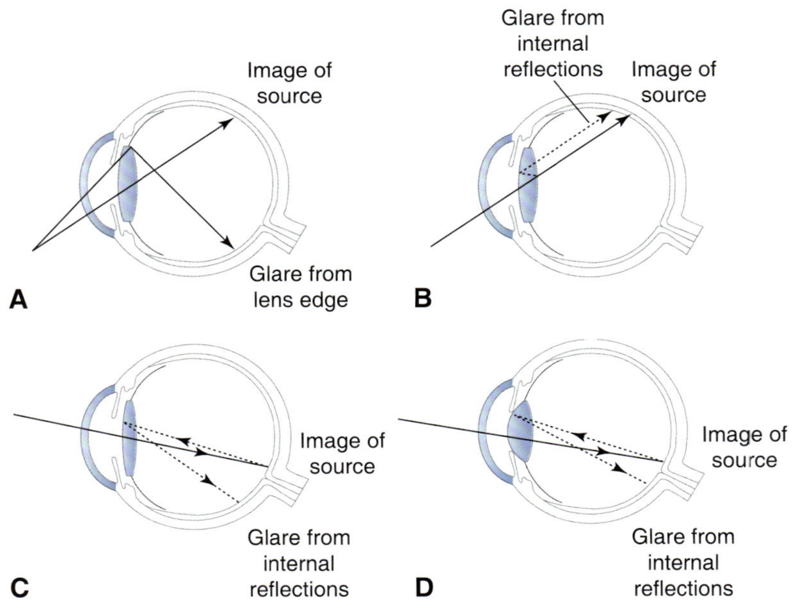

Figure 6-11 Lens-related vision disturbances. **A**, Light striking the edge of the intraocular lens (IOL) (not drawn to scale) may be reflected to another site on the retina, resulting in undesirable dysphotopsias. These problems arise less often with smoother-edged IOLs. **B**, Light may be internally re-reflected within an IOL, producing an undesirable second image or halo. Such re-reflection may be more likely to occur as the index of refraction of the IOL increases. **C**, Light may reflect back from the surface of the retina and reach the anterior surface of the IOL. The IOL acts as a concave mirror, reflecting back an undesirable dysphotopsic image. When the anterior surface of the IOL is more curved, the annoying image is displaced relatively far from the fovea. **D**, When the anterior IOL surface is less steeply curved, the annoying image appears closer to the true image and is likely to be more distracting. *(Redrawn by C. H. Wooley.)*

Davison JA. Positive and negative dysphotopsia in patients with acrylic intraocular lenses. *J Cataract Refract Surg*. 2000;26(9):1346–1355.

Erie JC, Bandhauer MH. Intraocular lens surfaces and their relationship to postoperative glare. *J Cataract Refract Surg*. 2003;29(2):336–341.

Franchini A, Gallarati BZ, Vaccari E. Computerized analysis of the effects of intraocular lens edge design on the quality of vision in pseudophakic patients. *J Cataract Refract Surg*. 2003; 29(2):342–347.

Henderson BA, Geneva II. Negative dysphotopsia: A perfect storm. J Cataract Refract Surg. 2015;41(10):2291–2312.

Holladay JT, Zhao H, Reisin CR. Negative dysphotopsia: the enigmatic penumbra. *J Cataract Refract Surg*. 2012;38(7):1251–1265.

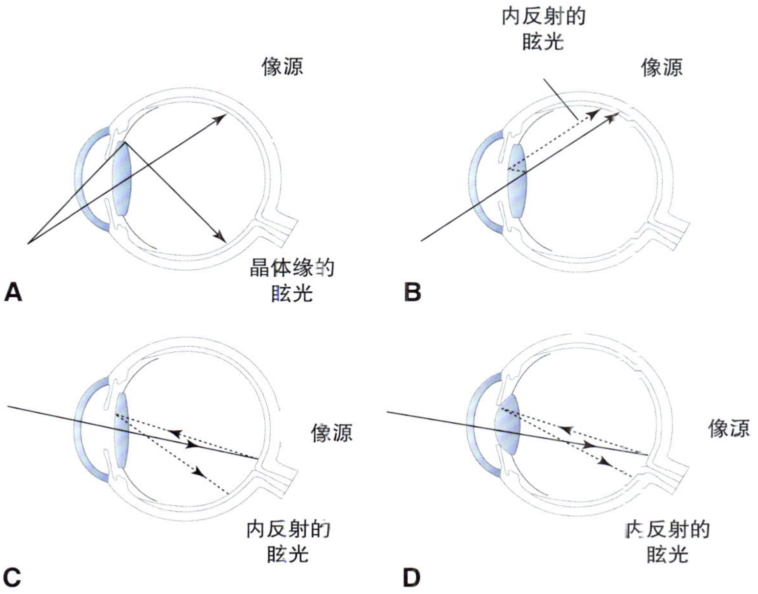

图 6–11　晶体相关视觉干扰现象。**A.** 光线遇到 IOL 的边缘（不作为计算），反射回视网膜的另一点，导致的失能性炫光。这些问题在光滑边缘的人工晶体上出现较少。**B.** 光线可能在人工晶体内部再反射，产生不良的第二个图像或光晕。随着 IOL 折射率增加，这些再反射更易发生。**C.** 光学可能反射回视网膜表面，再到达晶体的前表面。此时，人工晶体起到了凹面镜的效果，把光线反射回来，产生失能性炫光的像。当 IOL 前表面更弯曲时，干扰的图像会出现在离中心凹相对较远的位置。**D.** 当 IOL 前表面不太陡峭弯曲时，干扰的图像会出现在离真实物象更近的位置，从而更可能导致不适。*（译者注：资料来源见前页原文。）*

Davison JA. Positive and negative dysphotopsia in patients with acrylic intraocular lenses. *J Cataract Refract Surg*. 2000;26(9):1346–1355.

Erie JC, Bandhauer MH. Intraocular lens surfaces and their relationship to postoperative glare. *J Cataract Refract Surg*. 2003;29(2):336–341.

Franchini A, Gallarati BZ, Vaccari E. Computerized analysis of the effects of intraocular lens edge design on the quality of vision in pseudophakic patients. *J Cataract Refract Surg*. 2003; 29(2):342–347.

Henderson BA, Geneva II. Negative dysphotopsia: A perfect storm. J Cataract Refract Surg 2015;41(10):2291–2312.

Holladay JT, Zhao H, Reisin CR. Negative dysphotopsia: the enigmatic penumbra. *J Cataract Refract Surg*. 2012;38(7):1251–1265.

Nonspherical Optics

IOLs with more complex optical designs are now available. It may be possible to offset the positive spherical aberration of the cornea in pseudophakic patients by implanting an IOL with the appropriate negative asphericity on its anterior surface. IOLs with a *toric* surface may be used to correct astigmatism. Rotational stability may be of greater concern when plate-haptic toric lenses are implanted in the vertical axis than when they are implanted in the horizontal axis. As a toric lens rotates from the optimal desired angular orientation, the benefit of the toric correction diminishes. Misalignment of a toric lens may occur because of excyclotorsion or incyclotorsion of the eye as the patient moves from a vertical position to a recumbent position during surgery. Therefore, it is important to mark the eye for purposes of orientation while the patient is standing or sitting up. For the same reason, optical registration systems obtain their orientation data while the patient is sitting up. A misalignment of a properly powered toric IOL of only 10° reduces its efficacy by 30% and a misalignment of more than 30° off-axis increases the residual astigmatism of an eye; if it is 90° off-axis, the residual astigmatism doubles. Fortunately, some benefit remains even with lesser degrees of axis error, although the axis of residual cylinder changes. Newer designs are more stable than earlier ones.

Toric IOLs do not correct lenticular astigmatism and correct only that portion of corneal astigmatism that is regular. Although toric IOLs may hold benefit for patients with irregular, nonorthogonal, asymmetric, or unstable astigmatism, as may occur with keratoconus, caution should be exercised with the degree of astigmatic correction to be attempted.

Investigators have developed an IOL in which the optical power can be altered by laser after lens implantation. Similarly, a laser system in development may alter the optical power of a conventional acrylic lens after implantation. These technologies would be useful for correcting both IOL power calculation errors and residual astigmatism.

Mester U, Dillinger P, Anterist N. Impact of a modified optic design on visual function: clinical comparative study. *J Cataract Refract Surg*. 2003;29(4):652–660.

Sahler R, Bille JF, Enright S, Chhoeung S, Chan K. Creation of a refractive lens within an existing intraocular lens using a femtosecond laser.*J Cataract Refract Surg*. 2016;42(8):1207–1215.

Multifocal Intraocular Lenses

Conventional IOLs are *monofocal* and correct the refractive ametropia associated with removal of the crystalline lens. Because a standard IOL has no accommodative power, it provides a clear focus for visual targets at a single distance only. However, the improved visual acuity resulting from IOL implantation may allow a patient to see with acceptable clarity over a range of distances. If the patient is left with a residual refractive error of simple myopic astigmatism, the ability to see with acceptable clarity over a range of distances may be further augmented. In this situation, one endpoint of the astigmatic conoid of Sturm corresponds to the distance focus and the other endpoint represents myopia and, thus, a near focus; satisfactory clarity of vision may be possible if the object in view is focused between these 2 endpoints. In bilateral, asymmetric, and oblique myopic astigmatism, the blurred axis images are ignored and the clearest axis images are chosen to form one clear image for distance vision; the opposite images are selected for near vision. Thus, even standard IOLs may provide some degree of depth of focus and "bifocal" capabilities.

非球面光学

目前有光学设计更复杂的 IOL。前表面具有适量负性非球面的 IOL 被植入眼内，可抵消患者角膜的正球差。*复曲*面设计的 IOL 可用于矫正散光。当板形襻的复曲面人工晶体以垂直方向植入时，相较于水平方向的植入，更需要注意其旋转稳定性。当复曲面人工晶体发生旋转远离最优角度时，散光矫正效果就消失了。在手术过程中，患者从坐位转换为平卧位，眼球的外旋或内旋可能会造成复曲面人工晶体轴位的偏差。因此，在患者直立位或坐位时给眼球做标记定向是很重要的。出于同样的原因，光学注册系统也应该在患者坐位时获取定向数据。一定屈光度的复曲面 IOL 人工晶体轴位偏差仅 10° 即可减弱 30% 的矫正效果，超过 30° 的偏差会增加残余散光。如果旋转偏离 90°，则残余散光加倍。较小的轴位误差，虽然残余散光的轴位会改变，但仍然能保有一部分矫正散光效应。目前新的设计已比早期设计更加稳定。

复曲面人工晶体不矫正晶状体散光，仅矫正规则的角膜散光。虽然对于不规则、非相互垂直（非正交的）、不对称或不稳定散光的患者，如圆锥角膜，使用复曲面人工晶体可能有益，但尝试矫正散光度数时仍应谨慎。

研究人员发明了一种人工晶体，可以在植入后通过激光改变其光学焦度。同样有一种激光系统尚在研发中，可用于改变植入眼内的传统丙烯酸酯人工晶体的光学焦度。对于矫正 IOL 焦度计算误差和矫正残余散光，这些技术是有用的。

Mester U, Dillinger P, Anterist N. Impact of a modified optic design on visual function: clinical comparative study. *J Cataract Refract Surg*. 2003;29(4):652–660.

Sahler R, Bille JF, Enright S, Chhoeung S, Chan K. Creation of a refractive lens within an existing intraocular lens using a femtosecond laser.*J Cataract Refract Surg*. 2016;42(8):1207–1215.

多焦点人工晶体

传统的人工晶体是*单焦点的*，用于矫正晶状体摘除造成的屈光不正。由于常规的人工晶体无调节能力，只能清晰聚焦于一个固定的距离。当然，人工晶体植入后的视力改善可使患者的视力在一定范围内是清晰的。如果患者残留单纯近视散光，清晰范围可能扩大。在这种情况下，散光 Sturm 锥的一个端点对应视远聚焦，而另一个端点表示视近聚焦，当物体位于 2 点之间时，患者可以获得满意的清晰视觉。在双侧不对称的斜轴近视散光中，大脑会忽略模糊轴位上的像，选择最清晰轴位上的像来形成远用的清晰像，选择相反轴位上的像作为近用。临床上很难复制这个过程。因此，即使是常规的人工晶体也可以提供一定程度的焦深和“双焦”功能。

An alternate approach to this problem is to correct one eye for distance and the other for near vision; this approach is called *monovision*—this approach is also used with contact lenses. Nevertheless, most patients who receive IOLs are corrected for distance vision and wear reading glasses as needed.

Multifocal IOLs are designed to improve both near and distance vision to decrease patients' dependence on glasses. With a multifocal IOL, the correcting lens is placed in a fixed location within the eye, and the patient cannot voluntarily change the focus. Because object rays encounter both the distance and near portions of the optic, both near and far images are presented to the eye at the same time. The brain then processes the clearest image, ignoring the other(s). Most patients, but not all, can adapt to the use of multifocal IOLs.

The performance of certain types of IOLs is greatly impaired by decentration if the visual axis does not pass through the center of the IOL. On the one hand, the use of modern surgical techniques generally results in adequate lens centration. Pupil size, on the other hand, is an active variable, but it can be employed in some situations to improve multifocal function. Other disadvantages of multifocal IOLs are image degradation, "ghost" images (or *monocular diplopia*), decreased contrast sensitivity, and reduced performance in lower light (eg, decreased night vision). (See Videos 6-1 and 6-2.) These potential problems make multifocal IOLs less desirable for use in eyes with impending macular disease.

Accuracy of IOL power calculation is very important for multifocal IOLs because their purpose is to reduce the patient's dependence on glasses. Postoperative astigmatism should be low, given that visual acuity and contrast sensitivity are degraded with greater degrees of residual astigmatism.

VIDEO 6-1 Multifocal IOLs.
Courtesy of Mark Packer, MD, FACS, CPI.
Access all Section 3 videos at www.aao.org/bcscvideo_section03.

VIDEO 6-2 The optical cost of multifocal IOLs.
Animation developed by Joshua A. Young, MD.

Types of Multifocal Intraocular Lenses

Bifocal intraocular lenses

Of the various IOL designs, the bifocal IOL is conceptually the simplest. The bifocal concept is based on the idea that when there are 2 superimposed images on the retina, the brain always selects the clearer image and suppresses the blurred one. The first bifocal IOL implanted in a human was invented by Hoffer in 1982. The *split bifocal* was implanted in a patient in Santa Monica, Callifornia, in 1990. In this simple design, which was independent of pupil size, half the optic was focused for distance vision and the other half for near vision (Fig 6-12A). This design was reintroduced in 2010 as the Lentis Mplus (Oculentis,Berlin, Germany) and is now showing encouraging results in Europe.

替代方法是矫正一眼远用，另一眼近用，这被称为*单眼视*——这种方法也用于接触镜中。然而，大多数植入人工晶体的患者采取“矫正至视远清晰、根据需要配戴阅读镜”的方案。

多焦点人工晶体的设计是为了给患者提供良好的远、近视力，减少对眼镜的依赖。多焦点人工晶体在眼内的固定位置，患者不能自主改变焦点。因为物体的光线会同时经过光学部的视远区和视近区，远近的像可同时呈递给眼睛。然后大脑处理最清晰的像，而忽略其他的像。大多数患者可以适应这种情况，但并非所有人。

如果人工晶体的中心不在视轴上，某些类型人工晶体的功能会大大降低。一方面，现代手术技术可使人工晶体达到居中。另一方面，瞳孔大小也是一个重要的影响因素，可以用于改善多焦功能。多焦点 IOL 的其他缺点有成像质量下降、鬼影（或*单眼复视*）、对比敏感度下降、低照明时性能下降（如夜视困难）（见视频 6–1 和视频 6–2）。鉴于这些潜在的问题，对于可能患黄斑病变者，不宜选用多焦点人工晶体。

屈光度计算的精确性对多焦点人工晶体非常重要，因为其目的是减少患者对眼镜的依赖。由于较大的残余散光会降低视力和对比敏感度，因此力求较少的术后散光。

视频 6-1 多焦人工晶体.
Courtesy of Mark Packer, MD, FACS, CPI.
Access all Section 3 videos at www.aao.org/bcscvideo_section3.

视频 6-2 多焦人工晶体的光学意义.
Animation developed by Joshua A. Young, MD.

多焦点人工晶体的类型

双焦点人工晶体

在概念上，双焦点人工晶体设计是最简单的。双焦点的概念是，当有 2 个像叠加在视网膜上，大脑总是选择，而抑制模糊像。1982 年 Hoffer 发明的第 1 片双焦点人工晶体首次植入人眼。1990 年这种*分光双焦点*人工晶体被植入了加利福尼亚州圣莫尼卡的一位患者眼内。其设计与瞳孔大小无关，光学区的一半用于视远，另一半用于视近（图 6–12A）。2010 年 Lentis Mplus(Oculentis, 柏林，德国）再次引入了这种设计，目前在欧洲的应用结果令人满意。

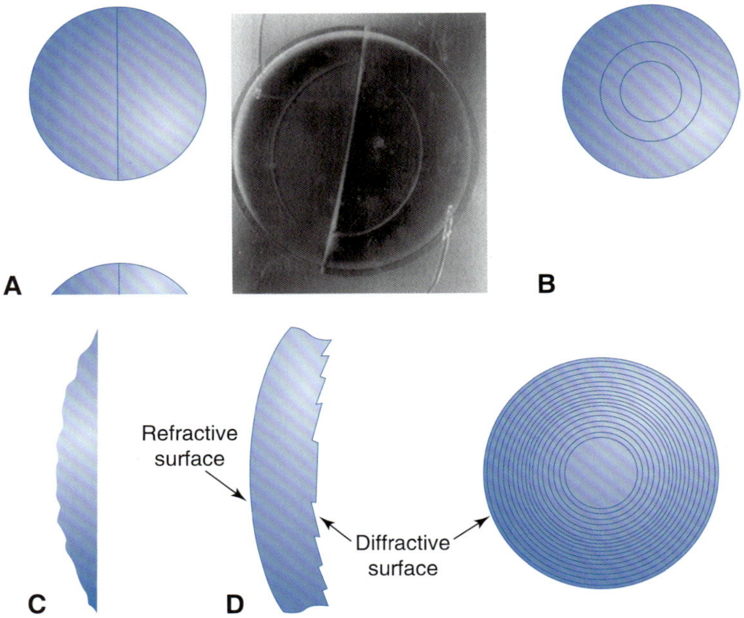

Figure 6-12 Multifocal intraocular lenses (IOLs). **A**, Hoffer split bifocal IOL (left) and photograph of a lens implanted in a patient in 1984 (right). **B**, Three-zone multifocal design. **C**, Multifocal IOL with several annular zones. **D**, Diffractive multifocal IOL; the cross section of the central portion is magnified (the depth of the grooves is exaggerated). *(Photograph courtesy of Kenneth J. Hoffer, MD; all illustrations redrawn by C. H. Wooley.)*

The additional power needed for near vision is not affected by the *AL* or by corneal power, but it is affected by the *ELP*. A posterior chamber IOL requires more near-addition power than does an anterior chamber IOL for the same focal distance. Approximately 3.75 D of added power is required to provide the necessary 2.75 D of myopia for a 14-inch(35 cm) reading distance.

Multiple-zone refractive intraocular lenses

These lenses use concentric refractive rings of different optical powers. In 3-zone bifocal lenses (Fig 6-12B) the central and outer zones are for distance vision; the inner annulus is for near vision. The diameters were selected to provide near correction for moderately small pupils and distance correction for both large and small pupils.

Another design uses several *annular zones* (Fig 6-12C), each of which varies continuously in power over a range of 3.50 D. The intention is that whatever the size, shape, or location of the pupil, all the focal distances are represented on the macula.

Diffractive multifocal intraocular lenses

Diffractive multifocal IOL designs (Fig 6-12D) use diffraction optics to achieve a multifocal effect. The overall spherical shape of the surfaces produces an image for distance vision. The posterior surface has a stepped structure, and the diffraction from these multiple rings produces a second image, with an effective add power. At a particular point along the axis, waves diffracted by the various zones add in phase, providing a focus for that wavelength. Approximately 20% of the light entering the pupil is dissipated in this process and does not reach the retina. Therefore, a variable decrease in contrast sensitivity should be expected when implanting these lenses. Diffractive IOLs are somewhat tolerant to decentration, but the optical aberrations that could develop due to IOL malposition can be troublesome for some patients.

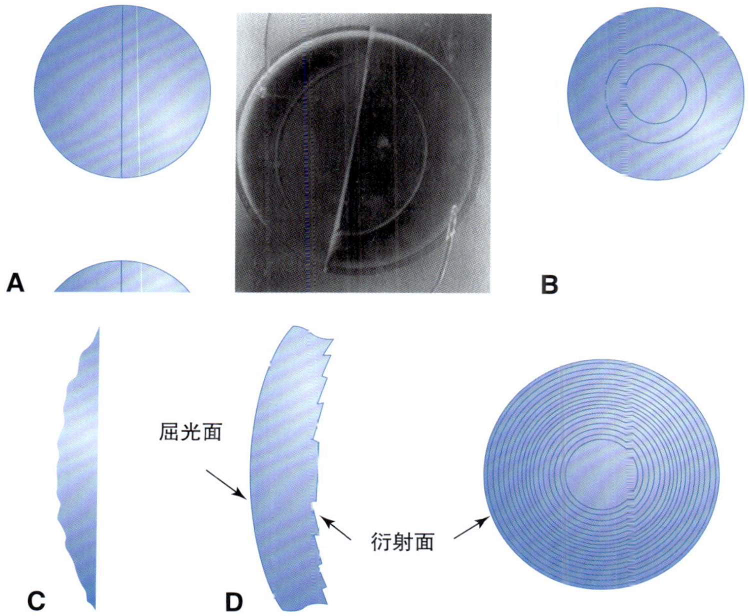

图 6–12　多焦点人工晶体。**A**. Hoffer 分光双焦点 IOL（左）和 1984 年植入的人工晶体照片（右）。**B**. 三区多焦点设计。**C**. 多环区的多焦点人工晶体设计。**D**. 衍射多焦人工晶体，放大的中央横截面（图示沟槽深度有夸大）。*（译者注：资料来源见前页原文。）*

近附加度不受*眼轴*和角膜屈光力的影响，但受 *ELP* 的影响。对于相同的聚焦距离，后房型人工晶体比前房型需要更多的近附加。阅读距离位于 14 in（35 cm）时，2.75 D 的近视需要约 3.75 D 的近附加度。

折射型多焦点人工晶体

这类人工晶体使用了具有不同光学焦度的同心折射环设计。在三区双焦人工晶体（图 6–12B）中，中央和最外区视远，内环视近。通过选择适当的小瞳孔提供视近的矫正，选择大瞳孔和小瞳孔提供视远的矫正。

另一个设计使用了*多个环形区*（图 6–12C），各环区的焦度在 3.5 D 范围连续变化。其优点是无论瞳孔大小、形状、位置如何，所有焦点都在黄斑成像。

衍射型多焦点人工晶体

衍射型多焦点人工晶体的设计（图 6–12D）是利用衍射光学实现多焦点效应。表面的整个球面产生视远的像，后表面有一个阶梯状结构，多环形区域的衍射产生有效的近附加度。在视轴的特定点上，不同区域的衍射波相位叠加，形成对应波长的焦点。在这个过程中，20% 进入瞳孔的光线弥散消耗，无法到达视网膜。因此，植入这类人工晶体会有对比敏感度不同程度的下降。一定程度的衍射型多焦点人工晶体偏中心可以耐受，但人工晶体偏位产生的像差却会令患者不适。

Second-generation diffractive multifocal intraocular lenses

The industry provides numerous refractive IOL designs, such as improvement in the rays taken to the intermediate focus providing some level of intermediate vision (trifocal IOLs), total eye asphericity control by adding negative asphericity to the IOL profile, and optical achromatization. These designs aim to decrease contrast sensitivity loss, extending at the same time the depth of focus to improve polyfocality.

Some of these IOLs incorporate an apodized diffractive lens. *Apodization* refers to the gradual tapering of the diffractive steps from the center to the outside edge of a lens to create a smooth transition of light between the distance, intermediate, and near vision focal points.

Clinical Results of Multifocal Intraocular Lenses

Some multifocal IOLs are designed to perform better for near vision; others, for intermediate. The performance targets of different multifocal IOLs is discussed in the section Modulation Transfer Function.

The best-corrected visual acuity (also called *corrected distance visual acuity*) may be less with a multifocal IOL than with a monofocal IOL; this difference increases in low-light situations. However, the need for additional spectacle correction for near vision is greatly reduced in patients with multifocal IOLs. Some patients are quite pleased with multifocal IOLs; others request their removal and replacement with monofocal IOLs. Interestingly, patients with a multifocal IOL in one eye and a monofocal IOL in the other often seem to be less tolerant of the multifocal IOLs than are patients with bilateral multifocal IOLs.

Patient selection is crucial for successful adaptation to multifocal IOLs. Selected patients must be willing to accept the trade-off–particularly in low-light situations—between decreased performance at distance vision (and at near vision, compared with that of a monofocal IOL and reading glasses) and the possibility of seeing well enough at all distances to be able to dispense with spectacles altogether. Patients with low contrast sensitivity function potential, such as those affected by glaucoma, retinal dystrophies, macular disease and advanced age, should be considered to be poor candidates for multifocal IOL implantation.

Alio JL, Plaza-PucheAB, Javaloy J, Ayala MJ, Moreno LJ, Piñero DP. Comparison of a new refractive multifocal intraocular lens with an inferior segmental near add and a diffractive multifocal intraocular lens. *Ophthalmology*. 2012;119(3):555–563.

Ford JG, Karp CL. *Cataract Surgery and Intraocular Lenses*: A *21st-Century Perspective*. 2nd ed. Ophthalmology Monograph 7. San Francisco: American Academy of Ophthalmology;2001.

Hoffer KJ. Personal history in bifocal intraocular lenses. In: Maxwell WA, Nordan LT, eds.Current Concepts of Multifocal *Intraocular Lenses*. Thorofare, NJ: Slack; 1991:chap 12,pp 127–132.

Muñoz G, Albarrán-Diego C, Javaloy J, Sakla HF, Cerviño A. Combining zonal refractive and diffractive aspheric multifocal intraocular lenses. *J Refract Surg*. 2012;28(3):174–181.

Ong HS, Evans JR, Allan BD. Accommodative intraocular lens versus standard monofocal intraocular lens implantation in cataract surgery. *Cochrane Database Syst Rev*. 2014;(5):CD009667.

Rosen E, Alió JL, Dick HB, Dell S, Slade S. Efficacy and safety of multifocal intraocular lenses following cataract and refractive lens exchange: Metaanalysis of peer-reviewed publications.*J Cataract Refract Surg*. 2016;42(2):310–328.

二代衍射型多焦点人工晶体

已经有多种多焦点人工晶体设计，例如改善中距焦点的光线以提高中距离视力（三焦点人工晶体）；增加人工晶体负球面性和光学消色像差，实现全眼非球面性控制。这些设计旨在减少对比敏感度损失，同时拓展焦深以提高多焦点性能。

其中一些人工晶体结合了变迹衍射透镜。*衍射控像法*是指衍射阶梯从人工晶体的中心向外边缘逐渐变细，从而实现远、中、近焦点的平滑过渡。

多焦点人工晶体的临床结果

一些多焦点人工晶体设计获得较好的近视力，而另一些则获得较好的中距视力。关于不同多焦点人工晶体的性能目标在调制传递函数一节中讨论。

使用多焦点人工晶体的最佳矫正视力（也称为矫正的远视力）较单焦点的差，在低照明的情况下更明显。但是，在植入多焦点人工晶体的患者中，需要额外眼镜矫正近视力的情况大大减少。一些患者对多焦点人工晶体很满意，也有一些要求取出并置换为单焦点人工晶体。有趣的是，与双眼都植入多焦点人工晶体的患者相比，一眼多焦点、另一眼单焦点的患者更不容易耐受多焦点人工晶体。

患者自己的选择是成功适应多焦点 IOL 的关键。患者必须愿意接受在视觉体验上的权衡，特别是在低照明的情况下——以视远（和视近）的视觉功能下降（与使用单焦点 IOL 辅助阅读镜相比较），换取在各距离都能看清、且丢弃框架眼镜。低对比敏感度的患者，如有青光眼、视网膜营养不良、黄斑疾病和高龄者，都不宜植入多焦点人工晶体。

Alio JL, Plaza-PucheAB, Javaloy J, Ayala MJ, Moreno LJ, Piñero DP. Comparison of a new refractive multifocal intraocular lens with an inferior segmental near add and a diffractive multifocal intraocular lens. *Ophthalmology*. 2012;119(3):555–563.

Ford JG, Karp CL. *Cataract Surgery and Intraocular Lenses: A 21st-Century Perspective*. 2nd ed. Ophthalmology Monograph 7. San Francisco: American Academy of Ophthalmology;2001.

Hoffer KJ. Personal history in bifocal intraocular lenses. In: Maxwell WA, Nordan LT, eds.*Current Concepts of Multifocal Intraocular Lenses*. Thorofare, NJ: Slack; 1991:chap 12,pp 127–132.

Muñoz G, Albarrán-Diego C, Javaloy J, Sakla HF, Cerviño A. Combining zonal refractive and diffractive aspheric multifocal intraocular lenses. *J Refract Surg*. 2012;28(3):174–181.

Ong HS, Evans JR, Allan BD. Accommodative intraocular lens versus standard monofocal intraocular lens implantation in cataract surgery. *Cochrane Database Syst Rev*. 2014;(5):CD009667.

Rosen E, Alió JL, Dick HB, Dell S, Slade S. Efficacy and safety of multifocal intraocular lenses following cataract and refractive lens exchange: Metaanalysis of peer-reviewed publications.*J Cataract Refract Surg*. 2016;42(2):310–328.

Accommodating Intraocular Lenses

These lenses are essentially monofocal IOLs designed to allow some degree of improved near vision. Usually, such designs involve linking accommodative effort to an anterior movement of the IOL, thereby increasing its effective power in the eye. This mechanism may be more effective with higher-power IOLs because their effective powers are more sensitive to small changes in position than are those of lower-power IOLs. The United States Food and Drug Administration (FDA) has approved one design that has shown some degree of accommodation, and other designs are awaiting FDA approval. However, currently, there is no clinical evidence that "accommodating" IOLs change axial position in the eye during near-vision tasks.

Cumming JS, Colvard DM, Dell SJ, et al. Clinical evaluation of the Crystalens AT-45 accommodating intraocular lens: results of the U.S. Food and Drug Administration clinical trial.*J Cataract Refract Surg*. 2006;32(5):812–825.

Dhital A, Spalton DJ, Gala KB. Comparison of near vision, intraocular lens movement, and depth of focus with accommodating and monofocal intraocular lenses. *J Cataract Refract Surg*. 2013;39(12):1872–1878.

Findl O, Kiss B, Petternel V, et al. Intraocular lens movement caused by ciliary muscle contraction. *J Cataract Refract Surg*. 2003;29(4):669–676.

Kohl JC, Werner L, Ford JR, et al. Long-term uveal and capsular biocompatibility of a new accommodating intraocular lens. *J Cataract Refract Surg*. 2014;40(12):2113–2119.

Langenbucher A, Huber S, Nguyen NX, Seitz B, Gusek-Schneider GC, Küchle M. Measurement of accommodation after implantation of an accommodating posterior chamber intraocular lens. *J Cataract Refract Surg*. 2003;29(4):677–685.

Matthews MW, Eggleston HC, Hilmas GE. Development of a repeatedly adjustable intraocular lens. *J Cataract Refract Surg*. 2003;29(11):2204–2210.

Matthews MW, Eggleston HC, Pekarek SD, Hilmas GE. Magnetically adjustable intraocular lens. *J Cataract Refract Surg*. 2003;29(11):2211–2216.

Modulation Transfer Function

As IOLs are developed to provide vision over many distances, a quantitative measure of optical performance is required. One particularly useful measure is the modulation transfer function (MTF). The MTF is the Fourier transform of the point spread function, a parameter often used when discussing wavefront aberrations. In the context of intraocular lenses, the MTF describes contrast degradation of a sinusoidal pattern as it passes through the optical system as well as the cutoff special frequency beyond which fine detail will not be resolved. MTF data are generally presented in the form of a graph in which the MTF for a particular wavelength and spatial frequency is shown over diopters of defocus or over distance. A reasonable simplification would be to understand these graphs as describing an IOL's performance over a range of distances.

It is important for the surgeon to be able to evaluate differences in IOL designs by their respective MTF curves. Bifocal IOLs demonstrate 2 distinct peaks in their MTF curves, 1 at distance and 1 at a near focal point that differs depending on IOL design. Trifocal IOLs demonstrate 3 peaks of varying heights.

可调节人工晶体

这类人工晶体是单焦点 IOL，用于一定程度改善近视力。其设计是通过 IOL 前移带来的调节改变，增加眼的有效屈光力。这在高焦度 IOL 中更有效，相比低焦度 IOL，其有效屈光力对位置的变化较为敏感。美国食品及药物管理局（FDA）已经批准了一项具有某种程度调节的设计，其他设计也正在等待 FDA 批准。但目前来说，尚没有临床证据显示“可调节”IOL 在近距离工作中会改变其在眼内的前后位置。

Cumming JS, Colvard DM, Dell SJ, et al. Clinical evaluation of the Crystalens AT-45 accommodating intraocular lens: results of the U.S. Food and Drug Administration clinical trial. *J Cataract Refract Surg.* 2006;32(5):812–825.

Dhital A, Spalton DJ, Gala KB. Comparison of near vision, intraocular lens movement, and depth of focus with accommodating and monofocal intraocular lenses. *J Cataract Refract Surg.* 2013;39(12):1872–1878.

Findl O, Kiss B, Petternel V, et al. Intraocular lens movement caused by ciliary muscle contraction. *J Cataract Refract Surg.* 2003;29(4):669–676.

Kohl JC, Werner L, Ford JR, et al. Long-term uveal and capsular biocompatibility of a new accommodating intraocular lens. *J Cataract Refract Surg.* 2014;40(12):2113–2119.

Langenbucher A, Huber S, Nguyen NX, Seitz B, Gusek-Schneider GC, Küchle M. Measurement of accommodation after implantation of an accommodating posterior chamber intraocular lens. *J Cataract Refract Surg.* 2003;29(4):677–685.

Matthews MW, Eggleston HC, Hilmas GE. Development of a repeatedly adjustable intraocular lens. *J Cataract Refract Surg.* 2003;29(11):2204–2210.

Matthews MW, Eggleston HC, Pekarek SD, Hilmas GE. Magnetically adjustable intraocular lens. *J Cataract Refract Surg.* 2003;29(11):2211–2216.

调制传递函数

随着多焦点人工晶体的发展，需要找出能够定量评估其光学性能的方法。一个特别有用的方法是调制传递函数（MTF）。MTF 是点扩散函数的 Fourier 变换，是讨论波前像差时常用的参数。在讨论人工晶体时，MTF 描述了正弦波形通过光学系统后对比度降低的情况以及截止特别频率（超过这个频率就不能分辨出微小的细节）。MTF 数据一般以图表的形式呈现，即在特定波长和空间频率，MTF 表现为离焦度或距离。简单来说，这些图表可理解为对人工晶体在一定范围内性能的描述。

对于手术医生来说，通过 MTF 曲线了解 IOL 设计的差异是很重要的。双焦点人工晶体的 MTF 曲线根据不同的设计，显示 2 个峰值，1 个在远焦点，1 个在近焦点。3 个焦点人工晶体显示 3 个峰值。

The area under the MTF curve represents the total light employed in imaging. This is always less than the total amount of light entering the eye because of absorption and, in the case of diffractive IOLs, destructive interference. The area under the MTF curve can be thought of as a photon budget and different IOLs spend this budget differently. Bifocal IOLs with higher near peaks can only improve MTF at near at the expense of distance MTF. This is clearly demonstrated in the comparison of the MTF curves of the Acrysof ReSTOR +2.5 and ReSTOR +3.0 bifocal IOLs (Alcon; Fort Worth, TX; Fig 6-13). Not only does the Re-STOR +2.5 IOL have its near peak at a greater distance than the ReSTOR +3.0 IOL, but the value of the near peak is itself lower. We can interpret this as the ReSTOR +2.5 IOL spending more of its photon budget on distance than does the ReSTOR +3.0 IOL.

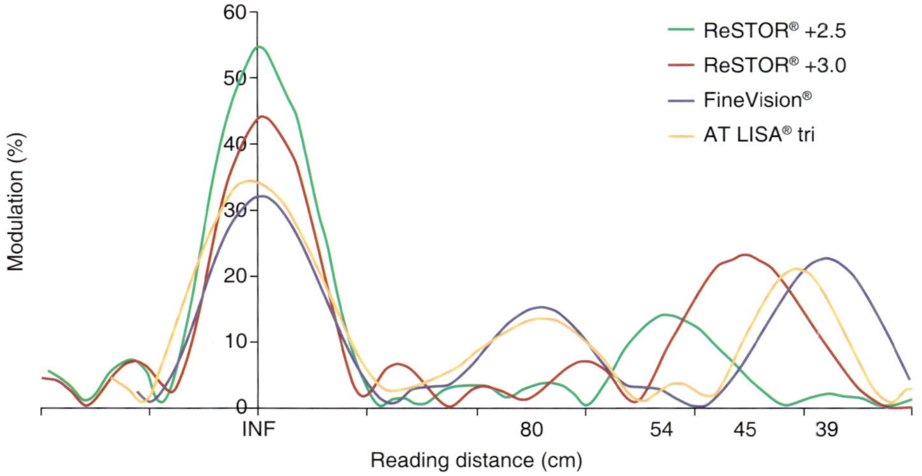

Figure 6-13 Through-focus MTF values of the AT LISA tri, FineVision, ReSTOR +2.5 D, and ReSTOR +3.0D IOLs, at 20/40 Snellen visual acuity equivalent (50 line pairs per mm). Manufacturers: AcrySof IQ ReSTOR IOLs, Alcon Laboratories, Fort Worth, TX, USA; AT LISA tri 839MP IOLs, Carl Zeiss Meditec AG, Jena, Germany; FineVision Micro F12 IOLs, PhysIOL SA, Liège,Belgium. Abbreviations: INF, infinity; IOL, intraocular lens; MTF, modulation transfer function. *(Reprinted from Carson D, Hill WE, Hong X, Karakelle M. Optical bench performance of AcrySof® IQ ReSTOR®, AT LISA® tri, and FineVision® intraocular lenses.* Clin Ophthalmol. *2014;8:2105–2115, with permission from Dove Medical Press Ltd.)*

MTF is of greatest utility in comparing conventional multifocal IOLs to newer extended-depth-of-focus (EDOF) lenses. A common feature of bifocal and trifocal IOLs is the very low MTF between the focal peaks, representing poor visual performance between the distance and near peaks. The MTF curves of EDOF lenses, like the TECNIS Symfony IOL (Johnson & Johnson Vision, Jacksonville, FL; Fig 6-14), do not have a precipitous drop between peaks and therefore demonstrate better performance at focal lengths between distance and near. However, it is important to remember that the total area under the MTF curve is not increased in EDOF lenses and the improvement in intermediate vision necessarily comes at the expense of performance at the peak focal distances.

MTF 曲线下的区域表示成像中使用的光线总量。由于眼内结构对光线的吸收，或者衍射型人工晶体对光线的破坏性干涉，MTF 曲线下光线总量小于进入眼内的光线总量。MTF 曲线下的面积可以看作是光子预算，不同的 IOL 消耗不同的预算。近峰较高的双焦 IOL 只能消耗远距离 MTF，以改善近距离 MTF。这在 Acrysof ReSTOR +2.5 和 ReSTOR +3.0 双焦人工晶体的 MTF 曲线对比中可以清晰地显示 (Alcon; Fort Worth, TX; 图 6–13)。Re–STOR+2.5 人工晶体的近峰距离比 ReSTOR+3.0 的近峰距离大，但近峰值较低。可以理解为 ReSTOR+2.5 人工晶体在远距离上比 ReSTOR+3.0 人工晶体消耗了更多的光子预算。

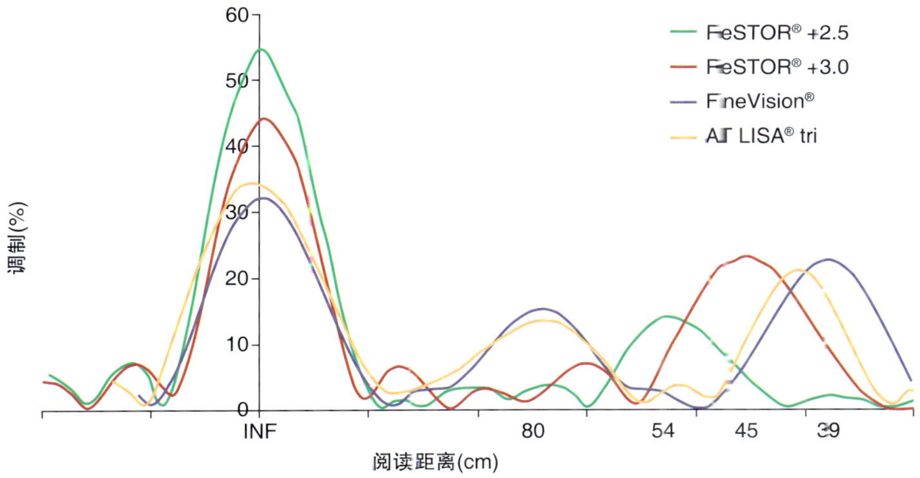

图 6–13　对应 Snellen 视力表 20/40(即 50 线对 /mm) 时，AT LISA tri、FineVision、ReSTOR +2.50 D 和 ReSTOR +3.00 D 人工晶体经焦点的 MTF 值。生产商 :AcrySof IQ ReSTOR IOLs, Alcon Laboratories, Fort Worth, TX, USA; AT LISA tri 839MP IOLs, Carl Zeiss Meditec AG, Jena, Germany; FineVision Micro F12 IOLs, PhysIOL SA, Liège, Belgium. 缩写 : INF, infinity; IOL, intraocular lens; MTF, 调制传递函数。*（译者注：资料来源见前页原文。）*

MTF 在对比传统多焦点人工晶体与新型扩展焦深（EDOF）人工晶体时最具实用性。双焦点和三焦点人工晶体的共同特征是焦点峰之间的 MTF 非常低，表示在远峰和近峰之间的视觉性能较差。EDOF 人工晶体的 MTF 曲线，如 TECNIS Symfony IOL(Johnson & Johnson Vision, Jacksonville, FL; 图 6–14)，在峰值之间没有急剧下降，因此在远近之间的焦距上显示出更好的视觉性能。然而，需要注意的是，在 EDOF 人工晶体中，MTF 曲线下的总面积没有增加，中间视力的改善是以消耗了远峰值焦点的视觉性能为代价的。

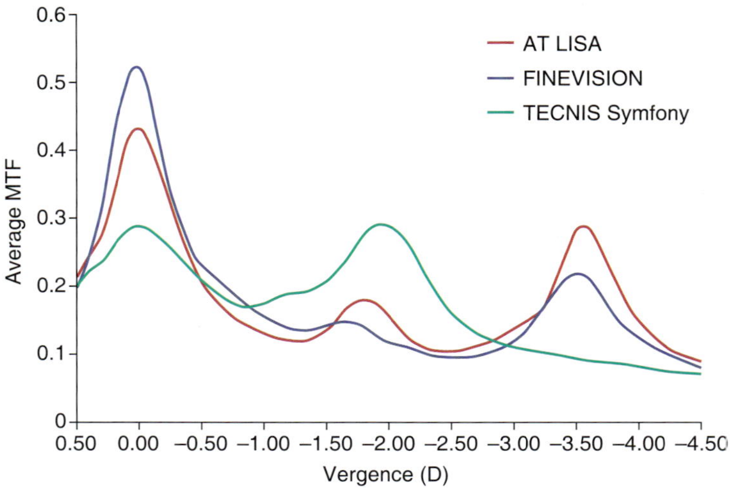

Figure 6-14 Through focus average modulation transfer function for all frequencies up to 100 cycles/mm of all intraocular lenses for the 4.5-mm optical aperture. Manufacturers: AT LISA, Carl Zeiss Meditec AG, Jena, Germany; FineVision, PhysIOL, Liège, Belgium; and TECNIS Symfony, Abbott Laboratories, Abbott Park, IL. *(Reprinted from Esteve-Taboada JJ, Domínguez-Vicent A, Del águila-Carrasco AJ, et al. Effect of large apertures on the optical quality of three multifocal lenses. J Refract Surg. 2015;31: 666–676. ©. 2015, with permission from Elsevier.)*

Artigas JM, Menezo JL, Peris C, Felipe A, Díaz-Llopis M. Image quality with multifocal intraocular lenses and the effect of pupil size: comparison of refractive and hybrid refractive-diffractive desig ns. *J Cataract Refract Surg.* 2007;33(12):2111–2117.

Carson D, Hill WE, Hong X, Karakelle M. Optical bench performance of AcrySof® IQ ReSTOR®, AT LISA®tri, and FineVision® intraocular lenses. *Clin Ophthalmol.* 2014;8:2105–2115.

Esteve-Taboada JJ, Domínguez-Vicent A, Del Águila-Carrasco AJ, Ferrer-Blasco T, Montés-Micó R. Effect of large apertures on the optical quality of three multifocal lenses. *J Refract Surg.* 2015;31(10):666-676.

Intraocular Lens Standards

The American National Standards Institute (ANSI) and the International Standards Organization (ISO) set standards for IOLs. Among these standards is one for IOL power labeling; it requires that IOLs with powers labeled as less than 25 D be within ±0.40 D of the labeled power and have no axial-power variations of more than 0.25 D. IOLs labeled 25-30 D must be within ±0.50 D of the labeled power, and those labeled greater than 30 D must be within ±1.0 D. Most ophthalmologists are unaware of this wide range allowed for the labeling of high-power IOLs. Although controversial, attempts are being made to narrow this allowed range so that all IOL powers would be within ±0.25 D of the labeled powers. Actual mislabeling of IOL power is rare but still occurs.

In addition to the labeling standards, the ANSI, ISO, and FDA have set various other IOL standards for *optical performance*, a term that refers broadly to the image quality produced by an IOL. Lenses are also tested for biocompatibility, the absence of cytotoxicity of their material, the presence of any additives (such as ultraviolet filters), genotoxicity, and photostability, as well as for their safety with YAG lasers. There are also standards for spectral transmission. Physical standards exist to ensure adherence to the labeled optic diameter, haptic angulation, strength, and mechanical fatigability of the components, as well as to ensure sterility and safety during injection.

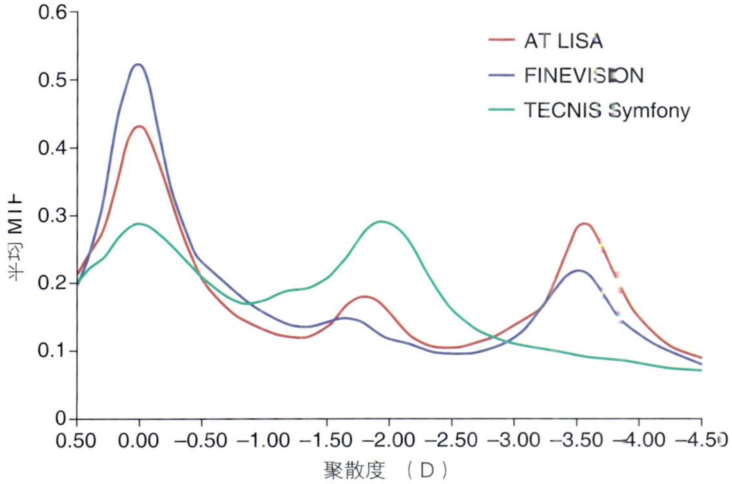

图 6–14　4.5mm 光圈、100cycles/mm 空间频率下，所有人工晶体经焦点的平均 MTF 表现。生产商：AT LISA, Carl Zeiss Meditec AG, Jena, Germany; FineVision, PhysIOL, Liège, Belgium; TECNIS Symfony, Abbott Laboratories, Abbott Park, IL. *（译者注：资料来源见前页原文。）*

Artigas JM, Menezo JL, Peris C, Felipe A, Díaz-Llopis M. Image quality with multifocal intraocular lenses and the effect of pupil size: comparison of refractive and hybrid refractive-diffractive designs. *J Cataract Refract Surg*. 2007;33(12):2111–2117.

Carson D, Hill WE, Hong X, Karakelle M. Optical bench performance of AcrySof ® IQ ReSTOR®, AT LISA®tri, and FineVision® intraocular lenses. *Clin Ophthalmol*. 2014;8:2105–2115.

Esteve-Taboada JJ, Domínguez-Vicent A, Del Águila-Carrasco AJ, Ferrer-Blasco T, Montés-Micó R. Effect of large apertures on the optical quality of three multifocal lenses. *J Refract Surg*. 2015;31(10):666-676.

人工晶体的标准

美国国家标准学会（ANSI）和国际标准组织（ISO）为人工晶体设定了标准。在这些标准中，有一项是针对 IOL 度数标识的；该标准要求标签上度数在 25.00 D 以内的 IOL，其度数误差在标识度数的 ±0.40 D 以内，且轴向度数的变化不超过 0.25 D。标签度数为 25.00~30.00 D 的，其误差在标识度数 ±0.50 D。标签度数大于 30.00 D 的，误差在 ±1.00 D 以内。大多数眼科医生不清楚对高度数 IOL 的容忍误差范围。尽管有争议，目前正在努力缩小这种允许误差范围，以便使所有 IOL 度数误差在标签度数的 ±0.25 D 以内。实际的人工晶体标签错误很少见，但仍会发生。

除了标签的标准，ANSI、ISO 和 FDA 也为人工晶体的*光学性能*设定了多种标准，这一术语是指广义上人工晶体的成像质量。人工晶体也会接受生物兼容性、材料的细胞毒性、添加剂（比如紫外线滤过物质）、基因毒性和光稳定能力，以及 YAG 激光安全性的测试。还有透过光谱的标准。物理标准应确保同标签上的说明一致，包括光学部直径、襻夹角、力度和晶体成分的机械易疲劳性，以及无菌状态和植入过程的安全性。

Chapter Exercises

Questions

6.1. Error in sound velocity. An ophthalmologist discovers that a measured axial length (*AL*) was taken using an incorrect *AL*. What should be the next course of action?

a. The patient should be scheduled for a return visit and the ultrasound repeated using the correct sound velocity.

b. A simple correction factor can be added algebraically to the incorrect-measure *AL* value.

c. The incorrect *AL* is likely due to an incorrect velocity. The incorrect *AL* can be corrected by dividing the *AL* by the incorrect velocity and multiplying by the correct velocity.

d. The sound velocity is so negligible that it does not need to be corrected.

6.2. The optical performance of monofocal, bifocal, and extended depth of focus (EDOF) IOLs necessarily differ in which way?

a. the acuities they produce at distance

b. the chromatic aberration induced

c. the contrast degradation induced at distance

d. the degree of accommodation each exhibits (ELP)

6.3. Which statement is the most characteristic of multifocal IOLs?

a. They offer increased image clarity and contrast for both near and far viewing.

b. They are independent of pupil size if they are well centered.

c. They offer a trade-off between decreased image quality and increased depth of focus.

d. They are indicated for all patients.

6.4. Which statement applies to piggyback IOLs?

a. Piggyback IOLs modify the vergence of light entering the eye after it exits the incorrectly powered primary IOL.

b. Piggyback IOLs can be used in a second operation only if the original IOL power was too low and additional dioptric strength is indicated.

c. A piggyback IOL may be useful after removal of an incorrectly powered IOL.

d. Piggyback IOLs may be less necessary as standard IOL power ranges increase.

6.5. What is the most relevant statement with respect to biometric formulas for IOL calculation?

a. The *AL* is the least important factor in the formula.

b. The refractive error resulting from an error in *AL* measurement is more consequential in long eyes than in short eyes.

c. Accuracy in *AL* measurement is relatively more important in short eyes than in long eyes.

d. During ultrasonic measurement of *AL* (A-scan), sound travels faster through the aqueous and vitreous than through the crystalline lens and cornea. Therefore, there is a need to make adjustment to the *AL* "measurement" by correcting for the incorrect velocity of sound.

e. The velocity of sound in an aphakic eye varies significantly between short and long eyes.

本章练习

问题

6.1 声速的误差。眼科医生发现，测得的*眼轴*长度是错误的。下一步应该采取的措施是？
a. 应安排患者回访，并使用正确的声速重新检查
b. 添加一个简单的修正系数进行算术上对错误 *AL* 值进行校准
c. 错误的 *AL* 值可能是源于选择了错误的声速进行测量。可以通过用测量值乘以正确的声速，再除以错误的声速进行矫正
d. 声速的影响微不足道，不需要被纠正

6.2 单焦点、双焦点和焦深拓展型（EDOF）人工晶体的光学表现必然的不同在何处？
a. 远视力
b. 产生的色像差
c. 远距离的对比度下降
d. 表现出的调节程度（ELP）

6.3 哪项表述是多焦点 IOL 最具特色的地方？
a. 视近和视远时，提供清晰度和对比度增高的成像
b. 如果位置居中，这些晶体是不依赖瞳孔大小的
c. 在成像质量下降和景深增加之间的权衡
d. 可用于所有患者

6.4 下列哪项描述适用于背驮人工晶体？
a. 背驮人工晶体是在第一个错误的人工晶体植入度数后，改变了光线进入眼内的会聚度
b. 只有当原始的 IOL 度数过低而需要额外的屈光力时，才在二次手术中使用背驮人工晶体
c. 在移除错误度数的 IOL 后，再使用背驮人工晶体可能是有用的
d. 随着标准人工晶体度数范围的增加，背驮人工晶体可能会变为不太必要

6.5 关于 IOL 计算的生物测量公式，哪项是最相关的表述？
a. *眼轴*长度是公式中最不重要的因素
b. *眼轴*长度测量误差引起的屈光不正对长眼轴眼球的影响比短眼轴更大
c. *眼轴*长度测量的准确性在短眼轴眼球中比在长眼轴眼球中的影响相对更大
d. 超声生物测量时（A 超），声波在房水和玻璃体中的传导速度快于晶状体和角膜内的速度。因此，需要用正确的声速对错误声速测量的结果进行校准
e. 无晶体眼内，声音在短眼轴和长眼轴中的传导速度差异很大

Answers

6.1. **c.** The formula to correct the *AL* is $AL \times V_C/V_I$, where V_C is the correct velocity and V_I is the incorrect velocity. This correction eliminates the need for the patient to undergo the procedure again. There is no factor that can be added to the *AL* to correct such an error, and the error is not negligible and thus cannot be ignored.

6.2. **c.** Multifocal IOLs, including bifocal and EDOF IOLs, necessarily trade contrast performance at distance for multifocality. Although distance acuity may be degraded in dim light in multifocal IOLs, acuity may be excellent at distance in all lenses. It is important to understand that acuity is not identical to optical performance.

6.3. **c.** Multifocal IOLs present both near and distant foci to the retina at the same time. This leads to an unavoidable decrease in image quality and contrast sensitivity, particularly at low levels of illumination. Pupil size may be a factor, particularly with certain types of multifocal IOLs.

6.4. **d.** Piggyback IOLs have been used to reach a total dioptric power that was unavailable in a single lens. As IOLs are becoming available in a wider range of powers, however, it is less likely that a piggyback IOL will be needed to reach an unusually high or low power. Piggyback IOLs are placed anterior to the primary lens and thus modify the light vergence before the light reaches the primary IOL.These IOLs may be used to correct inaccurate primary IOLs in a second operation if the original IOL power was too low or too high. They are not used after removal of an incorrectly powered IOL—"piggyback" implies that a second IOL is present in the eye.

6.5. **c.** Note the following comments for each option:

a. The axial length (*AL*) is the most important factor in the formula.

b. The refractive error resulting from an error in *AL* measurement is more consequential in short eyes than in long eyes.

c. Accuracy in *AL* measurement is relatively more important in short eyes than in long eyes. Correct answer.

d. During ultrasonic measurement of *AL* (A-scan),sound travels faster through the crystalline lens and cornea than through the aqueous and vitreous. Therefore,There is a need to make adjustment to the *AL* "measurement" by correcting for the incorrect velocity of sound.

e. The velocity of sound in an aphakic eye varies *insignificantly* between short and long eyes (ie, it is almost comparable).

答案

6.1 **c**。*眼轴*长的矫正公式是 $AL=AL\times V_C/V_I$，V_C 是校正的声速，V_I 是未校正的声速。这种校正可以使患者无须再进行重复的检查。无法通过对*眼轴*添加一个因子矫正该误差。这种误差不是微不足道，不可以被忽略。

6.2 **c**。多焦点人工晶体，包括双焦点和焦深拓展型 IOL，用远距离的对比度表现换取多焦点的视力。尽管在暗环境下多焦点 IOL 的远视力可能下降，但所有人工晶体的远视力表现都不错。要明白视力不等同于光学性能，这一点很重要。

6.3 **c**。多焦点晶体的远近焦点同时在视网膜上成像，这导致成像质量和对比敏感度不可避免的损失，尤其在暗照明环境下。瞳孔大小可能是一个因素，尤其是对于特定类型的多焦点人工晶体。

6.4 **d**。背驮被用于得到单片 IOL 无法提供的屈光力。随着人工晶体可以提供更宽广范围的屈光力，不太可能需要使用背驮晶体来获得少见的高焦度或低焦度。背驮 IOL 放置于最初 IOL 前面，因此可以改变到达最初 IOL 前光束的聚散度。如果最初 IOL 的度数过高或过低，这种晶体可通过二次手术植入眼内，校正不精确的最初 IOL。背驮人工晶体不是在取出第一片度数有误的 IOL 后再植入眼内的，"背驮"的意思是眼内的第二片人工晶体。

6.5 **c**。注意以下每一个选项的点评：

a. *眼轴*长度是晶体计算公式中最重要的因素。

b. *眼轴*长度测量误差引起的屈光不正，在短*眼轴*眼球中比在长*眼轴*眼球中更严重。

c. 与长眼轴眼球相比，眼轴测量的准确性在短眼轴眼球中相对更重要。

d. 超声生物测量*眼轴*时（A 超），声波在晶状体和角膜中的传导速度快于房水和玻璃体内的速度。因此，需要用正确的声速对错误声速测量的结果进行校准。

e. 在短眼轴和长眼轴的无晶体眼内的声速*差异不显著*（几乎是类似的）。

（翻译　卢淑杰　汪晓倩//审校　汪晓倩　石一宁//章节审校　杨亚军）

CHAPTER 7

Optical Considerations in Keratorefractive Surgery

Highlights

- The normal human cornea has a prolate shape that reduces spherical aberration.
- Keratorefractive surgical procedures modulate the shape of the cornea to reduce refractive error but can induce irregular astigmatism.
- New algorithms for excimer procedures have dramatically decreased the incidence and severity of night vision problems.
- The diagnosis of irregular astigmatism is made by meeting clinical and imaging criteria: loss of spectacle best-corrected vision but preservation of vision with the use of a gas-permeable contact lens, coupled with topographic corneal irregularity.
- Irregular astigmatism can frequently be understood in terms of basic aberration types, of which as few as 5 are of clinical interest. Aberrations are also conveniently described in terms of Zernike polynomials.
- Appropriate identification of preoperative irregular astigmatism is critical in keratorefractive surgery to optimize the visual result.

Glossary

Angle kappa Angle between the pupillary axis and the visual axis.

Irregular astigmatism In practice, astigmatism that decreases spectacle best-corrected vision but is improved with the use of a gas-permeable lens and shows topographic corneal irregularity.

Oblate A spheroidal shape whereby the curvature is flattest centrally and gradually steepens toward the periphery. An oblate shape is similar to grapefruit, or a sphere flattened at the poles.

Prolate A spheroidal shape whereby the curvature is steepest centrally and gradually flattens toward the periphery. A prolate shape is similar to the pole of an egg.

Q factor Value of the difference in corneal asphericity between peripheral and central rays.

Spherical aber ration Higher-order aberration where paraxial rays focus in a different plane than peripheral rays.

第 7 章

屈光手术中需要注意的光学问题

重点

- 正常人角膜呈椭球体的形态（中央陡周边平），可以减少屈光系统的球差。
- 角膜屈光手术通过改变角膜表面形态矫正屈光不正，但同时可引起不规则散光。
- 屈光手术的新算法大大降低了夜间视力异常的发生率和严重程度。
- 不规则散光的诊断需要同时满足临床和影像学标准：框架镜不能得到最佳矫正视力，但高透氧硬性接触镜下最佳矫正视力可提高，同时角膜地形图可见到明显的不规则形态。
- 不规则散光通常依照基本像差类型进行解释，至少有 5 种像差是和临床关系比较密切的。像差多用 Zernike 多项式表示。
- 正确辨识术前不规则散光是屈光手术成功的关键。

术语

k 角 瞳孔轴与视轴的夹角。

不规则散光 临床上这类散光多伴有角膜地形图形态的不规则改变，会明显降低框架眼镜最佳矫正视力，但高透氧硬性接触镜可提高此类患者的矫正视力。

扁球体状 一个中央扁平周边陡峭的类球面形状，有点像柚子或者是两极略平的球体。

椭球体状 一个中央陡峭周边扁平的类球面形状，有点像鸡蛋的顶部。

Q 值 角膜中央和周边部非球面程度的差异值。

球差 通过透镜近轴的光线与周边部的光线，两者焦点不在一个平面所导致的高阶像差。

Wavefront analysis Method to describe irregular astigmatism quantitatively, most frequently with Zernike polynomials.

Introduction

This chapter provides an overview of the optical considerations specific to keratorefractive surgery. Refractive surgical procedures performed with the intent to reduce refractive errors can be categorized as *corneal* (keratorefractive) or *intraocular*.

Keratorefractive surgical procedures can be divided into surgical-removal, surgical-neutral, and surgical-addition procedures. Surgical-removal procedures include photorefractive keratectomy (PRK), laser subepithelial keratomileusis (LASEK), epithelial laser in situ keratomileusis (epi-LASIK), laser in situ keratomileusis (LASIK), and small-incision lenticule extraction (SMILE). Surgical-neutral procedures include radial keratotomy (RK), astigmatic keratotomy (AK), laser thermal keratoplasty (LTK), and radiofrequency conductive keratoplasty (CK). Surgical- addition procedures include implantation of intracorneal ring segments and corneal inlays. Intraocular refractive procedures include implantation of a phakic intraocular lens (IOL), piggyback lens, and cataract and clear lens extraction with implantation of a monofocal, toric, multifocal, or accommodative intraocular lens.

Although these refractive surgical techniques alter the optical properties of the eye, keratorefractive surgery is generally more likely than lenticular refractive surgery to induce optical aberrations. This chapter discusses only keratorefractive procedures and their optical considerations. For a discussion of optical considerations in lenticular refractive surgery, see BCSC Section11, *Lens and Cataract*.

Various optical considerations are relevant to refractive surgery, both in screening patients for candidacy and in evaluating patients with vision complaints after surgery. The following sections address optical considerations related to the change in corneal shape after keratorefractive surgery, issues concerning the angle kappa and pupil size, and the various causes of irregular astigmatism.

Corneal Shape

A basic premise of refractive surgery is that the cornea's optical properties are intimately related to its shape. Consequently, manipulation of the corneal shape changes the eye's refractive status. Although this assumption is true, the relationship between corneal shape and the cornea's optical properties is more complex than is generally appreciated. .

波前像差分析　一种定量描述不规则散光的方法，常用 Zernike 多项式表示。

引言

本章主要讨论屈光手术中需要注意的光学问题。因为屈光手术的目的是降低或去除屈光不正，所以它分为*角膜*（角膜屈光手术）或*眼内手术*。

角膜屈光手术可分为手术去除、中和 / 保留组织和手术添加 3 大类。手术去除包括光学激光角膜切削术（PRK）、激光上皮下角膜磨镶术（LASEK）、上皮激光原位角膜磨镶术 (epi–LASIK)、激光原位角膜磨镶术（LASIK）和小切口透镜取出术（SMILE）。中和 / 保留手术包括放射状角膜切开术（RK）、散光性角膜切开术（也称角膜松解切开术）（AK）、激光角膜热成形术 (LTK)，和射频传导性角膜成形术 (CK)。手术添加包括角膜基质环植入术和角膜组织嵌入。眼内屈光手术包括有晶状体眼人工晶体植入术（IOL）、背驮人工晶体植入术（双联人工晶体植入术）、透明晶状体摘除联合眼内单焦、散光、多焦或调节型人工晶体植入术。

尽管这些屈光手术均能在一定程度上改变眼部的屈光状态，但相对于晶状体手术来讲，角膜的屈光手术更容易出现光学像差问题。这一章节主要讨论角膜屈光手术及其需考虑的光学问题。晶体手术的光学问题讨论请见第 11 册《*晶状体与白内障*》。

屈光手术在筛选患者和评估术后效果中需要考虑的光学问题很多，下面的章节着重讨论角膜屈光术后角膜形态的改变引起的光学问题、kappa 角和瞳孔直径的影响以及导致不规则散光的原因分析。

角膜形态

角膜屈光手术开展的前提是，角膜的光学特性与自身的形态息息相关。因此，改变角膜的形态就可以相应地改变眼睛的屈光状态。尽管这个假设是真实的，但角膜形态和角膜光学特性的关系远比我们通常所理解的要复杂得多。

The normal human cornea has a prolate shape (Fig 7-1), similar to that of the pole of an egg. The curvature of the human eye is steepest in the central cornea and gradually flattens toward the periphery. This configuration reduces the optical problems associated with simple spherical refracting surfaces, which produce a nearer point of focus for peripheral rays than for paraxial rays—a refractive condition known as *spherical aberration*. *Corneal asphericity*, the relative difference between the peripheral and central cornea, is represented by the Q factor. In an ideal visual system, the curvature at the center of the cornea would be steeper than at the periphery (ie, the cornea would be prolate), and the asphericity factor Q would have a value close to –0.50; at this value of negative Q, the degree of spherical aberration would approach zero. However, in the human eye, such a Q value is not anatomically possible (because of the junction between the cornea and the sclera). The Q factor for the human cornea has an average value of –0.26, allowing for a smooth transition at the limbus. The human visual system, therefore, suffers from minor spherical aberrations, which increase with increasing pupil size.

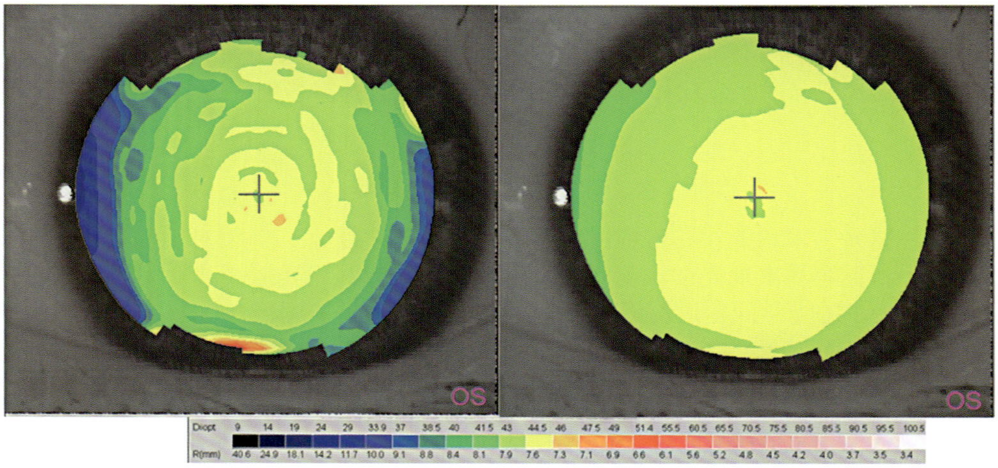

Figure 7-1 An example of meridional (tangential, left) and axial (right) maps of a normal cornea. *(Used with permission from Roberts C. Corneal topography. In: Azar DT, ed. Gatinel D, Hoang-Xuan T, associate eds. Refractive Surgery. 2nd ed. St Louis: Elsevier-Mosby; 2007:103–116.)*

Ablative procedures, incisional procedures, and intracorneal rings change the natural shape of the cornea to reduce refractive error. Keratometry readings in eyes conducted before they undergo keratorefractive surgery typically range from 38.0 D to 48.0 D. When refractive surgical procedures are being considered, it is important to avoid changes that may result in excessively flat (<33.0 D) or excessively steep (>50.0 D) corneal powers, which decrease vision quality and increase aberrations. A 0.8 D change in keratometry value (K) corresponds to approximately a 1.00 D change of refraction. The following equation is often used to predict corneal curvature after keratorefractive surgery:

$$K_{\text{postop}} = K_{\text{preop}} + (0.8 \cdot RE)$$

where K_{preop} and K_{postop} are preoperative and postoperative K readings, respectively, and RE is the refractive error to be corrected at the corneal plane. For example, if a patient's preoperative keratometry readings are 45.0 D (steepest meridian) and 43.0 D (flattest meridian), then the average K value is 44.0 D. If the amount of refractive correction at the corneal plane is –8.50D, then the predicted average postoperative K reading is 44.00 + (0.8 × –8.50) = 37.2 D, which is acceptable.

正常人的角膜是椭球体（图 7–1），像鸡蛋的顶端一样，角膜中央是最陡的地方，越往周边越平。角膜的这种形态可以减轻这种单透镜系统可能出现的光学问题。当平行光线通过单凸透镜折射后，周边区域的光线形成的焦点会比中央区域光线的焦点更靠近透镜（更靠前），这种屈光状态称为*球差*。*角膜的非球面性*在角膜中央与周边存在差异，用 Q 值来表示。在理想视觉系统中，角膜中央的曲率比周边曲率陡（角膜是椭球形），非球面性 Q 值接近 –0.5，Q 值呈负值时，球差接近 0。但在真实人眼中，这样的 Q 值从解剖学角度来说是不可能出现的（因为有角膜缘结构的存在），人类角膜的平均 Q 值是 –0.26，这样才能保证角膜平滑过渡到巩膜组织。因此，人眼屈光系统存在少量的球差，并且随瞳孔扩大而增加。

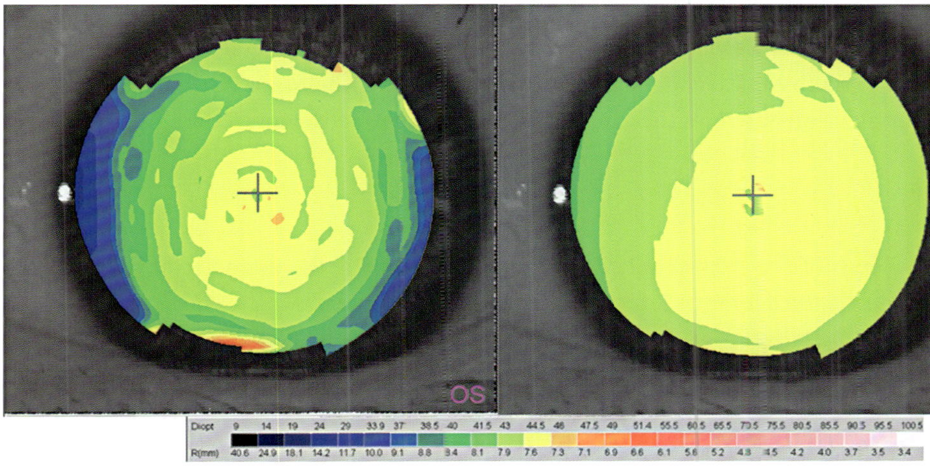

图 7–1　正常人角膜地形切线图（左）和轴向图（右）。*（译者注：资料来源见前页英文原文。）*

切削术、切开术和基质环植入术等技术通过改变角膜形态达到矫正屈光不正的目的。手术前，大多数人的角膜曲率在 38.00~48.00 D 之间。角膜屈光手术时为了避免视觉质量下降和像差增加，应尽量避免术后角膜过平（＜ 33.00 D）或过陡（＞ 50.00 D）。常规来讲，角膜曲率值 K 变化 0.80 D 可使眼部屈光变化 1.00 D，所以我们经常使用下面的公式预测术后角膜曲率情况：

$$K_{\text{postop}} = K_{\text{preop}} + (0.8 \cdot RE)$$

公式中 K_{preop} 指术前角膜 K 值，K_{postop} 指术后角膜 K 值，RE 是角膜平面的屈光不正矫正度数。比如，患者术前的角膜 K 值为 45.00 D（最陡子午线）和 43.00 D（最平子午线），平均 K 值即为 44.00 D 角膜面的屈光矫正量为 –8.50 D，术后预测的 K 值为 44 .00+（0.8 × –8.50）= 37.2 D。

The ratio of dioptric change in refractive error to dioptric change in keratometry approximates 0.8:1 owing to the change in posterior corneal surface power after excimer ablation. The anterior corneal surface produces most of the eye's refractive power. In the Gullstrand model eye (see Table 3-1), the anterior corneal surface has a power of +48.8 D and the posterior corneal surface has a power of –5.8 D, so the overall corneal refractive power is +43.0 D. Importantly, standard corneal topography instruments and keratometers do not measure corneal power precisely because they do not assess the posterior corneal surface. Instead, these instruments estimate total corneal power by assuming a constant relationship between the anterior and posterior corneal surfaces. This constancy is disrupted with surgical removal or surgical addition procedures, causing a change in the effective refractive index of the cornea. For example, after myopic excimer surgery, the anterior corneal curvature is flattened. At the same time, the posterior corneal surface remains unchanged or, owing to the reduction in corneal pachymetry and weakening of the cornea, the posterior corneal surface may become slightly steeper than the preoperative posterior corneal curvature, increasing its negative power.

The removal of even a small amount of tissue (eg, a few micrometers) during keratorefractive surgery may cause a substantial change in refraction (Fig 7-2). The Munnerlyn formula approximates the depth of the ablation based on the optical zone and the refractive correction:

$$t = \frac{S^2 D}{3}$$

where t is the depth of the central ablation in micrometers, S is the diameter of the optical zone in millimeters, and D is the degree of refractive correction in diopters.

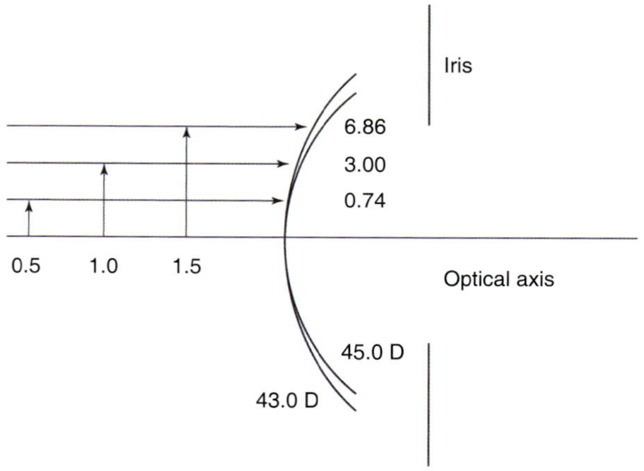

Figure 7-2 Comparison of a 43 D cornea with a 45 D cornea. Numbers below the *vertical arrows* indicate distance from the optical axis in millimeters; numbers to the right of the *horizontal arrows* indicate the separation between the corneas in micrometers. A typical pupil size of 3.0 mm is indicated. A typical red blood cell has a diameter of 7 µm. Within the pupillary space (ie, the optical zone of the cornea), the separation between the corneas is less than the diameter of a red blood cell. *(Courtesy of Edmond H. Thall, MD. Modified by C. H. Wooley.)*

屈光手术中屈光不正眼的屈光变化量与角膜屈光变化量之比约为 0.8:1，这与术后角膜后表面的变化有关。角膜前表面决定了眼的大部分屈光力。在 Gullstrand 模型眼中（见第 3 章人眼屈光 表 3–1），角膜前表面的屈光力是 +48.80 D，后表面屈光力为 –5.80 D，所以角膜总的屈光力为 +43.00 D。需要注意的是，常规的角膜地形图和角膜曲率计并不能准确测量出角膜真正的屈光力，因为它们不能测量角膜后表面。相反，这些仪器通过假设角膜前表面和角膜后表面之间的恒定关系来估算角膜的总屈光力。但由于切除性或植入性的角膜屈光术，这种常数相关关系就被打破了，导致角膜的有效折射率改变。例如，矫正近视的准分子屈光术后，角膜前表面的曲率降低，同时后表面不变，或者因为角膜厚度变薄和抵抗力减低，后表面会向前凸，这样后表面的负性屈光力会增加。

即使角膜屈光手术仅去掉角膜表面少量组织（例如，几微米）也能导致角膜屈光力的明显变化。根据光学区和屈光矫正，用 Munnerlyn 方程来估算切削深度。

$$t = \frac{S^2 D}{3}$$

t 是中央角膜的切削深度（μm），S 是光学区直径（mm），D 是屈光矫正量（D）。

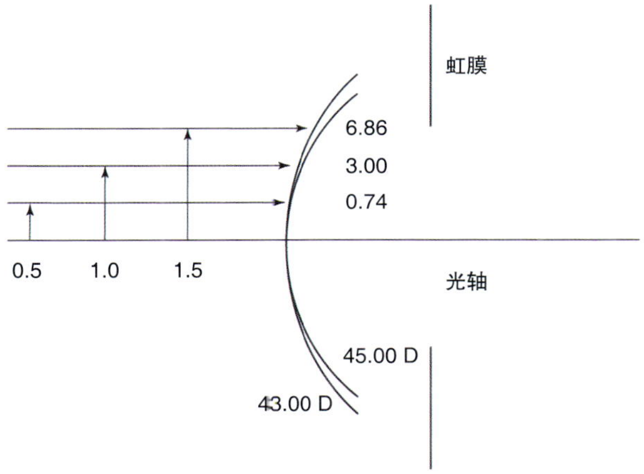

图 7–2　43.00 D 和 45.00 D 角膜的对比图，*垂直箭头*下面的数字代表距光轴的距离（mm），*水平箭头*右侧的数字代表与角膜的距离（μm），瞳孔直径为 3 mm，红细胞直径是 7 μm。在瞳孔区内（即指角膜光学区），2 种曲率的角膜间距不足一个血细胞直径。（*译者注：资料来源见前页英文原文。*）

An ideal LASIK ablation or PRK removes a convex positive meniscus in corrections of myopia (Fig 7-3A) and a concave positive meniscus in simple corrections of hyperopia (Fig 7-3B). Intracorneal rings flatten the corneal surface to correct myopia while arcuate incisional procedures cause localized flattening to reduce myopic astigmatism. LTK and CK cause focal stromal contraction and central steepening, correcting hyperopia. Finally, pinhole corneal inlays, like the KAMRA corneal inlay (AcuFocus Inc, Irvine, CA), do not change the shape but increase depth of focus on the retina by decreasing the size of the entrance pupil.

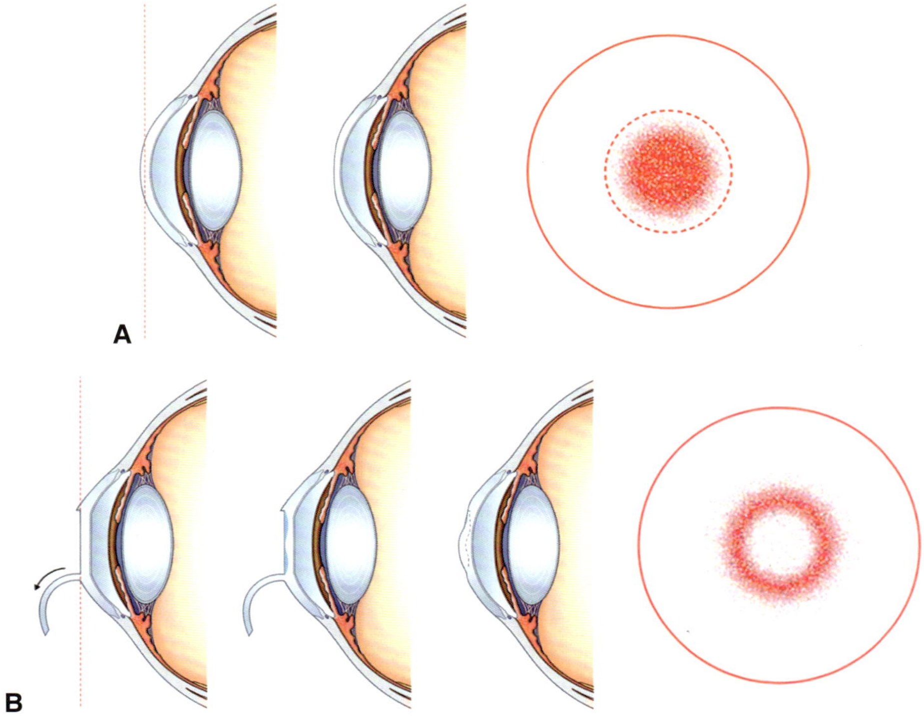

Figure 7-3 Myopic photorefractive keratectomy (PRK) and hyperopic laser in situ keratomileusis (LASIK). **A,** Schematic illustration of myopic PRK. The shaded area refers to the location of tissue subtraction. More stromal tissue is removed in the central than in the paracentral region (convex positive meniscus). **B,** Schematic illustration of hyperopic LASIK. A superficial corneal flap is raised. The shaded area refers to the location of tissue subtraction under the thin flap (concave positive meniscus). After treatment, the flap is repositioned. *(Used with permission from Poothullil AM, Azar DT. Terminology, classification, and history of refractive surgery. In: Azar DT, ed. Gatinel D, Hoang-Xuan T, associate eds. Refractive Surgery. 2nd ed. St Louis: Elsevier-Mosby; 2007:5–6. Figs 1-4, 1-5.)*

Azar DT, Primack JD. Theoretical analy sis of ablation depths and profiles in laser in situ keratomileusis for compound hyperopic and mixed astigmatism. *J Cataract Refract Surg*. 2000;26(8):1123–1136.

Holladay JT, Janes JA. Topographic changes in corneal asphericity and effective optical zone after laser in situ keratomileusis. *J Cataract Refract Surg*. 2002;28(6):942–947.

Koller T, Iseli HP, Hafezi F, Mrochen M, Seiler T. Q- factor customized ablation profile for the correction of myopic astigmatism. *J Cataract Refract Surg*. 2006;32(4):584–589.

一个完美的 LASIK 或 PRK 手术会在矫正近视时，从角膜前表面切除掉一个凸的正新月形（图 7-3A）；矫正单纯远视时，会切除掉一个凹的负新月形（图 7-3B）。角膜基质环，使角膜表面变平矫正近视；而周边环形切开，使局部曲率变平矫正近视散光。激光角膜热成形术（LTK）和射频传导性角膜成形术（CK）引起局限性角膜基质收缩使中央变陡以矫正远视。最后，中央带针孔的角膜嵌体，比如 KAMRA 角膜嵌体（AcuFocus Inc, Irvine, CA），并不改变角膜形态，但会通过减小入射光瞳大小的方法增加视网膜成像的焦深。

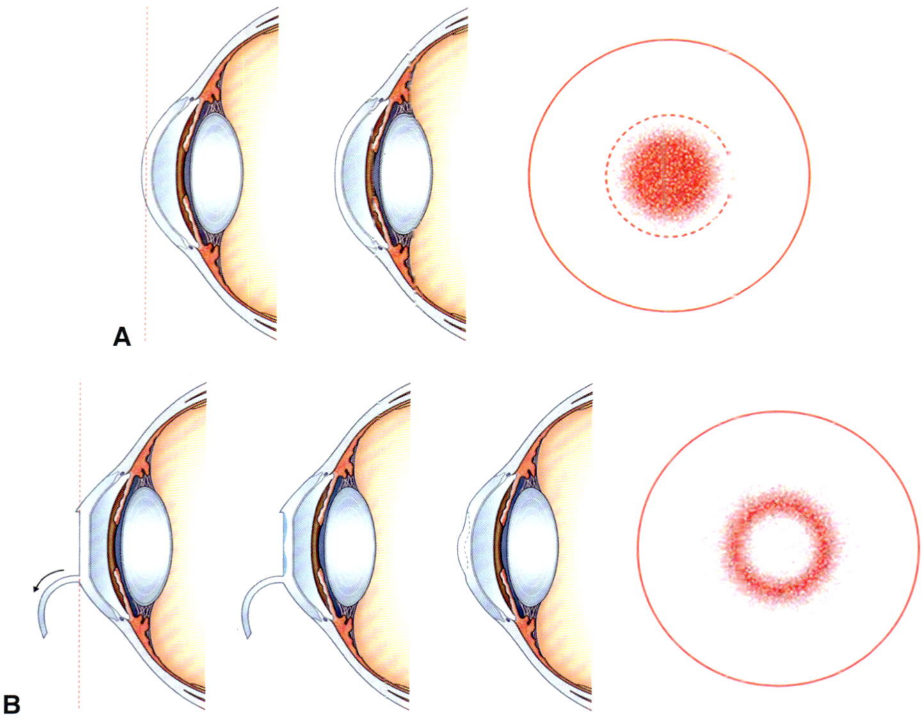

图 7-3　近视性光学激光角膜切削术（PRK）和远视性激光原位角膜磨镶术（LASIK）。**A.** 图示近视性 PRK，阴影部分为组织切削部位。中央区基质去除的比旁中心区多（凸透镜弯月形态）。**B.** 图示远视性 LASIK。掀起角膜瓣后，阴影区是薄瓣下组织切削部位（凹透镜弯月形态），然后复瓣。（*译者注：资料来源见前页英文原文。*）

Azar DT, Primack JD. Theoretical analy sis of ablation depths and profiles in laser in situ keratomileusis for compound hyperopic and mixed astigmatism. *J Cataract Refract Surg*. 2000;26(8):1123–1136.

Holladay JT, Janes JA. Topographic changes in corneal asphericity and effective optical zone after laser in situ keratomileusis. *J Cataract Refract Surg*. 2002;28(6):942–947.

Koller T, Iseli HP, Hafezi F, Mrochen M, Seiler T. Q- factor customized ablation profile for the correction of myopic astigmatism. *J Cataract Refract Surg*. 2006;32(4):584–589.

Angle Kappa

As discussed in Chapter 3, the pupillary axis is the imaginary line that is perpendicular to the corneal surface and passes through the midpoint of the entrance pupil (see Fig 3-3). The visual axis is the imaginary line that connects the point of fixation to the fovea. The angle Kappa (κ) is defined as the angle between the pupillary axis and the visual axis (which intersects the corneal surface very near the corneal apex in a regular cornea) and is measured by observing the difference between the apparent center of the pupil and the penlight reflex during monocular fixation of the light source. A large angle kappa results from a significant difference between these two. If the angle kappa is large, centering an excimer ablation over the geometric center of the cornea will effectively result in a decentered ablation. This can be particularly problematic in a hyperopic correction, in which a large angle kappa can result in a refractively significant "second corneal apex," causing monocular diplopia and decreased quality of vision. A large angle kappa must be identified before surgery to reduce the likelihood of a poor visual outcome.

Reinstein DZ, Gobbe M, Archer TJ. Coaxially sighted corneal light reflex versus entrance pupil center centration of moderate to high hyperopic corneal ablations in eyes with small and large angle kappa. *J Refract Surg*. 2013;29(8):518–525.

Wachler BS, Korn TS, Chandra NS, Michel FK. Decentration of the optical zone: centering on the pupil versus the coaxially sighted corneal light reflex in LASIK for hyperopia. *J Refract Surg*. 2003;19(4):464–465.

Pupil Size

Pupil size measurement has been an important factor in preoperative evaluations, prompted by observations that some patients with large pupils ($>$8mm) reported difficulties with night vision after undergoing keratorefractive surgery. Typical symptoms included the appearance of glare, starbursts, and halos; decreased contrast sensitivity; and poor overall quality of vision. Night-vision problems tended to occur in patients with both large pupils and small treatment zones ($\leqslant$ 6mm). The algorithms used in third-generation lasers, however, incorporate larger optical and transition zones, enabling surgeons to perform refractive procedures on patients with larger pupils. Use of these algorithms has dramatically decreased the incidence and severity of night- vision problems.

Many surgeons use default ablation zones during excimer procedures. The accepted standard transition zone between ablated and unablated cornea is 0.5–1.0 mm larger than the pupil; use of this zone helps minimize night-vision problems. To conserve corneal tissue, smaller optical zones are typically used in higher myopic corrections. In patients who require such corrections, the incidence of night- vision problems increases in part because of the mismatch between the size of the pupil and that of the optical zone. Modern transition zones aim to minimize this mismatch.

Patients with extremely large pupils ($\geqslant$8mm) should be identified and counseled about the potential for increased risk of complications. Spherical aberration may be increased in these patients. Clinical management of postoperative night-vision problems includes the use of a miotic such as brimonidine (0.2%) or pilocarpine (0.5%–1%).

Chan A, Manche EE. Effect of preoperative pupil size on quality of vision after wavefront- guided LASIK. *Ophthalmology*. 2011;118(4):736–741.

Myung D, Schallhorn S, Manche EE. Pupil size and LASIK: a review. *J Refract Surg*. 2013; 29(11):734–741.

kappa 角

在第 3 章中我们已经讨论过，瞳孔轴是垂直角膜平面并且通过瞳孔中心的光轴 (见图 3-3)，视轴是注视点和黄斑的连线。kappa（κ）角就是瞳孔轴和视轴的交角（在规则角膜中 2 个轴的交点非常接近角膜顶点），测量方法是观察瞳孔中心点和注视笔灯时角膜反光点间的位置差别。2 个点的位置差别明显时，去掉 kappa 角偏大。如果 kappa 角较大，角膜几何中心的中心定位切削会导致明显的偏心切削。这个问题在远视矫正中特别突出。kappa 角偏大可以造成角膜出现第二个角膜顶点，导致单眼复视和视觉质量下降。所以术前筛查时必须注意大 kappa 角的检查，以便减少术后矫正视力差问题的发生。

Reinstein DZ, Gobbe M, Archer TJ. Coaxially sighted corneal light reflex versus entrance pupil center centration of moderate to high hyperopic corneal ablations in eyes with small and large angle kappa. *J Refract Surg*. 2013;29(8):518–525.

Wachler BS, Korn TS, Chandra NS, Michel FK. Decentration of the optical zone: centering on the pupil versus the coaxially sighted corneal light reflex in LASIK for hyperopia. *J Refract Surg*. 2003;19(4):464–465.

瞳孔直径

瞳孔直径是术前评估患者眼睛状况的一个重要参数，临床上发现，瞳孔直径偏大（＞ 8mm）的患者角膜屈光手术后夜间视觉质量差。常见的症状有眩光、光芒、光晕，对比敏感度下降，以及整体视觉质量下降。瞳孔大且治疗区小（≤ 6 mm）的患者更容易出现上述夜间视觉问题。第三代激光机的计算程序采用了大光学区和过渡区切削，将大瞳孔也纳入手术适应证，使用这些手术计算程序可明显降低夜间视力不良的发生率和严重程度。

许多医生在准分子激光手术中切削区默认设置。为了减少夜间视觉质量问题，切削与非切削的过渡区，公认的标准是比瞳孔直径大 0.5~1.0 mm，这个过渡区有助于减少夜间视觉质量问题。为了保存角膜组织，较小的光学区域通常用于较高的近视矫正。瞳孔大小和光学区和的不匹配导致部分手术患者发生夜间视觉质量问题。现代的过渡区技术就是为了减少这类情况的发生。

大瞳孔 (≥ 8 mm) 的患者需要做出确认，告知其可能存在的并发症风险。这类患者术后球差会明显增加。对于术后夜间视觉问题，临床上可使用缩瞳剂，如溴莫尼定（0.2%）或者毛果芸香碱（0.5%~1%）。

Chan A, Manche EE. Effect of preoperative pupil size on quality of vision after wavefront- guided LASIK. *Ophthalmology*. 2011;118(4):736–741.

Myung D, Schallhorn S, Manche EE. Pupil size and LASIK: a review. *J Refract Surg*. 2013; 29(11):734–741.

Irregular Astigmatism

The treatment of postoperative irregular corneal astigmatism is a substantial challenge in refractive surgery. The diagnosis of irregular astigmatism is made by meeting clinical and imaging criteria: loss of spectacle best-corrected vision but preservation of vision with the use of a gas-permeable contact lens, coupled with topographic corneal irregularity. An important sign of postsurgical irregular astigmatism is a refraction that is inconsistent with the uncorrected visual acuity. For example, consider a patient who has −3.50D myopia with essentially no astigmatism before the operation. After keratorefractive surgery, the patient has an uncorrected visual acuity of 20/25 but a refraction of +2.00 −3.00 × 60. Ordinarily, such a refraction would be inconsistent with an uncorrected visual acuity of 20/25, but it can occur in patients who have irregular astigmatism after keratorefractive surgery.

Another important sign is the difficulty of determining axis location during manifest refraction in patients with a high degree of astigmatism. Normally, determining the correcting cylinder axis accurately in a patient with significant cylinder is easy; however, patients with irregular astigmatism after keratorefractive surgery often have difficulty choosing an axis. Automated refractors may identify high degrees of astigmatism that are rejected by patients on manifest refraction. Because their astigmatism is irregular (and thus has no definite axis), these patients may achieve almost the same visual acuity with high powers of cylinder at various axes. Streak retinoscopy often demonstrates irregular "scissoring" in patients with irregular astigmatism.

Typically, an AK incision will decrease regular astigmatism while maintaining the spherical equivalent (coupling); however, results of astigmatic enhancements can be unpredictable for patients with irregular astigmatism. For example, a surgeon may be tempted to perform an astigmatic enhancement on a patient who had little preexisting astigmatism but significant postoperative astigmatism despite good uncorrected visual acuity. In such cases, the astigmatic enhancement may cause the axis to change dramatically without substantially reducing cylinder power due to irregular astigmatism.

Irregular astigmatism can be quantified in much the same way as is regular astigmatism. We think of regular astigmatism as a cylinder superimposed on a sphere. Irregular astigmatism, then, can be thought of as additional shapes superimposed on cylinders and spheres. This corneal irregularity is then measured and quantified by wavefront analysis.

Application of Wavefront Analysis in Irregular Astigmatism

Refractive surgeons derive some benefit from having a thorough understanding of irregular astigmatism, for 2 reasons. First, keratorefractive surgery may lead to visually significant irregular astigmatism in a small percentage of cases. Second, keratorefractive surgery may also be able to treat it. For irregular astigmatism to be studied effectively, it must be described quantitatively. Wavefront analysis is an effective method for such descriptions of irregular astigmatism.

An understanding of irregular astigmatism and wavefront analysis begins with stigmatic imaging. A stigmatic imaging system brings all rays from a single object point to a perfect point focus. According to the Fermat principle, a stigmatic focus is possible only when the time required for light to travel from an object point to an image point is identical for all the possible paths the light might take.

不规则散光

角膜屈光手术后残留角膜不规则散光是一个比较棘手的问题。角膜不规则散光的诊断需要满足临床和形态诊断指标：框架镜不能得到最佳矫正视力，但改用高透氧硬性接触镜后最佳矫正视力可提高，并且角膜地形图呈不规则形。术后角膜不规则散光有一个重要的体征是屈光状态和裸眼视力不一致。比如，一个患者术前有 –3.50 D 的单纯近视，做角膜屈光手术后，患者的裸眼视力是 0.8，但屈光状态是 +2.00 /–3.00 × 60。一般来讲，这样一个屈光状态是不可能有 0.8 的裸眼视力的，但如果做角膜屈光手术后存在角膜不规则散光，则有这种可能。

另一个重要体征是患者的角膜散光很高，但主观验光很难确定散光轴位。一般来讲，大散光的散光轴位是很好确定的，但是对于角膜屈光手术后存在的不规则散光，散光轴位就不易确定了。尽管自动验光仪可以测出很明显的散光，但在主观验光中，患者很难接受这部分散光。因为散光是不规则的（所以轴位就不确定），无论将散光轴调整到什么位置上，患者的矫正视力都没有太大差别。使用带状光检影镜时可以见到不规则散光的“剪刀影”。

原则上，在维持原等效球镜的前提下，散光性角膜切开术（AK）可以减少规则散光，对于不规则散光则可能出现无法预知的散光增加。比如，先前几乎没有散光的患者，手术以后，虽然裸眼视力很好，但散光增加了。对于这种情况，如果不大幅度地减少不规则散光引起的柱镜度数，术后的散光增加会引起散光轴位显著的改变。

不规则散光能以规则散光一样的方式量化。我们认为规则散光像一个柱镜与一个球镜的叠加，然而，不规则散光能被认为是一个附加的形状与柱镜和球镜的叠加。这种角膜的不规则散光通过波前像差分析来测量和量化。

波前像差技术应用于不规则散光分析

基于 2 个原因，屈光手术医生会从彻底理解不规则散光中受益。第一，角膜屈光手术会导致少数患者外表显著的不规则散光。第二，角膜屈光手术也能治疗不规则散光。要有效地研究不规则散光，必须对其进行定量描述。波前分析是描述不规则散光的一种有效方法。

对不规则散光和波前分析的认识始于消散光成像。消散光成像系统使所有来自物点的光线形成完善的点像。依照 Fermat 原理，一个物点发出的所有光线、经过各种路径聚焦成像，仅当时长相同时，才能形成共轭像点。

An analogy to a footrace is helpful. Suppose that several runners simultaneously depart from an object point (A). Each runner follows a different path, represented by a ray. In this case, all the runners travel at the same speed on the ground, but slow down when running through water. Similarly, light rays will travel at the same speed in air but slow down in the lens. If all the runners reach the image point (B) simultaneously, the "image" is stigmatic. If the rays do not meet at point B , then the "image"is astigmatic.

Wavefront analysis is based on the Fermat principle. Construct a circular arc centered on the paraxial image point and intersecting the center of the exit pupil (Fig 7-4A). This arc is called the *reference sphere*. Again, consider the analogy of a footrace, but now think of the reference sphere rather than a point as the finish line. If the image is stigmatic, all runners starting from a single point will cross the reference sphere simultaneously. If the image is astigmatic, the runners will cross the reference sphere at slightly different times (Fig 7-4B). The *geometric wavefront* is analogous to a photo finish of the race. It represents the position of each runner shortly after the fastest runner crosses the finish line. The *wavefront aberration* of each runner is the time at which the runner finishes minus the time of the fastest runner. In other words, it is the difference between the reference sphere and the wavefront. When the focus is stigmatic, the reference sphere and the wavefront coincide, so that the wavefront aberration is zero.

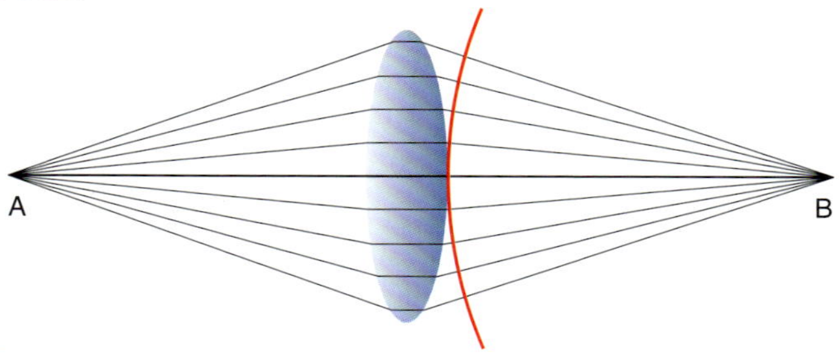

A

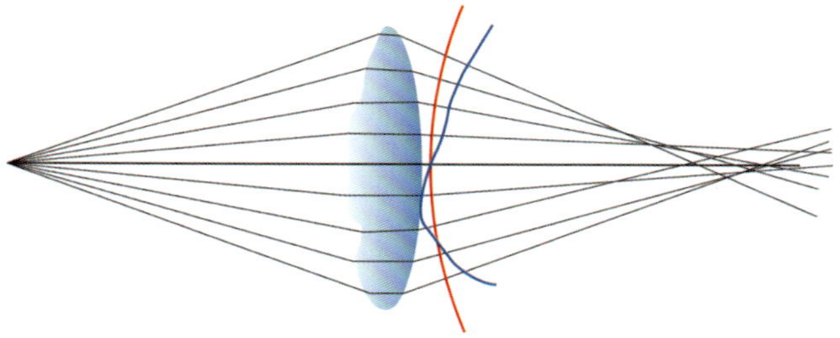

B

Fig 7-4 **A**, The reference sphere (in red) is represented in 2 dimensions by a circular arc centered on point B and drawn through the center of the exit pupil of the lens. If the image is stigmatic, all light from point A crosses the reference sphere simultaneously. **B**, When the image is astigmatic, light rays from the object point cross the wavefront (in blue), not the reference sphere. *(Courtesy of Edmond H .Thall, MD ;part B modified by C. H .Wooley.)*

类似于竞走运动一样，假设几个“竞赛者”同时从目标点（A 点）出发。每一个竞赛者的路线都不同（代表了不同的光路），竞赛者们在陆地的前进速度是相同的，但在水中的前进速度减慢。与此类似，光线在空气中以相同速度前进，但进入晶状体速度减慢减速。如果所有的竞赛者同时到达成像点（B），像是消散光的。如果光线不能在 B 点相遇，像是有散光的。

波前分析就是基于 Fermat 原理。构建一个以近轴像点为中心的圆弧，并与入射光瞳中心相交 (图 7–4A)。这个圆弧称为*参考球面*。重复上述竞赛假设，但这次将终点线假设在参考球面（而不是点），如果像是消散光的，竞赛者们从一个点出发，同时通过参考球面。如果像有散光，则竞赛者们通过参考球面的时间不一致 (图 7–4B)。*几何波前*类似于跑道终点的照片。记录最快赛跑者到达终点以后，每一位赛跑者的位置。每一位赛跑者的*波前像差*就是与最快的赛跑者的时间差，即参考球面与波前的差值。当形成共点焦点时，参考球面和波前的位置重合，波前像差为 0。

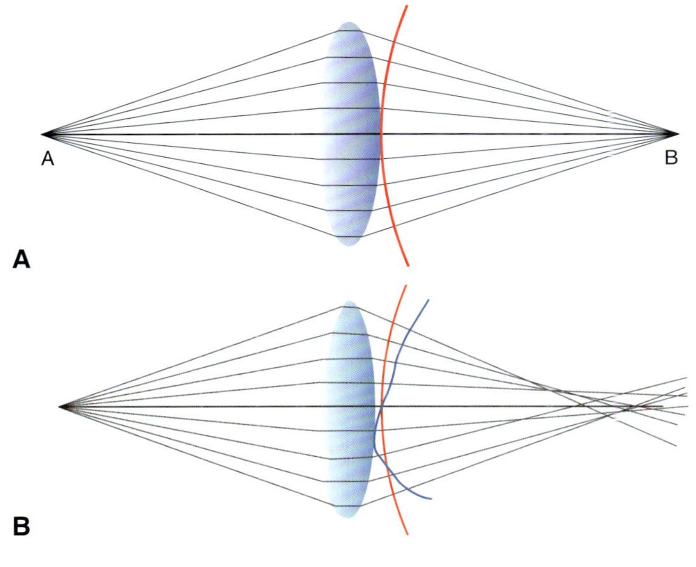

图 7–4　A. 参考球面（红线）用中心在 B 点的二维圆弧代表，画出时通过透镜的出射光瞳中心。如果像是消散光的，则来自 A 点的光线相交在参考球面。**B.** 如果图像有散光，那么从物体发出的光线通过波前（蓝色线），而不是通过参考平面。*（译者注：资料来源见前页英文原文。）*

Another interpretation of the Fermat principle is the point spread function produced by all rays that traverse the pupil from a single object point. This image is perpendicular to the geometric wavefront shown in Figure 7.5B. For example, keratorefractive surgery for myopia using surgical removal procedures reduces spherical refractive error and regular astigmatism, but it does so at the expense of increasing spherical aberration and irregular astigmatism (Fig 7-5).The cornea subsequently becomes less prolate, and its shape resembles an egg lying on its side. The central cornea become flatter than the periphery and results in an increase in the spherical aberration of the treated zone. Generally, keratorefractive surgery moves the location of the best focus closer to the retina but, at the same time, makes the focus less stigmatic. Such irregular astigmatism leads to decreased contrast sensitivity and underlies many visual complaints after refractive surgey.

Wavefront aberration is a function of pupil position. For example, coma is a partial deflection of spherical aberration. Figure 7-6 shows some typical wavefront aberrations. Myopia, hyperopia, and regular astigmatism can be expressed as wavefront aberrations. Myopia produces an aberration that optical engineers call *positive defocus*. Hyperopia is called *negative defocus*. Regular (cylindrical) astigmatism produces a wavefront aberration that resembles a saddle. Defocus(myopia and hyperopia) and regular astigmatism constitute the lower-order aberrations.

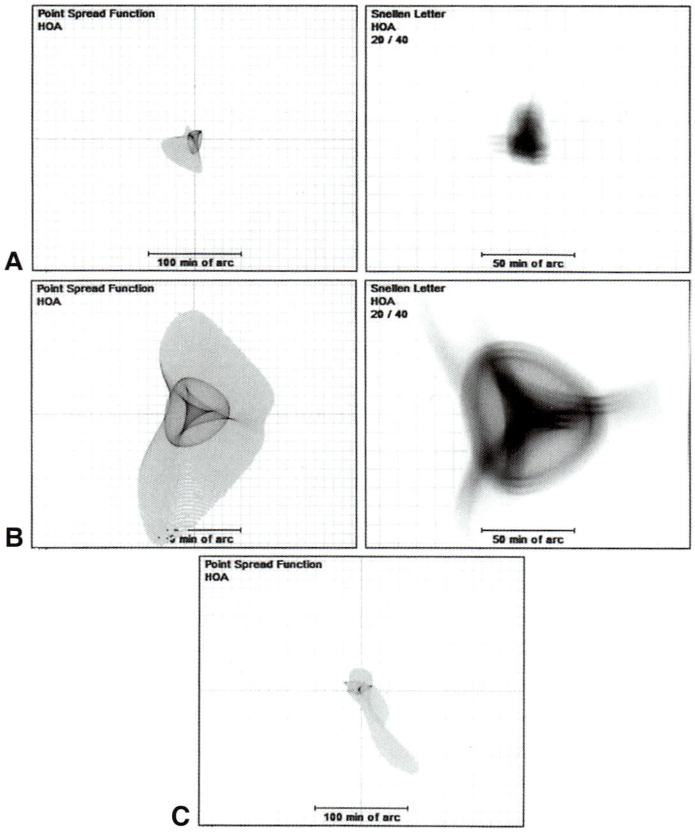

Figure 7-5 Examples of the effects of (**A**) coma, (**B**) spherical aberration, and (**C**) trefoil on the point spread functions of a light source. *(Courtesy of Ming Wang, MD.)*

Fermat 原理的另一个解释是点播散函数，它由一个物点通过瞳孔的全部光线产生。其成像与几何波前相互垂直，见图 7–5B。例如，角膜屈光手术治疗近视采用切削技术，减少球差和不规则散光(图 7–5)，结果角膜变成小椭圆，其形状近似于侧立的鸡蛋。角膜中央较周边平坦，导致治疗区球差增加。一般来说，角膜屈光手术将焦点位置移近视网膜，同时使焦点焦点小量消散光。不规则散光导致对比敏感度下降，呈现术后许多视觉问题。

波前像差是瞳孔位置的函数。例如，彗差是偏向的球差。图 7–6 是经典的波前像差。近视、远视和规则散光都可以用波前像差表达。近视会产生光学工程师称之为*正离焦像差*。远视产生负离焦，规则（柱镜）散光产生类似鞍形的波前像差。离焦（近视性及远视性）与规则散光共同组成了低阶像差。

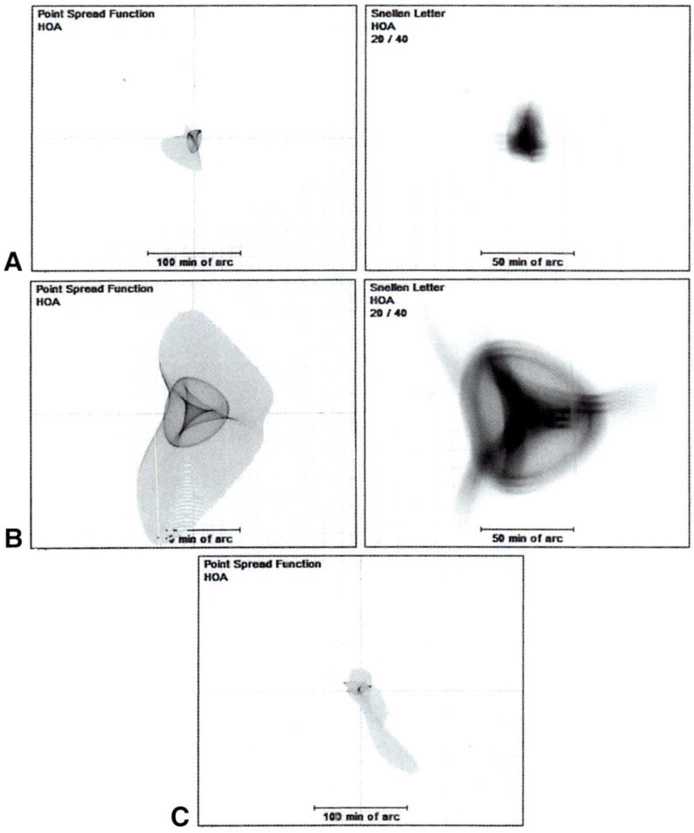

图 7–5　一光源的点播散函数。**A.** 彗星。**B.** 球差。**C.** 三叶草。*（译者注：资料来源见前页原文。）*

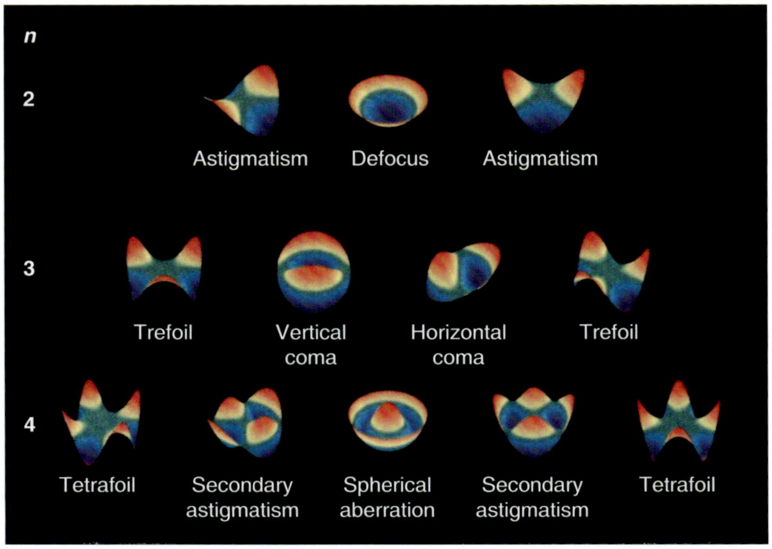

Figure 7-6 Second-, third-, and fourth-order wavefront aberrations (indicated by *n* values 2,3,and 4,respectively) are most pertinent to refractive surgery. *(Reproduced with permission from Applegate RA. Glenn Fry Award Lecture 2002: wavefront sensing, ideal corrections, and visual performance. Optom Vis Sci. 2004;81(3):169.)*

When peripheral rays focus in front of more central rays, the effect is termed *spherical aberration*. Clinically, spherical aberration is one of the main causes of night myopia following LASIK and PRK. After keratorefractive surgery, corneas that become more oblate (after myopic correction) will induce more-negative spherical aberration, while those that become more prolate (after hyperopic correction) will induce more-positive spherical aberration.

Another important aberration is *coma*. In this aberration, rays at one edge of the pupil cross the reference sphere first; rays at the opposite edge of the pupil cross last. The effect is that the image of each object point resembles a comet with a tail (one meaning of the word *coma* is "comet"). It is commoniy observed in the aiming beam during retinal laser photocoagulation; if the ophthalmologist tilts the lens too far off-axis, the aiming beam spot becomes coma shaped. Coma also arises in patients with decentered keratorefractive ablation or keratoconus. These situations may be treatable with intrastromal rings.

Higher-order aberrations tend to be less significant than lower-order aberrations , but the higher-order ones may worsen in diseased or surgically altered eyes. For example, if interrupted sutures are used to sew in a corneal graft during corneal transplant, they will produce higher-order , trefoil or tetrafoil aberrations. These can then be addressed with suture removal, suture addition, or *AK*. Also, in the manufacture of IOLs, the lens blank is sometimes improperly positioned on the lathe; such improper positioning can also produce higher-order aberrations.

Optical engineers have found approximateiy 18 basic types of astigmatism, of which only some—perhaps as few as 5—are of clinical interest. Most patients probably have a combination of all 5 types.

Wavefront aberrations can be represented in different ways. One approach is to show them as 3-dimensional shapes. Another is to represent them as contour plots. Irregular astigmatism can be described as a combination of a few basic shapes, just as conventional refractive error represents a combination of sphere and cylinder.

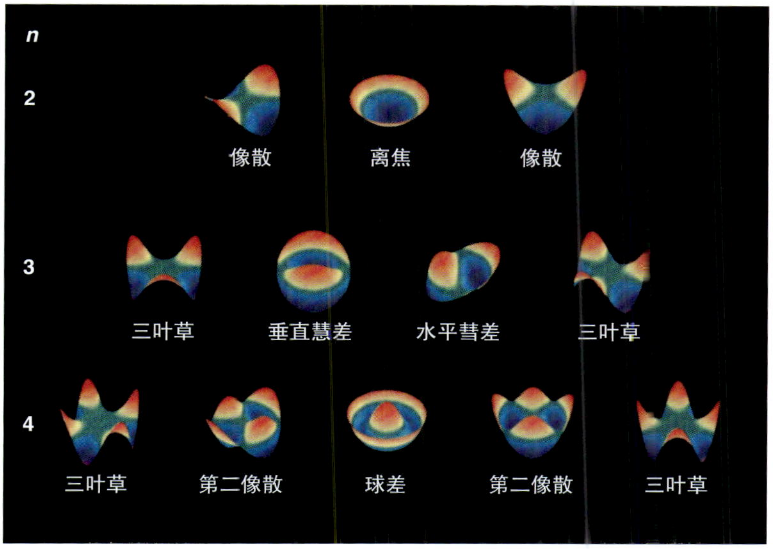

图 7–6　二阶、三阶和四阶像差（分别用 *n* 值代表 2,3,4）对于准分子手术最重要。（*译者注：资料来源见前页英文原文。*）

周边光线聚焦在更多的中央光线之前的效果称之为*球差*。临床上，球差是 LASIK 或 PRK 术后出现夜间近视的主要原因之一。在角膜屈光手术后，变得更加扁圆的角膜（近视矫正术后）会引起产生更多的负球差，而更加扁长的角膜（远视矫正术后）则会产生更多的正球差。

另一个重要的像差是*彗差*。这种像差，一侧瞳孔边缘光线首先经过参考球面，而对侧瞳孔边缘的光线最后经过参考球面，效果是一个物点的像类似一个拖着尾巴的彗星（单词 *coma* 的意思就是 comet）。如在视网膜光凝时的瞄准光，当医生将透镜倾斜的离轴太远时，瞄准光斑就会变成彗星状。彗差也可常见于偏心切削的角膜屈光手术患者，这一类状况可使用角膜基质内环治疗。

高阶像差没有低阶像差对视觉质量影响大，但在某些眼疾或术眼中影响会比较明显。比如，角膜移植中使用间断缝合的方法缝合植片，产生"三叶草"的高阶像差，可以通过移除缝线、增加缝线或散光性角膜切开术 AK 得到缓解。还有，在人工晶体的制作中，有时晶体毛坯放置的位置不当，也会产生高阶像差。

光学工程师已经发现了 18 种基本散光，其中只有一些（大概至少有 5 种）有临床意义。大多数患者的散光是这 5 种的混合。

波前像差可以用很多种方式表达。一种方式是三维图。另一种是轮廓图。不规则散光可以用几种基本形状组合而成，如屈光不正可以用球镜联合柱镜的方式表示。

Currently, wavefront aberrations are specified by *Zernike polynomials*, which are the mathematical formulas used to describe wavefront surfaces. *Wavefront aberration surfaces* are graphs generated using Zernike polynomials. There are several techniques for measuring wavefront aberrations clinically. The most popular is based on the *Hartmann-Shack wavefront sensor*. Which uses a low-power laser beam focused on the retina. A point on the retina then acts as a point source. In a perfect eye, all the rays would emerge in parallel and the wavefront would be a flat plane; however, in most eyes, the wavefront is not flat. Within the sensor is a grid of small lenses (lenslet array) that samples parts of the wavefront. The images formed are focused onto a charge-coupled-device chip, and the degree of deviation of the focused images from the expected focal points determines the aberration and thus the wavefront error (eg, see Fig 1-1 in BCSC Section 13, *Refractive Surgery*).

The most frequently used technology today are those based on measuring wavefront aberration via a ray-tracing method that projects detecting light beams sequentially rather than simultaneously, using a Hartmann-Shack wavefront sensor, further improving the resolution of wavefront aberration measurements. The application of Zernike polynomials' mathematical descriptions of aberrations to the human eye is less than perfect, however, and alternative methods, such as Fourier transforms, are being used in many wavefront aberrometers.

To normalize wavefront aberration measurements and improve postoperative visual quality in patients undergoing keratorefractive surgery, ophthalmologists are developing technologies to improve the accuracy of higher-order aberration measurements and treatment by using "flying spot" excimer lasers. Such lasers use small spot sizes (<1-mm diameter) to create smooth ablations, addressing the minute topographic changes associated with aberration errors.

For a more detailed discussion of the topics covered in this subsection, see BCSC Section 13, *Refractive Surgery*.

Causes of Irregular Astigmatism

Irregular astigmatism may be present before keratorefractive; it may be caused by surgery, or it may develop postoperatively. Preoperative causes include keratoconus, pellucid marginal degeneration, contact lens warpage, significant dry eye, corneal injury, microbial keratitis, and epithelial basement membrane dystrophy (Fig 7-7). All these conditions should be identified before surgery. Common intraoperative causes include decentered ablations and central islands, and, less commonly, poor laser optics, nonuniform stromal bed hydration, and LASIK flap complications (a thin, torn, irregular, incomplete, or buttonhole flap; folds or striae of the flap; and epithelial defects). Postoperative causes of irregular astigmatism include flap displacement, diffuse lamellar keratitis and its sequelae, flap striae, posterior corneal ectasia, irregular wound healing, dry eye, and flap edema.

Schallhorn SC, Farjo AA, Huang D, et al. Wavefront-guided LASIK for the correction of primary myopia and astigmatism: a report by the American Academy of Ophthalmology. *Ophthalmology.* 2008;115(7):12491261.

如今，波前像差主要用 *Zernike 多项式*表达，它是用数学公式描述波前阵面情况的方法。*每个像差面*使用 Zernike 多项式生成的图形来表达。临床上还有其他几种表达波前像差的方法，最广泛应用的是 *Hartmann-Shack 波前传感器*。它发射一束低功率激光投射到视网膜上，视网膜上的激光反射点就成为点光源。如果眼睛的屈光系统非常完美，那么所有的光线会平行射出并形成平面状的波前。实际上，大多数人眼的波前不是平面。传感器内的小透镜呈网格状（小透镜列阵组），是波前的标准模板，它产生的像聚焦在电荷耦合器件芯片上，从焦点产生的聚焦像的差异程度，可判断像差和波前像差 (见第 13 册《*屈光手术*》的图 1–1)。

目前最常用于描述波前像差的方法是光线追踪法，它按照时间顺序探测光束，采用 Hartmann–Shack 波前传感器，改进波前像差的分辨率。用 Zernike 多项式计算描述人眼像差并不精准，替代的方法有傅立叶变换用于多种波前像差仪。

为了让波前像差检查常规化，并提高角膜屈光手术的术后视觉质量，很多技术开始用于提高高阶像差检测的准确性，并使用“飞点”准分子激光。这种激光采用小光斑（直径 <1 mm），产生更加平滑的切削，并可以定位与像差有关的微小角膜表面改变。

关于这方面的细节，见 BCSC 第 13 册《*屈光手术*》。

不规则散光的原因

不规则散光可能在角膜屈光手术之前就已经存在，也可以手术后形成。术前原因有圆锥角膜、透明边缘角膜变性、接触镜翘曲、严重干眼、角膜外伤、感染性角膜炎和上皮基底膜营养不良 (图 7–7)。所有这些情况在术前都需要排除。术中引起角膜不规则散光的常见原因有偏心切削和中央岛，极少见的有光学区切削不良、角膜基质床脱水不均和 LASIK 角膜瓣并发症（角膜瓣过薄、撕裂、不规则、不全、纽扣瓣、瓣皱褶或条纹以及上皮缺损）。术后常见的原因包括瓣异位、弥漫性板层角膜炎及其后遗症、瓣条纹、角膜后扩张、不规则角膜创口愈合、干眼以及瓣水肿。

Schallhorn SC, Farjo AA, Huang D, et al. Wavefront-guided LASIK for the correction of primary myopia and astigmatism: a report by the American Academy of Ophthalmology. *Ophthalmology.* 2008;115(7):1249-1261.

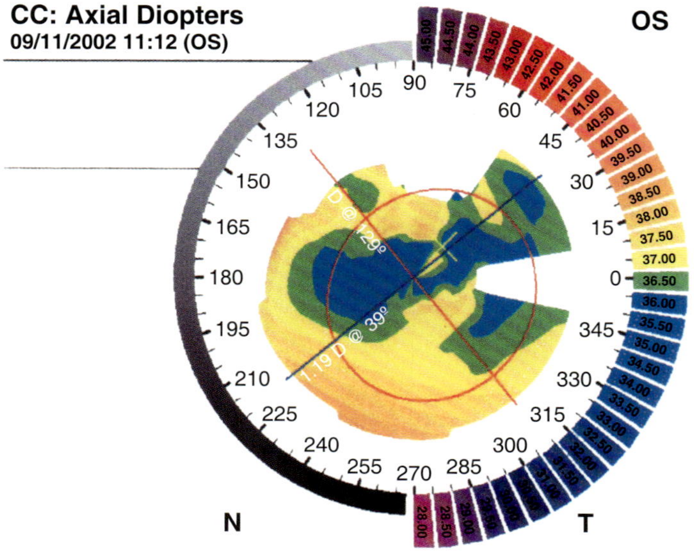

Figure 7-7 Irregular astigmatism in a corneal topographic map of the left eye of a patient with significant epithelial basement membrane dystrophy. The patient experienced glare and a general decline in quality of vision. Simulated *K* shows the flattest meridian at 39° and the steeper meridian at 129°. N = nasal; T = temporal. *(Courtesy of Ming Wang, MD.)*

Conclusion

Understanding and incorporating optical considerations into the treatment of patients undergoing keratorefractive surgery is important to enhance the visual results. Patient dissatisfaction after surgery, albeit rare, often stems from the subjective loss of visual acuity or quality, the source of which can usually be identified through a sound understanding of how keratorefractive surgery alters the optics of the eye. A good understanding of key parameters such as corneal shape, pupil size, the ocular surface, spherical and astigmatic errors, higher-order aberrations, laser centration and the angle kappa, and irregular corneal astigmatism can help optimize visual outcomes for keratorefractive surgery.

Chapter Exercises

Questions

7.1. The Munnerlyn formula approximates the depth of excimer laser tissue ablation:

$$t = \frac{S^2 D}{3}$$

where t is the central ablation depth in micrometers, S is the diameter of the optical zone in millimeters, and D is the degree of refractive correction in diopters. For a LASIK patient with a refractive correction of –6.00 –6.00 × 90 and a central corneal thickness of 520 μm, and for whom the LASIK flap thickness is 120 μm, an extremely conservative surgeon would not want to have a residual stromal bed (RSB) thickness of less than 300 μm. According to the Munnerlyn formula, what is the largest optical zone diameter that can be used for this treatment?

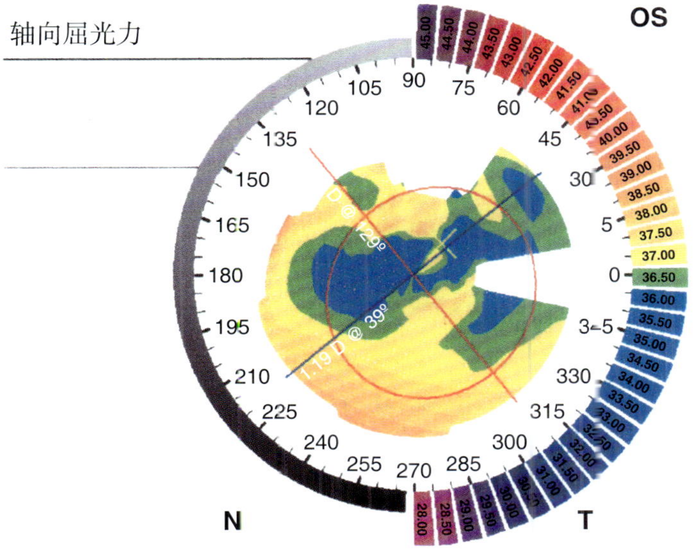

图 7–7　角膜地形图显示患者左眼不规则散光，患有上皮基底膜营养不良。患者有眩光和视觉质量严重下降。*K* 值 39° 最平坦，129° 最陡。*（译者注：资料来源见前页原文。）*

结论

理解和综合分析屈光状态，对于即将进行屈光手术的患者术后视觉质量的提升尤为重要。患者术后不满意的大多数原因与视觉质量下降有关，尽管很少见，但通过我们对角膜屈光手术如何改变人眼的屈光状态的全面理解，其不满意的原因显而易见。对关键参数的了解，包括角膜形态、瞳孔大小、眼表情况、球性屈光不正和散光、高阶像差，激光中心和 kappa 角，以及不规则角膜散光等，可以帮助我们优化角膜屈光术的视觉质量。

章节练习

问题

7.1　Munnerlyn 公式描述了准分子激光切削角膜组织的深度：

$$t = \frac{S^2 D}{3}$$

其中，t 是以微米为单位的中央角膜切削深度，S 是以 mm 为单位的光学区直径，D 是以 D 为单位的屈光矫正量。例如一位屈光矫正度数为 −6.00−6.00 × 90 的 LASIK 患者，而中央角膜厚度为 520 μm，拟行 LASIK 手术角膜瓣厚度为 120 μm，在非常谨慎的情况下，手术后角膜残余基质床应该不少于 300 μm。根据 Munnerlyn 公式，本例手术可以实施的最大光学直径是多少？

7.2. For the situation described in Question 7.1, what is the largest optical zone diameter. that can be used if PRK, rather than LASIK, is planned? Assume an epithelium thickness of 58 μm and an RSB thickness of 300 μm.

7.3. A patient with a preoperative manifest refraction of −3.50D, normal keratometry(K) readings, and a pachymetry measurement of 550 μm undergoes keratorefractive surgery. Three months postoperatively, the patient has an uncorrected visual acuity of 20/30 with a refraction of +2.00 −3.00 × 60 associated with postsurgical irregular astigmatism. What are the important signs that will aid in reaching a diagnosis?
a. difficulty in determining axis location during manifest refraction
b. discrepancy between automated refraction and manifest refraction
c. no improvement or change in visual acuity with large powers of cylinder at markedly different axes
d. all of the above

7.4. Corneal asphericity is represented by Q value. A spherical cornea with asphericity of $Q = 0$ is associated with
a. better visual acuity than a prolate cornea
b. improved optics if keratorefractive surgery results in postoperative $Q = -0.3$
c. improved optics if keratorefractive surgery results in postoperative $Q = 0$
d. improved optics if keratorefractive surgery results in postoperative $Q = +0.3$

7.5. A patient undergoing an evaluation for refractive surgery has K readings of 46.0 D/42.0 D. If LASIK were performed, what are the largest hyperopic and myopic spherical corrections tolerable?
a. +5.00 D, −11.25 D
b. +3.00 D, −11.25 D
c. +3.00 D, −6.25 D
d. +5.00 D, −7.00 D

Answers

7.1. Pachymetry value = t + LASIK flap thickness + RSB thickness = t + 120 μm + 300 μm. This implies that t = 100 μm. Then, $t = 100 = S^2 \times D/3$, where $D = 12$, the spherical component necessary to correct, which implies that $S^2 = 25$. Therefore, S = 5 mm; that is, the largest diameter that can be used for LASIK treatment in this situation by this surgeon is 5 mm.

7.2. Pachymetry value = t + epithelium thickness + RSB thickness. This implies that t = 520 μm − 58 μm − 300 μm = 162 μm. Because $t = S^2 \times 12/3$, this implies that $S^2 = 162/4 = 40.5$; thus, S = 6.4 mm, the largest diameter that can be used for PRK treatment in this situation by this surgeon.

7.3. **d.** all of the above.

7.4. **b.** improved optics if keratorefractive surgery results in postoperative $Q = -0.3$

7.5. **a.** +8.75 D, −11.25 D. The formula for keratometry change is approximately = 0.8 × refractive change. Here, the refractive change = (50 − 46)/0.8 = +5.00D and (33 − 42)/ 0.8 = −11.25 D based on maximum steepening of the steep axis and maximum flattening of the flat axis.

7.2　问题 7.1，假设上皮瓣厚度为 58 μm，而术后角膜残余基质床仍为 300 μm，如果用 PRK 术代替 LASIK 手术，最大光学区直径多大？

7.3　一位患者术前显然验光结果为 –3.50 D，角膜曲率 K 值正常，做准分子激光手术后测得的角膜厚度为 550 μm。手术 3 个月后，患者裸眼视力 20/30，验光度数 +2.00–3.00 × 60，伴有术后不规则散光。帮助我们做出诊断的重要线索为：

a. 显然验光时确定散光轴困难
b. 电脑验光与显然验光结果不符
c. 在截然不同的散光轴上用大度数柱镜矫正时矫正视力不提高
d. 上述都对

7.4　角膜非球性用 Q 值表示，Q 值为 0 的球形角膜，与哪个选项有关？
a. 球形角膜的视力比扁平角膜更好
b. 准分子激光术后 Q 值变为 –0.3，改进光学
c. 准分子激光术后 Q 值仍为 0，改进光学
d. 准分子激光术后 Q 值变为 +0.3，改进光学

7.5　一位患者术前角膜曲率 K 值的读数为 46.00 D/42.00 D，如果施行 LASIK，那么能矫正的最大球镜远视度数及近视度数能达到多少？
a. +5.00 D, –11.25 D
b. +3.00 D, –11.25 D
c. +3.00 D, –6.25 D
d. +5.00 D, –7.00 D

答案

7.1　角膜厚度算法 =t+LASIK 瓣厚度 + 术后角膜基质床厚度 =t +120 μm+300 μm。所以 t=100=$S^2 \times D/3$, 公式中 D=12，球镜部分充分矫正，所以 S^2=25，即 S=5 mm。答案即为 LASIK 手术能够做出的最大光学直径为 5 mm。

7.2　角膜厚度算法 = t+ 上皮瓣厚度 + 术后角膜基质床厚度。将病例数值代入公式，t=520 μm–58 μm–300 μm=162 μm。因为 t= $S^2 \times 12 \div 3$，所以 S^2=162 ÷ 4=40.5；所以 S=6.4 mm。答案即为 PRK 手术能够做出的最大光学直径为 6.4 mm。

7.3　**d**。以上都对。
7.4　**b**。准分子激光术后 Q 值变为 –0.3，改进光学。
7.5　**a**。 +8.75 D, –11.25 D。角膜曲率的计算公式 =0.8 × – 屈光度数变化，本例中屈光度数 =（50–46）÷ 0.8=+5.00D，以及（33–42）÷ 0.8=–11.25D。算法基于散光轴中陡 K 极限值和平 K 极限值。

（翻译　吴捷　王文军//审校　石一宁　吴捷//章节审校　白继）

CHAPTER 8

Optical Instruments

This chapter includes a related video, which can be accessed by scanning the QR code provided in the text or going to www.aao.org/bcscvideo_section03.

Highlights

- Instruments for refraction and topography: lensmeter, autorefractor, keratometer, corneal topographer, aberrometer
- Instruments for anterior- and posterior-segment examination: slit-lamp biomicroscope, applanation tonometer, surgical microscope, specular microscopy, ophthalmoscope, fundus camera, scanning laser ophthalmoscope, optical coherence tomography
- State-of-the-art technological advances in corneal topography, wavefront aberrometry, optical coherence tomography, and adaptive optics

Glossary

Adaptive optics A technique to compensate for irregularities (wavefront distortions) caused by imperfections (optical aberrations) in the ocular media, in particular the cornea and crystalline lens, when imaging the ocular fundus.

Autorefractor An automated system used to reveal the eye's refractive characteristics from a source of light reflected off the retina.

Corneal topography system An automated system used for producing a detailed map of the shape of the entire corneal surface. It is most useful in refractive surgery, after corneal transplant surgery, and in evaluating patients with keratoconus.

Direct ophthalmoscope A handheld instrument used to examine the posterior segment, using the optics of the patient's eye as a simple magnifier, and to assess the red reflex.

Indirect ophthalmoscope A device, worn on the head, that is used for the posterior segment examination in conjunction with auxiliary handheld diagnostic condensing lenses.

Instrument myopia A tendency for the eye to accommodate when looking into instruments.

第 8 章

光学仪器

本章包含一个相关视频，可以通过扫描本书提供的 QR 码或访问 www.aao.org/bcscvideo_section03。

重点

- 验光和地形图仪器：焦度仪，自动验光仪，角膜曲率计，角膜地形图仪，像差仪。
- 用于前段和后段检查的仪器：裂隙灯生物显微镜，压平眼压计，手术显微镜，角膜内皮显微镜，检眼镜，眼底照相机，扫描激光检眼镜，光学相干断层扫描。
- 角膜地形学、波前像差测量、光学相干断层扫描和自适应光学的最新技术进步。

术语

自适应光学　一种在眼底成像时补偿由眼部介质，特别是角膜和晶状体中的缺陷（光学像差）引起的波前畸变的技术。

自动验光仪　一种自动化系统，用于从视网膜反射的光源显示眼睛的屈光特征。

角膜地形图系统　一种自动化系统，用于生成整个角膜表面形状的详细图像。它在屈光手术、角膜移植手术后和评估圆锥角膜患者中很有用。

直接检眼镜　一种手持式仪器，可用于直接检查眼底，不必散大瞳孔，作为简单的放大镜用于患者眼的光学系统，并评估患者的红光反射功能。

间接检眼镜　一种戴在头部的仪器，使用时须充分散大瞳孔，结合手持式诊断聚光镜一起进行眼底的检查。

仪器性近视　在使用仪器时眼睛有发生调节的趋势。

Keratometer A device used to approximate the refracting power of the cornea by determining the curvature of the central outer corneal surface. It is typically used when fitting contact lenses and to diagnose disorders such as keratoconus.

Lensmeter A device that measures the power of spectacle or contact lenses.

Optical coherence tomography (OCT) A system based on low-coherence interferometry, using interference of broadband or tunable coherent light, that provides a high-resolution cross-sectional image of the retina or cornea.

Ray-deflection principle A method to infer the eye's refractive error employed in autorefractors and aberrometers. A stationary source of light "floods" the eye. The light emerging from the eye is then isolated into multiple beams. The deflection or deviation of each individual light beam is then compared with its ideal reference position.

Scanning laser ophthalmoscope A device that functions as both an ophthalmoscope and a fundus camera but requires significantly less light than those conventional flood illumination systems, thanks to the use of a rapidly scanning laser illuminating only a small spot of retina at a time.

Scheimpflug principle Also called *Scheimpflug camera*, in which a camera rotates perpendicular with the source of illumination, such as slit beams of light incident on the cornea. This configuration corrects for the nonplanar shape of the cornea and, thus, results in "distortion-free" cross sections.

Scheiner principle A method for detecting refractive errors using a double-pinhole aperture placed before the eye. Through such an aperture, an emmetropic eye forms a single point image of a distant point source on the retina; an ametropic eye forms a double image on the retina.

Slit-lamp biomicroscope Commonly called the *slit lamp*. The slit-lamp biomicroscope permits magnified examination of the eye, using various kinds of illumination. It is primarily used to perform anterior segment examinations. Several attachments for the slit lamp extend its use beyond these examination techniques, such as auxiliary lenses for slit-lamp examination of the retina.

Specular microscope A device used to evaluate the corneal endothelium. Contact specular microscopy allows for higher magnifications than slit-lamp biomicroscopy, demonstrates cell morphology, and calculates endothelial cell density.

Tonometer A device used to measure intraocular pressure. In Goldmann applanation tonometry specifically, performed with an attachment to the slit lamp, intraocular pressure is inferred from the amount of force required to flatten an area of 3.06 mm in diameter on the cornea.

Introduction

In this chapter, we discuss the basic principles and underlying concepts of various optical instruments that are commonly used to examine the eye. The discussion includes some recent state-of-the-art technological developments.

角膜曲率计　一种用于通过确定中央外角膜表面的曲率来近似计算角膜屈光力的仪器。它通常在配戴接触镜和诊断圆锥角膜等疾病时使用。

焦度计　一种用于测量眼镜或接触镜的屈光度的仪器。

光学相干断层扫描（OCT）　一种基于光学原理进行诊断成像的设备，利用宽带或可调相干光的干涉，提供视网膜或角膜的高分辨率横截面图像。

射线偏转原理　用自动验光仪和像差仪推断眼的屈光不正的方法。固定的光源"大量进入"眼睛，然后将从眼睛出射的光分离成多个光束，然后将每个单独光束的偏转或偏差与其理想参考位置进行比较。

扫描激光检眼镜　由于使用快速扫描激光一次仅照射一小部分视网膜，因此该装置既可用作检眼镜又可用作眼底照相机，但需要比传统泛光照明系统少得多的光。

Scheimpflug 原理　也称为 *Scheimpflug 相机*，它是相机垂直于照明源旋转的一种配置，例如入射在角膜上的狭缝光束。该构造矫正了角膜的非平面形状，因此导致"无变形"横截面。

Scheiner 原理　一种利用放置在眼前的双针孔来检测屈光不正的方法。通过这样的孔，对于远处点光源，正视眼在视网膜上形成的单个点像；屈光不正眼在视网膜上形成 2 个点像。

裂隙灯生物显微镜　通常称为*裂隙灯*。裂隙灯生物显微镜允许使用各种光源对眼睛进行放大检查。它主要用于进行前段检查。裂隙灯的几个附件将其用途扩展到这些检查技术之外，例如裂隙灯用于视网膜检查的辅助透镜。

角膜内皮显微镜　一种用于评估角膜内皮的仪器。接触角膜内皮显微镜比裂隙灯生物显微镜的放大倍数更高，可显示细胞形态，计算内皮细胞密度。

眼压计　一种用于测量眼压的仪器。具体而言，在 Goldmann 压平眼压计中，通过连接到裂隙灯来完成测量工作，依据在角膜上压平直径为 3.06 mm 的区域所需力的值来推断眼压。

引言

在本章中，我们将讨论通常用于检查眼睛的各种光学仪器的基本原理和基本概念。讨论内容包括一些最新的技术发展。

Refraction and Topography

Lensmeter

Manual lensmeter

The lensmeter measures the power of a spectacle or contact lens. It uses a fixed lens positioned a focal length away from the spectacle plane at the tip of the nose cone (Fig 8-1), by which the vergence induced in the spectacle plane becomes linearly related to moving a target.

In the lensmeter, an illuminated target is moved, varying the vergence at the tip of the nose cone, until it becomes focused on the reticle of a telescope. The target is focused only when parallel rays are entering the telescope (ie, when the light entering has zero vergence), which indicates that the "unknown" lens is exactly neutralizing the vergence that is coming out of the nose cone. The actual power of the lens can then be read from a dioptric scale, which is opposite of the power emerging from the nose cone.

The addition of the telescope facilitates the detection of zero vergence. This is because it magnifies vergence by the square of the power of the telescope, which enables the examiner to detect very small deviations from zero vergence without having his or her uncorrected refractive error cause significant error in the measurement. For best accuracy, the eyepiece can be adjusted beforehand, by focusing it on a reticle located inside the telescope, which eliminates any residual effect from the examiner's refractive error.

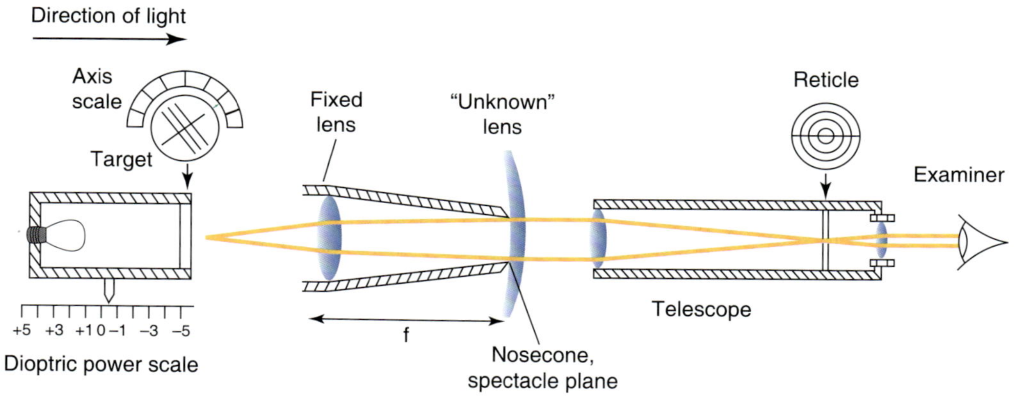

Figure 8-1 The lensmeter. An illuminated target is moved, varying the vergence at the tip of the nose cone, until it becomes focused on the reticle of a telescope. This is the case when the "unknown" spectacle lens is exactly neutralizing the vergence that is coming out of the nose cone. The light will then emerge from the spectacle lens with zero vergence (ie, collimated), and the target will be seen in sharp focus by the observer. The telescope magnifies vergence by the square of its power and thus facilitates the detection of zero vergence, increasing the precision of the measurement and reducing the effect of the observer's accommodation or refractive error. *(Reproduced from Guyton DL, et al. Ophthalmic Optics and Clinical Refraction. Baltimore: Prism Press; 1999. Illustration modified by Kristina Irsch, PhD.)*

Note that we cannot measure the true power of a lens with the lensmeter, as this would require us to measure from the lens's principal planes rather than from the lens's surface. To measure the distance correction using a lensmeter, we place the spectacle lens on the nose cone with the temples turned away from us, so the nose cone is against the back surface, because spectacle lenses are designated by their back vertex power (ie, the reciprocal of their back focal length).

验光和地形图

焦度计

手动焦度计

焦度计是用来测量眼镜或接触镜度数的一种仪器。它有一个固定位置的透镜，透镜至鼻锥尖托处待测眼镜平面的距离等于透镜的焦距（图 8–1），这样就会使眼镜平面的聚散度与移动靶标呈线性关系。

在焦度计中，移动受照靶标，改变对鼻锥的聚散度，直到它聚焦在望远镜的十字刻线上。只有当平行光线进入望远镜时（即光进入时具有零聚散度），靶标才能聚焦，这时表明“待测”镜片正好抵消了相对鼻锥的聚散度。于是可从焦度标盘中实际的镜片焦度，该焦度与从鼻锥形成的焦度相反。

附加的望远镜有助于检测零聚散度。这是因为望远镜中的聚散度呈焦度的二次方，这使得检查者能够检测到零聚散度的非常小的偏差，而不会因未矫正的屈光不正导致测量中的显著误差。为了获得最佳精准度，提前调整目镜，把靶标聚焦在望远镜内的分划板上，消除检查者屈光不正的残余影响。

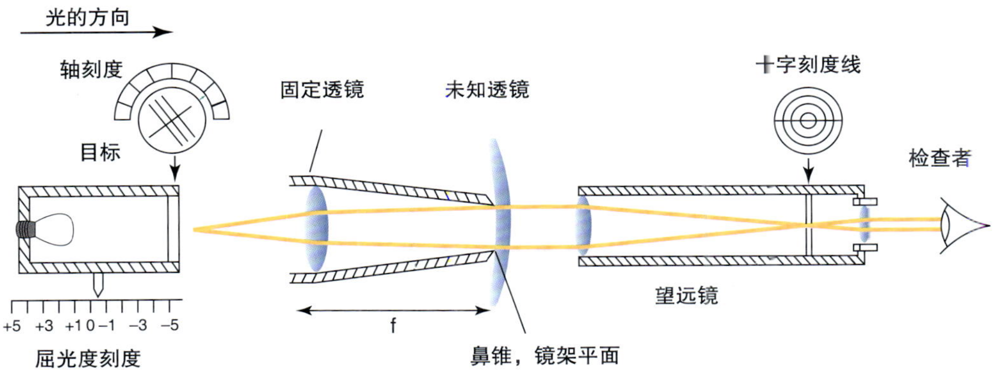

图 8–1　焦度计。移动受照靶标，改变对鼻锥尖的聚散度，直到它聚焦在望远镜的分划板上。这时“待测”眼镜的镜片正好抵消对鼻锥的聚散度。然后零聚散度的光将从眼镜镜片中出来（即校准），观察者将看到清晰聚焦的靶标。望远镜以焦度的二次方放大了它的聚散度，从而有助于检测零聚散度、提高测量精度并减少观察者的调节或屈光不正的影响。

请注意，我们无法用焦度仪测量镜片的真实焦度，因为这需要我们从镜片的主平面而不是从镜片的表面进行测量。为了焦度计测量的距离准确，我们将眼镜镜片放在鼻锥上，镜腿远离我们，鼻锥顶在后面，因为眼镜镜片由它们的后顶点焦度（即它们的后焦距的倒数）决定。

The target usually has a set of lines (eg, the American cross-line target as depicted in Fig 8-2) that permits the observer to determine whether the lens has cylindrical power. In the measurement of cylindrical power, as illustrated in Figure 8-2A, the cross-line target is first rotated, as well as moved forward or backward, until one set of lines is sharp. Then, it is moved forward or backward until the perpendicular set of lines is sharp. The difference in target settings is the cylindrical power. The cylindrical axis is read from a scale indicating the orientation of the cross-line target in degrees.

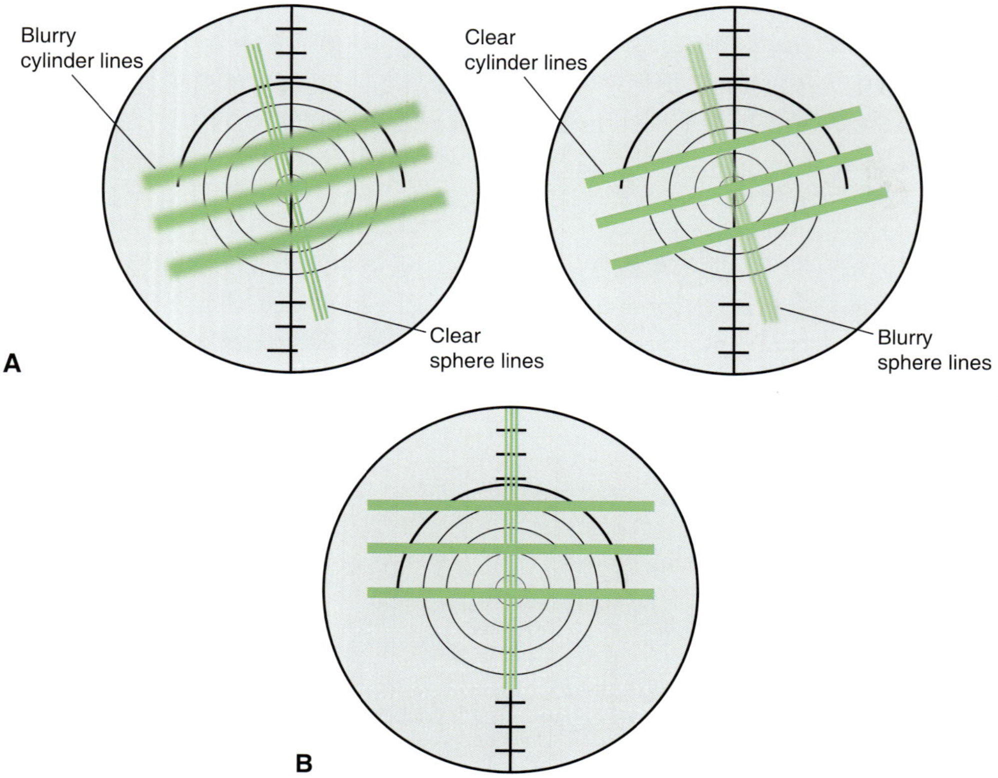

Figure 8-2 Illustration of view inside lensmeter. **A**, In the measurement of cylindrical power, the cross-line target is rotated, via the axis wheel, so that the lines are continuous and do not appear "broken," indicating the correct axis of the cylinder. The cross-line target is also moved forward or backward, via the power wheel, until 1 set of lines is clear (left). Then, it is moved forward or backward until the perpendicular set of lines is clear (right). The difference in target settings is the cylindrical power of the lens. **B,** Upward displacement of the target pattern indicates the presence of base-up prism. *(Modified from Gutmark R, Guyton DL, Irsch K. Prescribing Prisms.Focal Points: Clinical Modules for Ophthalmologists. San Francisco: American Academy of Ophthalmology; 2011, module 10:p4.)*

Prism in spectacles can also be detected by means of a lensmeter. If there is no prism present in the lens, the center of the cross-line target will be in the center of the lensmeter reticule. If, however, the intersection of the target lines is off-center (Fig 8-2B), and the lens must be shifted away from the patient's normal viewing position to recenter it in the reticule, then one knows that prism is present in the spectacle lens. If the intersection of the target lines is decentered horizontally, horizontal prismatic power is present, whereas a vertical shift indicates the presence of vertical prism power, with the shift in the direction of the prism base. In Figure 8-2B, the target lines are vertically displaced upward from the center, as is the case when vertical prism power, base-up, is present.

靶标通常具有一组线（例如图 8-2 中所示的美国十字线靶标），其允许观察者确定镜片是否具有柱镜焦度。在测量柱镜焦度时，如图 8-2A 所示，首先旋转十字线靶标，同时前后移动，直至一组线变得清晰。然后，将它向前或向后移动，直到垂直的一组线条变得清晰。靶标设置的差值就是柱镜焦度。从十字线靶标指示方向的刻度读取柱镜轴，单位为（°）。

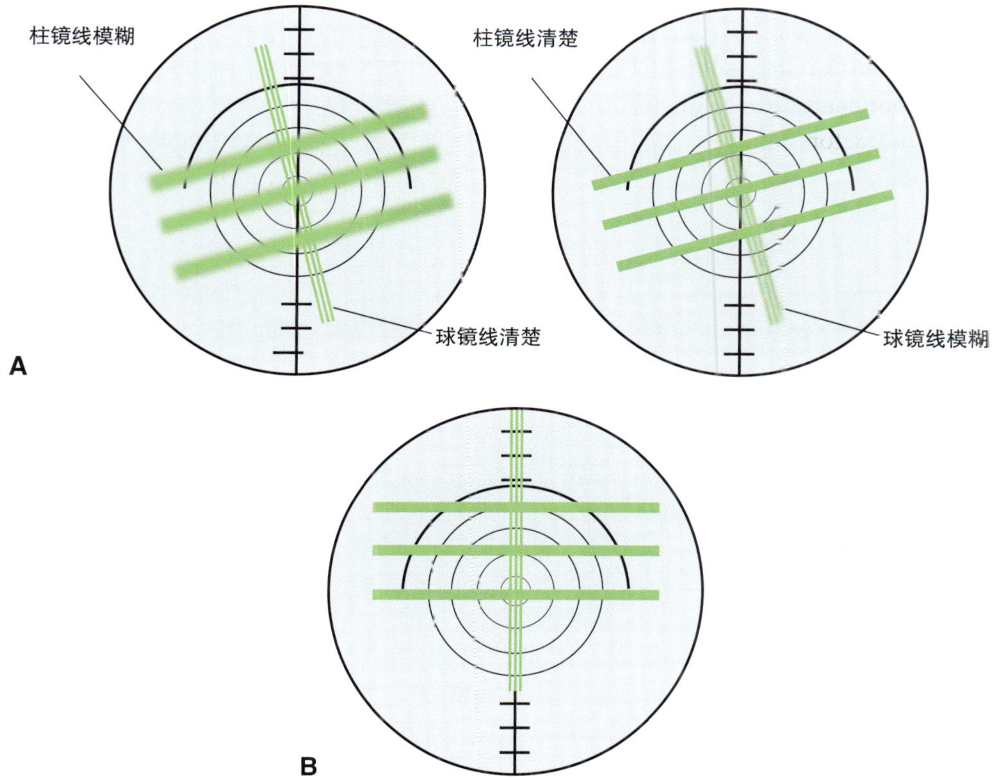

图 8-2　焦度计里的图例。**A.** 在测量柱镜焦度时，使用柱镜轴轮旋转十字线靶标，使得线条连续并且不会出现“断裂”，表示出正确的柱镜轴。使用焦度轮使十字线靶标前后移动，直到一组线条变得清晰（左）。然后，将它向前或向后移动，直到垂直的一组线条变得清晰（右）。靶标设置的差值就是柱镜的焦度。**B.** 靶标图案的向上位移表明存在基底向上棱镜。*（译者注：资料来源见前页英文原文。）*

眼镜中的棱镜也可以通过焦度计检测。如果镜片没有棱镜，则交叉线目标的中心将位于焦度计十字线的中心。如果目标线的交点偏离中心（图 8-2B），并且必须将镜片移离患者的正常观察位置，并重新定位十字线，则提示镜片存在棱镜焦度。如果目标线的交叉点水平偏移，则存在水平棱镜焦度，而垂直偏移表示垂直棱镜焦度的存在，并向棱镜基底的方向偏移。在图 8-2B 中，目标线从中心向上垂直移位，提示存在垂直棱镜焦度，且基底向上。

When determining a patient's reading add, the examiner places the spectacles on the nose cone with the temples turned around, toward the examiner, so that the front of the glasses rests on the nose cone. The front vertex power of the distance portion is measured, which will be significantly different from the back vertex power for high plus lenses (in cases other than a distance lens with strong plus power, there is usually little or no clinically significant difference in the measurements), and the front vertex power of the near portion is measured. The difference in power between the distance and near portions of the lens specifies the reading-add power.

Automatic lensmeter

The principles underlying automatic lensmeters differ from those of manual ones. Automated lensmeters do not neutralize the unknown lens but rather measure the deflection of light rays (similar to automated refractors) as they pass through various parts of the lens to calculate lens power and prismatic effect.

Autorefractors

Autorefractors project near-infrared or infrared light into the eye via a beam splitter and employ various optical principles to reveal the eye's refractive characteristics from the measured light reflected from the ocular fundus.

The foundation for most of the optical principles employed in modern autorefractors (including automated lensmeters), and aberrometers was laid by Christopher Scheiner nearly 400 years ago. Using an opaque disk perforated with 2 pinhole apertures (known as the *Scheiner disk*), he demonstrated that an eye's spherical error could be measured. This *Scheiner principle* relies on the fact that a double-pinhole aperture placed before the eye evokes different responses in an ametropic eye than in an emmetropic eye (Fig 8-3). When looking at a small, distant light source, a normal (emmetropic) eye will see a single spot of light with or without the double-pinhole aperture upfront. In case of either myopia or hyperopia, on the other hand, 2 separate spots are seen when the double-pinhole aperture is in place. This is because in a myopic eye (for example), the 2 bundles of light that have been created by the double-pinhole aperture come to focus in the vitreous, crossing over and creating 2 separate spots on the retina; in a hyperopic eye, the 2 bundles of light come to focus beyond the retina, which also leaves 2 separate spots on the retina. One can refract an eye by placing diverse lenses in front of the eye, or by moving the point source axially, until a single spot of light is achieved on the retina.

A modified, objective form of this principle is still used today in most autorefractors. For example, in some instruments, the pinhole apertures are effectively replaced by 2 light-emitting diodes (LEDs) imaged in the pupillary plane. From the axial position of the LEDs required to achieve a single image on a camera, the patient's refractive error is determined. This may be repeated in various meridians to determine any astigmatic component of the refractive error.

在确定患者的阅读近附加焦度时，检查者将眼镜放在鼻锥上，使镜腿转向检查者，使眼镜的前部靠在鼻锥上。测量远用部分的前顶点焦度，并且测量近用部分的前顶点焦度，但高度正透镜的后顶点焦度与其前顶点焦度明显不同（除了高度远用镜片以外，这个临床测量没有显著差异）。镜片远用和近用部分的焦度差确定了阅读近附加焦度。

自动焦度计

自动焦度计的基本原理与手动焦度计的原理不同。自动焦度计不中和未知镜片，而是当光线经过镜片的不同部位时，通过测量光线的偏转（类似于自动验光仪）来计算镜头焦度和棱镜度。

自动验光仪

自动验光仪是通过光线分束器将近红外或红外光投射到眼睛中，并根据各种光学原理，计算出从眼底反射出来的光的屈光特性。

现代自动验光仪（包括自动焦度计）和像差仪所采用的大多数光学原理都是在 400 年前由 Christopher Scheiner 奠定的。他使用 1 个带有 2 个针孔的不透明圆盘（称为 *Scheiner 圆盘*），证明可以测量眼球的球形误差。该 *Scheiner 原理*依赖于这样的事实：在眼睛前面放置的双针孔光圈在屈光不正的眼睛中引起不同的反应，而在正视眼中则不会出现这种现象（图 8–3）。当观察 1 个小的远距离光源时，正常眼（正视眼）会看到 1 个光点（有或没有双针孔光圈）。而在近视或远视的情况下，通过双针孔光圈，可以看到 2 个单独的光点。这是因为在近视眼中，由双针孔形成的 2 束光聚焦在玻璃体内交叉，并在视网膜上形成 2 个单独的光点；在远视眼中，2 束光聚焦在视网膜之外，视网膜上也是留下了 2 个独立的光点。人们可以通过在眼睛前方放置不同的镜片，或者通过轴向移动点光源来折射进入眼睛的光线，直到在视网膜上形成单个光点。

目前，大多数自动验光仪仍然是依据这种原理的改良而进行的客观检测。例如，在一些仪器中，针孔有效地由在瞳孔平面中成像的 2 个发光二极管（LED）代替，从在相机上获得单个图像所需的 LED 的轴向位置，来确定患者的屈光不正。这可以在各种子午线中重复，以确定屈光不正的任何散光度。

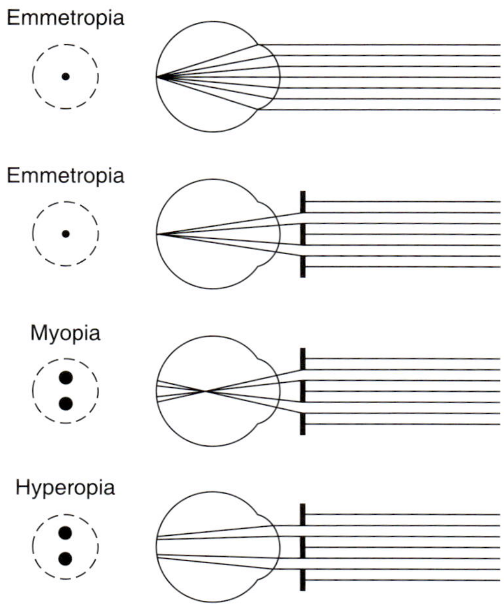

Figure 8–3 The Scheiner principle. Double pinhole apertures placed before the pupil isolate 2 small bundles of light. An object not conjugate to the retina appears doubled instead of blurred. (*Modified from Duane TD, ed. Clinical Ophthalmology. Vol 1. Hagerstown, MD: Harper & Row; 1983:2.*)

Many recent instruments use a stationary source of light to "flood" the eye and then isolate the light emerging from the eye into multiple beams (eg, via a Hartmann screen— essentially a Scheiner disk with multiple holes, or a multi-lenslet array, as described by Shack). They then measure the deflection or deviation from their ideal reference positions of the emerging individual light rays to infer the eye's refractive error. This method is commonly referred to as the *ray-deflection principle.* It enables, not just the measurement of spherocylindrical errors but also the measurement of higher-order aberrations, if multiple parts of the pupil are analyzed, as is done with aberrometers.

The main difficulties with autorefractors are the result of human factors, such as poor fixation and accommodative fluctuation, including so-called *instrument myopia*; that is, the tendency to accommodate when looking into instruments. Various methods of fogging and automatic tracking have been developed to overcome the latter, with some success.

Keratometer

The keratometer is used to approximate the refracting power of the cornea by determining the curvature of the central outer corneal surface. It does this by measuring the image size of a reflected mire in each of the principal meridians, accomplished by lining up prism-doubled images at a distance regulated by sharpness of focus. Note that doubling of the image is performed to avoid problems and inaccuracies from involuntary eye motion. There are 2 basic methods by which the doubled mire images are aligned with one another. For example, in the Javal-Schiøtz-style keratometer (Haag-Streit USA, Mason, OH), the mire separation is adjusted while the image doubling is constant (Fig 8-4A). In the Bausch + Lomb (Bridgewater, NJ) style of keratometer, on the other hand, the mire location is fixed and the image doubling is variable (Fig 8-4B). Corneal refractive power is inferred from the calculated radius of curvature using the formula for surface power $D = (n-1)/r$. In practice, a correction for the small refractive effect (minus power) of the corneal back surface is incorporated in the value for the refractive index of the cornea.

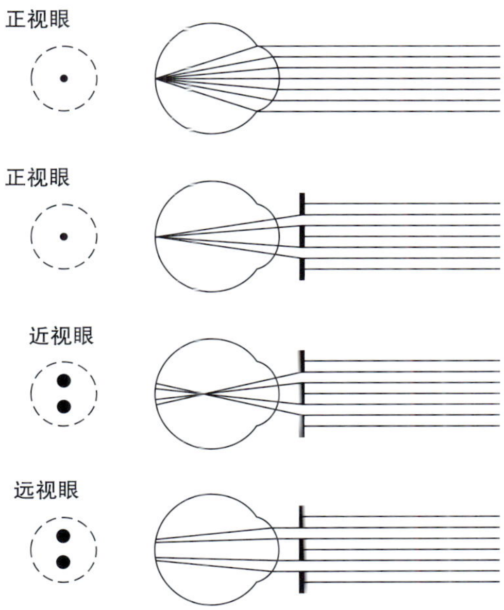

图 8–3　Scheiner 原理，在瞳孔之前放置双针孔，分离 2 小束光。未与视网膜共轭聚焦的物体形成双像，但不是模糊像。*（译者注：资料来源见前页英文原文。）*

新的仪器用固定光源“充满”眼睛，然后将从眼睛射出的光隔离成多个光束（例如，通过具有多个孔的 Hartmann 屏，最基础的是 Scheiner 盘，或多个小透镜阵列，如 Shack 所描述的）。然后，通过测量偏离或偏离其出现的单个光线的理想参考位置，以推断眼睛的屈光不正。该方法通常被称为*射线偏转原理*。如果分析瞳孔的各个部分，就会发现这种新仪器不仅可以测量球柱面屈光不正，还可以测量高阶像差，这与像差仪一样。

自动验光仪的主要问题是人为因素，如固定不良和调节波动，包括*仪器性近视*，也就是说，人在注视仪器时眼睛会产生调节。人们已经开发了各种雾视和自动跟踪方法来解决这个问题，并有一些改进。

角膜曲率计

角膜曲率计通过确定中央外角膜表面的曲率来计算近似角膜的屈光力。通过竖排棱镜双像在规定的距离处清晰聚焦来完成每个子午线反射像大小的测量。应该注意到，使用双像避免了无意识的眼球运动造成的问题和误差。有 2 种基本方法使视标双像彼此对齐。其中，一种方法是，在 Javal–Schiøtz 式角膜曲率计（Haag–Streit USA，Mason，OH）中，调整光标分离，而双像系统不变（图 8–4A）。另一种方法是，在 Bausch+Lomb 式角膜曲率计（Bridgewater，NJ）中，光标位置是固定的，双像系统是可变的（图 8–4B）。使用面屈光力 $D = (n-1)/r$ 的公式，通过曲率半径推断出角膜屈光力。实际上，角膜内面的小屈光力（负焦度）的矫正已包含在角膜折射率中。

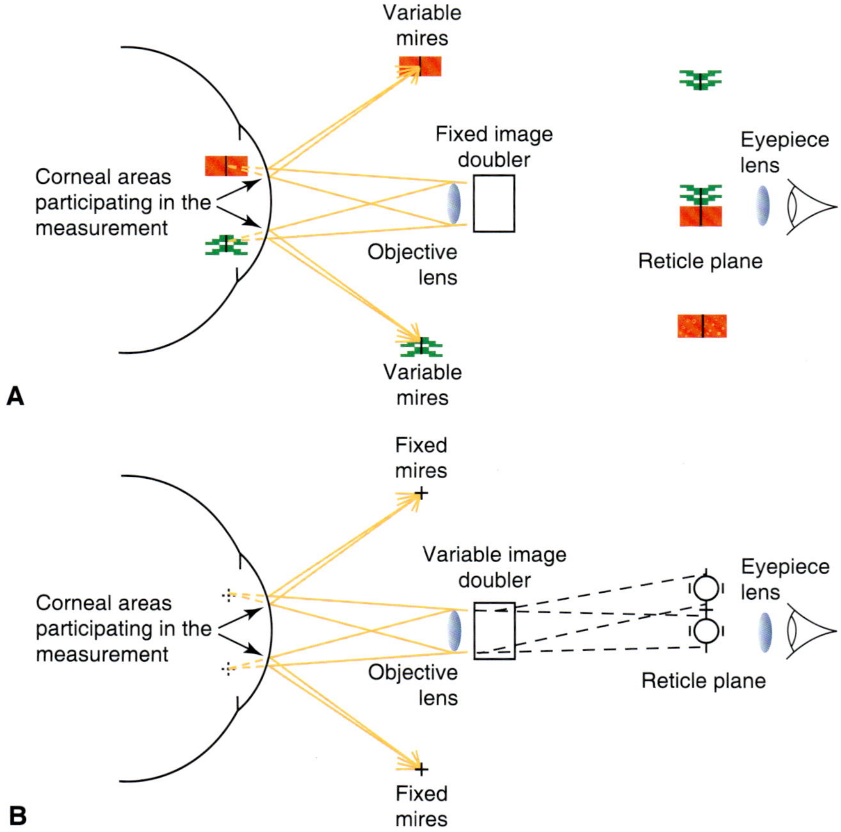

Figure 8-4 Keratometer principle. The curvature of an annulus of the cornea about 3 mm in diameter is determined by measuring the image size of reflected mires in each of the principal meridians. This is accomplished by the examiner lining up the prism-doubled images. Corneal refractive power is inferred from the obtained radius of curvature using the formula for surface power $D = (n - 1)/r$, where D is the corneal power in diopters, n is the keratometric refractive index at 1.3375, an empirically derived "standardized" refractive index for the cornea that takes the minus power of the corneal back surface into account, and r is the radius of the corneal curvature (in meters). **A**, The Javal–Schiøtz style keratometer employs a fixed-image doubling device, and the mire separation is variable. **B**, The Bausch + Lomb style of keratometer employs a variable image doubling device, and the mire dimensions are constant. *(Reproduced from Guyton DL,et al. Ophthalmic Optics and Clinical Refraction. Baltimore: Prism Press; 1999. Illustration modified by Kristina Irsch, PhD.)*

Conventional keratometry is performed at only 1 diameter, approximately 3 mm, and is therefore lacking the detail provided by more elaborate topography.

Automatic keratometers use principles similar to those used in automated lensmeters and refractors, measuring the amount of deflection of the reflected light.

Corneal Topography

Unlike keratometry instruments, corneal topography instruments produce a detailed map of the shape of the entire corneal surface. Originally, corneal topography was limited to analysis of the anterior corneal surface, with the predominant technique being based on the Placido-disk principle (Fig 8-5). Computerized Placido disk–based topographers assess the reflection of a circular mire of concentric lighted rings (Fig 8-6). More precisely, the distance between the rings is measured, from which the height of the cornea is calculated and commonly displayed as dioptric color maps of the corneal surface (see also BCSC Section 13, *Refractive Surgery*).

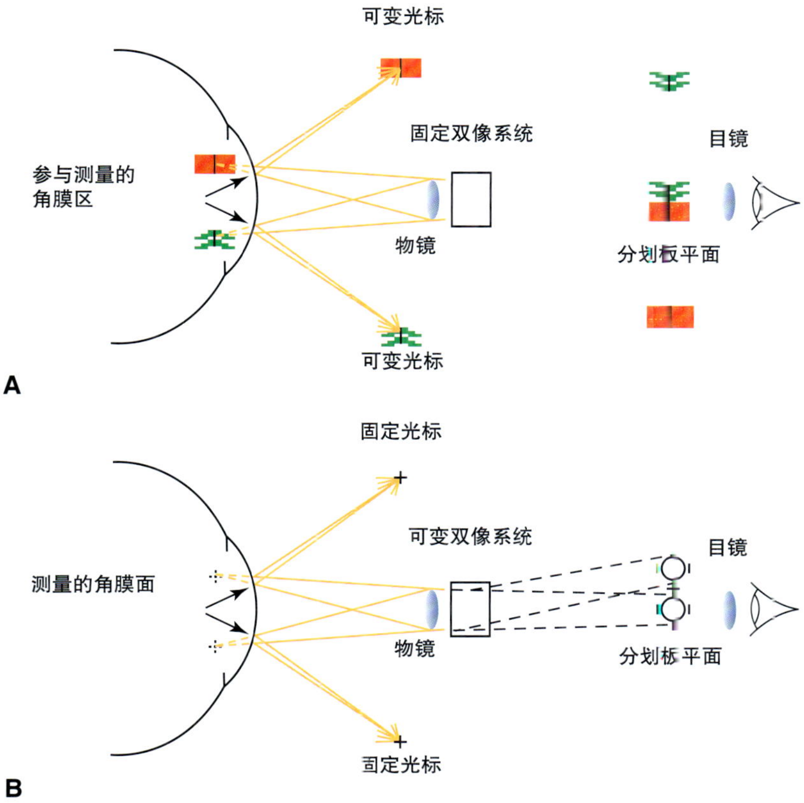

图 8-4　角膜曲率计原理。直径约为 3mm 的角膜曲率，通过测量每个主要子午线中反射的光标像大小来确定。这是由检查者排列棱镜双像来完成的。根据表面屈光力 $D = (n-1)/r$ 的公式，从所获得的角膜曲率半径推断角膜屈光力。其中 D 是以屈光度为单位的角膜屈光力；n 是角膜折射率，其值为 1.3375，经验导出的"标准化"角膜折射率考虑到了角膜内面负屈光力；r 是角膜曲率半径（以 m 为单位）。**A.**Javal-Schiøtz 式角膜曲率计采用固定双像系统，并且光标分离是可变的。**B.**Bausch + Lomb 式角膜曲率计采用可变双像系统，并且光标大小是恒定的。*（译者注：资料来源见前页英文原文。）*

传统的角膜曲率仅测量角膜的 1 个子午线的直径约为 3mm 的区域，没有地形图所提供的精细细节。

自动角膜曲率计与自动焦度计和自动验光仪的原理类似，测量的是反射光的偏转量。

角膜地形图

与角膜曲率计不同，角膜地形图是整个角膜表面形状的详细图。最初，角膜地形图仅限于角膜前表面的分析，其主要技术是基于 Placido 盘原理（图 8-5）。计算机化的 Placido 盘式角膜地形图，评估同心发光环的环形光标的反射（图 8-6）。更准确地说，它通过测量环之间的距离，可以计算角膜的高度，并且显示为角膜表面的彩色屈光彩图（也参见 BCSC 第 13 册《*屈光手术*》）。

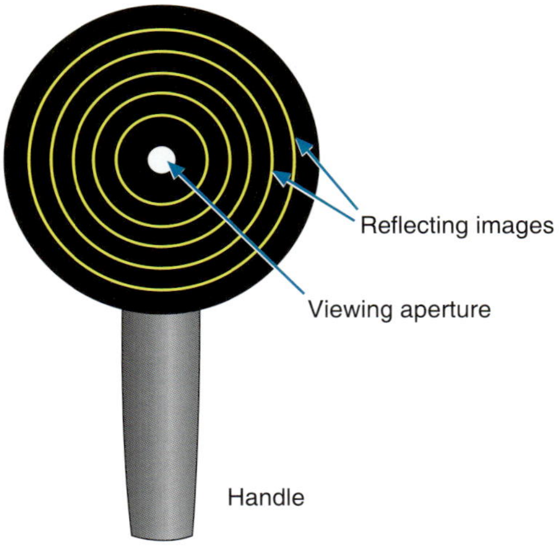

Figure 8-5 A Placido disk. *(Courtesy of Neal H. Atebara, MD. Redrawn by C. H. Wooley.).*

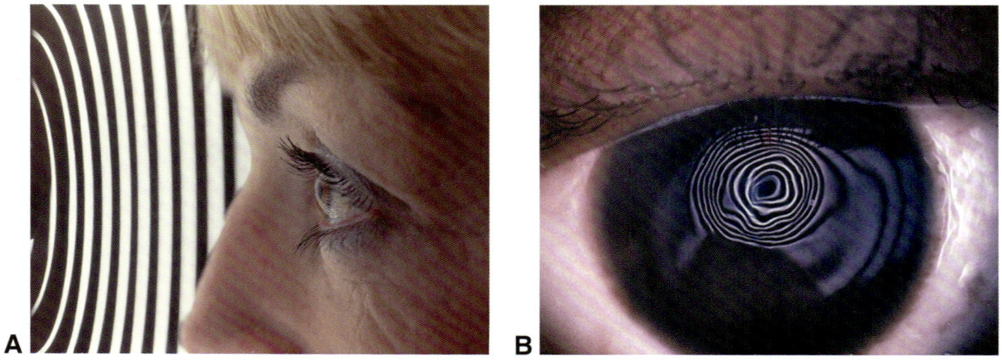

Figure 8-6 Computerized Placido disk–based topography of the cornea. **A**, The ring reflections of the Placido disk–based topographer can be seen on this patient's cornea. This image is then captured and analyzed. **B**, Image of distorted mires on a cornea with keratoconus. *(Courtesy of M. Bowes Hamill, MD.)*

Technological advances enable the characterization of both the anterior and posterior corneal surfaces. These alternative techniques are actually "tomography"-based (and therefore are also suited for corneal pachymetry) and derive topography information via elevation measurements from cross-sectional images of the cornea obtained photographically. They involve the projection of slit beams of light that scan the cornea and either use a stereo-triangulation method (slit-scanning technique), or a camera that rotates perpendicular with the slit beams, to capture the illuminated corneal cross sections. The latter, known as the *Scheimpflug principle or Scheimpflug camera*, corrects for the nonplanar shape of the cornea and, thus, enables "distortion-free" imaging.

Wavefront Aberrometers

Corneal topography can measure the shape of the surface of an irregular cornea, but it cannot measure the actual refractive topography of the entire lens–cornea optical system. For such measurements, instruments traditionally used in astronomy to measure optical distortions, or *wavefront aberrations*, induced by the inhomogeneous and turbulent earth atmosphere, have been applied to the examination of the human eye. These instruments are called *wavefront* aberrometers or simply *aberrometers*.

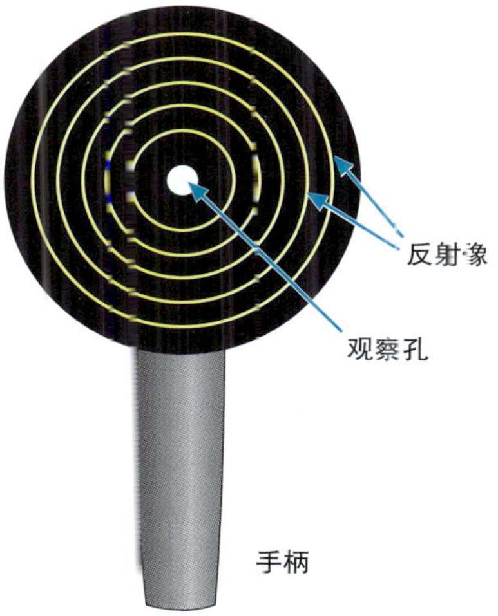

图 8–5　Placido 盘 *（译者注：资料来源见前页原文。）*

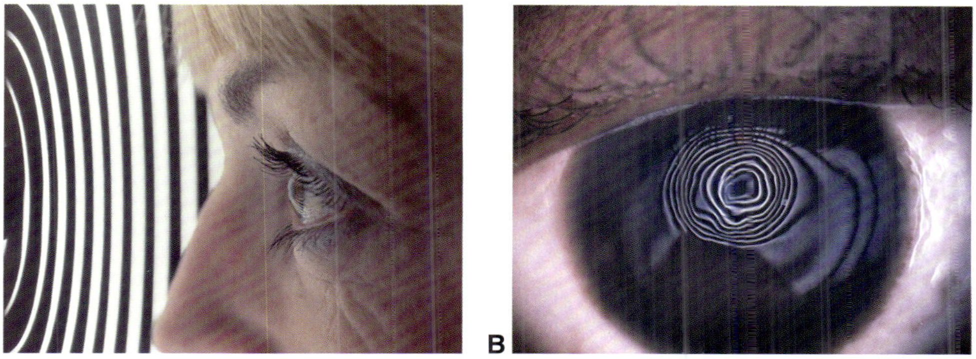

图 8–6　计算机化的 Placido 盘式角膜地形图。**A.** 可以在该患者的角膜上看到 Placido 盘式地形图的环形反射，然后捕获并分析该图像。**B.** 圆锥角膜上的扭曲的光标像。*（译者注：资料来源见前页英文原文。）*

技术的进步使角膜前表面和角膜后表面的特征得以显现。这些替代技术实际上是基于“断层扫描”的原理（因此也是适用于角膜厚度测量的方法），并且通过照相获得的角膜横截面图像的高度，测量得出角膜地形图信息。通过投射的狭缝光束，扫描角膜；采用立体三角测量方法（狭缝扫描技术），或者与狭缝光束垂直旋转的相机，以捕获照射的角膜横截面。后者称为 *Scheimpflug 原理*或 *Scheimpflug 相机*，可矫正角膜的非平面形状，从而实现“无失真”成像。

波前像差仪

角膜地形图可以测量不规则角膜表面的形状，但它不能测量整个晶状体－角膜光学系统的实际屈光地形图。为此，人们将天文学测量地球大气不均匀和湍流引起的光学畸变或*波前像差*的仪器，应用于人眼检查。这些仪器被称为*波前像差仪*或简称为*像差仪*。

Wavefront aberrometers are essentially ray-deflection autorefractors (the prototype of which was the Scheiner disk) that measure the deflection of light rays passing through many pupil locations, rather than just a few locations sufficient to determine only spherocylindrical errors of the eye, as described previously in the section on autorefractors.

For ophthalmic applications, the most popular method employed for wavefront aberrometry is Hartmann-Shack aberrometry, which was first demonstrated by Josef Bille and colleagues in 1994.

Before getting into the details of the underlying principles, let us first review the nature of a wavefront. It is an artificial construct connecting points in a light ray bundle of equal travel time from a common source. This is perhaps best understood in the example of water waves, as illustrated in Figure 8-7. The perfect wavefront shown on the top nicely illustrates that, in general, wavefronts are perpendicular to the ray direction. The concept of wavefront aberrations is simulated on the bottom, where we can see an irregular wavefront that becomes distorted by a floating twig.

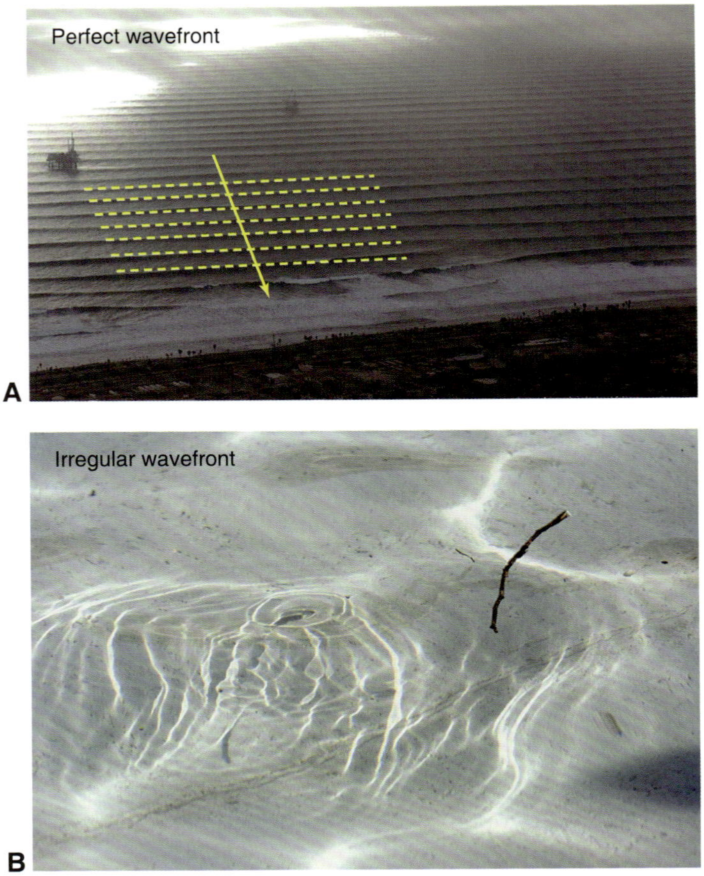

Figure 8-7 Pictorial explanation of wavefront aberrations by means of water waves. **A**, A perfect, regular wavefront is shown. **B**, An irregular wavefront is shown that became distorted by a floating twig. *(Part A by Sang Pak, modified by Kristina Irsch, PhD. Part B by Alain Vagner.)*

波前像差仪基本上是射线偏转自动验光仪（其原型是 Scheiner 盘），其测量穿过瞳孔位置的多束光线的偏转，而不是仅以几个位置确定眼睛的球柱屈光误差，如“自动验光仪”一节所述。

对于眼科应用，最常用的波前像差测量方法是 Hartmann–Shack 像差测量法，这是 Josef Bille 及其同事在 1994 年首次证明的方法。

在深入了解基本原理之前，让我们首先回顾一下波前的本质。它是一种认为的构想，将来自同源的、行进时间相同的光线束中的点连接起来。在水波的例子中可以最好地理解这一点，如图 8–7 所示。A 图中显示的理想波前很好地说明了波前通常垂直于光线方向。在 B 图中模拟波前像差的概念，在那里我们可以看到被浮动树枝扭曲变形的不规则波前。

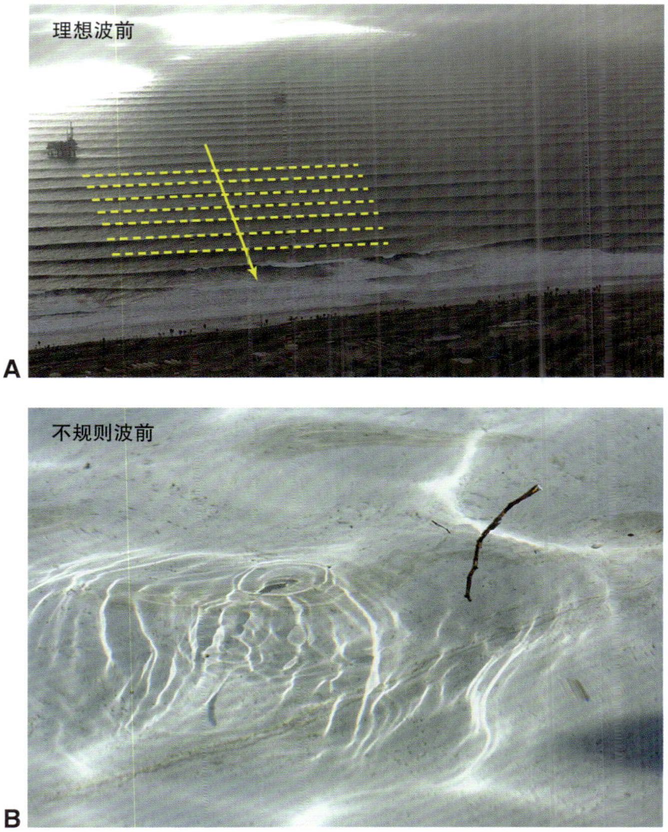

图 8–7 通过水波对波前像差进行的图解说明。**A.** 显示了理想的规则波前。**B.** 显示出不规则的波前，它被浮动的树枝扭曲。*（译者注：资料来源见前页英文原文。）*

In Hartmann-Shack aberrometry, ocular wavefront distortions are measured using a Hartmann-Shack wavefront sensor (Fig 8-8), which consists of a micro-lenslet array and a charge-coupled device (CCD) camera. A micro-lenslet array is a lattice of tiny lenses that can be thought of as a multifaceted lens, like an insect eye (Fig 8-9). An object imaged through such a lens results in multiple images of the same object arranged in an array. For example, in aberrometry, the light reflected out of the eye is partitioned into multiple beams by the micro-lenslet array, forming multiple images of the same retinal spot on the CCD camera. An ideal eye produces a perfect emerging wavefront and thus a regular array of spot images, with each image falling on the grid produced by the optical center of each facet of the multi-lenslet array (Fig 8-10A). An eye with aberrations, however, produces an irregular wavefront and thus an irregular array of spot images, displaced from where they should otherwise fall on the grid (Fig 8-10B). From the displacement of each spot, the shape of the wavefront can be reconstructed and represented in the form of a 2-dimensional wavefront map.

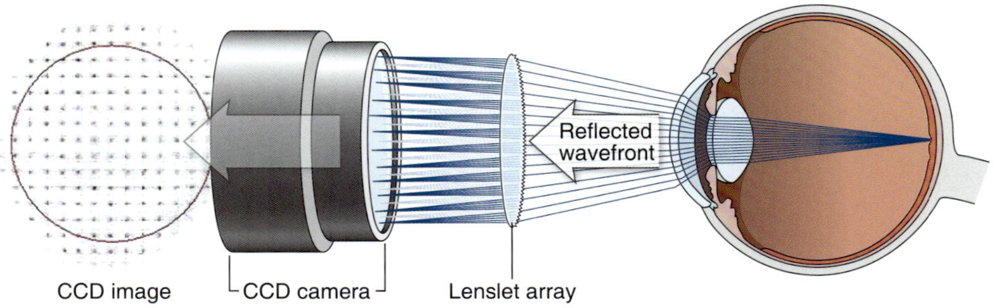

Figure 8-8 Schematic of a Hartmann-Shack wavefront sensor. In Hartmann-Shack aberrometry, wavefront distortions are measured using a Hartmann-Shack sensor (HSS) that consists of a micro-lenslet array and a charge-coupled device (CCD) camera. *(Redrawn by Mark Miller from a schematic image courtesy of Abbott Medical Optics.)*

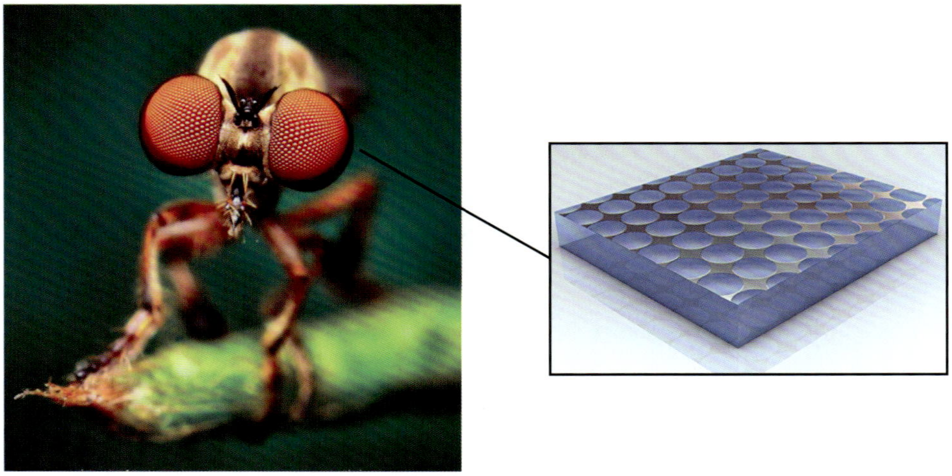

Figure 8-9 Pictorial explanation of a micro-lenslet array (*right*) by means of an insect eye (*left*). *(Courtesy of Thomas Shahan, modified by Kristina Irsch, PhD; inset reproduced with permission from Axetris AG.)*

在 Hartmann–Shack 像差测量中，使用 Hartmann–Shack 波前传感器（图 8–8）测量眼波前畸变，该传感器由微小透镜阵列和电荷耦合器件（CCD）相机组成。微小透镜阵列是微小透镜的晶格，可以被认为是多面透镜，如昆虫眼（图 8–9）。通过这种透镜成像的物体形成了以阵列排列的相同物体的多个像。例如，在像差测量中，通过微小透镜阵列将从眼睛反射的光分割成多个光束，从而在 CCD 照相机上形成有相同视网膜斑点的多个像。理想的眼睛产生理想的新波前，因此产生规则的点像阵列，每个像落在由多小透镜阵列的每个小平面的光学中心产生的网格上（图 8–10A）。然而，具有像差的眼睛产生不规则的波前，因此产生不规则的点像阵列，从它们应该落在网格上的位置处移位（图 8–10B）。根据每个光斑的位移，可以重建波前的形状并以二维波前图的形式表示。

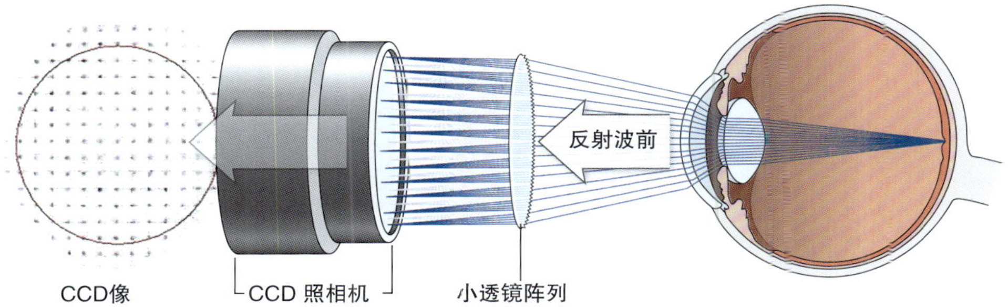

图 8–8　Hartmann–Shack 波前传感器的示意图。在 Hartmann–Shack 像差测量中，使用 Hartmann–Shack 传感器（HSS）测量波前畸变，该传感器由微小透镜阵列和电荷耦合器件（CCD）相机组成。*（译者注：资料来源见前页英文原文。）*

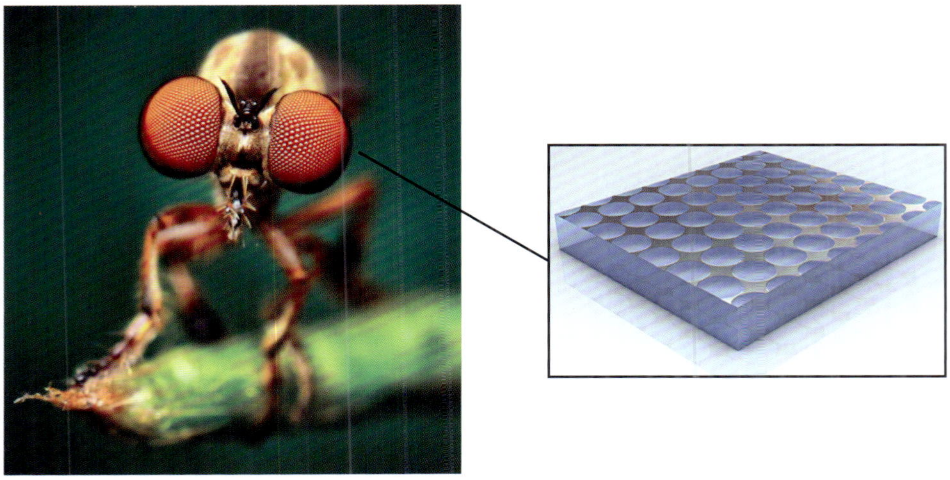

图 8–9　通过昆虫眼 *（左）* 对微小透镜阵列 *（右）* 进行图解说明。*（译者注：资料来源见前页英文原文。）*

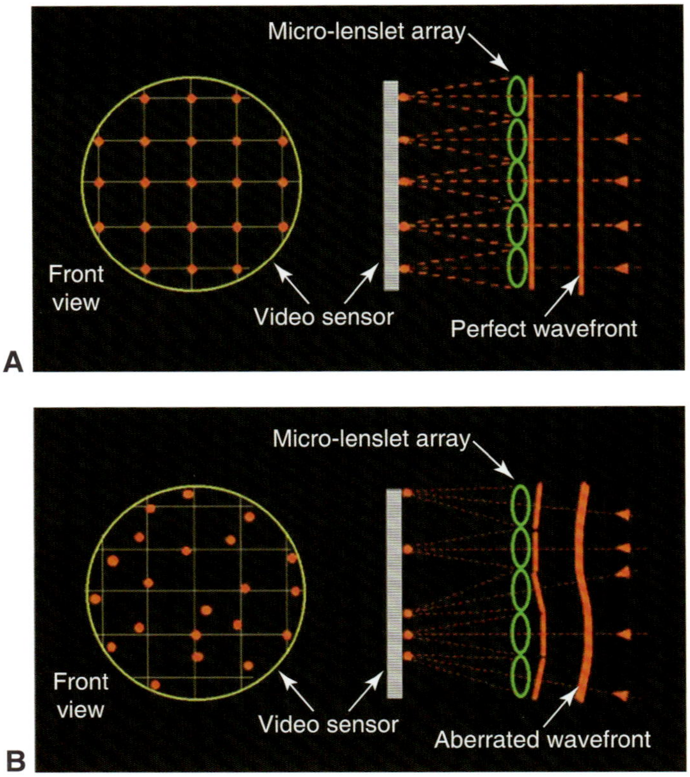

Figure 8-10 An object imaged through a multi-lenslet array. In aberrometry, the light reflected out of the eye is divided into multiple beams by the micro-lenslet array, forming multiple images of the same retinal spot on the charge-coupled device (CCD) camera or video sensor. **A**, An ideal eye produces a perfect undistorted emerging wavefront and thus a regular array of spot images, with each image falling on the grid produced by the center of each facet of the multi-lenslet array. **B**, An aberrated eye produces a distorted wavefront and thus an irregular array of spot images, displaced from where they should otherwise fall on the grid. *(Illustration reproduced from Thibos LN. Principles of Hartmann-Shack aberrometry. J Refract Surg. 2000;16(5):S563–S65.)*

Liang J, Grimm B, Goelz S, Bille JF. Objective measurement of wave aberrations of the human eye with the use of a Hartmann–Shack wave-front sensor. *J Opt Soc Am A Opt Image Sci Vis.* 1994;11(7):1949–1957.

Anterior- and Posterior-Segment Imaging

Slit-Lamp Biomicroscope

As with many ophthalmic instruments, it is instructive to consider the illumination and viewing systems of the slit-lamp biomicroscope separately. The illumination system is a light source that is restricted by an adjustable aperture producing a slit of variable height, width, and orientation, to produce an optical section through the eye. The viewing system is a binocular stereomicroscope with individually focusable eyepieces. To vary the magnification of the viewing system, there may be a Galilean magnification changer, a rotating drum of Galilean telescopes that can be oriented either forward to provide higher magnification or backward to provide lower magnification. Alternatively, there may be 2 sets of eyepieces or objective lenses, or a zoom system in which lenses are moved back and forth to change the magnification.

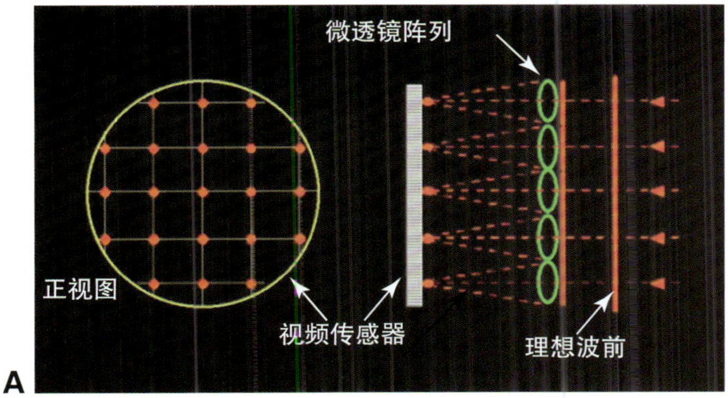

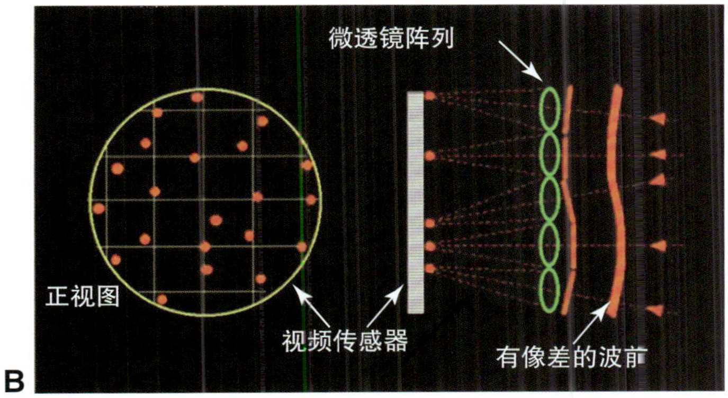

图 8–10　通过多小透镜阵列成像的物体。在像差测量中，通过微小透镜阵列将从眼睛反射的光分成多个光束，在电荷耦合器件（CCD）照相机或视频传感器上形成有相同视网膜斑点的多个像。**A.** 理想的眼睛产生理想的无畸变波前，因此产生规则的点像阵列，每个像落在由多小透镜阵列的每个小平面的中心产生的网格上。**B.** 具有像差的眼睛产生扭曲波前，因此产生不规则的点像阵列，从它们应该落在网格上的位置处移位。*（译者注：资料来源见前页英文原文。）*

Liang J, Grimm B, Goelz S, Bille JF. Objective measurement of wave aberrations of the human eye with the use of a Hartmann–Shack wave-front sensor. *J Opt Soc Am A Opt Image Sci Vis.* 1994;11(7):1949–1957.

前段和后段成像

裂隙灯生物显微镜

与许多眼科仪器一样，分别从裂隙灯生物显微镜的照明和观察系统来了解裂隙灯生物显微镜。照明系统是可调节孔径的限制光源，产生高度、宽度和方向可变的狭缝光源，形成透过眼睛的光学切面。观察系统是双目立体显微镜，具有可单独聚焦的目镜。Galileo 放大率变换器和 Galileo 望远镜的旋转鼓可以改变观察系统的放大倍数，后者向前转动时放大率增高，向后转动时放大率降低。还有 2 组目镜或物镜，或变焦系统，使其前后移动镜头来改变放大率。

The illumination system and the viewing system with its various levels of magnification are mounted on separate arms. In ordinary usage, these rotate about the same vertical axis in a parfocal arrangement, so that they both focus precisely over a common pivot point. This arrangement allows the examiner to study the eye in *direct illumination*. Purposefully separating the illumination and viewing arms from their coupled alignment to horizontally and/or vertically decenter the beam allows for *indirect illumination*. Variations of these illumination techniques allow for examination of the anterior segment in a variety of ways, some of which are described next and illustrated in Figure 8-11 (see also BCSC Section 8, *External Disease and Cornea*).

Examination Techniques

- *Direct focal illumination*. This is the most commonly used examination technique, in which the examiner focuses on the area directly illuminated by the slit (Fig 8-11A).
- *Retroillumination*. The beam can be decentered, so that it is striking the iris, with the examiner focusing with the microscope in front, on the cornea, for example. This enables the observer to see corneal opacities illuminated against the black pupil by the reflected light from the iris (iris retroillumination). As another example, by shining the beam through the edge of the pupil, one can observe opacities in the cornea, iris, and lens retroilluminated by the reflected light from the fundus (fundus retroillumination; Fig 8-11B).
- *Sclerotic scatter*. The slit beam is decentered so that it strikes the junction between sclera and cornea, causing light to be totally internally reflected, like a fiberoptic light pipe (Fig 8-11C). In this manner, light follows its longest possible path through the cornea and makes nebular opacities more visible against a dark pupil background.
- *Specular reflection*. By looking directly at the bright reflection of the slit beam under high magnification, the examiner can observe irregularities in the corneal surface and see the endothelial cell pattern (Fig 8-11D; this is the principle underlying specular microscopy).

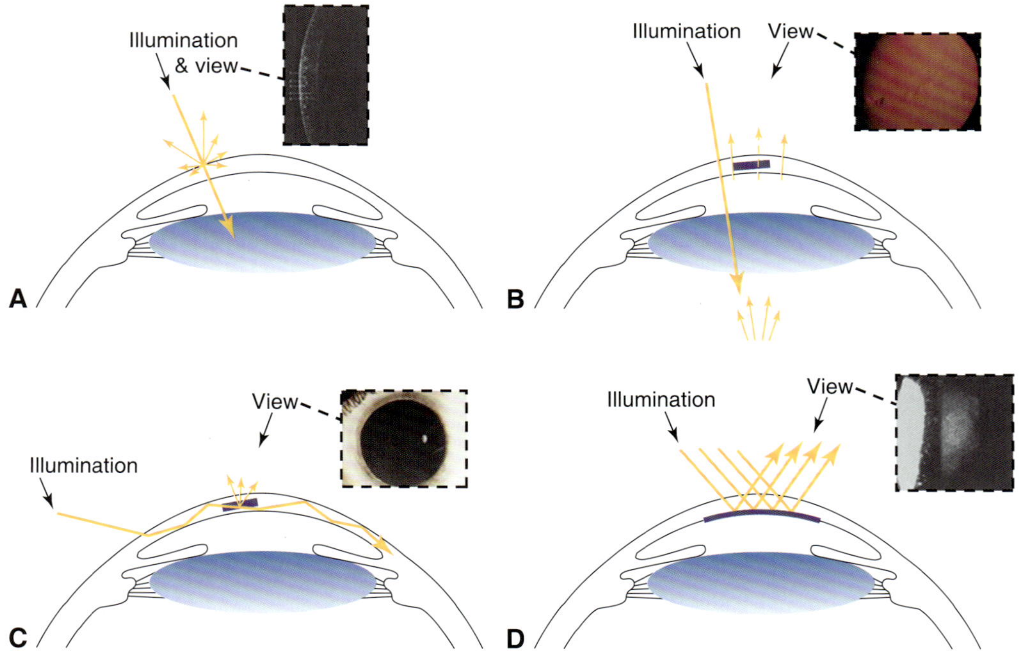

Figure 8-11 Examination techniques with the slit-lamp biomicroscope. **A**, Direct illumination. **B**, Retroillumination. **C**, Sclerotic scatter. **D**, Specular reflection. *(Illustration by Kristina Irsch, PhD.Insets in A–D reproduced with permission from Krachmer JH, Mannis MJ, Holland EJ, eds. Cornea. 2nd ed. Vol 1. Philadelphia: Elsevier/Mosby; 2005:201-217. © CL Mártonyi, WK Kellogg Eye Center, University of Michigan.)*

具有各种放大水平的照明系统和观察系统安装在单独的臂上，通常以等焦面的方式围绕相同的垂直轴旋转，可精确地聚焦在共同的轴心点上。这样，检查者可以用*直接照明*观察眼睛。有目的地将照明和观察臂从它们的耦合对齐分开，呈水平和（或）垂直偏心，进行*间接照明*。这些照明技术的变化便于各种方式的前段检查，如下所述。在图 8–11 中示出（也参见 ECSC 第 8 册《*外眼疾病与角膜*》）。

检查技巧

- *直接焦点照明*。这是最常用的检查技术，检查者专注于狭缝直接照射的区域（图 8–11A）。
- *后映照*。光束可以偏心，照射到虹膜上，检查者用显微镜聚焦在角膜上，通过来自虹膜（虹膜逆向照射）的反射光看到黑瞳孔背景下的角膜混浊。另一种方法是，将光束照射在瞳孔边缘，可以观察到眼底后映照光背景下（眼底逆向照射，见图 8–11B）的角膜、虹膜和晶状体的混浊。
- *巩膜散射*。狭缝光束偏心照射在巩膜和角膜的连接处，使光线完全内部反射，就像光纤光管一样（图 8–11C）。光沿着角膜到达混浊部位，使其在瞳孔暗背景下清晰可见。
- *镜面反射*。通过在高放大倍数下直接观察狭缝光束的明亮反射，检查者可以观察角膜表面的不规则性，以及内皮细胞形态（见图 8–11D，这是内皮显微镜的原理）。

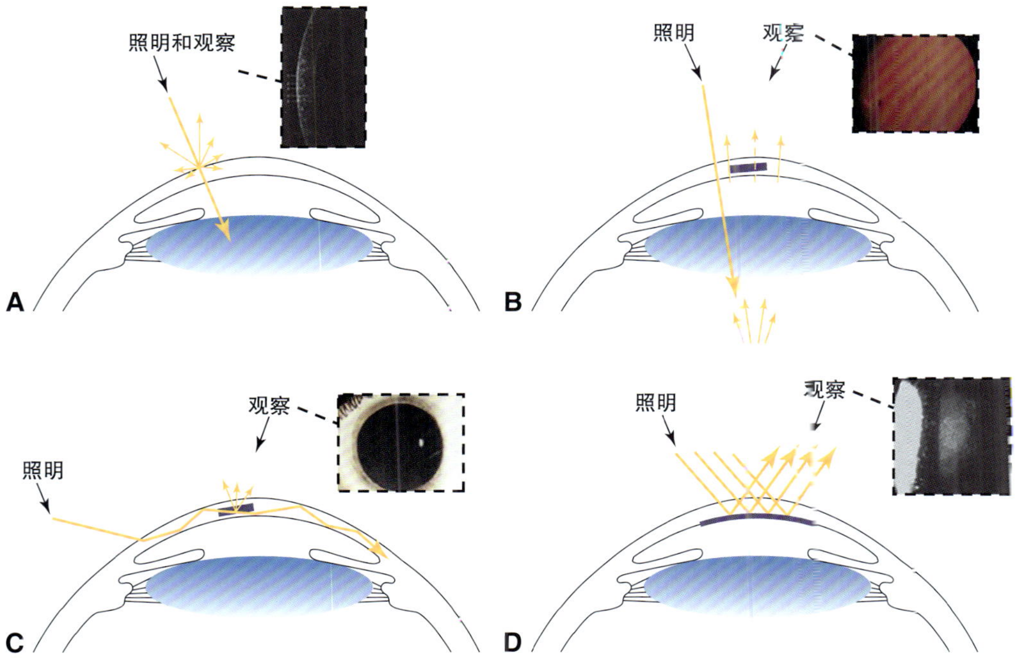

图 8–11　裂隙灯生物显微镜检查技术。**A.** 直接照明。**B.** 后映照。**C.** 巩膜散射。**D.** 镜面反射。*（译者注：资料来源见前页英文原文。）*

There are several attachments for the slit lamp that extend its use beyond these examination techniques,some of which are described below.

Applanation Tonometry

In tonometry, the intraocular pressure (IOP) of an eye is measured. In Goldmann applanation tonometry specifically, performed with an attachment to the slit lamp, IOP is inferred from the amount of force required to flatten an area of 3.06 mm in diameter on the cornea.

Applanation tonometry is based on Newton's third law of motion, in particular that the pressure (ie, force per surface area) inside the eyeball equals the force applied to its surface divided by the area of contact. This assumes that the eye is infinitely thin-walled, perfectly elastic, and dry, none of which hold true, producing 2 confounding forces: (1) a force generated by the eye's corneal rigidity (because the eye is not infinitely thin-walled or perfectly elastic), which is directed away from the globe; and (2) a force generated by the surface tension of the tear film (because the eye is not dry), which is directed toward the globe. Hans Goldmann determined empirically that if enough force is applied to produce a circular area of flattening 3.06 mm in diameter, the opposing forces caused by scleral rigidity and surface tension cancel each other out, allowing the pressure in the eye to be inferred from the force applied.

The head of the applanation tonometer, which is placed against the patient's cornea, creating a tear film meniscus, contains split-field prisms that split the magnified image of tear film meniscus into 2 (like the image doubling associated with keratometry) separated by exactly 3.06 mm. The tear film is often stained with fluorescein dye and viewed under a cobalt blue light to enhance the visibility of the resultant yellow/green circle of tears. The examiner adjusts the applanation pressure until the half circles are aligned so that their inner margins just touch one another (Fig 8-12). At this point, the circle is exactly 3.06 mm in diameter, and the reading on the tonometer (multiplied by a factor of 10, as it is measured in dynes of force) represents the IOP in millimeters of mercury.

Several factors, especially central corneal thickness, can substantially affect the accuracy of applanation tonometry (see BCSC Section 10, *Glaucoma*).

Surgical Microscope

The operating microscope works on principles similar to those of the slit-lamp biomicroscope. The illumination source of the operating microscope, unlike that of the slit-lamp biomicroscope, is not slit-shaped, and the working distance for the operating microscope is longer to accommodate the specific requirements of ocular surgery. The illumination is said to be "coaxial." However, it is technically paraxial rather than coaxial (Fig 8-13), as the viewing apertures and illumination path are separated in modern operating microscopes.

裂隙灯有几个附件，其使用范围超出了这些检查技术，其中一些如下所述。

压平眼压计

眼压计用于测量眼内压（IOP）。将 Goldmann 压平眼压计连接到裂隙灯上，眼内压是通过在角膜上压平直径为 3.06 mm 的区域所需的力推断的。

压平眼压计的工作原理是基于 Newton 第三运动定律，特别是眼球内部的压力（即每表面积所受的力）等于施加于其表面的力除以接触面积，这里假设眼球壁无限薄、全弹性和干燥。但对于人眼而言这种假设并没有真实存在，并且会产生 2 个混淆力：①由眼睛角膜刚性所产生的力（因为眼睛不是无限薄壁或完全弹性的），这个力离开眼球；②由泪膜的表面张力（因为眼睛并不是干燥的）所产生的力，其朝向眼球。Hans Goldmann 根据经验确定，如果施加足够的力以产生直径为 3.06 mm 的圆形平坦区域，则由巩膜刚性和表面张力引起的相反力将相互抵消，进而可以从施加的力推断眼内压力。

压平眼压计的头部，靠着患者的角膜放置，形成泪膜半月板，包含分裂区域棱镜，将泪膜半月板的放大图像分成 2 个（就像与角膜曲率测量相关的图像倍增一样），并正好相隔 3.06 mm，泪膜通常用荧光素染料染色并在钴蓝光下观察，以增强所得的黄色 / 绿色泪环的可见度。检查者调整压平压力，直到半圆对齐，使其内边缘恰好相互接触（图 8–12）。此时，圆的直径正好为 3.06 mm，而眼压计上的读数［乘以系数为 10，因为它以力的达因数来衡量（1dyn=10^{-5}N）］表示以 mmHg 为单位的眼内压。

多个因素，尤其是中央角膜厚度影响压平眼压测量的准确性（参见 BCSC 第 10 册《*青光眼*》）。

手术显微镜

手术显微镜的工作原理类似于裂隙灯生物显微镜。与裂隙灯生物显微镜不同的是，手术显微镜的照明源不是裂隙的，并且手术显微镜的工作距离更长，以适应眼科手术的特定要求。照明路径被称为“同轴”，但在技术上是近轴的（图 8–13），因为观察孔和照明路径在现代手术显微镜中是分开的。

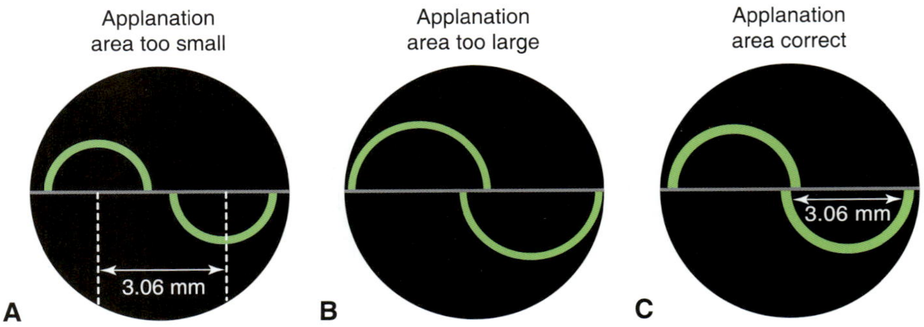

Figure 8-12 The split prism in the applanation head creates 2 offset images. **A**, When the area of applanation is smaller than 3.06 mm, the arms of the inner semicircles remain some distance apart. **B**, When the area of applanation is greater than 3.06 mm, the arms of the inner semicircles overlap. **C**, When the area of applanation is exactly 3.06 mm, the arms of the inner semicircles just touch each other. This is the endpoint for measuring intraocular pressure. The value of 3.06 mm was chosen to approximately balance tear-film surface tension and corneal rigidity. *(Courtesy of Neal H. Atebara, MD. Redrawn by C. H. Wooley.)*

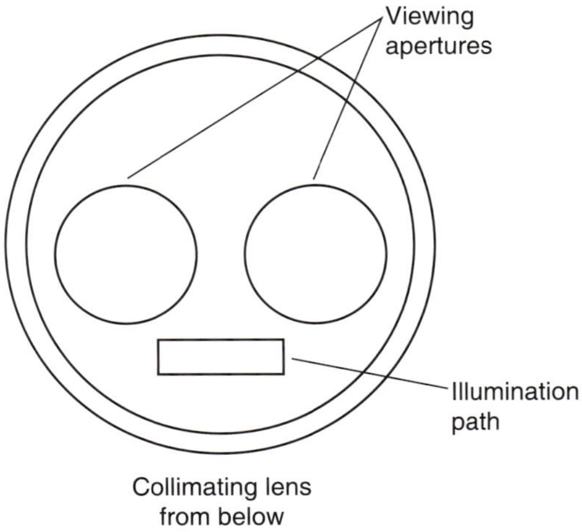

Figure 8-13 Illumination and viewing paths of the surgical microscope as seen from below the collimating lens, demonstrating paraxial rather than coaxial illumination. *(Reproduced from Guyton DL, et al. Ophthalmic Optics and Clinical Refraction. Baltimore: Prism Press; 1999. Illustration modified by Kristina Irsch, PhD.)*

Specular Microscopy

Specular microscopy is a modality for examining endothelial cells that uses specular reflection from the interface between the endothelial cells and the aqueous humor. The technique can be performed using contact or noncontact methods. In both methods, the instruments are designed to separate the illumination and viewing paths so that reflections from the anterior corneal surface do not obscure the weak reflection arising from the endothelial cell surface.

As we learned earlier, endothelial cells can also be visualized through a slit-lamp biomicroscope, if the illumination and viewing axes are symmetrically displaced on either side of the normal line to the cornea (see Fig 8-11D). A narrow illumination slit must be used; hence, the field of view is narrow.

Contact specular microscopy allows for higher magnifications than slit-lamp biomicroscopy, making cellular detail and endothelial abnormalities more discernible and allowing for cell counting as well as the study of morphology (see also BCSC Section 8, *External Disease and Cornea*).

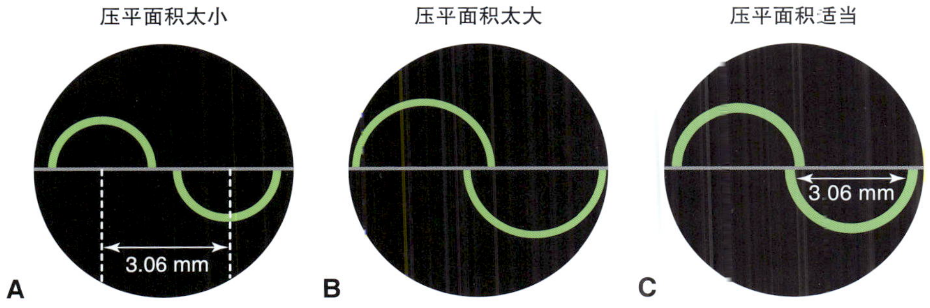

图 8–12　压平眼压计头部的分裂棱镜产生的 2 个偏移图像。**A.** 当压平直径小于 3.06 mm 时，内半圆的臂保持一定距离。**B.** 当压平直径大于 3.06 mm 时，内半圆的臂重叠。**C.** 当压平直径正好为 3.06 mm 时，内半圆的臂部恰好相互接触。这是测量眼压的终点。应选择压平直径为 3.06 mm 的值以近似平衡泪膜表面张力和角膜刚度。*（译者注：资料来源见前页英文原文。）*

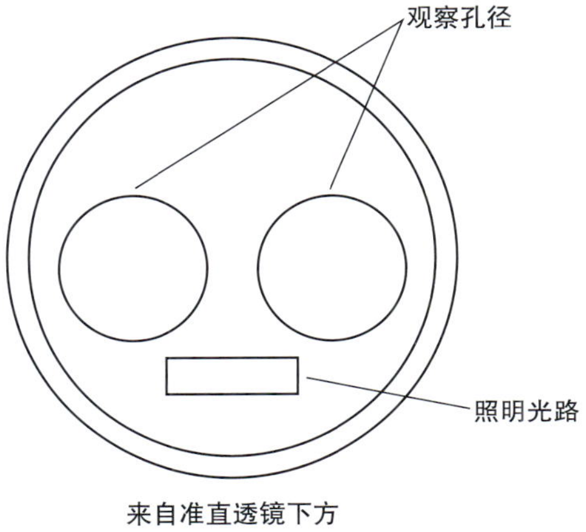

图 8–13　从准直透镜下方看到的手术显微镜的照明和观察路径，证明了照明路径是近轴的而不是同轴的。*（译者注：资料来源见前页英文原文。）*

镜面反射显微镜（内皮镜）

镜面反射显微镜是检查内皮细胞的仪器，其使用来自内皮细胞和房水之间界面的镜面反射来检查内皮细胞，可以使用接触或非接触方法来实现该技术。在这 2 种方法中，仪器被设计成分离照明和观察路径，使得来自前角膜表面的反射不会影响内皮细胞表面的弱反射。

如前所述，如果光照和视轴在角膜法线的两侧对称位移，也可以通过裂隙灯生物显微镜观察内皮细胞（图 8–11D），须用狭窄的照明，因而其获得的视野较狭窄。

接触镜面反射显微镜比裂隙灯生物显微镜的放大倍数更高，可使细胞的细微结构和异常更加明显，并可以进行细胞计数以及形态学研究（另见 BCSC 第 8 册《外眼疾病与角膜》）。

Auxiliary Lenses for Slit-Lamp Examination of the Retina

The cornea and lens together provide so much convergence that ordinarily we cannot see the retina using a slit-lamp biomicroscope. At most, the slit lamp could view about half of the way back from the crystalline lens to the retina, and usually no more than one third of the way. Auxiliary lenses for slit-lamp examination of the retina can be placed in front of the eye to overcome this problem. Table 8-1 lists common auxiliary lenses for slit-lamp examination of the retina.

The Goldmann 3-mirror contact gonioscopy lens is a special viewing lens that is widely used for looking at the eye with the slit lamp. With a power of about −64 D, it essentially nullifies the power of the eye (recall that the eye itself has about 60 D of plus power) and provides an upright view of the posterior pole. The mirrors inside the contact lens enable alternative (left-right reversed) views of more and less peripheral portions of the eye, and even of the angle of the anterior chamber (Fig 8-14; gonioscopy). The main disadvantage of the Goldmann lens is its limited field of view requiring rotation of the lens to visualize more than a small patch of the fundus.

Table 8-1 Auxiliary Lenses for Slit-Lamp Examination of the Retina

Lens	Field of View	Image Magnification	Laser Beam Magnification
Goldmann-style 3-mirror contact lens	60°/66°/76°	1.06×	0.94×
Posterior pole contact contact lens[a]	70°/84°	1.06×	0.94×
Wide field contact lens[b]	110°/132°	0.7×	1.4×
Very wide field contact lens[c]	120°/144°	0.51×	1.97×
60D noncontact lens	68°/81°	1.15×	0.87×
90D noncontact lens	74°/89°	0.76×	1.32×

[a] For example, Volk Area Centralis, Mainster Focal Grid.
[b] For example, Volk TransEquator, Mainster Wide Field.
[c] For example, Volk QuadrAspheric, Mainster PRP 165.

Other examples of contact lenses for the slit-lamp biomicroscope are the fundus contact lenses from manufacturers such as Volk (Mentor, OH) or Ocular Instruments (Bellevue, WA). Examples include the Area Centralis lens for viewing the central fundus, and the QuadrAspheric and TransEquator lenses that enable peripheral wide-angle views of the retina.

Holding a high-power plus lens (eg, 60 D or 90 D fundus lenses) in front of the eye, produces an inverted aerial image of the retina,which can be viewed with the slit lamp in a manner similar to performing "indirect ophthalmoscopy" (Fig 8-15).

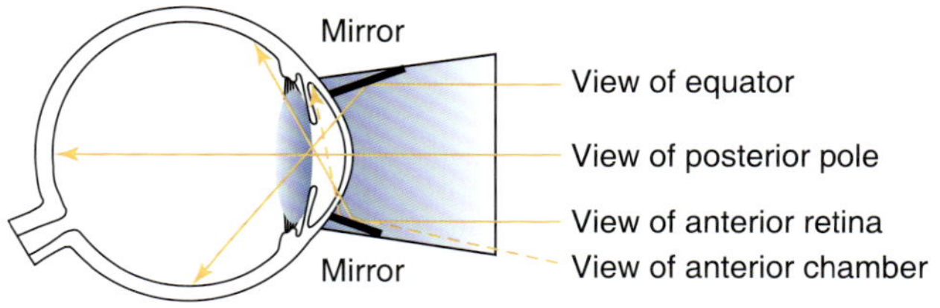

Figure 8-14 Goldmann 3-mirror contact lens. The flat-front contact lens essentially nullifies the power of the eye and provides an upright view of the posterior pole. The mirrors at various angles inside enable alternative (inverted) views of different parts of the retina and the anterior chamber angle (gonioscopy). *(Reproduced from Guyton DL, et al. Ophthalmic Optics and Clinical Refraction.Baltimore: Prism Press; 1999. Illustration modified by Kristina Irsch, PhD.)*

用于视网膜裂隙灯检查的辅助镜片

由于角膜和晶状体会产生很强的光线会聚，我们无法使用裂隙灯生物显微镜观察视网膜，仅可以观察晶状体到视网膜的 1/2 深度，通常不超过 1/3。可将视网膜裂隙灯检查的辅助镜片置于眼睛前方观察视网膜。表 8–1 列出了用于视网膜裂隙灯检查的常用辅助镜片。

接触式 Goldmann 三面镜房角镜是一种特殊的观察镜，广泛用于裂隙灯。有约为 –64 D 的屈光力，基本上中和了眼屈光力（回想一下，眼睛本身具有约 60 D 的正屈光力），并且后极成直立像；接触镜内的镜面的眼周边成像则是替代视图（左右反转），还有前房角视图（见图 8–14，前房角镜检查）。Goldmann 镜的主要缺点是其视野有限，需要转动镜子来观察一小块眼底。

表8–1　裂隙灯下观察视网膜所需的辅助镜

镜片	视野	放大率	照射放大率
接触式Goldmann三面镜	60°/66°/76°	1.06×	0.94×
后极接触镜[a]	70°/84°	1.06×	0.94×
广角接触镜[b]	110°/132°	0.7×	1.4×
超广角接触镜[c]	120°/144°	0.51×	1.97×
60D 非接触镜	68°/81°	1.15×	0.87×
90D 非接触镜	74°/89°	0.76×	1.32×

a.例如，Volk Area Centralis, Mainster Focal Grid.
b.例如，Volk Trans Equator, Mainster Wide Field.
c.例如，Volk Quadr Aspheric, Mainster PRP165.

用于裂隙灯生物显微镜的接触镜还有 Volk（Mentor，OH）或 Ocular Instruments（Bellevue，WA）等制造商生产的接触镜，包括用于观察中央眼底的 Area Centralis 透镜，以及 QuadrAspheric 透镜和 TransEquator 透镜，能够对视网膜进行周边广角观察。

眼前置高度数正透镜（例如 60 D 或 90 D 的接触镜），产生视网膜倒像，可以进行裂隙灯下的“间接检眼镜”检查（图 8–15）。

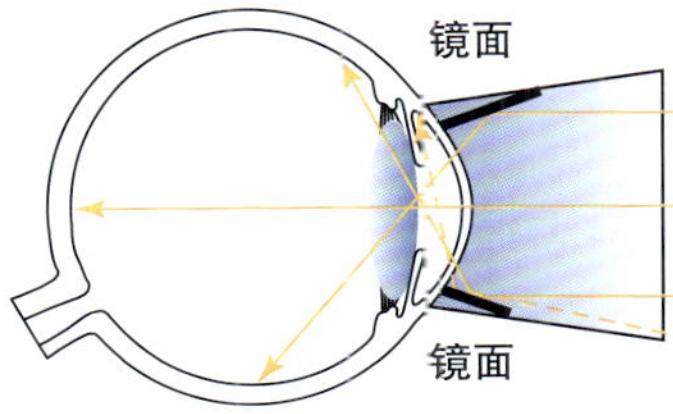

图 8–14　Goldmann 三面镜。前平面镜基本上抵消了眼睛的屈光力，并且可得到后极的直立正像。可以用不同角度内置镜（倒置）变换观察视网膜和前房角（房角镜）。*（译者注：资料来源见前页英文原文。）*

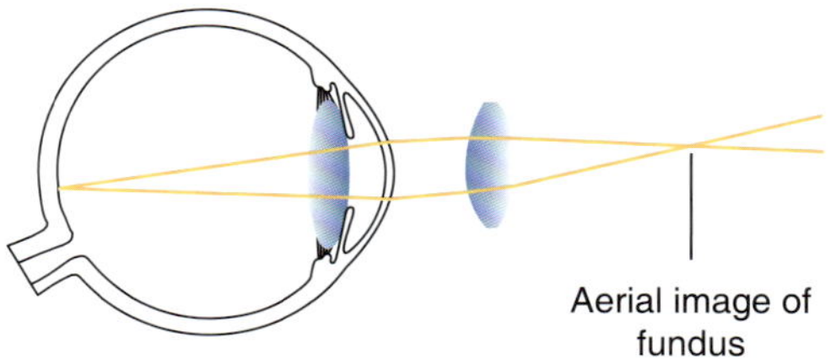

Figure 8-15 High-power plus lenses for slit-lamp indirect ophthalmoscopy (eg, 60 D and 90 D fundus lenses) held in front of the eye produce an inverted aerial image of the retina within the focal range of a slit-lamp biomicroscope. *(Reproduced from Guyton DL, et al. Ophthalmic Optics and Clinical Refraction. Baltimore: Prism Press; 1999. Illustration modified by Kristina Irsch, PhD.)*

Ophthalmoscopy

An ophthalmoscope is an instrument for viewing the retina and associated tissues—the ocular fundus. It consists of 3 essential elements: a source of illumination, a method of reflecting the light into the eye, and an optical means of correcting an unsharp image of the fundus. Imaging of the fundus is carried out either by direct or indirect ophthalmoscopy.

Direct ophthalmoscope

With direct ophthalmoscopy, the examiner uses the optics of the patient's eye as a simple magnifier to look at the retina. If both the examiner and patient have emmetropic vision and are not accommodating, rays of light coming from a point on the patient's retina exit parallel, with zero vergence, and continue through the empty peephole of the direct ophthalmoscope. These parallel rays of light are then focused onto the examiner's retina. Thus, the examiner's retina becomes conjugate to the patient's retina when a direct ophthalmoscope is used.

When the examiner looks through the peephole of a direct ophthalmoscope, with no lenses in place, just past the edge of (or aperture in) a mirror that reflects light into the patient's eye, almost coaxial to the examiner's view, an upright, virtual, magnified retinal image is seen. The optics of the emmetropic normal eye are approximately +60D, so using the formula for a simple magnifier, the magnification is 60/4, or 15× (Fig 8-16). This means that the patient's retina appears 15 times larger than if the retina were removed from the eye and held at 25 cm. Only a small field of view is seen with the direct ophthalmoscope (about 7°) because, even when being as close to the patient as possible, the peripheral rays that are coming from the peripheral part of the patient's retina cannot be captured, as they do not enter the examiner's pupil (Fig 8-17).

If the patient or examiner has an uncorrected spherical refractive error, a series of auxiliary lenses is available to dial into the path of the direct ophthalmoscope for compensation. If the patient's eye is myopic, a minus lens is dialed in, to overcome the extra plus power "error lens" inside the patient's eye. Those 2 lenses create a Galilean telescope effect, increasing magnification and decreasing the field of view. Similarly, the retina of a hyperopic eye will be magnified less than 15× because of the reverse Galilean telescope created by the minus power error lens inside the patient's eye and the plus lens of the direct ophthalmoscope.

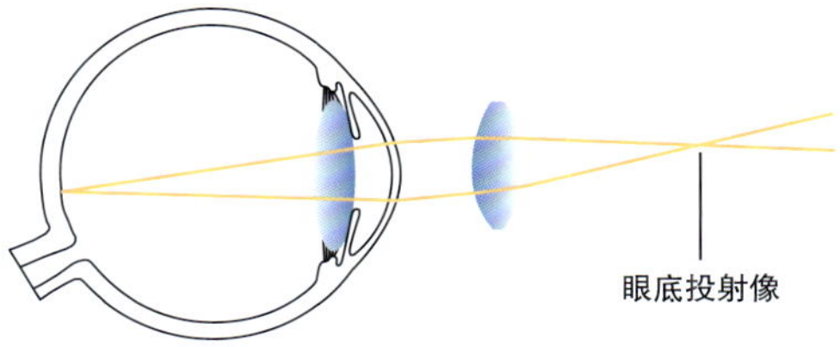

图 8–15　高度数的凸透镜（例如 60D 和 90D 的检眼镜）。将高度数的凸透镜加在眼前，在裂隙灯的焦距范围下式倒立的视网膜像。*（译者注：资料来源见前页英文原文。）*

检眼镜

检眼镜是一种观察眼底视网膜及相关组织的仪器。它由 3 个基本要素组成：一个光源，一种将光线重新反射到眼睛中的方法，以及一种矫正眼底非清晰前的像的光学方法。眼底的成像是通过直接或间接检眼镜检查进行的。

直接检眼镜

直接检眼镜如同一个放大镜，使得检查者可以直接观察患者的视网膜。如果检查者和患者都是正视眼，并且无调节，那么从患者的视网膜上的一点发出光线呈平行、无会聚光线，通过直接检眼镜的窥视孔，这些平行的光学将直接聚焦到检查者的视网膜上。因此，检查者的视网膜和患者的视网膜成为共轭关系。

当检查者从直接检眼镜的窥视孔看过去的时候，在没有矫正镜片的情况下，正好经过镜子的边缘（或孔径）反射光进入患者的眼睛，几乎与检查者同轴，检查者可以看到一个直立的放大虚像。一个正视眼的光学度数约为 +60 D，所以用公式表达这个简单的放大镜，其放大率为 60/4（15 ×）（图 8–16）。这就是说当直接检眼镜在离患者的眼 25 cm 的距离时，患者的视网膜被放大了约 15 倍。通过直接检眼镜，只能观察到很小的视野（约为 7°），因为即使检查者尽量靠近患者的眼睛，从患者视网膜周边部发出的平行光线，也不能通过检查者的瞳孔而被捕捉到（图 8–17）。

如果患者或检查者有未矫正的屈光不正，可将一组辅助透镜组成的刻度盘置于直接检眼镜检视路作为矫正补偿。如果患者是近视，可以拨入负镜片，矫正患者过多“错误的”正屈光力。这 2 个镜片将产生 Galileo 远镜效应，即增加放大率、减少视野。同理，根据反向 Galileo 望远镜效应，远视眼的视网膜放大率小于 15 ×，因为患者眼睛的负屈光力中和了部分直接检眼镜的正透镜度数。

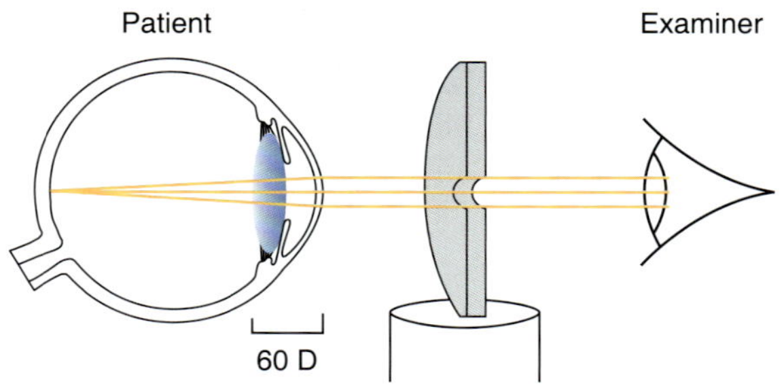

Figure 8-16 Magnification of direct ophthalmoscopy. With direct ophthalmoscopy the examiner basically uses the optics of the patient's eye as a simple magnifier to look at the retina. The optics of the emmetropic eye are approximately +60 D, thus the magnification is 60/4, or 15×, according to the formula for a simple magnifier. *(Reproduced from Guyton DL, et al. Ophthalmic Optics and Clinical Refraction. Baltimore: Prism Press; 1999. Illustration modified by Kristina Irsch, PhD.)*

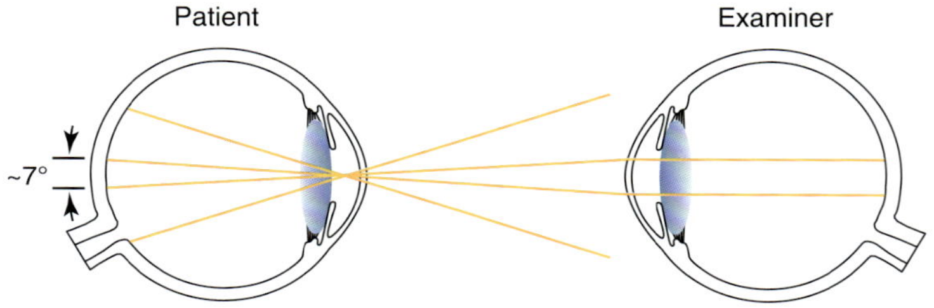

Figure 8-17 Field of view with direct ophthalmoscopy. Even when being as close to the patient as possible, the peripheral rays that are coming from the peripheral part of the patient's retina do not enter the examiner's pupil, restricting the field of view to about 7°. *(Reproduced from Guyton DL,et al. Ophthalmic Optics and Clinical Refraction. Baltimore: Prism Press; 1999. Illustration modified by Kristina Irsch, PhD.)*

Indirect ophthalmoscope

In indirect ophthalmoscopy, an ophthalmic "condensing" lens is used to increase the field of view, by capturing the peripheral rays (that are lost in direct ophthalmoscopy) and bringing them into the examiner's pupil (Fig 8-18). Thus, a much wider field of view is seen with the indirect ophthalmoscope (eg, about 25° with an ordinary 20 D condensing lens).

Assuming that the patient's eye has normal vision, rays of light coming from a point on the patient's retina leave the eye with zero vergence and are gathered and focused by the condensing lens into what is called an intermediate *aerial image*; that is, an image of the patient's retina in space. In case of a 20 D condensing lens, this image is located one-twentieth of a meter closer to the examiner, who therefore sees an optically real, inverted image of the patient's retina that appears to be 5 cm closer to the examiner's eye than the 20 D lens. With the examiner looking at that aerial image, it will be focused on the examiner's retina. Thus, in indirect ophthalmoscopy, the patient's retina, the aerial image, and the examiner's retina are all conjugate to each other.

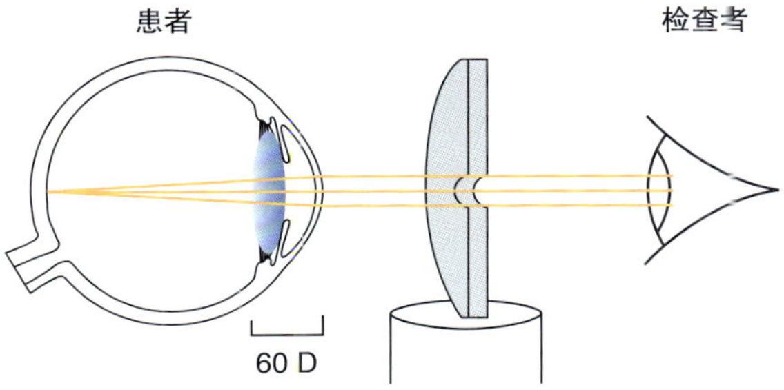

图 8–16　直接检眼镜的放大倍数。直接检眼镜的原理是检查者将患者的眼睛作为一个简单的光学放大镜，观察患者视网膜。一个正视眼的光学度数约 +60 D，用一个简单的计算公式可以得到其放大度数为 60/4（15x）。*（译者注：资料来源见前页英文原文。）*

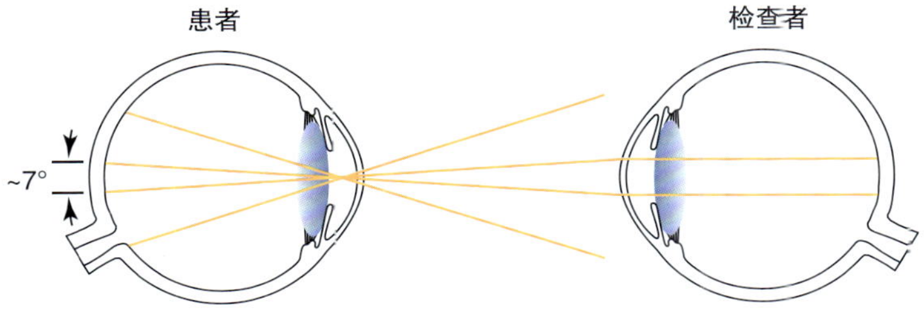

图 8–17　直接检眼镜检查的视野。即使尽可能地靠近患者，来自患者视网膜周边部分的周边光线也不会进入检查者的瞳孔，这将视野限制在了大约 7° 的范围内。*（译者注：资料来源见前页英文原文。）*

间接检眼镜

在间接检眼镜中，使用眼科“聚光”透镜增加视野，它通过捕获周边光线（在直接检眼镜中丢失的），并将其带入检查者的瞳孔（图 8–18）。因此，间接检眼镜可以观察到更大的视野（例如，20 D 的聚光透镜可形成大约为 25° 的视野）。

假设患者的眼睛视觉正常，从患者视网膜上的某一点射出的光线会以零聚散度离开眼睛，通过聚光透镜形成*中间投射像*，即患者视网膜在空间形成的像。20 D 透镜的像位于检查者 1/20m 处，因此检查者能够看到患者视网膜的倒立实像，该像比 20 D 的透镜离检查者眼睛的距离近 5cm。当检查者看那个投影像时，它会聚焦在检查者的视网膜上。因此，在使用间接检眼镜进行检查时，患者的视网膜、空间中的视网膜像和检查者的视网膜都是相互共轭的。

The most important conjugate planes in indirect ophthalmoscopy, however, are the cornea and the faceplate of the indirect ophthalmoscope (Fig 8-19). The main purpose of the condensing lens, other than the purpose of forming the aerial image, is to make the faceplate of the indirect ophthalmoscope conjugate to the patient's cornea, so that the bright illumination light passes at a different place through the cornea, offset from where the examiner's pupils are looking, to avoid reflections back from the cornea into the examiner's eyes. This is very important because the cornea reflects about 2% of the light, but the observed retinal image is only 0.1% of the light. Thus, the retina cannot be seen if any light from the cornea is reflected back into the observation pathway. Therefore, in indirect ophthalmoscopy, the light pathway is separated from the observation pathway by imaging the faceplate on the cornea with the condensing lens, so that the aerial image of the retina can be seen. The images of the observer's pupils in the plane of the cornea are very small circle—about 10% of the observer's pupil's diameters—and thus form virtual pinholes (the drawing in Figure 8-19 shows these images much larger than they are in practice). These tiny entrance pupils limit the light available for the observer to view the fundus, but also allow very clear images to be appreciated even in the presence of imperfect ocular media, such as cataracts or vitreous debris. This is a mixed blessing—it allows for better views of the fundus than can be obtained in many cases, for example, with the direct ophthalmoscope, but prevents the observer from appreciating the visual impairments caused by the media imperfections.

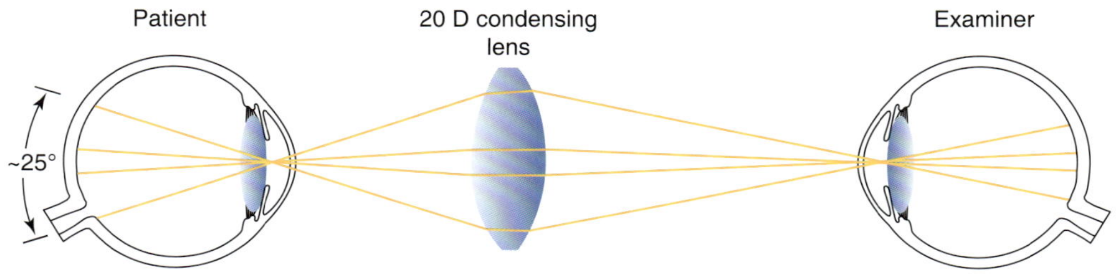

Figure 8-18 Field of view with indirect ophthalmoscopy. Unlike in direct ophthalmoscopy, the condensing lens captures the peripheral rays, enlarging the field of view to about 25° with an ordinary 20 D condensing lens. *(Reproduced from Guyton DL, et al. Ophthalmic Optics and Clinical Refraction.Baltimore: Prism Press; 1999. Illustration modified by Kristina Irsch, PhD.)*

The binocular eyepieces in the indirect ophthalmoscope, via mirrors and/or prisms, reduce the interpupillary distance from about 60 mm to 15 mm, to fit the images of examiner's pupils along with the light source within the patient's pupil, allowing for binocular viewing. (If the patient's pupil is small, the illuminating and observation pathways can be brought closer by varying the positions of mirrors or prisms in the eyepieces). This causes a reduction of the examiner's stereoscopic vision by 60/15, or 4×, which fortunately is compensated for by the axial magnification of the aerial image.

然而，间接检眼镜中最重要的共轭面板是角膜和间接检眼镜面板（图 8–19）。使用聚光透镜的主要目的是使间接检眼镜的面板与患者的角膜共轭，而不是形成投射像，因此，要使明亮的照明光通过角膜的不同位置，与检查者的瞳孔所看到的位置偏离，以避免光从角膜反射回检查者的眼睛。这是非常重要的，因为角膜反射大约 2% 的光，但是观察到的视网膜像仅占光的 0.1%。因此，如果从角膜中有任何光反射回观察路径，就无法看到视网膜。因此，在间接检眼镜中，利用聚光透镜对角膜上的面板成像，将光路与观察光路分离，从而可以看到视网膜的投射像。观察者在角膜平面上的瞳孔像是个非常小的圆，大约是观察者瞳孔直径的 10%，因此形成了虚的针孔（图 8–19 中的图显示的这些图像比实际的图像要大得多）。这些微小的入口使瞳孔限制了观察者观察眼底的光线，但也使得眼屈光介质混浊（如白内障或玻璃体碎片）的情况下可以看到非常清晰的像。这具有双重优点——与直接检影镜等许多其他情况相比，可以更好地观察眼底，还可以不受屈光介质混浊的影响来观察眼底。

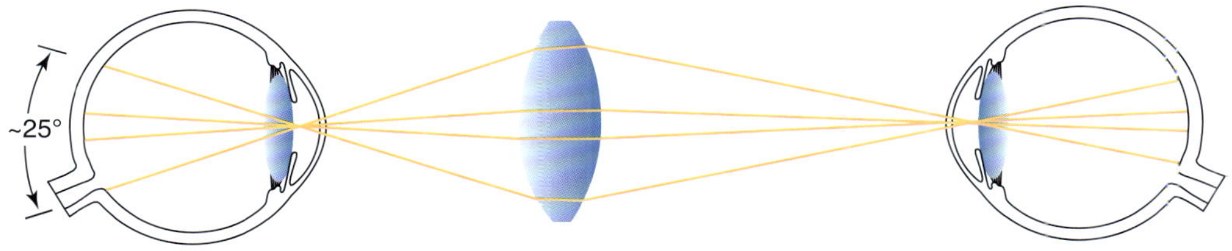

图 8–18　间接检眼镜的视野。不同于直接检眼镜，聚光透镜捕捉周边光线，普通的 20 D 透镜的视野扩大到约为 25°。*（译者注：资料来源见前页英文原文。）*

间接检眼镜中的目镜，通过反射镜和（或）棱镜将瞳孔间距离从约为 60 mm 减少到 15 mm，以适应检查者的瞳孔像以及患者瞳孔内的光源，从而允许其双目观看。（如果患者的瞳孔小，可以通过改变镜或棱镜在目镜中的位置使照明和观察路径更近）。这导致了检查者的立体视觉减少 60/15（4 ×），但可以通过投射像的轴向放大来补偿。

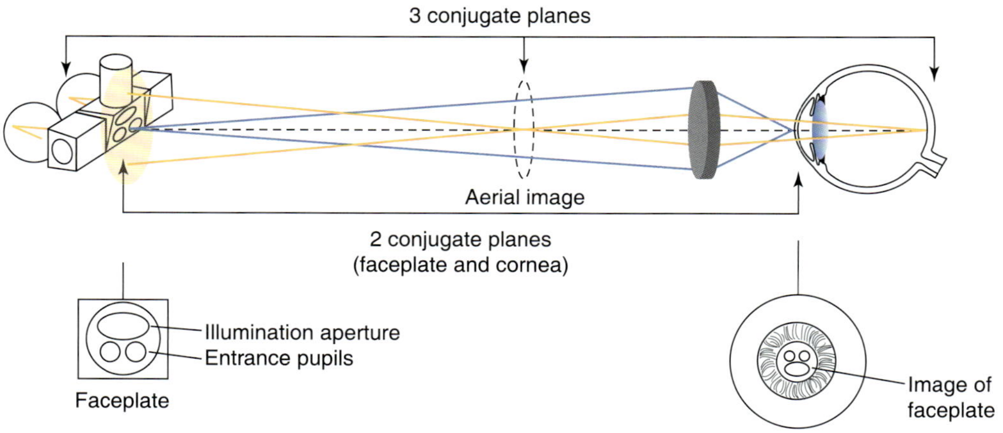

Figure 8-19 Conjugate planes in indirect ophthalmoscopy. The patient's retina, the aerial image, and the examiner's retina, as well as the faceplate of the indirect ophthalmoscope and the patient's cornea, are conjugate to each other when performing indirect ophthalmoscopy. *(Reproduced from Guyton DL, et al. Ophthalmic Optics and Clinical Refraction. Baltimore: Prism Press; 1999. Illustration redrawn by Kristina Irsch, PhD.)*

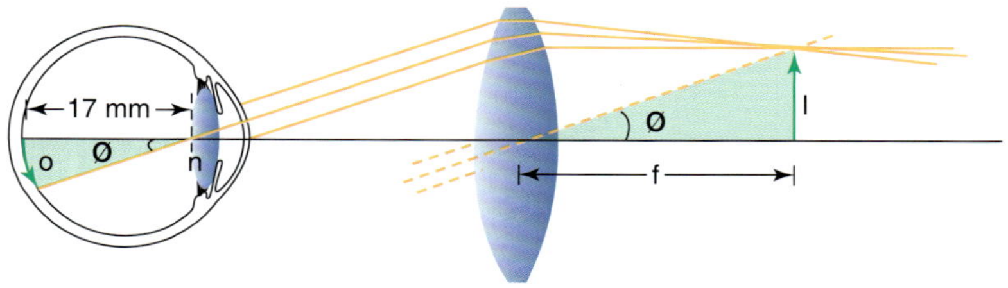

Figure 8-20 Magnification of the aerial image in indirect ophthalmoscopy. For an emmetropic eye, by similar triangles, transverse magnification equals the focal length of the condensing lens divided by the focal length of the eye in air, and therefore the power of the eye divided by the power of the condensing lens. *(Reproduced from Guyton DL, et al. Ophthalmic Optics and Clinical Refraction. Baltimore: Prism Press; 1999. Illustration modified by Kristina Irsch, PhD.)*

To appreciate this, let's look at the transverse magnification of the aerial image, which turns out to be the power of the eye divided by the power of the condensing lens (see Fig 8-20), that is 60/20, or 3×, for an emmetropic eye and a 20 D condensing lens. The aerial image is thus wider than the actual object on the retina. Recall that the axial magnification is the square of the transverse (lateral or linear) magnification, that is, in our case 9×. The image that is observed is thus greatly distorted in depth, which helps make up for the loss in stereoacuity due to the reduced interpupillary distance. The eyepieces reduce depth fourfold, so the overall axial magnification is 9/4, or 2.25×. Thus, things are observed 3 times wider and 2.25 times increased in depth. Other choices of condensing lens power result in different ratios of transverse and lateral magnification.

However, the threefold transverse magnification of the aerial image is not the overall transverse magnification of indirect ophthalmoscopy. The overall transverse magnification depends upon the distance from which the aerial image is observed. From about 40 cm, from where it is usually observed, the overall transverse magnification is about 3×25/40, or 1.87, with the 20 D condensing lens (Fig 8-21), much less compared to a direct ophthalmoscope, which provided 15× magnification (see Fig 8-16). In summary, small details are observed with the direct ophthalmoscope that cannot be seen with the indirect ophthalmoscope.

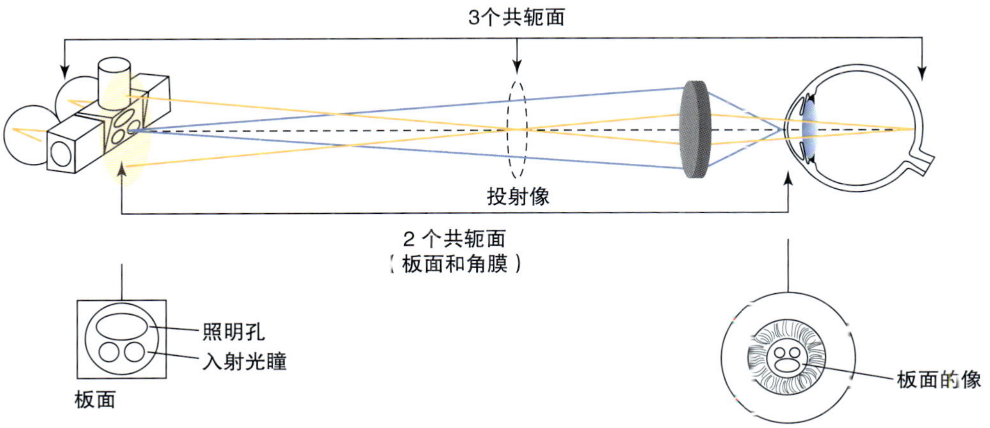

图 8-19　间接检眼镜的共轭平面。在进行间接检眼镜检查时，患者的视网膜、投射像和检查者的视网膜以及间接检眼镜面板和患者的角膜彼此共轭。*（译者注：资料来源见前页原文。）*

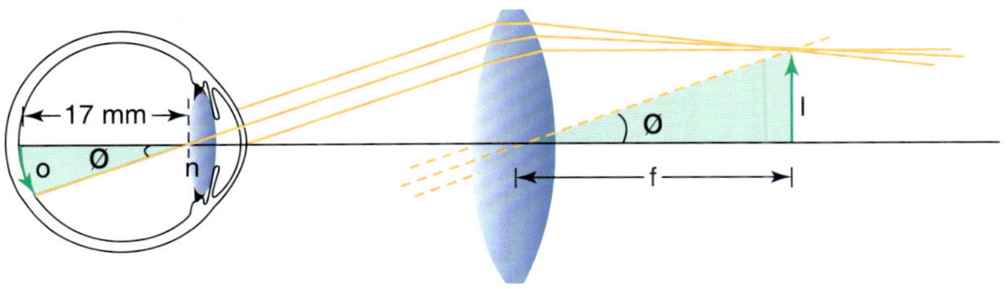

图 8-20　间接检眼镜检查中投射像的放大倍数。对于正视眼，通过类似的三角形，横向放大率等于聚光透镜的焦距除以眼睛在空气中的焦距，因此眼睛的焦距除以聚光透镜的焦距。*（译者注：资料来源见前页原文。）*

为了理解这一点，让我们来看看投射像的横向放大率，即是眼睛的屈光力除以透镜的屈光力（参见图 8-20），对于正视眼（60 D）和使用 20D 凸透镜，相对于 60/20（3×）。因此，投射像比视网膜上的实际物体更宽。回想一下，轴向放大率是横向（侧向或线性）放大倍数的二次方，也就是说，在这种情况下是 9×。因此，所观察的像在深度上严重失真，这有助于弥补由于瞳孔间距离减小而造成的立体视觉损失。目镜深度减少至 1/4，因此轴向放大倍数为 9/4（2.25×）。因此，观察到的东西的宽度增加至 3 倍，深度增加至 2.25 倍。另外，聚光透镜的屈光力的选择导致横向放大倍率和侧向放大倍数的比率不同。

然而，投射像的 3 倍横向放大率不是间接检影镜总的横向放大倍数。总的横向放大率取决于观察投射像的距离。距观察的地方大约为 40 cm，用 20 D 凸透镜，总的横向放大率大约为 3×25/40（1.87×）（图 8-21），相比而言，远小于直接检影镜提供了 15 倍的放大倍数（图 8-16）。综上所述，用间接检眼镜观察不到直接检眼镜的细节。

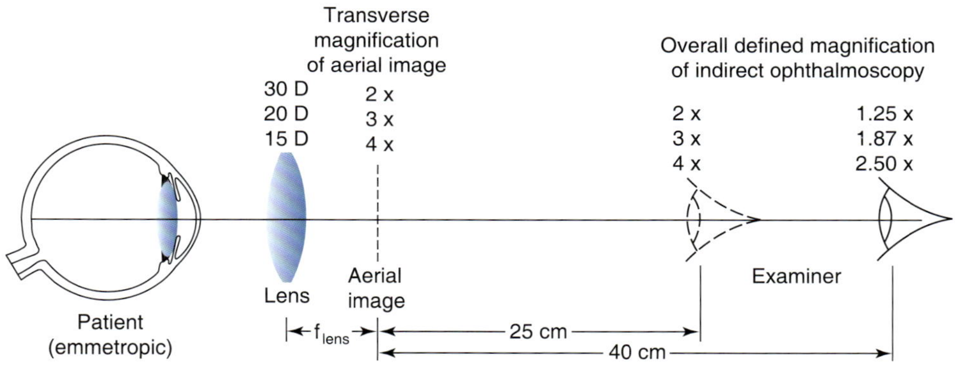

Figure 8-21 Overall magnification of indirect ophthalmoscopy with different condensing lenses depends on the distance from which the aerial image is observed. From about 40 cm, from where it is usually observed, the overall magnification is about 1.87×, with the 20D condensing lens. *(Reproduced from Guyton DL, et al. Ophthalmic Optics and Clinical Refraction. Baltimore: Prism Press;1999. Illustration modified by Kristina Irsch, PhD.)*

Fundus Camera

The fundus camera uses the optical principles of indirect ophthalmoscopy. It is essentially an indirect ophthalmoscope with a perforated mirror taking the place of the faceplate of the indirect ophthalmoscope that separates the observation and illumination pathways, and the aerial image is simply reimaged onto the camera's film or sensor array.

With the addition of different filters, *fluorescein angiography* can be performed with the fundus camera. Fluorescein has its absorption maximum at about 490 nm, in the blue part of the spectrum, whereas the emission maximum is at about 530 nm, in the green part of the spectrum. In fluorescein angiography, an "excitation filter" permits blue light to pass and excite the fluorescein; on the return path, a "barrier filter" allows the green light to pass, but blocks the background blue light, allowing the fluorescent image to be recorded with high-resolution monochrome film or sensor array.

Scanning Laser Ophthalmoscope

The scanning laser ophthalmoscope functions as both an ophthalmoscope and a fundus camera but requires significantly less light than those conventional flood illumination systems. This is because in the scanning laser ophthalmoscope, the use of a rapidly scanning laser (eg, a 670-nm diode laser) illuminating only a small spot of retina, allows inversion of the allocation of illumination and viewing apertures used in conventional systems. In other words, unlike the ophthalmoscope or fundus camera, where illumination uses most of the pupillary area with a separate small area reserved for viewing (Fig 8-22A), the scanning laser ophthalmoscope uses the larger area for light collection ("viewing") and the smaller one for illumination (Fig 8-22B). It is this inversion that improves the optical collection efficiency, allowing lower light intensity levels to be used.

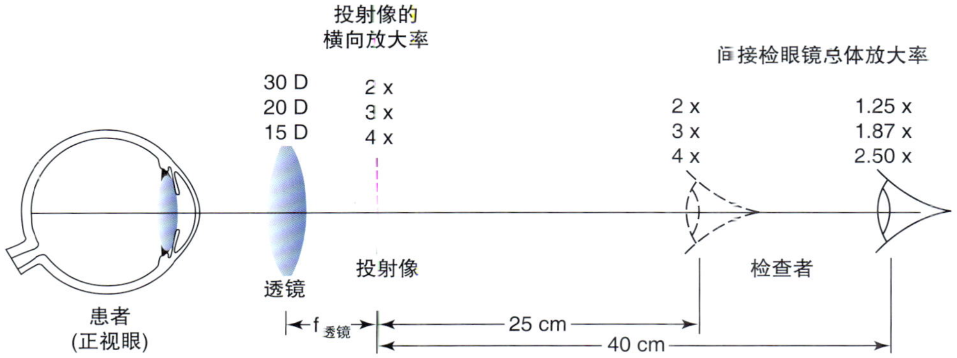

图 8–21　使用不同聚光透镜的间接检影镜的整体放大率取决于观察投射像的距离。从大约 40 cm 处，即从通常观察到投射像的地方，用 20 D 凸透镜进行检查，则整体放大率约为 1.87 ×。*（译者注：资料来源见前页英文原文。）*

眼底照相机

眼底照相机运用间接检眼镜检查的光学原理。它本质上是一种带有穿孔镜的间接检眼镜，取代了间接检眼镜的面板，从而将观察和照明路径分开，并且简单地将投射像重新成像到照相机的胶片或传感器阵列上。

使用不同的附加滤光镜，眼底照相机可以进行*荧光血管造影*。荧光素在光谱的蓝色部分的吸收峰大约为 490 nm，而在光谱的绿色部分的发射峰大约为 530 nm。在荧光血管造影中，“激发滤光片”允许蓝光通过并激发荧光素；在回路中，“阻挡滤光片”允许绿光通过，但是阻挡背景蓝光，采用高分辨率单色胶片或传感器阵列，记录荧光图像。

激光扫描检眼镜

扫描式激光检眼镜兼有检眼镜和眼底照相机的功能，但与传统的泛光照明系统相比，它需要更少的光线。这是因为在扫描激光检眼镜使用快速扫描激光（例如，670 nm 二极管激光器）只照射一小块视网膜，可以反转传统系统中使用的照明和观察孔径的分配。换句话说，与检眼镜或眼底照相机的照明灯照亮瞳孔区域的大部分，只留有单独的小区域供观看（图 8–22A）不同，扫描激光检眼镜使用较大的区域进行光收集（“观看”），而只把较小的区域用于照明（图 8–22B）。正是这种反转提高了光收集效率，允许使用较低光强的照明。

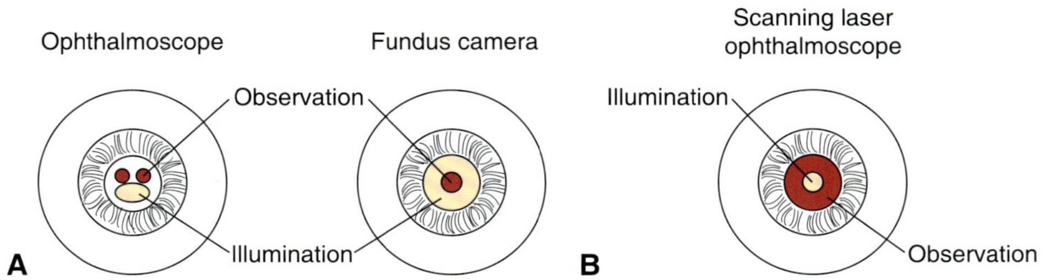

Figure 8-22 Illumination and observation path in conventional ophthalmoscopy and fundus imaging versus scanning laser ophthalmoscopy. Unlike the ophthalmoscope or fundus camera, where illumination uses most of the pupillary area with a separate small area reserved for observation **(A)**, the scanning laser ophthalmoscope uses the larger pupillary area for observation and the smaller one for illumination **(B).** *(Illustration modified by Kristina Irsch, PhD.)*

The following sections describe a few types of scanning laser ophthalmoscopes.

In a scanning laser ophthalmoscope, a highly collimated laser beam is physically moved via scanning mirrors over the retina in a grid pattern, delivering all its energy to a very small spot for a very short time. Light returned from each point is detected and synchronously decoded to produce an ocular fundus image.

Confocal scanning laser ophthalmoscope

In confocal scanning laser ophthalmoscopy, a pinhole is placed in front of the detector to cut off scattered or defocused light coming from outside the point of illumination or interest, which otherwise can blur the image (Fig 8-23). This results in a focused, high-contrast image of a single tissue layer located at the focal plane.

The position of the confocal aperture determines from which layer in the fundus the reflected light is collected, and it enables tomographic information to be extracted. More precisely, by moving the plane of the pinhole, multiple optical sections through the tissue of interest can be acquired.

The series of optical section images forms a layered 3-dimensional image and can be used to construct topography and reflectance images of the fundus. The topography image is constructed by identifying the peak intensity (reflectance) along the z-axis from all optical sections at each pixel location. The reflectance image is constructed as a summation of intensities along the z-axis from all of the optical sections at each pixel location.

Confocal scanning laser microscope

With the use of objective lenses, usually put in contact with the patient's corneal surface, the confocal scanning laser ophthalmoscope can be turned into a confocal laser scanning microscope, enabling tomography through different depths of the cornea at cellular resolution (see BCSC Section 8, *External Disease and Cornea*).

Angiography and autofluorescence imaging

The use of various wavelengths allows for additional applications with the confocal scanning laser ophthalmoscope, such as fluorescein angiography, indocyanine green angiography, and autofluorescence imaging (see also BCSC Section 12, *Retina and Vitreous*).

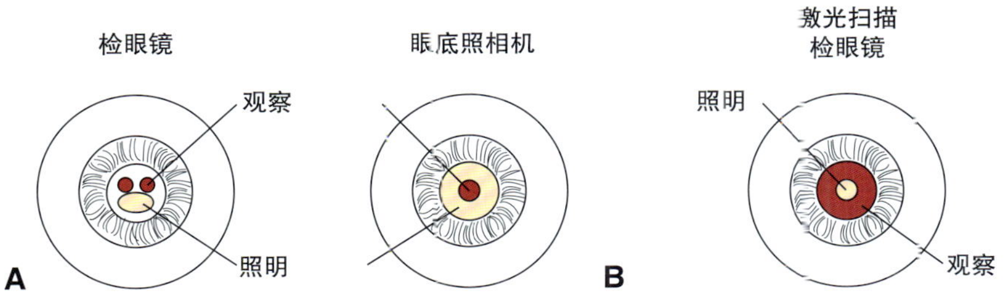

图 8–22　常规眼底检查和眼底成像与扫描激光检眼镜检查的光照和观察路径。与检眼镜或眼底照相机不同，其瞳孔区域的大部分用于照明，只保留单独的小区域用于观察（**A**），而扫描激光检眼镜则不同，其使用较大的瞳孔区域进行观察，而把较小的瞳孔区域用于照明（**B**）。*（译者注：资料来源见前页英文原文。）*

以下是部分描述扫描激光检眼镜的几种类型：

在扫描激光检眼镜中，高度准直的激光束通过扫描镜以网格图案的形式将图像物理移动在视网膜上，并将其所有能量以光斑点的形式在短时间内传送到每个网格上。每个光斑点返回的光被检测到并同步解码，再产生眼底图像。

共焦扫描激光检眼镜

在共焦扫描激光检眼镜检查中，在探测器的前面放置 1 个针孔用来切断来自照明光的散射、离焦或变形，避免产生模糊像（图 8–23）。在聚焦平面上的单个组织层可获得聚焦的高对比度像。

从眼底的哪一层收集反射光，决定了共焦孔的位置，并且它能够提取断层信息。更确切地说，通过移动针孔的平面，可以获得多层人们感兴趣的组织的光学切片。

该系列光学断层图像构成 1 个分层的三维图像，可用于构建眼底地形图和反射率图像。眼底地形图像是通过识别在光截面的每个像素沿着 z 轴的形成峰值强度（反射率）而构造的。来自光截面的每个像素沿 z 轴的光强度总和构造成反射率图像。

共焦扫描激光显微镜

通过与患者角膜表面接触的物镜，共焦扫描激光检眼镜可以变成共焦激光扫描显微镜，从而能够对不同深度的角膜形态进行细胞级的高分辨率成像（见 BCSC 第 8 册《*外眼疾病与角膜*》）。

血管造影与自荧光成像

各种波长的使用拓展了共聚焦扫描激光检眼镜的应用，例如荧光血管造影、吲哚青绿血管造影和自荧光成像（参见 BCSC 第 12 册《*视网膜与玻璃体*》）。

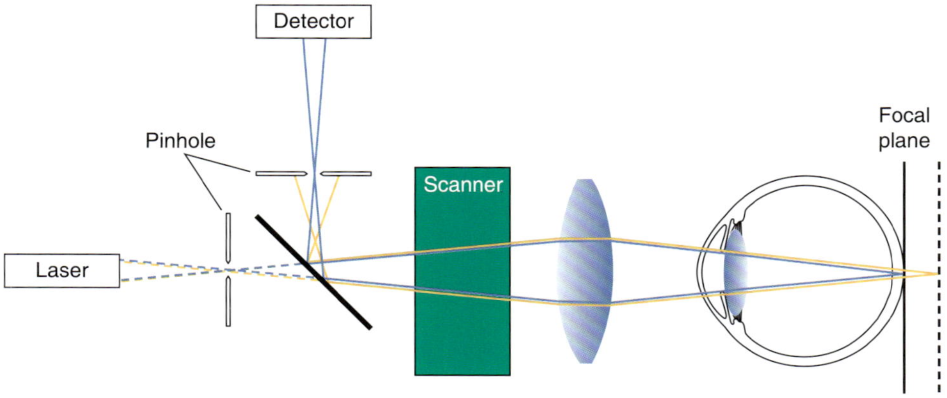

Figure 8-23 Principle of confocal laser scanning ophthalmoscopy. A pinhole aperture prevents defocused or scattered light coming from outside the focal plane, which otherwise can blur the image, from entering the detector. *(Illustration modified by Kristina Irsch, PhD.)*

For *fluorescein angiography* with the scanning laser ophthalmoscope, a blue argon laser at 488 nm is used to excite the dye, while a barrier filter at about 500 nm edge wave-length separates the excitation and fluorescent light.

The same laser is also used to generate fundus *autofluorescence* images, relying on the natural fluorescence occurring from the retinal layers, such as lipofuscin that accumulates in the retinal pigment epithelium. It may also be used (but without the use of the barrier filter) to create "red-free" or blue reflectance images, which can aid in the visualization of pathologies that have low contrast to the red color.

For *indocyanine green angiography*, on the other hand, a diode laser at 790 nm wave length is used to excite the dye, while a barrier filter at 810 nm edge wavelength separates excitation and fluorescent light.

Scanning laser polarimeter

The retinal nerve fiber layer is birefringent, which means that polarized light travels through it at different speeds depending on whether the polarization is along or across the fibers (see Chapter 2). The scanning laser polarimeter is a confocal scanning laser ophthalmoscope with an integrated ellipsometer that enables the measurement of this retardation. There is a linear relationship between the thickness of a birefringent medium and its retardation. By measuring the total retardation of the human retina point by point in a raster pattern, from the change in polarization state in the light retroreflected from the fundus, a "topographic map" of the birefringent nerve fiber layer thickness in the eye's retina can be created. This provides a quantitative method for detecting evidence of eye diseases such as glaucoma, which is characterized by loss of nerve fibers in its early state.

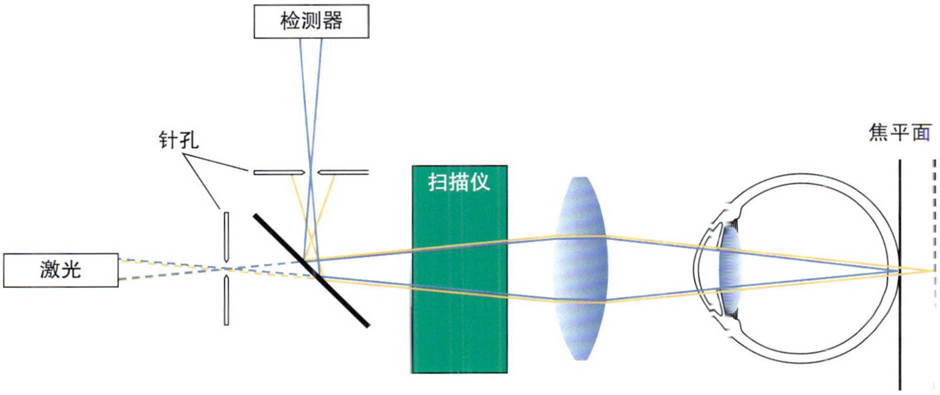

图 8 – 23　激光共聚焦检眼镜原理。针孔防止来自焦平面外部的散焦或散射光进入探测器，否则会产生模糊图像。*（译者注：资料来源见前页英文原文。）*

对于扫描激光检眼镜的*荧光血管造影*，可使用 488 nm 波长的蓝色氩激光激发荧光染料，而阻挡滤光片可将 500 nm 边缘波长的激发荧光分离。

同样的激光也被用来产生*眼底自荧光*图像，这依赖于视网膜层产生的自然荧光。例如视网膜色素上皮中积累的脂褐素。它也可以被用来（但不使用屏障过滤器）创建“无赤光”或蓝色反射率图像，这有助于与红色对比度低的病理的可视化。

另一方面，对于*吲哚青绿血管造影*，使用 790 nm 波长的二极管激光器来激发荧光染料，而阻挡滤波器可将 810 nm 边缘波长的激发荧光分离。

扫描式激光偏振仪

视网膜神经纤维层是双折射的，这意味着偏振光以不同的速度通过视网膜神经纤维层，这取决于偏振光是沿着纤维还是横过纤维（见第 2 章）。扫描激光偏振仪是一种具有集成椭圆仪的共焦扫描激光检眼镜，能够测量神经纤维的延迟。双折射介质的厚度与其延迟之间存在线性关系。通过以光栅图案逐点测量人视网膜的总延迟，从眼底反射后的光的偏振态变化中，可以形成眼视网膜双折射神经纤维层厚度的“地形图”。这为青光眼等眼部疾病提供了定量检测方法，而青光眼的早期特点是神经纤维丢失。

Optical Coherence Tomography

Optical coherence tomography (OCT) is an optical analogue to ultrasound imaging, using infrared light instead of sound. The much higher speed of light compared with sound allows for finer resolution, but direct electronic measurement of the shorter "echo" times it takes light to travel from different structures at axial distances within the eye is not feasible. Interferometry enables us to overcome this difficulty in the following manner. Light is split into 2 beams, and the beam backscattered from the ocular tissue is then compared (interfered) with the beam that has traveled a known time from the reference mirror. Interference patterns are observable when the optical distances traveled by the 2 beams match to within the coherence length of the light. In OCT, broadband (ie, low coherent) light sources are used (eg, a superluminescent diode emitting a beam of light with long [red] wavelengths —reds being chosen because they are scattered in tissue less than is blue light), rather than narrow -band (ie, high coherent) light sources, such as a laser, because it gives the instrument greater sensitivity to the differences in time the 2 beams have traveled (see Video 2-2).

In time-domain OCT (TD-OCT; Fig 8-24), the position of the mirror is adjusted so that interference patterns show up, as a function of time, whenever the 2 beams have traveled almost the same amount of time. Results similar to the ultrasound's A-scan are generated, as light is reflected at interfaces between layers of tissue. Cross-sectional images are generated by performing successive A-scans at different transverse positions on the retina or cornea, yielding 2-dimensional results like an ultrasound's B-scan (see BCSC Section 12, *Retina and Vitreous* and BCSC Section 8, *External Disease and Cornea*). By acquiring sequential cross-sectional images, 3-dimensional, volumetric results are obtained.

In Fourier-domain OCT (FD-OCT), also called *spectral domain OCT* or *frequency domain OCT*, the reference beam mirror is fixed at one position. Interference fringe patterns, all mixed together, arise from the various tissue interfaces, but Fourier analysis enables them to be dissected apart. When the pattern arises from closer tissue interfaces, the fringe patterns' undulations are spaced farther apart than those arising from deeper tissue planes, which yield fringes spaced more closely together. The more highly reflective tissue plane interfaces yield higher-amplitude fringe patterns. Thus, the spacing of the fringe pattern tells us how deep in the tissue it comes from, and its amplitude tells us how much the light is reflected by that tissue plane interface. In this manner, the A-scan of all the depths is obtained instantly without moving the reference mirror. Scanning across the retina (or cornea) yields 2-and 3-dimensional images. Thus, FD-OCT is much more efficient than TDOCT, resulting in both greater speed and higher signal-to-noise ratio, and therefore higher-resolution images.

There are 2 implementations of FD-OCT: spectrometer-based or swept-source implementation. A spectrometer-based version of FD-OCT uses a prism or grating in front of the detector to separate light into its spectral components, whereas a swept-source version of the FD-OCT replaces the super luminescent diode's band of frequencies with a tunable laser. The laser sequentially sweeps through different frequencies, one at a time, and the A-scan is performed for each frequency at each location. Unlike spectrometer based FD-OCT systems, swept-source-based systems are not limited by spectrometer resolutions and thereby support larger axial depth measurement ranges. Also, commonly available swept sources have a wavelength centered at about 1 μm, thereby enabling imaging deeper into the tissue. This allows us to see the vitreous, retina, and choroid more easily in a single image.

光学相干断层扫描技术

光学相干断层扫描技术（OCT）是一种使用红外光代替声波的光学模拟超声成像技术。与声波相比，高速的光波可形成更精细的分辨率，但是想要以轴向距离传播所需的极短的“回声”时间，用直接电子测量光来观察眼内的不同结构，则是无法实现的。而干涉法用以下方式可以解决这个问题。将光分成 2 束，然后将从眼组织向后散射的光束与从后视镜经过了已知时间的光束进行比较（干涉）。当 2 束光的光学距离与光的相干长度相匹配时，就可以观测到干涉图案。在 OCT 中，使用宽的（即低相干）光源（例如，选择发射具有长的红波长的光束的超发光二极管，因为它们在组织中的散射小于蓝光，而不是窄的（即高相干）光源（例如激光器，因为它使仪器对 2 束光束传播的时间差异更敏感了）。见视频 2-2。

在时域 OCT（TD-OCT，见图 8-24）中，调整反射镜的位置，使得每当 2 束光传播了几乎相同的时间量时，干涉图案就作为时间的函数出现。其结果与 A 超声波的扫描结果相似，因为光在组织层之间存在界面反射。截面图像是通过在视网膜上或角度不同的横向位置进行连续 A 扫描产生的，产生的 2 维图像如同 B 超扫描。（见 BCSC 第 12 册《*视网膜与玻璃体*》和 BCSC 第 8 册《*外眼疾病与角膜*》）。通过获得连续截面图像，可以得到 3 维体积的图像。

Fourier 域 OCT（FD-OCT），也称为*谱域 OCT* 或*频域 OCT*。在 FD-OCT 中，基准光束镜被固定在 1 个位置上，产生于不同的组织界面的干涉条纹图案全都混合在一起，但是 Fourier 分析使它们能够被分开。当图案产生于较近的组织界面时，条纹图案起伏的间隔更远，产生于较深的组织界面的起伏的间隔更紧密。即更高的反射性界面形成更大的波动条纹，所以，从条纹图案的间距可得知其来自多深的组织，从它的振幅可知光被该组织界面反射了多少。以这种方式，在不移动参考镜的情况下可立即获得所有深度的 A 型扫描。视网膜（或角膜）断面的扫描可产生 2 维和 3 维图像。因此，FD-OCT 比 TD-OCT 更有效，有更快的速度和更高的信噪比，从而可获得更高分辨率的图像。

有 2 种方式可以实现 Fourier 域 OCT：基于光谱仪或扫频源的。基于光谱仪的 FD-OCT 使用探测器前面的棱镜或光栅将光分离为其光谱分量，而基于扫频源的 FD-OCT 用可调谐激光器代替超发光二极管的频带。激光顺序地扫过不同的频率，在每个位置 1 次扫 1 个，对每个频率进行 A 型扫描。与基于光谱仪的 FD-OCT 系统不同，基于扫频源的系统不受光谱仪分辨率的限制，从而可支持更大的轴向深度测量范围。此外，通常用的扫频源具有以大约直径为 1 μm 的圆形区域为中心的波长，因此能够到更深层的组织中成像。这使得我们能够更容易地在单个图像中看到玻璃体、视网膜和脉络膜。

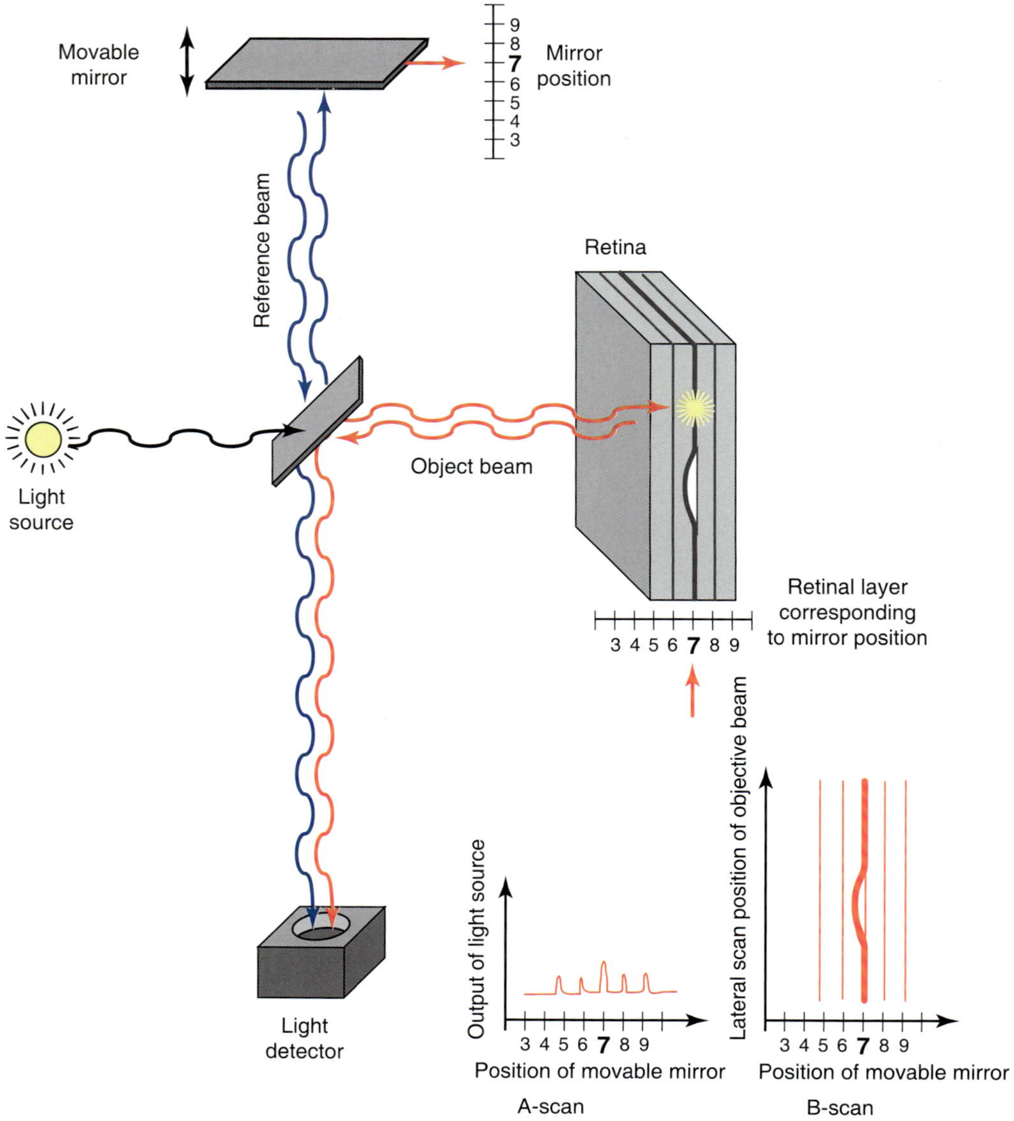

Figure 8-24 Optical coherence tomography based on the principle of low-coherence interferometry. *(Courtesy of Neal H. Atebara, MD. Redrawn by C. H. Wooley.)*

Adaptive Optics

Adaptive optics (AO) refers to a technique to compensate for distortions caused by optical aberrations in the media between the camera and the object being imaged. It was originally developed for use in astronomical telescopes to compensate for optical distortions induced by the inhomogeneous earth atmosphere. It has since evolved to become a powerful clinical tool in ophthalmology.

In an ophthalmic AO system, a wavefront sensor, such as the Hartmann-Shack wave front sensor, measures the distorted wavefront emerging from the eye, made irregular by aberrations of the cornea and crystalline lens.

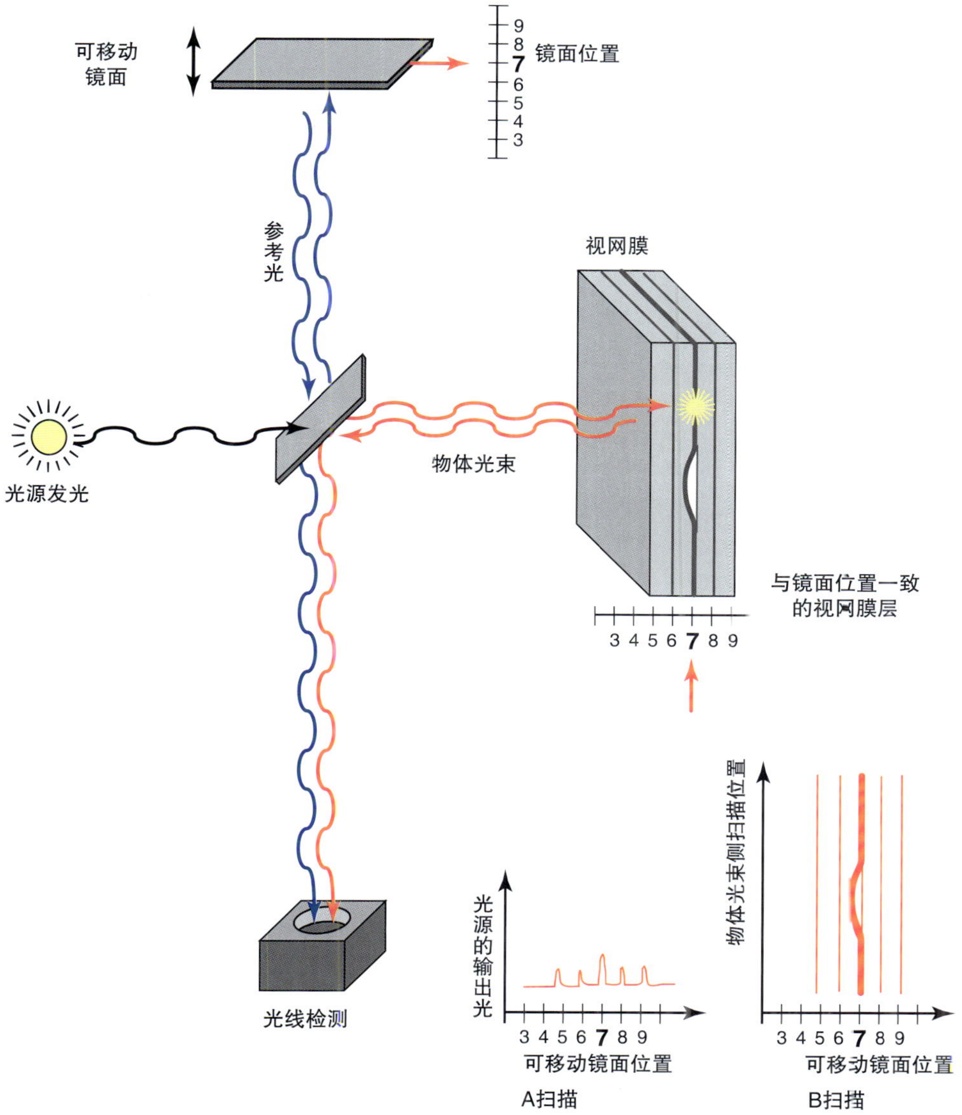

图 8—24　基于低相干干涉原理的光学相干层析断层扫描技术。*（译者注：资料来源见前页英文原文。）*

自适应光学

自适应光学（AO）是一种对在照相机和成像物体之间的介质中，由于光学像差产生的畸变的补偿技术。它最初被用于天文望远镜，补偿由不均匀的地球大气引起的光学畸变。现在已经发展成为眼科的一个强有力的临床工具。

在眼科 AO 系统中，波前传感器，例如 Hartmann Shack 波前传感器，用来测量角膜和晶状体的像差造成不规则的畸变波前。

Note that even for a normal eye, as the pupil enlarges, optical aberrations in the peripheral areas of the anterior segment come into play and may result in considerable distortions to the retinal image. For example, under low lighting conditions, the pupil dilates to approximately 5–7 mm in diameter. Higher-order aberrations become significant and lead to broadening of the point spread function (PSF, the image of a point source of light; see Chapter 2).

After measuring the distortion of the retina-reflected light, the AO system "undistorts" the beam via reflection by a deformable mirror. This is a very special mirror with a flexible surface and multiple electric actuators that can rapidly deform the mirror surface to modify the impinging aberrated wavefront accordingly, thereby effectively removing the distortions, as represented in Video 8-1.

VIDEO 8-1 Correction of aberrations via reflection of a deformable mirror.
Animation developed by Kristina Irsch, PhD.
Access all Section 3 videos at www.aao.org/bcscvideo_section03.

AO thus enables imaging of the human retina with unprecedented resolution, such as revealing individual photoreceptors or the walls of blood vessels. One should note that AO by itself does not provide an image; rather an AO subsystem is incorporated into an existing imaging device, as indicated in Figure 8-25. AO subsystems have thus far been successfully integrated into three ophthalmic imaging devices: fundus cameras, scanning laser ophthalmoscopes, and the OCT device.

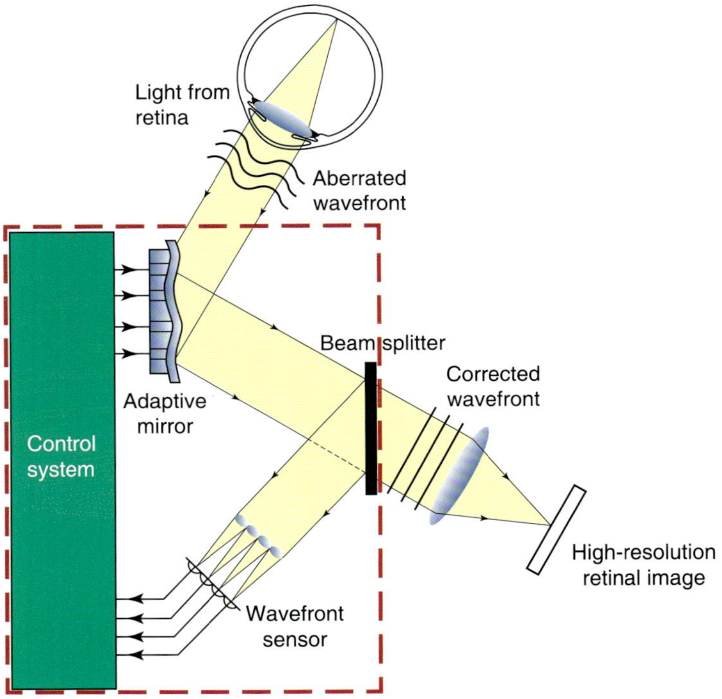

Figure 8-25 Basic principle of adaptive optics. The distorted emerging wavefront from the eye, made irregular by aberrations of the cornea and lens, gives a blurred retinal image at the start. The irregularities in the pattern of multiple images of the object produced by a micro-lenslet array allows us to determine what exactly are the distortions produced by the interfering ocular media, and then with a deformable mirror, we can modify the beam accordingly, so as to remove the distortions, which results in a high resolution retinal image. Note that adaptive optics by itself does not provide an image; rather an AO subsystem is incorporated into an existing imaging device, as indicated in red. *(Courtesy of Christopher Dainty, National University of Ireland, Galway.)*

注意，即使是正常的眼睛，在瞳孔放大时，AO 系统对其前部周边区域的光学像差也起作用，并且可能导致视网膜像的相当大的畸变。例如，在低光照条件下，瞳孔扩大到直径约为 5~7mm。高阶像差增加，并导致点播散函数（PSF，点光源的图像）的扩大。参见第 2 章。

在测量了视网膜反射光的畸变之后，AO 系统通过可变形反射镜的反射来获得“不失真”光束。这是一种非常特殊的反射镜，具有柔性表面和多个电动执行器，可以快速地使反射镜表面变形，从而相应地修改碰撞畸变波前，从而有效地消除畸变，如视频 8–1 所示。

视频8–1　通过变形镜的反射矫正像差。
由Kristina Irsch 哲学博士提供模拟模型。
访问所有第3册视频在www.aao.org/bcscvideo_section03.

因此，AO 能够以前所未有的分辨率，实现人的视网膜成像，可以显示单个光感受器或血管壁。应当注意，AO 本身并不提供像，而只是将 AO 子系统合并到现有成像设备中，如图 8–25 所示。到目前为止，AO 子系统已经被成功地集成到 3 个眼科成像设备中：眼底照相机、扫描激光检眼镜和 OCT 设备。

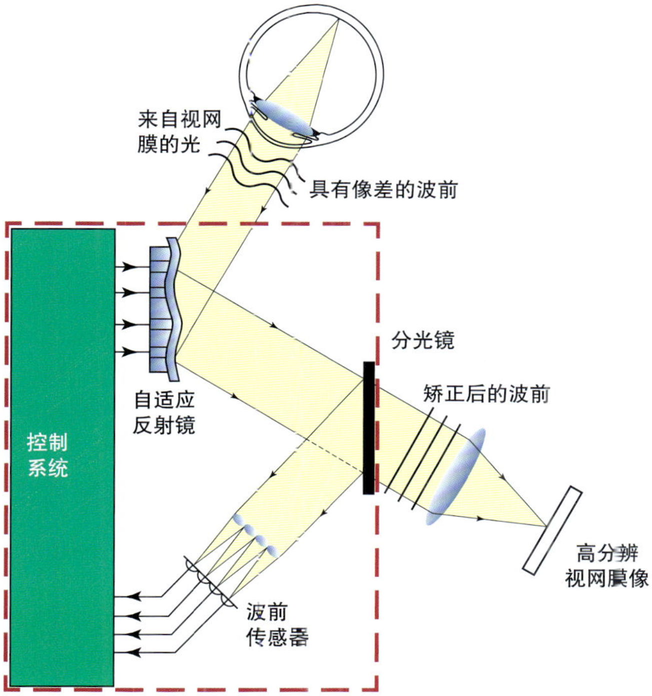

图 8–25　自适应光学的基本原理。来自眼睛的畸变波前，由于角膜和晶状体的像差而变得不规则，给出最初的模糊的视网膜像。由微透镜阵列产生的物体的多个图像中，不规则性使我们精确地确定通过干扰眼介质产生畸变，然后利用可变反射镜，我们可以相应地修饰光束，以去除畸变，从而产生具有高分辨率的视网膜图像。注意，自适应光学本身并不提供像，而只是将 AO 子系统并入现有的成像设备中，如图中红色所示。*（译者注：资料来源见前页原文。）*

Chapter Exercises

Questions

8.1 Slit-lamp biomicroscopy enables viewing of the corneal endothelium using which technique?
   a. retroillumination
   b. specular reflection
   c. direct focal illumination
   d. sclerotic scatter

8.2 Which statement does not characterize how keratometers work?
   a. They measure the radius of curvature of the central cornea.
   b. They assume the cornea to be a convex mirror.
   c. They directly measure the refractive power of the cornea.
   d. They use a mathematical formula to convert radius of curvature to approximate refractive power.

8.3 In what way is the manual keratometer inaccurate for determining corneal power in intraocular lens calculations following myopic laser vision correction?
   a. the keratometry measurement of the posterior surface does not change and is still accurate.
   b. The keratometer mire cannot be imaged at all following laser vision correction.
   c. The assumed relationship between the anterior and posterior surfaces, which is the basis of the assumed index of refraction, is no longer accurate.
   d. Significant irregular astigmatism is present in all corneas that have under gone keratorefractive surgery, and the keratometer is no longer accurate.

8.4 The indirect ophthalmoscope employs one of the brightest light sources used in clinical ophthalmology. Why is such a bright light necessary?

8.5 Which statement is inaccurate for fundus examination with the direct ophthalmoscope?
   a. The optic disc will appear larger in a myopic eye than a normal or hyperopic eye.
   b. The optic disc will appear smaller in a myopic eye than a normal or hyperopic eye.
   c. The optic disc will appear smaller in a hyperopic eye than a normal or myopic eye.
   d. Smaller details can be observed than with the indirect ophthalmoscope.

8.6 When a binocular indirect ophthalmoscope is used with a patient with small pupils, binocular visualization can be improved by which technique?
   a. moving the ophthalmoscope's mirrors or prisms closer to the observer
   b. narrowing the observer's effective interpupillary distance
   c. moving the ophthalmoscope's eyepieces farther apart
   d. increasing the distance between the observer's head and the patient
   e. all of the above

Answers

8.1 **b.** With an ordinary slit lamp, the outlines of individual endothelial cells are best seen by viewing the specular reflection of a narrow slit beam at high magnification. A wider field can be viewed using a specular microscope, with a contact optical system to decrease surface reflections.

章节练习

问题

8.1 裂隙灯生物显微镜能用何种技术观察角膜内皮细胞？
- a. 后映照
- b. 镜面反射
- c. 直接聚焦照明
- d. 巩膜散射

8.2 下面哪种说法不能描述角膜曲率计是如何工作的？
- a. 它们测量中心角膜的曲率半径
- b. 它们认为角膜是一个凸面镜
- c. 它们直接测量角膜的屈光力
- d. 它们用一个数学公式把曲率半径转换成近似的屈光力。

8.3 在近视激光矫正后的人工晶状体计算中，手动角膜测量仪采用何种方式不能准确测量角膜屈光力？
- a. 角膜后表面的角膜曲率测量没有改变，一直都是准确的
- b. 在激光视觉矫正之后，角膜曲率计不能完全成像
- c. 作为假定折射率的基础的前表面和后表面之间的假定关系不再精确
- d. 所有进行过角膜屈光手术的角膜都存在明显的不规则散光，角膜曲率计也不再精确

8.4 间接检眼镜采用的光源是临床眼科最明亮的光源之一。为什么需要这样明亮的灯光？

8.5 用直接检眼镜进行眼底检查时，下面表述中不准确的是哪一项？
- a. 近视眼的视盘比正常眼或远视眼更大
- b. 与正常眼或远视眼相比，近视眼的视盘会更小
- c. 与正常眼或近视眼相比，远视眼的视盘会更小
- d. 与间接检眼镜相比，可以观察到更小的细节

8.6 当双目间接检眼镜用于小瞳孔患者时，下面哪种技术可以提高双目视觉效果？
- a. 将检眼镜的面镜或棱镜移向观察者
- b. 缩小观察者的有效瞳孔间距
- c. 将检眼镜的目镜移动得更远
- d. 增加观察者头部与患者之间的距离
- e. 上述所有选项均可

答案

8.1 **b**。在使用普通的裂隙灯时再配合使用窄缝的光束高倍镜，可以清楚地看到单个内皮细胞的轮廓。可以使用角膜内皮显微镜的接触光学系统来减少表面反射，从而可观察到更宽的视野。

8.2 **c.** Keratometers approximate the refractive power of the cornea by measuring the radius of curvature of the central cornea and assuming the cornea to be a convex mirror. The formula $D=(n-1)/r$ is then used to convert this radius of curvature into an approximate refractive power, where r is the radius of curvature of the reflective cornea, and n is the keratomeric refractive index at 1.3375.

8.3 **c.** The 1.3375 index of refraction is calculated to compensate for the minus-powered posterior corneal surface that cannot be measured with the keratometer. Myopic keratorefractive surgery primarily flattens the anterior surface, and therefore the assumed index of refraction is no longer correct. Another problem following myopic keratorefractive surgery is that the extreme center of the cornea is usually flattened substantially more than the annulus measured by the manual keratometer (approximately 3 mm). Both errors will lead to overestimating the power of the cornea and a hyperopic postoperative result, if not corrected for in the calculation.

8.4 The condensing lens images the observer's entrance pupils as 2 very small discs that fall within the patient's entrance pupil (along with the image of the ophthalmoscope bulb's filament, which must not coincide with the images of the observer's pupils, to avoid obscuring the fundus with reflections from the patient's cornea). Of all the light the ophthalmoscope shines into the patient's eye, only the emergent light that passes through these pupillary images enters the eyes of the observer and is available for viewing the fundus. As these image discs occupy far less than 1% of the area of the patient's entrance pupil, and only about 0.1% of the light is reflected from the fundus, the ophthalmoscope "wastes" over 99% of the light that enters the patient's eye in forming the image visible to the observer, requiring a very bright light source.

8.5. **b.** With direct ophthalmoscopy, the examiner uses the optics of the patient's eye as a simple magnifier to look at the retina. The optics of the normal eye are approximately +60 D, so using the formula for a simple magnifier, the magnification is 60/4, or 15×. If the patient's eye is myopic, a minus lens is dialed in, to overcome the extra plus power "error lens" inside the patient's eye. Those 2 lenses create a Galilean telescope effect, increasing magnification and decreasing the field of view. Similarly, the retina of a hyperopic eye will be magnified less than 15× because of the reverse Galilean telescope effect created by the minus power error lens inside the patient's eye and the plus lens of the direct ophthalmoscope. Thus, the size of the optic disc will appear larger (and not smaller) in a myopic eye than in a hyperopic or a normal eye.

8.6 **e.** When looking through a small pupil, the observer can improve visualization by narrowing his or her effective interpupillary distance. This can be accomplished by several means. Moving the ophthalmoscope's mirrors or prisms closer to the observer (the "small-pupil feature" available on some ophthalmoscopes) decreases the distance between the light paths to the observer's left and right eyes, effectively narrowing the observer's interpupillary distance. Moving the ophthalmoscope's eyepieces farther apart also decreases the distance between the light paths to the observer's eyes, similarly narrowing the observer's effective interpupillary distance. Increasing the distance between the observer and the patient decreases the angle formed by the observer's eyes and the patient's eye, thereby allowing the light paths from the observer's eyes to "squeeze through" a smaller pupil.

8.2 **c**。角膜曲率仪通过测量中央角膜的曲率半径，并假设角膜是凸面镜来近似得到角膜的折射能力。然后使用公式 $D=(n-1)/r$ 将该曲率半径转换成近似屈光力，其中 r 是反射性角膜的曲率半径，n 是角膜折射率，其值为 1.3375。

8.3 **c**。计算折射率为 1.3375，以补偿用角膜曲率计无法测量的角膜后表面的负度数。因为近视性角膜屈光手术主要是使前表面变平，因此原先的折射率不再正确。近视性角膜屈光手术后的另一个问题是角膜的极中心的曲率通常比手动角膜曲率计（直径约为 3 mm）测量的环形空间平得多。如果在计算中没有得到矫正，则这 2 个错误将导致过度估计角膜的屈光度和术后的远视结果。

8.4 聚光透镜将观察者的入射光瞳成像为 2 个非常小的圆盘，它们落在患者的入射光瞳中（连同检眼镜灯丝泡的像，它们必须与观察者瞳孔的像不一致，以避免由于患者角膜的反光而使眼底成像模糊）。在所有的光中，检眼镜的光照射到患者的眼睛中时，只有出射光通过这些瞳孔像进入观察者的眼睛，并且可用于观察眼底。由于这些像占据患者瞳孔入口的面积远小于 1%，并且只有约 0.1% 的光从眼底反射，所以在形成观察者可见的图像时，检眼镜"浪费"了进入患者眼睛的光的 99% 以上，因此需要使用非常明亮的光源。

8.5 **b**。通过直接检眼镜检查时，检查者将患者眼睛的光学系统当作一个简单的放大镜通过其来观察视网膜。普通眼睛的光学系数约为 +60 D，所以用一个简单的放大倍数公式可以计算得到其放大倍数是 60/4 （15×）。如果患者的眼睛是近视的，则拨入负透镜，以抵消患者眼睛内多余的加权"误差透镜"。这 2 个透镜产生 Galileo 望远镜效应，增加放大率并减少视野。同样，远视眼的视网膜放大率小于 15×，这是由于患者眼内的负度数误差透镜和直接检眼镜的正透镜产生的反向 Galileo 望远镜效应。因此，近视眼的视盘大小比远视眼或正常眼大。

8.6 **e**。当观察 1 个小瞳孔时，观察者可以通过缩小他（或她）的有效瞳孔间距来提高视觉效果。这可以通过几种方法来完成。将检眼镜的镜面或棱镜移近观察者（类似某些检眼镜上的"小瞳孔特征"）可以减少光路到观察者左眼和右眼之间的距离，有效地缩小观察者的瞳孔间距离。将检眼镜的眼镜移得更远也会减少到观察者眼睛的光路之间的距离，同样可缩小观察者的有效瞳孔间距离。增加观察者和患者之间的距离减小了观察者的眼睛和患者眼睛形成的角度，从而允许来自观察者的眼睛的光路"挤入"较小的瞳孔。

（翻译　胡笳　王西欧 // 审校　石一宁　李易 // 章节审校　朱丹）

CHAPTER 9

Vision Rehabilitation

Highlights

- Patients with visual acuities less than 20/40 or scotomas, field loss, or contrast sensitivity loss will benefit from low vision evaluation and multidisciplinary vision rehabilitation to assist them to achieve their goals and maintain quality of life despite vision loss.
- An evaluation of visual acuity, contrast sensitivity, location and size of scotomas relative to fixation, and extent of midperipheral and peripheral field loss allows clinicians to appreciate the impact of vision loss on patients' function and informs effective rehabilitation interventions.
- Multidisciplinary vision rehabilitation addresses reading (eg, magnification requirements), daily activities (eg computer accessibility or doing kitchen tasks), safety (eg, fall prevention or ability to take medications), participation (eg, driving) and psychosocial well-being (eg, adjustment to vision loss or depression).
- The range of devices that patients can benefit from includes optical devices, such as reading adds and illuminated magnifiers; electronic devices, such as smartphones, e-readers, video magnifiers, or audio books; and nonoptical devices, such as large-format telephones or television remote controls.
- Medicare and some insurance companies fund training by occupational therapists for patients with vision loss, just as rehabilitation is funded for patients who have had strokes or hip fractures.
- Patients with any level of vision loss may experience vivid, recurrent visual hallucinations, such as seeing patterns, faces, flowers, or people. When patients have full insight that these images are not real and no other neurologic symptoms or diagnosis to explain the hallucinations, it is attributed to the Charles Bonnet syndrome.

Glossary

Bioptic telescope Spectacle-mounted devices that are typically placed above the visual axis for spotting distance targets, such as traffic lights in jurisdictions where bioptic driving is allowed.

第 9 章

视觉康复

重点

- 视力低于 20/40，或有盲点、视野缺损，或对比敏感度缺失的患者将得益于低视力评估和各种学科的视觉康复，尽管有视觉缺失，但也能帮助他们达到希望的目标和维持生活质量。
- 视力，对比敏感度、盲点的位置和大小与注视的关系，周边和中周部视野缺失程度的评估，可让医生理解视觉缺失对患者功能的影响，并影响有效的康复干预。

- 多学科的视觉康复包括阅读（例如放大需求）、日常活动（例如计算机或厨房工作）、安全（例如预防跌倒或能够获得药物）、参与（例如驾驶）和社会心理健康（例如适应视觉缺失或抑郁）。

- 患者能获益的设备范围包括光学设备，例如阅读附加镜和带照明的放大镜；电子设备，例如智能手机、电子阅读器、视频放大，或有声读本；非光学设备，例如大字体电话或电视遥控器。

- 医疗保险和一些商业保险公司为视觉缺失患者的职业治疗师的培训提供资金，就像为中风或髋部骨折患者的康复提供资金一样。

- 任何程度视觉缺失的患者都可能经历活生生的、反复出现的视觉幻觉，例如，看到图案、面孔、花或人。当患者完全明白这些影像不是真实的，也没有其他的神经症状或诊断来解释这种幻觉时，可以诊断为 Charles Bonnet 综合征。

术语

双光望远镜　安装在眼镜上的设备，通常装在视轴上方区域，用来注视远距离目标，例如在允许配戴双光设备驾驶的辖区内，注视远处目标，如交通信号灯。

Charles Bonnet syndrome A condition in individuals who have some degree of vision loss that is characterized by vivid recurrent hallucinations and insight that what is being seen is not real. Individuals may see patterns or formed images such as people, faces, or landscapes. The degree of vision loss may be moderate or severe, and the vision loss can be acuity loss or visual field loss due to ocular or neurologic disease.

Eccentric fixation Using nonfoveal fixation to view the object of regard.

Legal blindness A level of vision loss at which patients are entitled to certain concessions or services in various jurisdictions. Legal blindness is typically defined in the United States as visual acuity less than or equal to best corrected visual acuity of 20/200 or a visual field of equal to or less than 20° around central fixation.

Low vision Vision loss that cannot be corrected by standard eyeglasses or by medical or surgical treatment. The cause may be ocular or neurologic disease.

Macular microperimeter A perimetry device that images the retina during visual field testing. This allows more reliable perimetry evaluation of patients with unstable fixation or eccentric fixation. The retina can be imaged with a camera or scanning laser ophthalmoscopy. Macular microperimetry is also called *fundus-related perimetry* or *macular perimetry*.

Preferred retinal locus The area of nonfoveal retina that a patient repeatedly uses for fixation, when the foveal area is impaired.

Scanning training Training to enhance compensatory visual search into nonseeing areas of the visual field, such as hemianopic field loss. Methods of training include search tasks on devices with displays of lights that can be programmed, computer training programs, and scanning training practice typically implemented by occupational therapists.

Video magnifiers Devices that combine digital cameras and viewing screens in handheld, desk, or head-mounted formats. They have also been referred to as *closed-circuit televisions* (CCTVs).

Vision rehabilitation A multidisciplinary clinical process aimed at enabling individuals with vision loss to reach their goals for visual tasks as well as optimal personal safety and psychological and social function. The American Academy of Ophthalmology's Preferred Practice Pattern Guideline *Vision Rehabilitation for Adults* outlines that comprehensive vision rehabilitation assesses and addresses 5 areas: reading, activities of daily living, safety, continued participation despite vision loss, and psychosocial well-being.

Visual prosthesis A device to provide vision substitution for individuals who are blind. Devices being implanted or under development stimulate the retina (epireintal, subretinal, suprachoroidal) or visual cortex. A device is available that places an lectrode array on the tongue.

Introduction

In this chapter, we discuss the approach to the patient with low vision. Topics cover the evaluation of the patient and rehabilitation interventions, including devices, training, discussion with patients, and referral to other resources.

Charles Bonnet 综合征　有某种程度视觉缺失的个人的一种状况，其特征是有活生生的、反复出现的幻觉，并意识到所看到的并不是真实的。这些人可能看到图案或形成的图像，如人、面孔或风景。视觉缺失的程度可以是中度或重度，视觉缺失可以是由于眼睛或神经疾病引起的视力缺失或视野缺失。

非中心注视　使用非黄斑区注视来观察注视的物体。

法定盲　视觉丧失的一个级别，那些患者在不同的司法管辖区内，有权获得某种特权或服务。法定盲通常在美国定义为最佳矫正视力低于或等于 20/200，或中央注视视野小于等于 20°　。

低视力　不能被常规的眼镜或药物手术治疗的视觉丧失。可以是眼部或神经疾病导致的。

黄斑微视野仪　在视野测试中成像于视网膜的一种视野测量设备。这使得对不稳定注视或非中心注视的患者进行的视野评估更可靠。可以用照相机或激光扫描检影镜成像于视网膜。黄斑微视野仪又称*眼底相关视野检查*或*黄斑视野检查*。

视网膜优先定位　当中心凹区域受损时，患者反复用来固视的非中心凹视网膜区域。

扫描训练　用来提高补偿性视觉搜索进入视野的无视力区域能力的训练，如偏盲视野缺失。训练方法包括：在带有可编程灯光显示设备上进行搜索任务、计算机训练程序和扫描训练练习，后者通常由职业治疗师执行。

视频放大器　包括数码相机和手持的观看屏幕设备、书桌或头戴式设备。它们也被称为*闭路电视*（CCTVs）。

视觉康复　一个多学科的临床过程，旨在使视觉缺失的个人能够达到他们视觉工作的需求目标，以及最佳的个人安全和心理及社会功能。美国眼科学会的临床指南（PPP）中，将*成人视觉康复*概括为综合性的视觉康复评估和 5 个重点领域：阅读、日常生活活动、安全、视觉缺失后的继续参与，以及社会心理健康。

视觉假体　为盲人提供替代视觉的装置。这种被植入或正在研发的装置用来刺激视网膜（视网膜上、视网膜下、脉络膜上腔）或视觉皮层。有一种装置已经被应用，它将电子阵列放在舌头上。

引言

这章中，我们讨论低视力患者的治疗方法，内容包括患者的评估和康复干预，后者有设备、训练、与患者的沟通和其他资源的推荐。

Approach to the Patient With Low Vision

In 2012, an estimated 4,195,966 Americans aged 40 and older were reported to have vision impairment and blindness—2.9 million individuals had less than 20/40 visual acuity and 1.3 million were estimated to be legally blind, with best-corrected visual acuity of 20/200 or less or a visual field of 20° or less around fixation. Most of these individuals were elderly, as prevalence of vision loss increases with age. Vision loss impacts patient safety, independence, quality of life, and psychosocial well-being. Seniors with vision loss are at risk for falls, injuries, medication errors, nutritional decline, social isolation, and depression at far higher rates than reported for sighted individuals.

The ophthalmologist is in a unique position to support patients with vision loss by "recognizing and responding": recognizing that vision loss, even moderate vision loss, impacts patients' ability to successfully accomplish the things they need and want to do, and responding by facilitating access to vision rehabilitation services. Although the ophthalmologist may not personally provide these services, appreciation of the strategies and options in the vision rehabilitation "toolbox" allows you to understand why referring patients to such services is important and beneficial, and to provide specific examples to your patients of what vision rehabilitation can offer. In addition, your empathy in recognizing a patient's reaction to vision loss, whether it be fear, anger, or sadness, and conveying that you understand the connection of their emotion to their loss, can be a brief, but important step in the continuum of care, from diagnosis to rehabilitation.

Any patient with eye disease that cannot be improved with medical or surgical treatment, and who is not able to successfully accomplish necessary visual tasks is a candidate for vision rehabilitation. Practitioners frequently err in referring only patients with severe vision loss for vision rehabilitation. In fact, rehabilitation can be very important even for patients with good acuity and eye disease that is associated with scotomas or with reduced contrast perception, such as patients receiving injections for exudative macular degeneration who may still have quite good visual acuity. The Academy's Preferred Practice Pattern Guideline *Vision Rehabilitation for Adults* recommends that patients with acuity less than 20/40, contrast sensitivity loss, and peripheral or central field loss be referred for low vision evaluation. Ophthalmologists are encouraged to ask patients what tasks they are having difficulty doing because of their decreased vision. Patients whose only difficulty is reading fine print can usually be assisted by routine eye-care services; however, when low vision impacts activities beyond the ability to read fine print, the many practical options of vision rehabilitation are useful.

A strategy for comprehensive vision rehabilitation begins with a low vision evaluation and is followed, as indicated, by training and referral to resources and specialized services.

Prevent Blindness America. Vision problems in the U.S. Available at www .visionproblemsus.org. Accessed November 5, 2017.

Low Vision Evaluation

The low vision evaluation includes a history, measurement of visual function, and creation of a vision rehabilitation plan. In contrast to an ophthalmic examination, in which visual function and ocular status are evaluated with the intent to diagnose and treat, the evaluation of the patient seeking vision rehabilitation aims to assess and address reading, valued activities of daily living, patient safety, continued participation despite vision loss, and psychosocial well-being.

低视力患者的治疗方法

2012 年，据报道 40 岁及以上的美国人中有 4,195,966 人经评估有视觉损害和眼盲——290 万人的视力低于 20/40，130 万人估计为法定盲，也就是最佳矫正视力≤ 20/200 或视野≤ 20° 。这些人中大多数为老年人，并且随着年龄的增加，视力缺失的患病率也在增加。视觉缺失影响患者的安全性、独立生存能力、生活质量和社会心理健康。视觉缺失的老年人发生跌倒、受伤、用药错误、营养下降、社会孤独和抑郁的风险比例远远高于有视力人群。

眼科医生在帮助视觉缺失患者方面处于一个独特的位置，即帮助他们“识别和响应”：识别就是认识到视觉缺失，因为即便是中等程度的视觉缺失，也会影响患者成功实现他们需要和想做事情的能力。响应就是促使患者接受视觉康复服务。虽然眼科医生可能不会亲自提供这些服务，但对视觉康复“工具箱”中的策略和选项的理解，使医生可以理解为什么将患者推荐给这些服务是重要的和有益的，并可以为患者提供帮助其视觉康复的具体方法。此外，当医生认识到患者对视觉缺失的反应，如恐惧、愤怒或是悲伤时，向患者表达医生的理解，在从诊断到康复的持续护理中，这是一个简明且重要的一步。

任何通过药物或手术治疗不能得到改善，且不能成功完成必要的视觉任务的眼病患者，都是视觉康复的候选人。医生经常错误地认为只有严重视觉缺失的患者才需要向其推荐视觉康复。事实上，即使对于那些视力虽然很好，但有盲点或对比敏感度下降的眼病患者来说，康复也是非常重要的，比如那些因渗出性黄斑变性接受注射治疗的患者，可能仍然有很好的视力。美国眼科协会的*成人视觉康复*指南建议，视力低于 20/40、对比度敏感度缺失、周围或中心视野缺失的患者应进行低视力评估。眼科医生应该询问患者，视觉下降给他们带来哪些工作困难。仅仅阅读小字困难的患者可通过常规眼保健服务得到改善，然而，当不仅仅是阅读小字受影响时，选择有效的视觉康复就很有帮助。

综合的视觉康复战略要从低视力评价开始，接着再进行培训和推荐给相关的专门服务机构。

Prevent Blindness America. Vision problems in the U.S. Available at www .vis onproblemsus.org. Accessed November 5, 2017.

低视力评估

低视力评估包括询问病史、视功能检查和建立视觉康复计划。眼科的检查是以诊断和治疗为目的来评估视觉功能和眼部状态，而在对于寻求视觉康复的患者低视力评估中，目的在于评估有效的阅读、日常生活活动、患者的安全、视觉缺失后的继续参与及社会心理健康。

Patient history

As with other clinical encounters, the history provides important information that directs the remainder of the examination. The low vision history focuses on the limitations the patient's vision imposes on their function: what they are having difficulty doing.

Ocular history The disease, rate of progression, and previous ocular treatments will typically correlate with the patient's functional complaints. For example, patients with macular degeneration would be anticipated to have different difficulties than patients with slowly progressive glaucoma.

General history The current living situation, supports, employment, hobbies, illnesses, and use of glasses, devices, cell phones, and computers are all relevant issues in the history. Systemic diseases can impact rehabilitation interventions, such as when arthritis or tremors impair a patient's ability to hold a book or a handheld magnifier.

Patient's subjective report of difficulties or goals The patient's goals and values help direct and prioritize rehabilitation efforts. Tasks may still be difficult after rehabilitation, but patients highly value success in accomplishing tasks that are important to them. The examiner should ask the patient about difficulties with (1) reading tasks, such as reading newspapers, mail, and handwritten notes; (2) activities of daily living, such as shopping, cooking, using a cell phone or computer, shaving, and watching television; (3) safety issues, including falls, reading medications, and kitchen safety; (4) barriers to participation, including driving status, transportation alternatives, and isolation; and (5) psychosocial status, such as anxieties, including worry about visual hallucinations experienced and depressive symptoms, and concerns about responsibilities, such as financial or caregiving responsibilities.

Charles Bonnet syndrome Patients with Charles Bonnet syndrome see images of objects that are not real. The condition affects up to one-third of visually impaired persons. Patients are often relieved to discuss their hallucinations. They may see vivid, recurrent formed images of patterns, such as wallpaper or barbed wire, or even images such as people or landscapes. Many patients are puzzled by this symptom. Some are anxious, as they do not understand what they are experiencing, and a small proportion are very upset. Most patients will not report the hallucinations unless the clinician inquires, for fear of being labeled as mentally unwell.

A diagnosis of Charles Bonnet syndrome can be made if the patient has 4 clinical characteristics: (1) vivid recurrent hallucinations; (2) some degree of vision loss; (3) insight into the unreality of the images, when it is explained to them; and (4) no other neurologic or psychiatric diagnosis to explain the hallucinations. Charles Bonnet syndrome is a diagnosis of exclusion, and patients should be referred for neurologic or psychiatric evaluation if they have any other neurologic signs or symptoms (see BCSC Section 5, *Neuro-Ophthalmology*).

Assessment of Visual Function

As in ophthalmology in general, visual acuity is an important and common measure of visual function in vision rehabilitation, as the task performance of a person with 20/70 visual acuity will likely differ from that of someone with 20/400 visual acuity. Other measures of visual function, however, are also important, especially contrast sensitivity and central visual field. Two patients with 20/40 visual acuity, for example, may have different contrast perception and different central visual field, and have very different reading performance and require different devices and training. In some disease settings, such as glaucoma or after stroke, peripheral visual field will also be important.

患者病史

与临床工作一样，病史提供了指导进一步检查的重要信息。低视力病史关注的是患者视力对其功能的限制：他们做什么事情会有困难。

眼部病史　疾病发展的速度和既往的眼科治疗都与患者的功能性症状相关。例如，可以预料到的是，黄斑变性患者与慢性进行性青光眼患者会遇到不同的困难。

一般病史　当前的生活状态、抚养状态、就业情况、爱好、疾病，以及眼镜、家用器具、手机和电脑的使用都是病史涉及的问题。系统性疾病影响康复干预，例如，当患关节炎或颤抖时，将会影响患者拿书或手持放大镜。

患者对困难或目标的主观报告　患者的目标和价值观有助于管理和考虑康复的优先努力方向。康复以后工作可能依然还是困难的，但患者会高度重视并成功地完成对他们非常重要的工作。检查者应该询问患者的有关困难有：① 阅读，例如读报、读信、手写笔记；② 日常生活的活动，例如购物、烹饪、使用手机或电脑、刮胡子、看电视；③ 安全问题，包括摔倒、辨认药物、厨房安全；④ 参与行为的障碍，包括驾驶状态、交通选择、独处情况；⑤ 社会心理状态，例如焦虑，包括对幻觉经历和抑郁症状的担心，以及对责任的担心，例如经济责任或看护责任。

Charles Bonnet 综合征　患有 Charles Bonnet 综合征的患者会看到并不真实存在的图像。这种状况会影响 1/3 视觉损害的人群。讨论幻觉的感受可以缓解患者的症状。他们可能会看到生动的、反复出现的图案图像，例如墙纸或铁丝网，甚至是人物或风景的图像。许多患者对这种症状感到困惑。有些人很焦虑，因为他们不明白自己在经历什么，一小部分人很沮丧。除非医生询问到这些问题，大部分患者不会主动述说这些幻觉，因为害怕被视为精神不正常。

患者如果有以下 4 个临床特征就可诊断为 Charles Bonnet 综合征：① 生动地反复出现幻视；② 一定程度的视觉损失；③ 当向他们解释的时候，能够认识到图像的不真实性；④ 没有其他神经病学或精神病学的诊断能解释这些幻视。Charles Bonnet 综合征的诊断是一种排除性诊断，如果患者有任何其他神经病学的症状或体征，应该推荐患者接受神经病学或精神病学评估（见 BCSC 第 5 册《*神经眼科学*》）。

视觉功能的评估

通常在眼科中，视力是视觉康复中重要而普通的视觉功能指标，视力为 20/70（0.3）的人的表现很可能与视力为 20/400（0.05）的人不同。然而其他的视觉功能检查也很重要，尤其是对比敏感度和中心视野。例如，2 个视力都是 20/40（0.5）的患者，他们可能有不同的对比感知和不同的中心视野，阅读表现也非常不同，需要不同的设备和训练。对于一些疾病，例如青光眼或中风后，此时对周边视野的检查也很重要。

Visual acuity Accurate visual acuity measurements can be made to very low levels. Charts can be brought to closer-than-standard viewing distances. An ETDRS chart is commonly used at 1 or 2 m (Fig 9-1). For patients with very poor vision, the Berkeley Rudimentary Vision Assessment, a set of 25-cm cards held at 25 cm, is available for quantifying visual acuity as low as 20/16,000. Care is taken to carefully measure acuity in patients with low vision by optimizing the refraction, allowing patients adequate time to respond, and often using different testing distances.

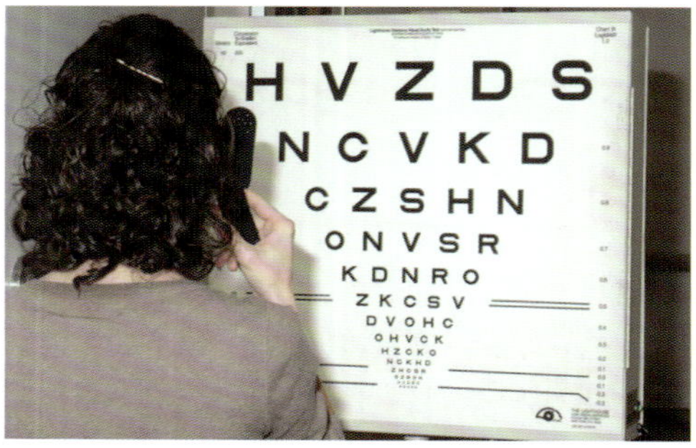

Figure 9-1 Measuring visual acuity with the ETDRS chart at 1 meter. *(Courtesy of Scott E. Brodie, MD, PhD.)*

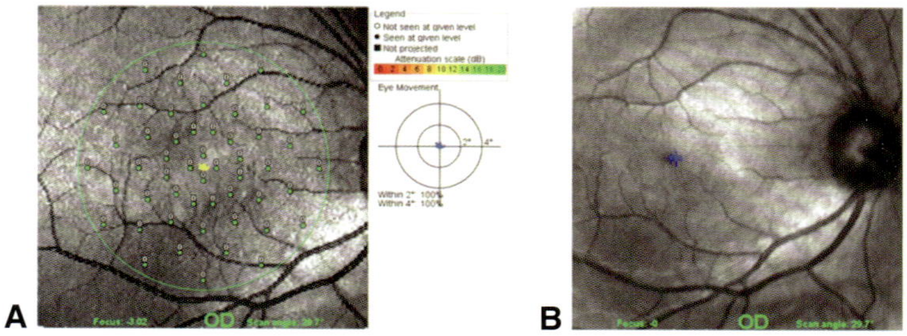

Figure 9-2 Macular microperimetry showing normal central field. **A**, All targets were responded to (green circles). **B**, The fixation is at the fovea (blue crosses). *(Courtesy of Mary Lou Jackson, MD.)*

Fixation Patients with normal vision fixate a visual acuity chart with their fovea (Fig 9-2). Patients with macular disease may fixate with eccentric areas of the retina, or preferred retinal loci (PRLs; Fig 9-3). Visual acuity can vary when using areas of differing retinal sensitivity. Clues to understanding fixation behavior include head and eye movement, patient subjective reports, and measured fixation with macular microperimetry.

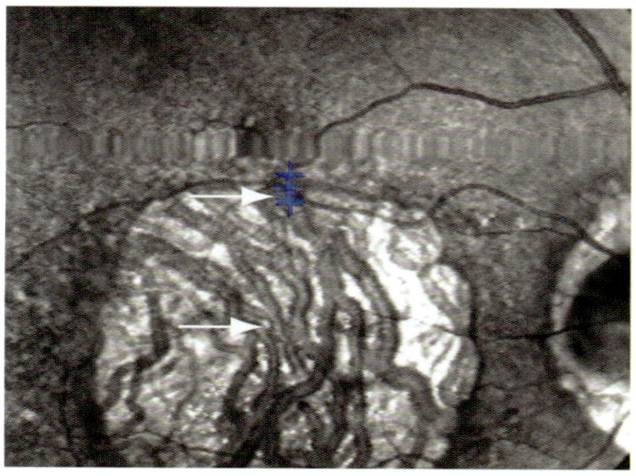

Figure 9-3 Macular photo showing anatomic fovea *(lower arrow)* and location of eccentric fixation with a preferred retinal locus (PRL) *(upper arrow)*. *(Courtesy of Mary Lou Jackson, MD.)*

视力　准确的视力测量可以测出非常低的视力水平。可以将视力表拿到比标准注视距离更近的距离。ETDRS 视力表通常在 1 m 或 2 m 处使用（图 9–1）。对于视力非常差的患者，Berkeley 大学的基本视觉评估中，手持一套 25 cm 卡片在 25 cm 处检查，可以有效量化 20/16,000 的视力。通过对屈光的最佳矫正，仔细检查低视力患者的视力，注意允许患者有足够的时间做出反应，并经常使用不同的检查距离。

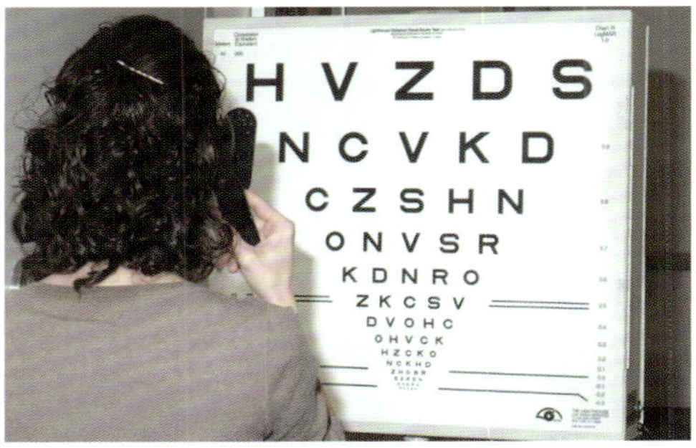

图 9–1　使用 ETDRS 视力表在 1 m 处检查视力 *（译者注：资料来源见前页英文原文。）*

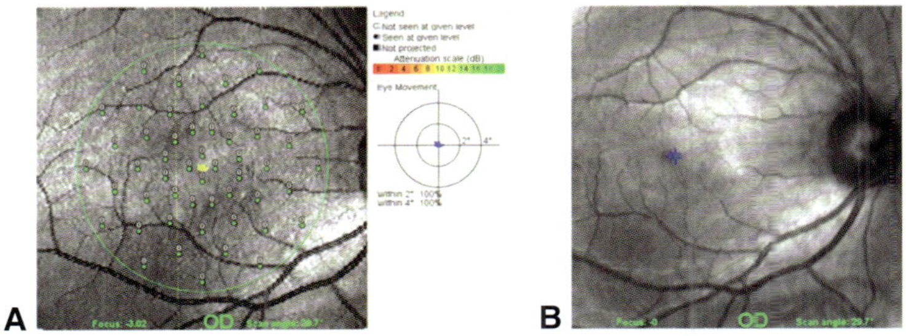

图 9–2　黄斑微视野检查仪显示正常的中心视野。**A.** 所有目标都有反应（绿色环）。**B.** 中心凹注视（蓝色十字）。*（译者注：资料来源见前页英文原文。）*

注视　正常视力的患者用他们的中心凹注视视力表（图 9–2）。黄斑病变的患者可能用视网膜的偏中心区域来注视，或优选视网膜定位点（PRLs；图 9–3）。当使用不同视网膜敏感度的区域时，视力会不同。了解注视行为的线索包括头部和眼部的运动、患者的主观报告和用黄斑微视野计检查注视状态。

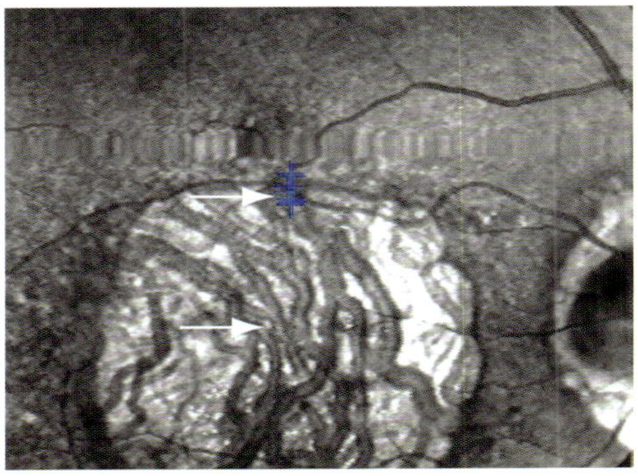

图 9–3　黄斑照片显示中心凹的解剖结构（*下方箭头*，和偏中心注视的位置及优选视网膜定位点（PRL）（*上方箭头*）*（译者注：资料来源见前页英文原文。）*

Crossland MD, Culham LE, Kabanarou SA, Rubin GS. Preferred retinal locus development in patients with macular disease. *Ophthalmology*. 2005;112(9):1579–1585.

Refraction The goal of refraction for patients with low vision is to check for significant uncorrected refractive errors; however, only about 10% of low vision patients will benefit from alternate refractive correction, as the source of their poor vision is typically ocular disease, not refractive error. The vision rehabilitation clinician must temper unreasonable expectations, such as the expectation that new glasses can solve vision problems associated with the eye disease, and ensure that patients do not deplete their financial resources on spectacles that offer little benefit, especially when they could put that money toward other devices that significantly improve function. Purchase of new glasses is often best delayed until the patient can compare the benefit of other rehabilitation options and devices to the benefit of spectacles.

Specific strategies can assist the low vision refraction including using a trial frame, retinoscopy at a shorter distance with greater working-distance lens power, using a +1.00/−1.00 cross cylinder for patients with poorer acuity to allow them to appreciate the differences between choices, or using an automated refractor. The vision rehabilitation clinician watches for fluctuating acuity in diabetic patients and balance corrections in an eye that may now be the better-seeing eye. Full corrections, rather than balance corrections, are encouraged. Polycarbonate lenses can be considered for ocular safety. It is not uncommon that patients with macular disease have very small areas of foveal retina surrounded by dense scotoma: foveal-sparing scotomas (Fig 9-4A). This is seen in both dry and treated wet macular degeneration, Stargardt disease, and other macular diseases. Such patients may be unable to read the larger letters on a visual acuity chart, causing the examiner to abandon the testing and record very low acuity. More careful testing, or testing at a closer distance, however, may reveal that the patient can in fact discern smaller letters when he or she is able to align the limited central field with the targets on the eye chart (Fig 9-4B).

Contrast sensitivity The ability to discern contrast is a separate visual function from visual acuity, and the functions are not directly correlated. Patients with poor contrast sensitivity have difficulty seeing the edges of steps, reading light-colored print, driving in foggy or snowy conditions, and recognizing faces. Contrast sensitivity varies with target size (spatial frequency), and the relationship between contrast threshold and spatial frequency may be displayed as a contrast sensitivity curve (see BCSC Section 3 Chapter 3). Formal tests of contrast sensitivity include paper charts and computer tests, the later allowing greater testing range. Paper charts may test a range of spatial frequencies (Fig 9-5A), or a single spatial frequency (Fig 9-5B).

Patients whose visual impairment includes loss of contrast sensitivity may benefit from illuminated magnifiers or electronic magnification, and nonoptical strategies, such as task lighting, or modification of contrast in tasks, such as using a black felt-tip marker.

Crossland MD, Culham LE, Kabanarou SA, Rubin GS. Preferred retinal locus development in patients with macular disease. *Ophthalmology*. 2005;112(9):1579–1585.

验光　为低视力患者验光的目的是检查出未矫正的屈光不正；然而，只有大约 10% 的低视力患者的视力通过不同的屈光矫正得以改善，因为他们的视力不良是源于眼病，而非屈光不正。从事视觉康复的临床医生必须降低患者不合理的期望，例如期望新眼镜能解决与眼病相关的视觉问题，不要让患者在收效甚微的眼镜上花费过多的费用，特别是当能显著提高视功能的设备需要花费时。最好让患者比较各种视觉康复手段和设备，不要急于先购买新眼镜。

能帮助低视力患者进行验光矫正的具体策略包括：试镜架；在较短的距离使用较大的工作距离透镜焦度进行检影；使用 ±1.00D 的交叉柱镜，使他们能体会 2 个选择之间的不同；或使用自动验光仪。视觉康复医生应注意糖尿病患者的视力波动，并权衡现在视力矫正较好的眼，鼓励全矫正，而不是权衡矫正。为了眼睛的安全应考虑聚碳酸酯镜片。黄斑病变患者常有非常小的中心凹视网膜区域被致密的盲点所围绕，此即中心凹回避盲点（图 9–4A）。干性黄斑变性和治疗后的湿性黄斑变性、Stargardt 病和其他黄斑病变患者都有这种表现。这类患者有可能看不见视力表上的大字母，使得检查者放弃检查，并记录非常低的视力。然而如果更加仔细地检查或者在更近的距离检查时则会发现，当患者能将有限的中心视野和视力表上的视标对齐时，他（或她）能识别更小的字母（图 9–4B）。

对比敏感度　辨别对比度的能力不同于视力的视觉功能，两者之间没有直接的联系。对比敏感度差的患者在看台阶的边缘、阅读浅色的字体、起雾或下雪时驾驶以及识别面孔时都有困难。对比敏感度随着视标尺寸（空间频率）而改变，而对比度阈值和空间频率两者间的关系用对比敏感度曲线来表示（见 BCSC 第 3 册的第 3 章）。对比敏感度的正式检查包括纸质图表和计算机检查，后者允许有更大的测试范围。纸质图表可测试一个范围内的空间频率（图 9–5A），或单一的空间频率（图 9–5B）。

带有照明的放大镜、电子放大以及非光学方法对伴有对比敏感度缺失的视觉损害患者是有益的，例如改变工作照明或改变工作中的对比度，例如使用黑色毡制粗头笔。

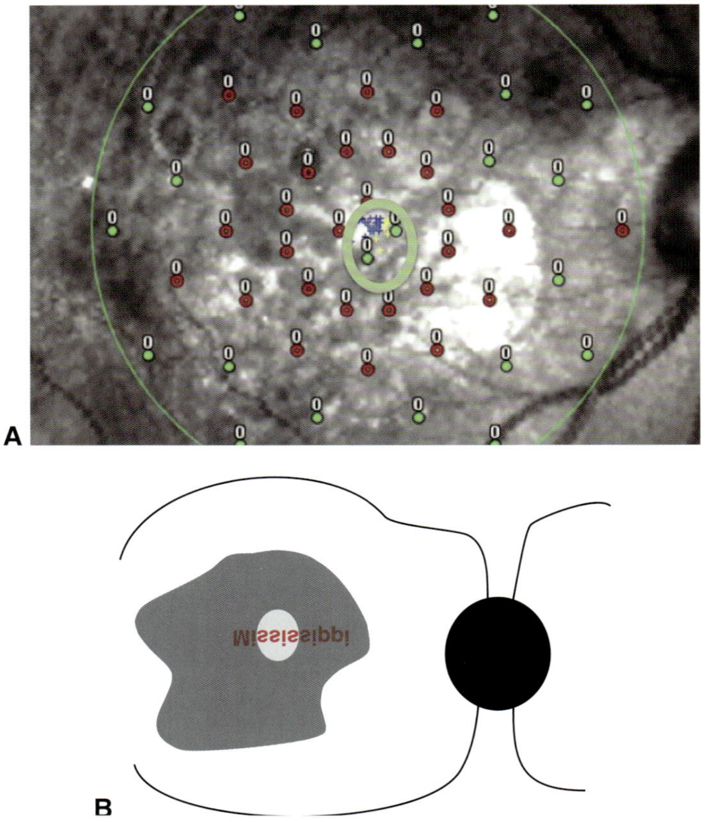

Figure 9-4 Foveal-sparing scotoma. **A**. Macular microperimetry of paracentral scotoma: green dots indicate targets that are seen by patient; red dots indicate missed targets. **B**. Effect of foveal-sparing scotoma on visualization of large print. *(Courtesy of Mary Lou Jackson, MD, and American Academy of Ophthalmology/Vision Rehabilitation Committee.)*

Central visual field The largest group of patients referred for vision rehabilitation are patients with central field loss due to age-related macular degeneration (AMD). Traditional field testing with Goldmann or Humphrey perimeters maps the visual field relative to a central fixation point. This is accurate in patients with stable central fixation, but results can be misleading in patients with unstable or eccentric fixation. Defects can be under-or overrepresented or displaced. Other nonautomated testing methods, such as Amsler grids, cannot assess fixation and will not detect approximately half of central or paracentral scotomas due to perceptual completion, or "filling in." The macular microperimeter monitors fundus location and then determines the patient's direction of gaze before each target is presented. Macular microperimetry (also called *fundus-related perimetry*), documents the patient's retinal point of fixation, scotomas, and the relationship of the fixation point to the scotomas. Most patients with central scotomas spontaneously develop eccentric fixation but may have poor oculomotor control at the eccentric area or preferred retinal loci (see Fig 9-3). They may use multiple PRLs, change fixation depending on target size or illumination, or develop a sense of "straight ahead" related to their PRL, rather than their fovea.

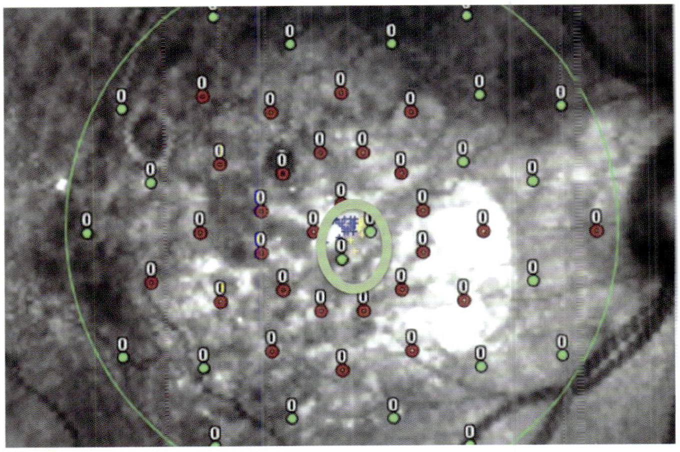
A

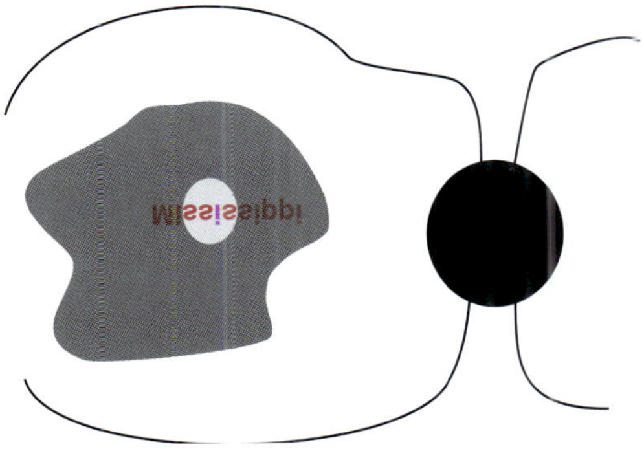

B

图 9-4　中心凹回避盲点。**A.** 旁中心盲点的黄斑微视野检查：绿色点表示被患者看到的视标，红色点表示遗漏的视标。**B.** 中心凹回避盲点在大字体显示中的效果。*（译者注：资料来源见前页英文原文。）*

中心视野　被推荐进行视觉康复的患者多数是由于年龄相关性黄斑变性（AMD）引起的中心视野缺失。传统视野检查用的 Goldmann 视野计或 Humphrey 视野计，绘制的是相对于中心注视点的视野图。这对于有稳定中心注视的患者来说是精确的，但对于不稳定的或非中心注视的患者来说，结果可能是有误导性的，损伤可能是不完全表现或过度的表现，或者偏移。其他的非自动检查方法，例如 Amsler 表，由于知觉完成或“填充”的原因，不能察觉近乎一半的中心或旁中心盲点，所以不能用来评估注视。黄斑微视野计监控眼底的位置，在每一个视标出现之前，先确定患者的固视方向，所以黄斑微视野计（也被称为*眼底相关视野计*）可以记录患者视网膜的注视点、盲点，以及注视点与盲点之间的关系。大部分有中心盲点的患者自动形成非中心注视，但在非中心区域或优选视网膜位点可能眼球运动控制较差（见图 9-3）。他们可能会使用多个优选视网膜定位点（PRLs），依照视标大小和光照度来改变注视，或者发展成一种与他们的优选视网膜定位点“直接相关的注视”，而不是他们的中心凹相关的注视。

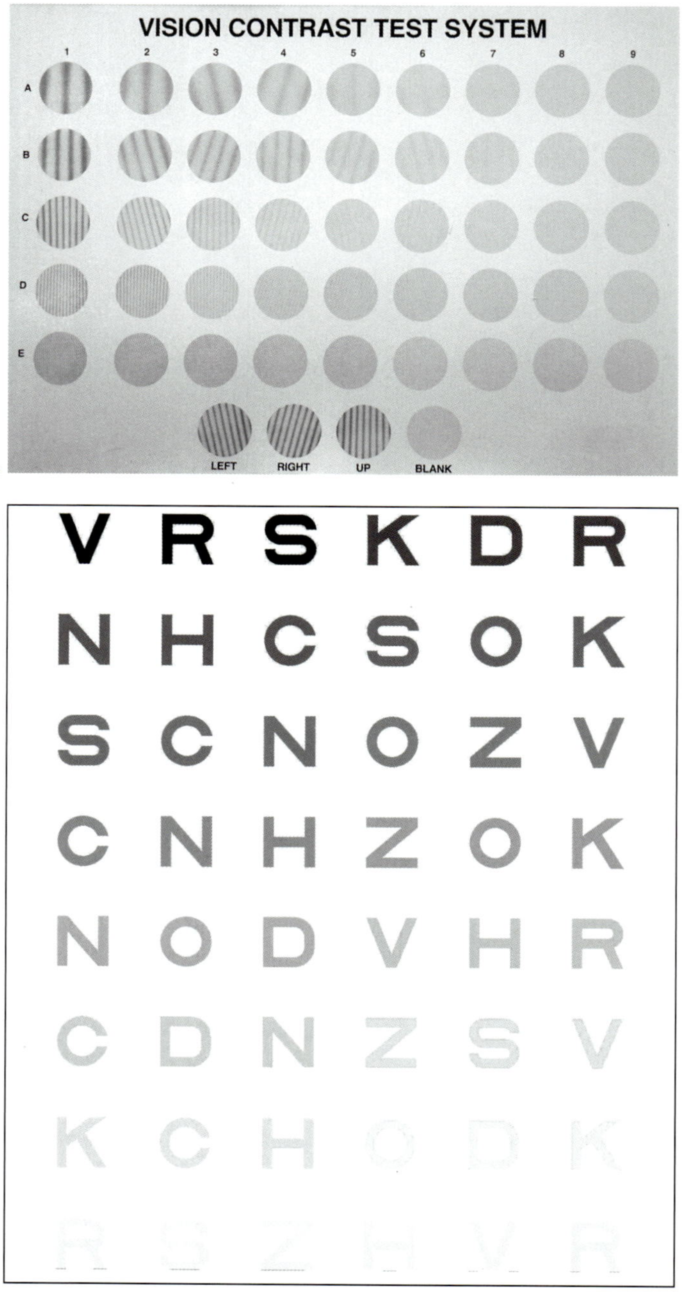

A

B

Figure 9-5 Eye charts for measuring contrast sensitivity. **A**, Vistech chart. Spatial frequency increases from top to bottom; contrast decreases in each row from left to right. Patient must detect whether grating pattern is tilted to left, vertical, or tilted to right; see samples in bottom row. **B**, Pelli-Robson chart. Contrast of large Sloan letters decreases in groups of 3 from top to bottom and left to right within each line. *(Part A courtesy of Scott E. Brodie, MD, PhD; part B reprinted with permission from Pelli DG, Robson JG, Wilkins AJ. The design of a new letter chart for measuring contrast sensitivity. Clin Vision Sci. 1988;2(3):187–199. Copyright © 2002, Pelli DG, Robson JG. Distributed by Haag-Streit.)*

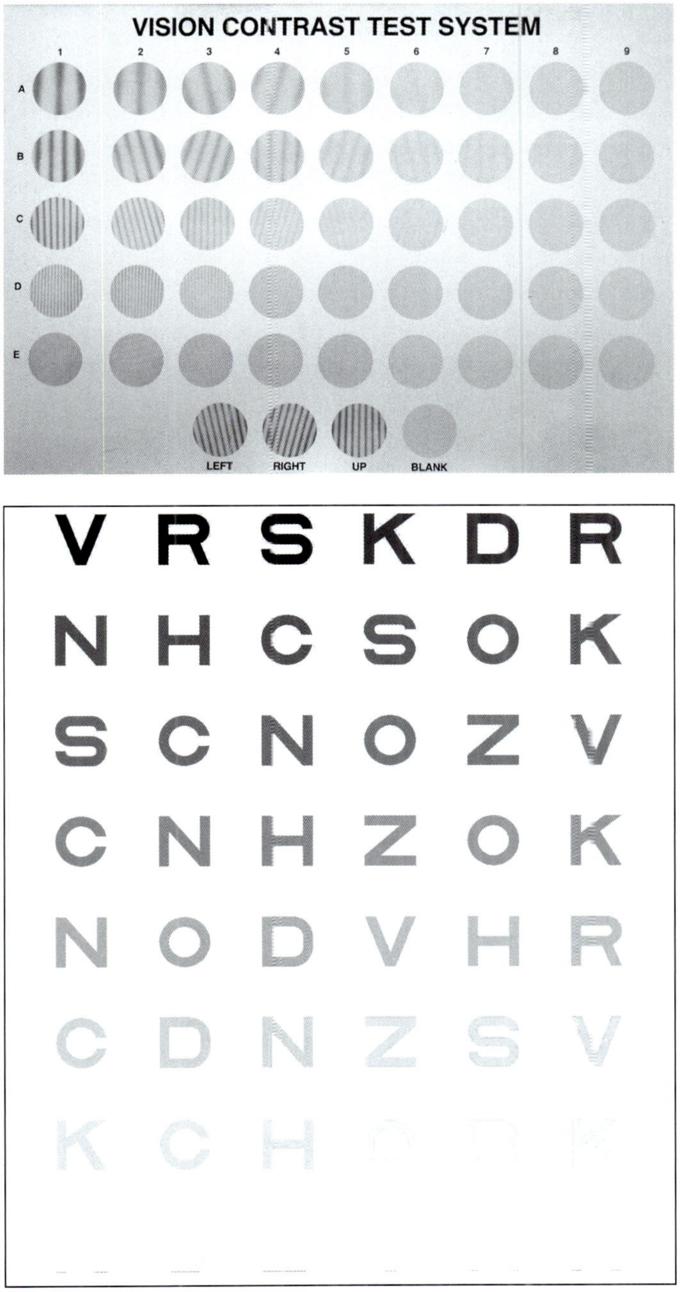

A

B

图 9-5　检查对比敏感度的图表。**A.** Vistech 图表。空间频率从上往下增加；每一行的对比敏感度从左到右减低。参考看最后一行的样板，患者必须辨认光栅图案是斜向左、垂直、还是斜向右的。**B.** Pelli-Robson 图表。3 个一组的大的 Sloan 字母的对比度在每一行中从上往下和从左往右下降。*（译者注：资料来源见前页原文。）*

The vision rehabilitation clinician needs to appreciate the nature of the patient's fixation (foveal or eccentric), the presence and nature of scotomas (central or paracentral), and the relationship of fixation and scotoma. For example a scotoma may surround fixation, as in foveal-sparing scotomas (see Fig 9-4A), be right of fixation (Fig 9-6A) and obscure next words (Fig 9-6B), or be left of fixation (Fig 9-7) and make it difficult to carry out an accurate saccade to the beginning of the next line of print. Although some believe that a PRL looking up (Fig 9-8) is optimal, as it would allow a horizontal span for left-to-right readers, no difference in reading speed with PRL location has been determined. Scotomas that surround seeing retina may interfere with the recognition of large objects, fluent reading, or using magnification, depending on the size of the central seeing field (see Fig 9-4B).

Scotomas can vary widely in size, shape, number, and density, and they may not correspond to the fundus appearance of atrophy, scarring, or pigment alteration. This lack of correspondence is particularly important to consider in patients with wet AMD who receive anti–vascular endothelial growth factor (anti-VEGF) injections. Such patients may not exhibit obvious scars yet still have significant scotomas in their central field.

Crossland MD, Jackson ML, Seiple WH. Microperimetry: a review of fundus related perimetry. *Optometry Reports*. 2012; 2:11–15.

A

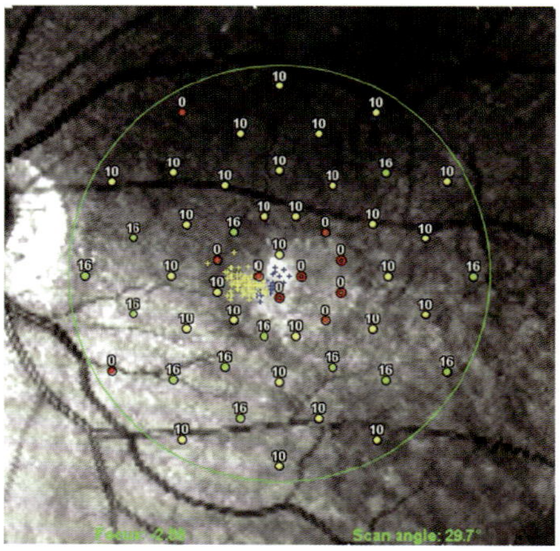

B

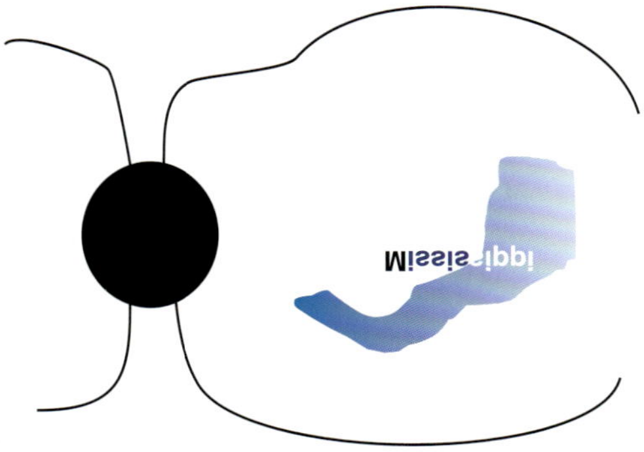

Figure 9-6 Macular microperimetry. **A**, A scotoma (red targets) right of fixation (yellow crosses). **B**, This pattern of scotoma would decrease the horizontal perceptual span when reading, obscure the next word, and be anticipated to interrupt normal reading saccades. *(Courtesy of Mary Lou Jackson, MD.)*

视觉康复医生需要了解患者的注视性质（中心凹或非中心）、盲点的存在与性质（中心或旁中心），以及注视点和盲点的关系。例如一个环绕注视点的盲点，就像中心凹回避盲点一样（见图 9-4A），在注视点的右边（图 9-6A），会遮挡下一个文字（图 9-6B），或者在注视点的左边（图 9-7），使得准确地扫视到下一行文字的开始很困难。虽然一些人认为 PRL 查找是最佳的，当为从左到右阅读的人给予了一个水平区域的时候，PRL 位置已经被确定，在阅读速度上没有不同。环绕有视觉视网膜的盲点会干扰大目标的识别、流畅的阅读以及放大镜的使用，但它取决于中心有视觉区域的大小（见图 9-4B）。

盲点在大小、形状、数量和密度上可以有很大的差异，它们可能与眼底萎缩、疤痕或色素紊乱的表现不一致。对于接受了抗血管内皮生长因子（anti-VEGF）注射的湿性 AMD 患者，考虑到这种缺乏一致性尤为重要。这些患者可能没有明显的疤痕，但他们的中心视野已经有了明显的盲点。

Crossland MD, Jackson ML, Seiple WH. Microperimetry: a review of fundus related perimetry. *Optometry Reports*. 2012; 2:11–15.

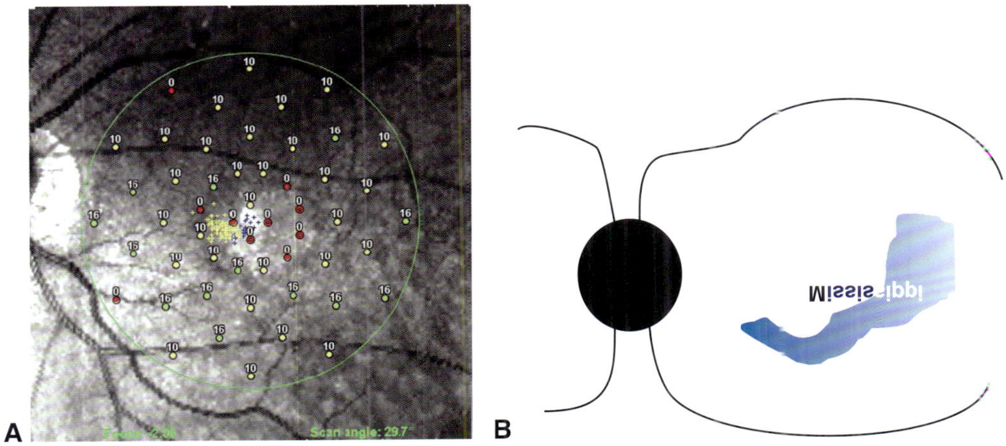

图 9-6 水黄斑微视野计。**A.** 盲点（红色指标）在注视点（黄色指标）的右边。**B.** 在阅读的时候盲点的图案将会使平知觉广度减低，遮挡下一个文字，可能会干扰正常的阅读扫视。*（译者注：资料来源见前页英文原文。）*

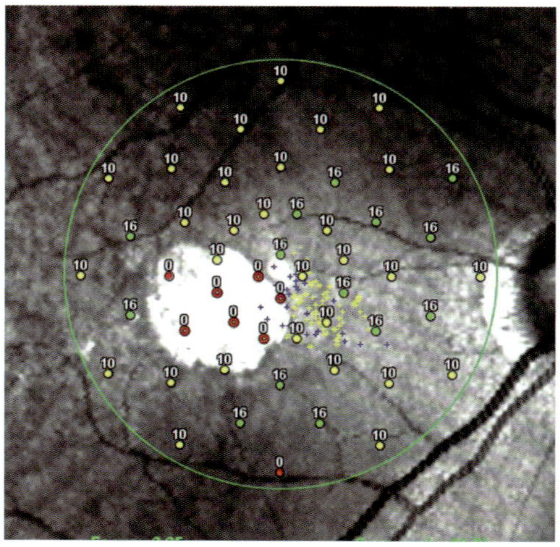

Figure 9-7 The scotoma is left of fixation and may cause difficulty finding the beginning of the next line of text. *(Courtesy of Mary Lou Jackson, MD.)*

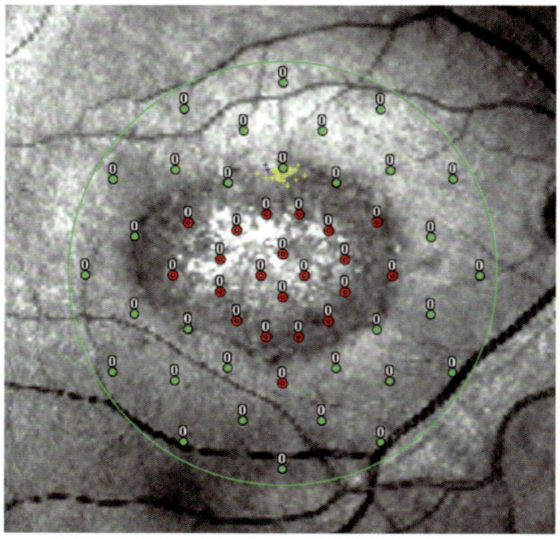

Figure 9-8 The patient has moved the eye up to use a preferred retinal loci looking up. *(Courtesy of Mary Lou Jackson, MD.)*

Peripheral visual field Peripheral visual field defects cause patients to bump into objects or people, trip over objects and curbs, and lose their orientation particularly in unfamiliar areas. Goldmann fields, automated peripheral fields, or carefully conducted confrontational fields can be informative in the setting of patients with glaucoma, peripheral retinal disease, or optic nerve or neurologic disease affecting visual pathways.

Assessments of other visual functions Glare, color vision (discussed in BCSC Section 5, *Neuro-Ophthalmology* and in BCSC Section 12, *Retina and Vitreous*), binocularity (see BCSC Section 6, *Pediatric Ophthalmology and Strabismus*), eye movements and accommodation (see BCSC Section 6, *Pediatric Ophthalmology and Strabismus*) may be considered in some situations. Glare is the discomfort or impairment of vision caused by scattered light (mainly Mie-type scattering in the forward direction; see Chapter 2). It occurs commonly in ocular conditions such as corneal disease, cataracts, macular dystrophy, and albinism, and somewhat less commonly in AMD or glaucoma. Patients with reduced contrast sensitivity often require increased illumination, which may, in turn, exacerbate glare. Therefore, determining sensitivity to glare is important so that you can advise patients about optimal lighting.

The simplest way to assess glare is through the history; however, formal testing can be done with a brightness acuity tester, a handheld device that allows the patient to view a distant target through a small dome that floods the eye with off-axis illumination.

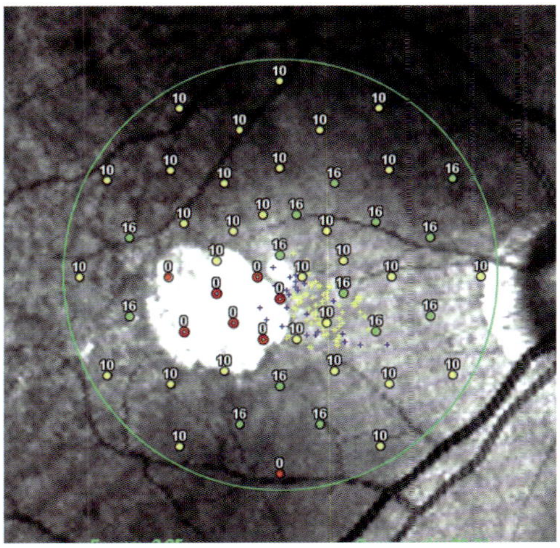

图 9–7　在注视点左边的盲点可能很难找到下一行文字的开始。*(译者注：资料来源见前页英文原文。)*

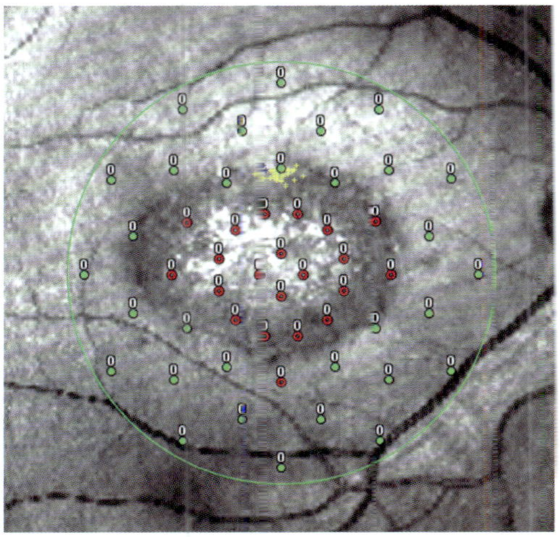

图 9–8　患者将眼睛向上移动，使用优选视网膜定位点去注视。*(译者注：资料来源见前页英文原文。)*

周边视野　周边视野缺失会导致患者撞到物体或人，被物体或在路边绊倒，尤其是在不熟悉的区域容易迷失方向。对于患有青光眼、周边视网膜疾病、视神经疾病或影响视路的神经疾病的患者，Goldmann 视野检测、自动周边视野检测以及有仔细引导的相对视野检查都能获得有用信息。

其他视觉功能的评估　在某些情况下应该考虑眩光、色觉（在 BCSC 第 5 册《*神经眼科学*》和 BCSC 第 12 册《*视网膜与玻璃体*》）、双眼视觉（见 BCSC 第 6 册《*小儿眼科与斜视*》）、眼球运动和调节 (见 BCSC 第 6 册《*小儿眼科与斜视*》)。眩光是由于光线散射引起的视觉不适或损害（主要是在向前方的 Mie 散射，见第 2 章）。这通常源于眼部疾病，例如角膜疾病、白内障、黄斑营养不良和白化病，而 AMD 或青光眼少见。对比敏感度减低的患者通常需要增加照明，但这样反过来可能会加剧眩光。因此，测定眩光的敏感性很重要，可以建议患者选择最佳照明。

最简单的评估眩光的方法是回顾病史，然而，正规检查法常用亮度锐度检查仪，这是一款手持的设备，让患者通过一个小的圆顶仪器来观察远处的目标，这个圆顶仪器会有非视轴的光照涌入眼睛。

Performance of visual tasks

To assess patients' current success with visual tasks, they can be observed doing tasks such as reading, using their cell phone or computer, writing, or ambulating. Reading tests vary and include tests to assess reading single numbers or words (spot reading), paragraphs (continuous print reading; eg, the International Reading Speed Texts [iReST]) or sentences with decreasing size of text (eg, the Minnesota Low-Vision Reading Test MNREAD, Fig 9-9). Useful variables include the minimum size of print that can be read with current glasses or devices (reading acuity), reading errors, and the optimal size text for reading fluency (critical print size). The latter can inform magnification goals. It is important to note that different patients with the same distance visual acuity will read different sizes of near print if they are using different powers of reading add. The reading add power used and the distance from the eye to the text should always be documented when measuring near vision (eg, 0.4 M at 40 cm, with +2.50 add). For purposes of vision rehabilitation, it is often convenient to describe the print size of reading materials using M notation. Note: the M size of an optotype is the distance (in meters) at which the sample can be read by a person with normal acuity—thus, "1 M" print is normally legible at 1.0 m.

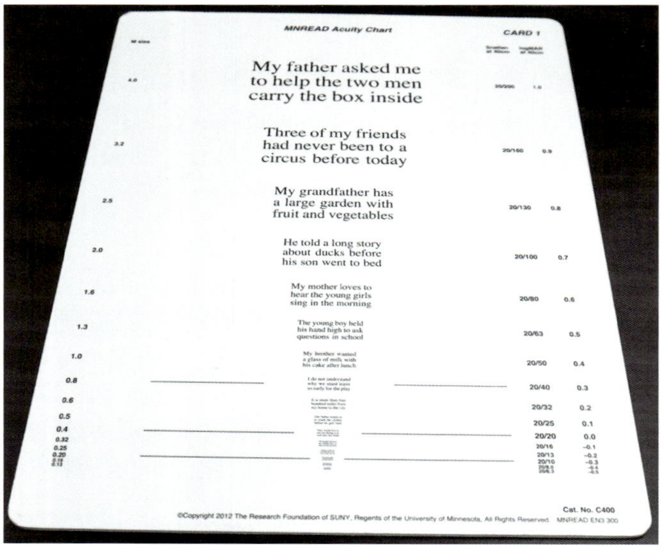

Figure 9-9 The MNREAD reading test has a range of text sizes. Patients may have difficulty reading the larger text yet find it easier to read smaller text when they have a limited area of central seeing retina. *(Courtesy of Mary Lou Jackson, MD.)*

Observing a patient reading the actual material that he or she normally reads—such as the newspaper or medication labels, or doing a task that they value such as using a cell phone, writing, reading prices at arm's length or walking independently—can reveal not only difficulties or successes, but also current adaptive strategies, such as head posture, manipulation of the material, or attempts to use current devices. Computer and cell phone difficulties may include losing the cursor into surrounding areas of field loss, misdialing phone numbers, or having difficulty with keyboards.

Observing a patient ambulate provides valuable insight into the need for orientation and mobility training, white-cane or support-cane use, or scanning training.

Many different questionnaires have been used to elicit patient reports of difficulties with visual tasks.

实施视觉工作

为了评估患者能否胜任目前的视觉工作，可以观察他们正在做的一些工作，例如阅读、使用手机或电脑、书写或走动。阅读测试是多种多样的，包括阅读单个数字或单词（点阅读）、段落［连续文字的阅读，例如国际阅读速度文本（iReST）］，或文本字体越来越小的句子［例如明尼苏纳州低视力阅读测试（MNREAD），图 9-9］的评估。有用的变量包括使用当前眼镜或设备所能阅读的最小印刷字体（阅读视力）、阅读错误，以及阅读流畅的最佳文本大小（临界印刷大小）。后者可以为放大目标提供信息。值得注意的是，不同患者虽然有相同的远距离视力，如果使用不同度数的阅读近附加，他们将可以阅读不同大小的近距离的印刷字体。当测量近处视力时，所用的阅读附加度数和眼睛到文本的距离都应该被记录下来（例如，在 40cm 处，用 +2.50D 近附加视力 0.4M）。为了视觉康复，使用 M 标记法描述阅读材料的字体大小通常比较方便。注意：视标的 M 大小是指这个视标能被正常视力的人读出的距离（以 m 为单位），因此，“1M”的字体正常在 1m 的距离内是能被辨认的。

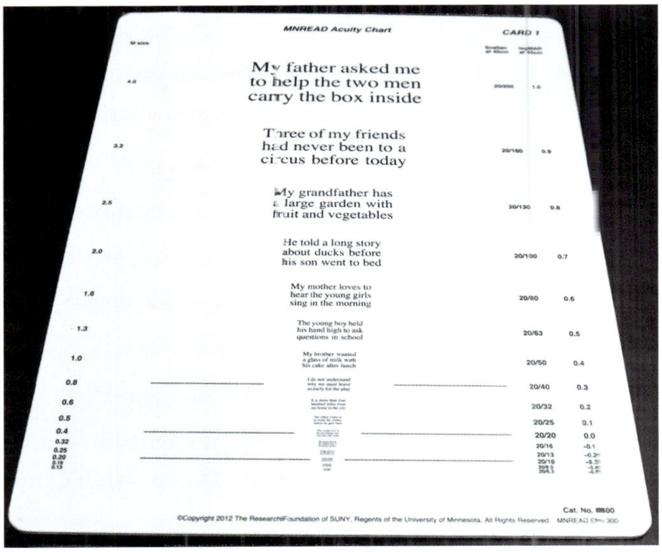

图 9-9　MNREAD 阅读检查有系列的文本大小。当患者有一个有限的中心可见视网膜区域时，他们可能阅读大视标文本有困难，但发现阅读小视标更容易。*（译者注：资料来源见前页英文原文。）*

观察患者真实的阅读材料，即他（或她）平时的阅读物，例如报纸或药品标签，或做一件他们认为有价值的工作，例如使用电话、书写、在一臂长的距离看价格，或自己行走，这样不仅能发现他们在现实生活中是否存在困难，也可以发现可行的方法，例如头位、对物品的操作方法，或努力使用现有的设备。计算机和手机的操作问题可能包括光标落在视野缺失的周边区域而找不到、错拨电话号码或使用键盘困难。

观察患者的行走，对定向和行走训练、白色拐杖或支持拐杖的使用或扫视训练的需求提供了有价值的认识。

许多不同的问卷常常被用来引导患者表述自身的视觉困难。

Interventions

Devices

Traditional options for magnification include higher adds, high-plus reading glasses, magnifiers, and telescopes. (Magnification is discussed in Chapter 1). Other practical solutions to difficulties include modifying a task, such as by moving closer to distant targets; using larger formats, such as large-print checks; or substituting with audio, such as digital audio books available through libraries or online. There is increasing interest in devices such as e-readers, cell phones, computers and electronic magnification as excellent options for patients with low vision. Other technologies include head-worn devices, devices that read text aloud, detect objects, or assist patients with low vision or blindness by giving audio directions. Implantable devices include the implantable miniature telescope and retinal prosthesis.

Higher adds The simplest intervention for a patient with moderate low vision is to increase the reading add. Ophthalmologists should be strongly encouraged to consider +4.00 adds or simple over-the-counter readers, such as +4.00 readers, as long as patients can learn to maintain the closer focal distance and use supplemental lighting if beneficial. This can be attempted prior to referral for comprehensive vision rehabilitation. Patients will often accept higher adds, such as readers in powers from +6.00 to +12.00 with appropriate base-in prism and the appropriate focal distance. A +10.00 reading add will require a reading distance at the focal point of the lens, which will be 1/10 m (ie, 10 cm, or 4 in). In binocular patients, prism is required to assist convergence and relax accommodation. The recommended prism strength is 2 prism diopters (Δ) more base-in (BI) than the numerical add power, in each eye. For example, if the distance prescription is plano OU and the appropriate add power for reading is +8.00D, then the prescription should read as follows: OD: +8.00 sphere with 10Δ BI; OS: +8.00 sphere with 10Δ BI. Prism is not required in adds up to +4.00 D.

Readers with prism are available ready-made in powers from +6.00 D to +14.00 D and allow a wide field of view. Monocular aspheric spectacles, available from +6.00 D to +32.00 D, are used less often. Computer glasses with intermediate-strength add powers are useful and can be prescribed as a bifocal with the intermediate power in the upper segment. In general, reading glasses allow hands-free magnification and a large field of vision; however, there is a shortened working distance, and supplemental lighting is required.

Historically an add was calculated as the inverse of the visual acuity (Kestenbaum rule: the inverse of the visual acuity fraction is the add power, in diopters, to read 1 M type—about 8 points, corresponding to the 20/50 line on a standard near-vision card calibrated for use at 14 inches), and this calculation may provide a general starting point; however, it is now appreciated that many other factors influence reading fluency, such as fixation location, scotomas, perceptual span, crowding, and contrast sensitivity. The Kestenbaum rule would estimate that a patient with 20/200 acuity would require 200/20, or 10 D of add. For fluent reading, patients with 20/200 acuity may actually require higher add than calculated.

干预

设备

传统的放大镜包括高度数的近附加、高度数正镜度阅读镜、放大镜和望远镜（放大在第 1 章已讨论）。其他解决困难的实际方法包括：调整目标，例如移近远距离目标；或使用大字本，例如大字支票；或用音频替代，例如图书馆或在线提供的数码音频书籍。患者对设备的兴趣在不断增长，例如电子阅读器、手机、计算机和电子放大器等，因为它们是低视力患者极好的选择。其他技术包括头戴设备、大声读出文本的设备、探测物体的设备，或通过音频方向来帮助低视力患者或盲人。植入设备包括植入微型望远镜和人工视网膜技术。

高度数的近附加　对于中度低视力的患者最简单的干预就是增加阅读近附加。建议眼科医生考虑 +4.00 D 的近附加或简单的不需处方的阅读镜，例如 +4.00 D 的阅读镜，只要患者能学习维持更近的焦距，并使用补充照明。在推荐进行综合视觉康复之前，可以试用这些方法。患者通常接受更高的近附加，例如 +6.00 D~+12.00 D 的阅读镜，附带适当的底向内的三棱镜，并有合适的焦距。一个 +10.00 D 的阅读近附加，阅读距离在镜片的焦点处，即 1/10m（即 10cm，或 4 in）。在双眼视的患者中，需要棱镜帮助集合和放松调节。推荐的棱镜度数是在每一只眼比附加度数的数字多 2 的底向内（BI）的棱镜度（Δ）。例如，如果双眼的远距离处方是平光，合适的近附加阅读度数是 +8.00 D，阅读的处方是：OD 为 +8.00 球镜带 10ΔBI，OS 为 +8.00 球镜带 10ΔBI。近附加低于 +4.00 D 的不需要加棱镜。

市场上有现成的带有棱镜的阅读镜，度数从 +6.00 D 到 +14.00 D，并有宽阔的视野。还有单眼非球面镜，从 +6.00 D 到 +32.00 D，但通常较少使用。中距离近附加的电脑眼镜很有用，如双光镜，中距离度数在眼镜的上半部分。一般的阅读镜是非手持大视野放大镜，但工作距离短，需要有补充照明。

历史上近附加是用视力的倒数来计算的（Kestenbaum 法则：视力分数的倒数是近附加的度数，以 D 为单位，为了阅读 1M 的字体——大约 8 点，与已校准在 14in 处使用的标准近距离视力表上的 20/50 一行视标相一致），这个计算方法提供了一个大体的起点。然而，现在认识到还有许多因素影响到阅读流畅度，例如注视位置、盲点、知觉广度、拥挤度和对比敏感度。Kestenbaum 法则预计一个 20/200 视力的患者将需要 200/20 或者 10 D 的近附加，而为了实现流畅阅读，20/200 视力的患者可能实际需要比计算更高的近附加。

Magnifiers Handheld and stand magnifiers are available in illuminated or nonilluminated formats. A simple handheld or illuminated stand magnifier in low-to-medium power can allow continuous text reading for patients with mild-to-moderate vision loss. Patients with tremors or difficulty holding a magnifier may find success with a stand magnifier that rests directly on the page (Fig 9-10). Stand magnifiers are set in a frame that sits on the material and keeps the lens at the appropriate distance. Higher-powered magnifiers (higher than 20 D) have a limited field of view and allow one to read short text, but are seldom comfortable for extended reading of continuous print because of the requirement of continuous movement along the line of text. Low-powered magnifiers (+5 to +12 D) with light-emitting-diode illumination are the most common handheld magnifiers (Fig 9-11).

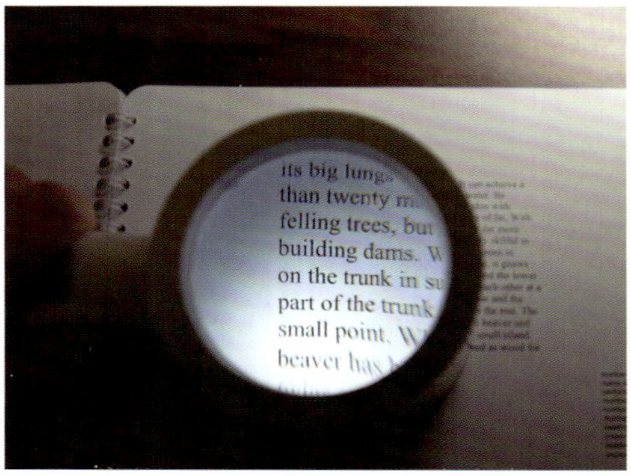

Figures 9-10 An illuminated stand magnifier placed flat against the page provides magnification, illumination, and stability. As with all magnifiers, the field of view decreases with increased magnification. *(Courtesy of Mary Lou Jackson, MD.)*

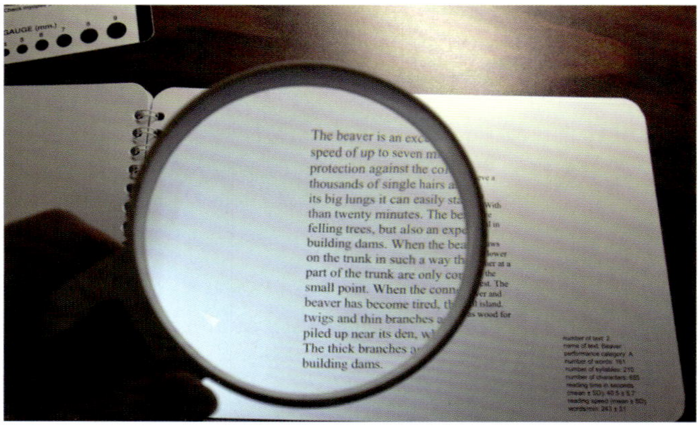

Figure 9-11 Illuminated hand magnifier. *(Courtesy of Mary Lou Jackson, MD.)*

放大镜　手持式和立式放大镜都有带照明或不带照明的款式。用一个低中度手持式或带照明的立式放大镜，轻中度视觉缺失的患者就可以持续阅读。患者有颤抖症状或手持放大镜困难时，可以使用直接放在页面上的立式放大镜（图 9–10）。立式放大镜通常安装在一个框架上，立在材料上并使镜片保持在一个合适的距离。高度数放大镜（高于 20 D）的视野有限，可以用来读短文，但不能舒适地进行长时间的连续阅读，因为需要沿着一行文本不断移动。带有发光二极管照明的低度放大镜（+5~+12 D）是最常用的手持式放大镜（图 9–11）。

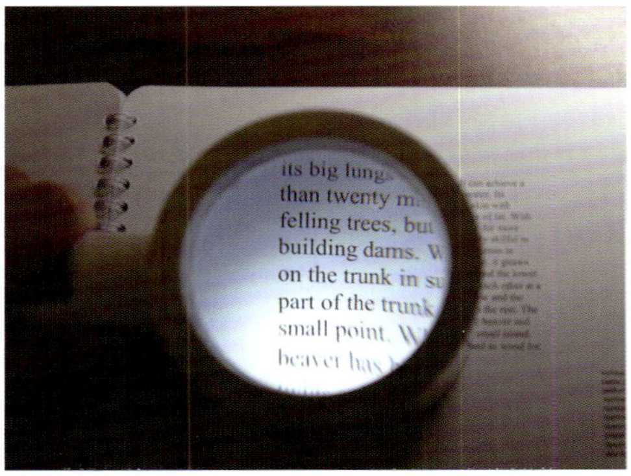

图 9–10　带照明的立式放大镜平放在页面上，具有放大、照明和稳定的功能与特点。与所有的放大镜一样，视野随放大率的增加而减少。*（译者注：资料来源见前页原文。）*

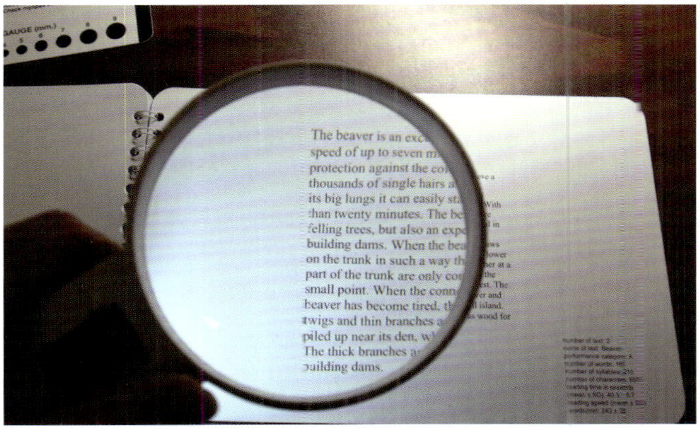

图 9–11　带照明的手持放大镜。*（译者注：资料来源见前页原文。）*

The "power" or "magnification factor" or "enlargement ratio" of a magnifier is usually specified in terms of the relative angular size of the magnified image compared with the angular size of the original object at a standard reading distance (see Chapter 1). Most commonly, the reference distance is taken as 25 cm. In general, the maximal magnification will be obtained when the object to be viewed is placed at the anterior focal point of the magnifier. When the magnifier is used this way, the magnification factor is equal to the dioptric power of the lens divided by 4 (the dioptric equivalent of the reference distance of 25 cm). For example, the power of a +24 D magnifier is 6× (24 D/4 D); however, magnifiers are used in different manners and held at different distances. Simple low-power magnifiers (eg, +4 D) are rarely used by holding the object at the anterior focal point of the magnifier, because it is difficult to hold a lens steady so far from the page; therefore, the previous magnification factor convention is no longer appropriate. Magnifiers are often labeled with a "trade magnification" power. Trade magnification is calculated as the (diopter power of the hand magnifier)/4 +1, so the trade magnification of +4 D handheld lens is 2×.

Telescopes There are 2 types of telescopes; astronomical (also called *Keplerian*) telescopes and Galilean telescopes (optics of telescopes are discussed in Chapter 1). Their features are compared in Table 9-1. Telescopes are much less commonly used than magnifiers, as tasks that require magnification for distance viewing are less-frequent goals than those for near viewing. Handheld monoculars, binoculars, and spectacle-mounted telescopes allow the benefit of magnification at a greater distance, with the drawback of reduction in field of view, a narrow depth of field, and reduced contrast. (Fig 9-12A). The latter is particularly limiting in patients with significant loss of contrast sensitivity. Autofocus telescope models are available. A simple telescopic spectacle without a casing has become popular, as it is lightweight and relatively inexpensive (Fig 9-12B).

Loupes (telemicroscopes) are spectacle-mounted close-focusing telescopes set to focus at near points. They allow a greater working distance than high-add reading glasses; however, as with all telescopes, the visual field is narrow and the depth of field small. Bioptic telescopes are spectacle-mounted telescopes set to focus at distance, mounted in the upper portion of the lenses of carrier spectacles. Many states, and the Netherlands in Europe, allow driving with bioptic telescopes. The telescopic portion of the spectacles is positioned superior to the line of sight and used only briefly to read signs or look into the distance. The rest of the time, the individual drives looking through the regular prescription portion of his or her spectacles. Driving with a bioptic telescope requires prescription of the device as well as device training, driver training and, in some states, on-road evaluation. Patients with good contrast sensitivity and intact central field are optimal candidates for bioptic driving.

Table 9-1 Comparison of Galilean and Astronomical Telescopes

Feature	Astronomical Telescope	Galilean Telescope
Enlargement range	1.5–4.0×	2.0–10.0×
Length[a]	Longer	Shorter
Field of view[a]	Smaller	Wider
Focusing range[a]	Greater	Smaller
Image quality[a]	Better	Poorer
Weight[a]	Heavier	Lighter
Complexity	More complex	Simpler

[a] Indicates comparison matched for enlargement.

放大镜的“度数”或“放大倍数”或“放大率”，通常是指放大像形成的相对角度与在标准阅读距离处原物体的角度之比（见第 1 章）。大多数情况下的参考距离为 25cm，一般当观察的物体放在放大镜的前焦点时，可获得最大的放大。当以这种方式使用放大镜时，放大倍数等于镜片的度数除以 4（参考距离 25cm 的等效度数）。例如，度数为 –24D 的放大镜是 6×（24D/4D）。然而，放大镜是以不同的方式、拿在不同的距离使用的，很少将物体拿在低度数放大镜（例如 +4D）的前焦点处使用，因为很难在离页面这么远的地方保持放大镜的稳定，因此，前面的放大倍率约定不再合适。放大镜通常被贴上“商用放大率”度数的标签。商用放大率是这样计算的：（手持放大镜的度数 /4）+1，即 +4D 手持放大镜的商用放大率是 2×。

望远镜　望远镜有 2 种：天文望远镜（也称 *Kepler* 望远镜）和 Galileo 望远镜（望远镜的光学在第 1 章已讨论）。两者特点的比较见表 9–1。望远镜不常用，因为与近距离注视相比，远距离注视需要放大的工作目标较少。手持单目、双目和安装在眼镜上的望远镜能获得较好的远距离放大效果，伴随的缺点是视野缩小、景深狭小和对比度下降（图 9–12A）。后者（指 Galileo 望远镜）尤其限制了有明显对比敏感度缺失的患者。市场上有一款自动聚焦望远镜。还有一款无壳望远镜很流行，因为它重量轻，相对便宜（图 9–12B）。

Loupes（显微望远镜）是安装在眼镜上的近聚焦的望远镜，其将近点设为焦点。与高度近附加的阅读眼镜相比，它有更大的工作距离。然而，像所有的望远镜一样，它的视野窄、景深小。双光望远镜是安装在眼镜上的望远镜，设远距离为焦点，安装在镜片的上部分。美国的许多州以及欧洲的荷兰允许使用双光望远镜的人驾驶。眼镜的望远镜部分安装在视线的上部，只在看标识或看远距离时短暂使用，其余的时间都是使用他（或她）的眼镜常规处方部分。使用双光望远镜驾驶，要求医生给出设备处方和进行使用设备训练、驾驶员的训练，在某些州还需要进行道路评估。具有好的对比敏感度和完整的中心视野的患者，是双光望远镜驾驶的最佳候选人。

表9–1　Galileo和天文望远镜的对比

特征	天文望远镜	Galileo望远镜
放大范围	1.5~4.0 ×	2.0~10.0 ×
长度[a]	较长	较短
视野[a]	较小	较大
聚焦范围[a]	较大	较小
成像质量[a]	较好	较差
重量[a]	较重	较轻
复杂性	较复杂	简单

注：[a]指相同放大率下的比较。

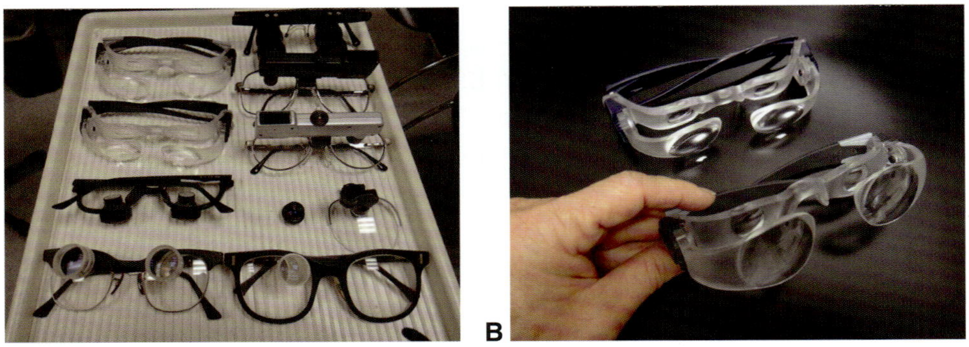

A B

Figures 9-12 Telescopic devices. **A**, This range of telescopic devices includes monocular and binocular telescopes. **B**, The spectacle telescope is lightweight and binocular and can be used for stationary distance viewing such as watching television. *(Courtesy of Mary Lou Jackson, MD.)*

Electronic devices Electronic devices allow magnification, contrast enhancement, and text-to-speech conversion. Magnification using video magnifiers (video cameras combined with screens; also referred to as *CCTVs*), computers, or tablets is now used very extensively by patients with low vision (Fig 9-13). Video magnifiers are available in various formats, including handheld versions, desk versions, or devices worn on the head. They allow variable magnification, comfortable reading positions, and enhanced or reversed contrast, features not available with optical magnifiers. Desk and head-mounted video magnifiers can use optical character recognition to read text aloud. Computer accessibility options on Windows and Macintosh computers provide magnification, modified contrast, and audio screen readers. Large monitors and larger-format keyboards assist, and televisions are often used as large monitors. The major difficulties with electronic devices are cost and training requirements; however, in some jurisdictions, and for certain individuals, devices are provided at no or reduced cost. For example, devices are provided by some state societies and are also provided to veterans.

When the accessibility features of the computer operating system are not adequate, additional magnification, screen reading (eg, AI Squared's ZoomText; see Fig 9-13I), or speech-to-text software can be considered. These require training. Smartphones provide very impressive utility for patients with vision loss as they allow not only magnification, but also text-to-speech and audio interaction for voice dialing phone numbers, searching the internet, and sending voice texts or email. Many additional cell phone applications can identify colors, currency, or objects. New and emerging voice-directed devices accomplish tasks such as setting thermostats or selecting music. Services available using cell phone applications can offer audible directions, object identification, or identification of objects in one's path. Audio books, most often in DAISY digital format (Digital Accessible Information System) are used widely by patients with vision loss and are available free through the Library of Congress in the US, the Center for Equitable Library Access in Canada, and from online libraries such as Bookshare. These are extensive libraries. The Bookshare accessible library, for example, has more than 500,000 titles that can be accessed via audio, by listening while seeing highlighted text, by using digital braille, or converting to large print or paper braille format. Many applications and devices exist to play audio books.

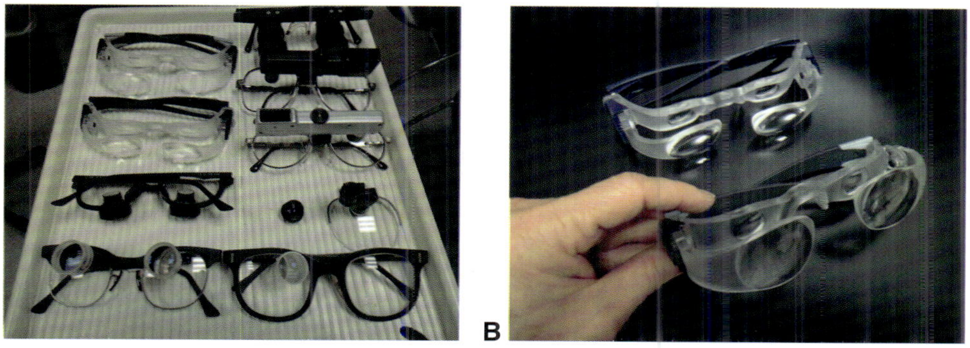

图 9-12　望远镜设备。**A.** 一系列望远镜设备 – 单目和双目望远镜。**B.** 眼镜式望远镜 – 轻型双目，用于远距离稳定观看，例如看电视。*（译者注：资料来源见前页原文。）*

电子设备 电子设备可以放大、增强对比度和进行文本的语音转换。现在低视力患者已经广泛使用视频放大镜进行放大（摄像机联合屏幕，也被称为 *CCTVs*），例如在计算机或平板电脑上的阅读（图 9-13）。视频放大镜有多种形式，包括手持版、桌面版或头戴式装置，具有可变放大、舒适的阅读位置以及增强或反转的对比度等功能，这些是光学放大镜所不具备的特点。桌上和头戴视频放大镜能使用光学特征来识别朗读文字。Windows 和 Macintosh 计算机的计算机辅助功能选项可提供放大、对比度调整和屏幕的音频朗读，还有大显示器和大字体键盘辅助。电视机常常被用作大显示器。电子设备的主要问题在于成本和需要训练，一些行政管辖区或者个人会提供免费或低价的设备，例如，一些州立社团提供设备或为退役军人提供设备。

当电脑操作系统的辅助功能不够的时候，可以考虑附加的放大率、读屏（例如，AI Squared's ZoomText；见图 9-13I）或者具有从语音到文本转换功能的软件，而使用这些功能需要进行训练。智能手机为视觉损害的患者提供了非常好的实用软件，因为它们不仅有放大功能，还有从文本到语音的转换、语音拨号、搜索网络、发送语音短信和语音电子邮件等功能。许多附加的手机应用程序能识别颜色、货币或物体。新兴的声控设备能完成恒温调节器设定或音乐的选择。手机应用程序还能提供的服务，包括声音定向、物体识别或行走路途中的物体识别。有声图书通常为 DAISY 数码格式（数字无障碍信息系统），已经为视觉缺失患者广泛使用，并且可以通过美国的国会图书馆、加拿大的公平图书馆访问中心、在线图书馆免费获得，如 Bookshare。这些是扩展的图书馆。例如 Bookshare 图书馆，有 50 多万册书可以通过音频阅读，边听边看标注的文本，使用数码 Braille 盲文，或转化为大字印刷，或纸质 Braille 盲文形式。许多应用程序和设备都能播放有声书。

Nonoptical aids The armamentarium of tools to assist patients with impaired vision extends beyond electronic and optical devices. Simple, practical devices include large-format watches, telephones, remote controls, playing cards, and checks. Talking clocks, scales and timers, bold-lettered computer keyboards, needle threaders, dark-lined writing paper, and felt-tip pens with black ink are a partial list of items that are often useful.

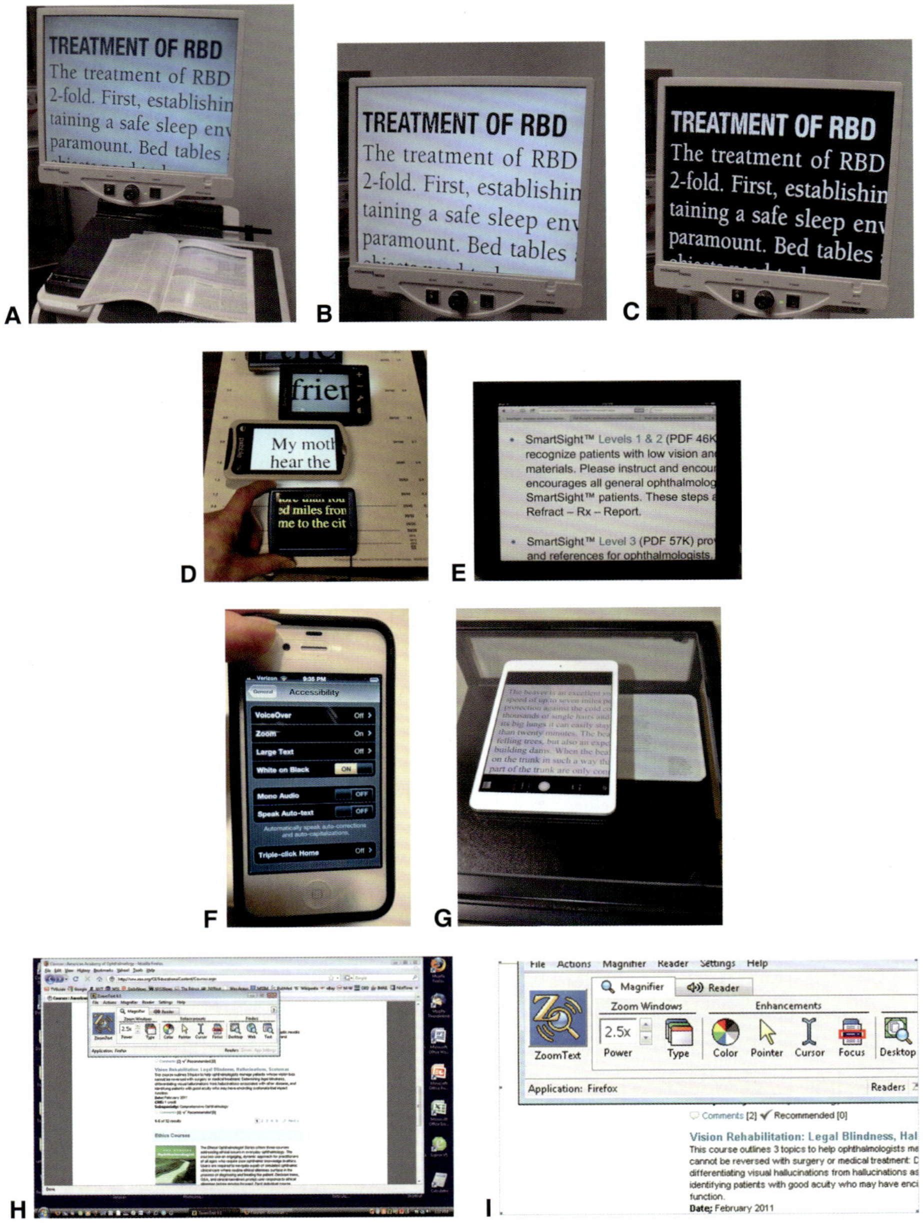

Figure 9-13 Electronic low vision aids. **A**, Desktop video magnifier. **B**, Same magnifier as in part A, in high-contrast mode. **C**, Same magnifier as in A, in reverse-contrast mode. **D**, Portable handheld video magnifiers. **E**, Tablet device used as a large-print e-reader. **F**, Smartphone accessibility features. **G**, Tablet device used as a video magnifier by placing on a glass desk. **H**, Standard-format Windows computer screen. **I**, Same computer screen as in part H, magnified using screen enlargement tools. *(Courtesy of Scott E. Brodie, MD, PhD; Mary Lou Jackson MD.)*

非光学助视器　辅助视觉损害患者的医疗设备已经超出了电子和光学设备的范畴。简单、实用的设备包括大字体手表、电话、遥控器、扑克牌和支票，说话时钟、磅秤和计时器，粗体字的电脑键盘、穿针器、黑色线的信纸、黑色墨水毡笔都是常用物品，这些仅是部分清单。

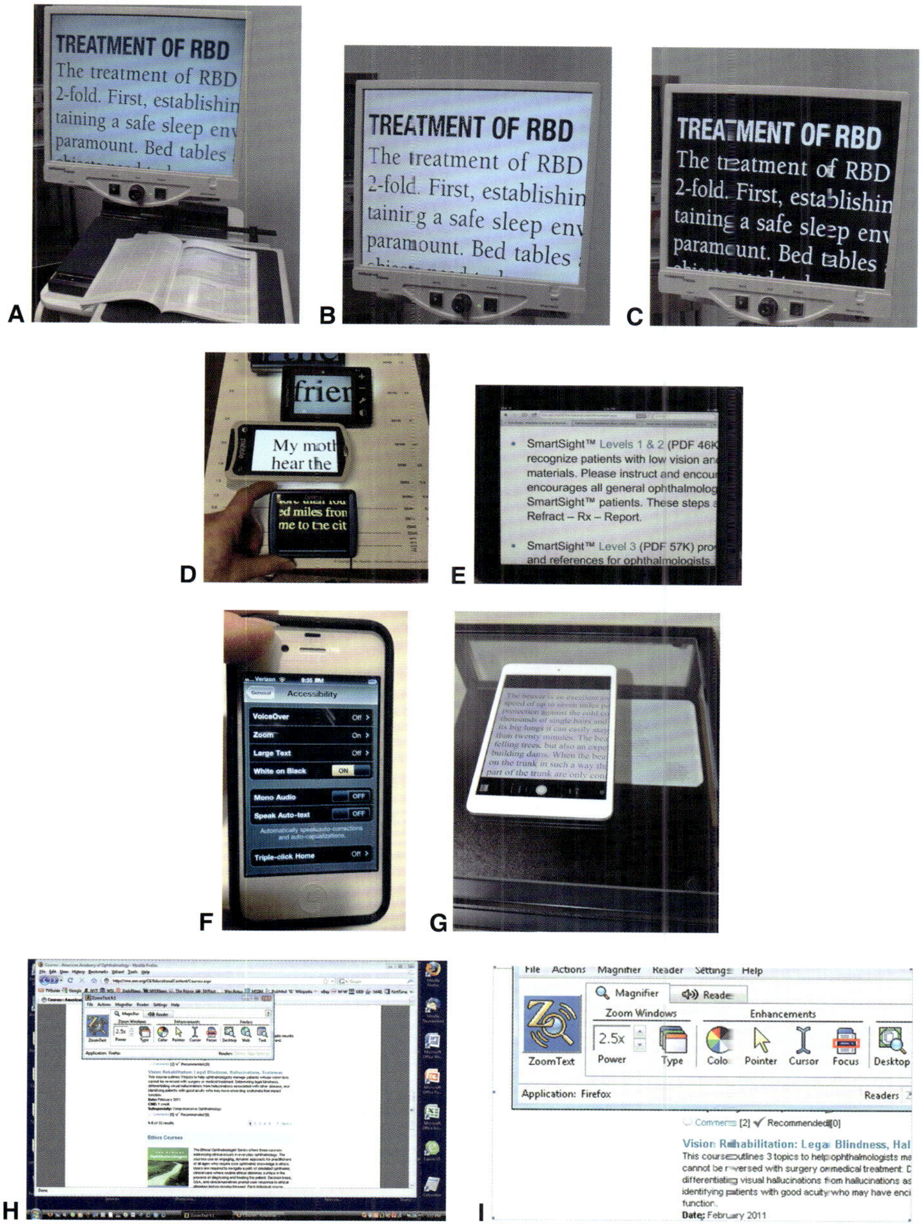

图 9–13　电子低视力助视器。**A.** 桌面视频放大器。**B.** 与图 A 相同的放大器，高对比度模式。**C.** 与图 A 相同的放大器，翻转对比模式。**D.** 便携式手持式视频放大器。**E.** 用作大字印刷电子阅读的平板电脑。**F.** 智能手机辅助功能。**G.** 放在玻璃桌面用作视频放大的平板电脑设备。**H.** 标准格式的 Windows 系统电脑屏幕。**I.** 与 **H** 相同的电脑屏幕，使用屏幕放大工具。*（译者注：资料来源见前页原文。）*

Blind rehabilitation and sight substitution devices Patients with no or very limited vision, particularly those who lose vision quickly, will require blind rehabilitation with sight substitutes that may include electronic text-to-speech or braille. Refreshable braille displays can be connected to computers and tablet devices. They have small, moving pins that rise or lower to create braille patterns that can be read tactilely. Short-term residential blind rehabilitation services, available in some areas, can offer great benefit for patients faced with the daunting task of adjusting to sudden and profound loss of vision. Prosthetic retinal implants are being developed, and many groups around the world are working on subretinal, suprachoroidal, or epiretinal devices in addition to cortical visual prostheses that stimulate the brain directly. Currently, devices allow patients to see outlines or contrast.

Training

After the low vision evaluation and creation of a vision rehabilitation plan for interventions, patients should be trained to accomplish tasks with modifications and use of appropriate devices. Medicare and some other health insurers in the US fund occupational therapists to train patients, just as rehabilitation is provided for other disabilities such as neurological or orthopedic conditions. Occupational therapists, or other state or privately funded vision rehabilitation therapists or technology specialists, can assess home safety, modify lighting, provide labels for appliances or dials, assist with strategies to manage glare, and instruct in accessibility features with computers, tablets, or cell phones. Physical, cognitive, psychosocial, and environmental factors that may impact performance must be considered. Although eccentric fixation can develop spontaneously in patients with central field loss, training may improve the efficiency of using the PRL. Approaches to training include perceptual training, oculomotor training, practice reading magnified text, and training a new direction of fixation (trained retinal locus). Currently, research has not identified a single recommended method. Prisms for assisting eccentric viewing in maculopathy are controversial and infrequently used. A large sample randomized controlled trial showed little benefit.

Gaffney AJ, Margrain TH, Bunce CV, et al. How effective is eccentric viewing training? A systematic literature review. *Ophthalmic Physiol Optics*. 2014(34):427–437.

Pijnacker J, Verstraten P, van Damme W, Vandermeulen J, Steenbergen B. Rehabilitation of reading in older individuals with macular degeneration: a review of effective training programs. *Neuropsychol Dev Cogn B Aging Neuropsychol Cogn*. 2011, 18(6):708–732.

Smith HJ, Dickinson CM, Cacho I, et al randomized controlled trial to determine the effectiveness of prism spectacles for patients with age-related macular degeneration. *Arch Ophthalmol*. 2005, 123(8):1042–1050.

Vision Rehabilitation for Field loss

Patients with neurologic disease often have field loss, processing deficits, or ocular symp- toms that can be assisted by vision rehabilitation. Scanning, sector prisms to displace im- ages to the seeing field, and vision restoration with computer training are rehabilitation strategies proposed for patients with hemianopia. A comparative trial of scanning and prisms showed improvement in vision-related quality of life with scanning training. Scanning training can be provided by Medicare-funded occupational therapists. Stroke management guidelines include reviews of evidence for interventions for visual neglect.

盲人康复和视觉替代设备 没有视力或视力非常有限的患者，尤其是快速视觉缺失的患者，需要视觉替代来实现盲人康复，包括电子的文本到语音转换或 Braille 盲文。将可更新的 Braille 显示器连接到电脑和平板电脑上，它们有小的可移动的针脚，能升起来或降下去形成 Braille 图案，从而实现触觉阅读。有些区域为短期居住盲人提供康复服务，这有助于突然严重视力丧失的患者缓和艰巨的调整处境。人工视网膜植入技术正在开发中，世界上很多团体都在研究视网膜上、脉络膜上或视网膜前的设备，除此之外，还有直接刺激大脑视皮质的视觉假体。目前，患者用这些设备可以看到轮廓或形成对比度。

训练

在对低视力评估后，就要建立视觉康复干预计划。经过训练调整、使用合适的设备，帮助患者最终完成工作目标。美国联邦医疗保险和其他健康保险资助职业治疗师训练患者，提供针对如神经或骨科疾病等残疾的康复服务。职业治疗师或其他州或私人资助的视觉康复治疗师或技术专家，能评估家庭安全、修改照明、为电气用具或电话做标签、控制眩光，并指导学习运用计算机、平板电脑或手机的辅助功能。还必须考虑生理的、认知的、社会心理的和环境的因素对视觉康复的影响。非中心注视可以在中心视野缺失的患者中自然形成，训练可能改善 PRL 的使用效率。训练的方法包括知觉训练、眼球运动训练、阅读放大文字的练习和新注视方向的训练（训练视网膜定位）。目前，尚没有公认的方法推荐。在黄斑病变中，用棱镜协助改善非中心视觉仍存争议，并不常使用。一个大样本的随机对照试验显示其并无益处。

Gaffney AJ, Margrain TH, Bunce CV, et al. How effective is eccentric viewing training? A systematic literature review. *Ophthalmic Physiol Optics*. 2014(34):427–437.

Pijnacker J, Verstraten P, van Damme W, Vandermeulen J, Steenbergen B. Rehabilitation of reading in older individuals with macular degeneration: a review of effective training programs. *Neuropsychol Dev Cogn B Aging Neuropsychol Cogn*. 2011, 18(6):708–732.

Smith HJ, Dickinson CM, Cacho I, et al randomized controlled trial to determine the effectiveness of prism spectacles for patients with age-related macular degeneration. *Arch Ophthalmol*. 2005, 123(8):1042–1050.

视野缺损的视觉康复

神经系统疾病的患者通常有视野缺损、进行性视野缩小或眼部症状，这些均可以通过视觉康复获得改善。扫视训练、使用可移动物像至有效视野范围的棱镜以及进行可改善视力的电脑训练，这些都是偏盲患者的视觉康复策略。有一项研究比较了扫视训练和辅助棱镜 2 种方法的视力恢复情况，结果显示：患者进行扫视训练后，与视觉相关的生活质量有所改善。医疗机构资助的职业治疗师可以为患者提供扫视训练。中风患者康复指南中包括视觉忽略对视觉干预的情况。

Rowe FJ, Conroy EJ, Bedson E, et al. A pilot randomized controlled trial comparing effective- ness of prism glasses, visual search training and standard care in hemianopia. *Acta Neurol Scand*. 2017;136(4)310–321.

Trauzettel-Klosinski S. Rehabilitation for visual disorders. *J Neuroophthalmol*. 2010;30(1): 73–84.

Discussion With Patients

Often physicians must communicate information to patients with low vision that patients will perceive as "bad news," such as that they are not able to drive or that vision will not improve. Communication techniques have been conceptualized in different communication models (Fig 9-14); however, keys to delivering bad news include allowing sufficient time for the discussion, acknowledging patient emotions and conveying that the physician appreciates that the emotions are connected to the negative news. A helpful resource is the free Guide to Assessing and Counseling Older Drivers, which includes a chapter about counseling patients who can no longer drive.

The SPIKES Health Care Communication Model

S—*Setting:* The clinician is seated, appears comfortable, and does not interrupt when the patient speaks.

P—*Perception:* "What have you been told about your driving up to now?"

I—*Invitation:* "How much detail would you like to know about the licensing requirements?"

K—*Knowledge:* "Today I do need to discuss your driving with you." (Warning shot)

E—*Empathy:* "Hearing that you do not meet the licensing requirements is clearly a major shock to you. I wish the news were better."

(The patient cries, and the clinician pauses and looks away.) "I see that this news upsets you. Let's just take a break now until you're ready to start again."

S—*Strategy and summary:* "So the summary of all this is that your vision does not meet the requirements to maintain a valid driver's license, and, unfortunately, you will now not be able to drive. Is that your understanding?"

A

The Four E's Model of health care communication

Engagement: "Would you like to take your coat off? We talked about your vision and the diagnosis of age-related macular degeneration in your last visit. Is there anything else you were wondering about?"

Empathy: "It is tough to have to think about alternate ways to get around if you cannot drive the way you used to."

Education: "What would you like to know about licensing requirements and vision standards?"

Enlistment: "I believe we have common ground here, since neither of us wants you to be involved in an accident. We both want to keep you driving safely as long as possible and make the decision not to drive at the right time."

B

Figure 9-14 Communication models. **A**, The SPIKES Healthcare Model of Communication was authored by Robert Buchman. **B**, The Four-E Model of Health Care Communication was developed by the Institute for Healthcare Communication. *(Part B from Buchman R. Breaking bad news: the SPIKES strategy. Community Oncology. 2005;Mr:138–142.)*

Rowe FJ, Conroy EJ, Bedson E, et al. A pilot randomized controlled trial comparing effective- ness of prism glasses, visual search training and standard care in hemianopia. *Acta Neurol Scand*. 2017;136(4)310–321.
Trauzettel-Klosinski S. Rehabilitation for visual disorders. *J Neuroophthalmol*. 2010;30(1): 73–84.

与患者的沟通

患者通常认为低视力是“坏消息”，因为这使得他们不能开车，也可能意味着视力无法提高等，而医生必须与低视力患者沟通这一病情。观察不同的沟通模型，我们将沟通技巧概念化（图9–14）。传达坏消息的关键包括：留出足够的讨论时间、辨别患者的情绪、医生要能理解患者的情绪与坏消息有关。有一个免费资源很实用，即《老年司机咨询和评估指南》，其中一章有关于不能继续驾驶的患者的咨询服务。

SPIKES 医患沟通模型

S（*setting*）——设置面谈：医生坐位，态度和蔼，聆听患者叙述，不打断。

P（*perception*）——评估认知：“到目前为止，有人告诉过您关于开车的事吗?”

I（*invitation*）——明确邀请：“关于驾驶证视力的要求您想了解多少？”

K（*knowledge*）——给予信息：“今天我需要讨论您开车的事情了。”（避免过于直白）

E（*empathy*）——移情：“听说您不符合驾驶证视力检查要求，我知道这对您来说是一个很大的打击。我真心希望情况能好一些！”(患者哭了，医生停止说话，移开目光)“我知道这个消息让您很难过。我们休息一下，等您准备好了，我们再继续。”

S（*strategy and summary*）——策略与总结：“总之，不幸的是，您目前的视力不符合继续持有驾驶执照的体检要求，从现在开始您将不能再驾驶。您能理解吗?”

A

4E医患沟通模型

交流（engagement）：“您想脱掉外套吗?您上次就诊时诊断为老年性黄斑变性，您还有其他疑问吗?”

移情（empathy）：“我知道，如果不能像以前那样开车出行的话，您很难有其他的出行方式选择。”

教育（education）：“您想了解关于驾驶证视力的要求吗?”

认同（enlistment）：我不想让您卷入一场交通事故，相信您也不希望如此，在这一点上，我们目标一致，都希望尽可能地安全驾驶，希望您做出决定：目前阶段将不再自己开车。

B

图 9–14　沟通模型。　**A.** SPIKES 医患沟通模型，由 Robert Buchman 提出。　**B.** 4E 医患沟通模型，由医疗沟通协会提出。*（译者注：资料来源见前页原文。）*

Other Services

Many other agencies and services are involved in multidisciplinary vision rehabilitation including optometric practices, state services, services for veterans, driving rehabilitation services, talking-book libraries, transportation services, counseling and support groups. Devices are provided in some jurisdictions, such as certain European countries, and by some agencies such as the US Department of Veterans Affairs. Orientation and mobility training is offered by some agencies to provide instruction in using visual cues, telescopes, long white canes, and GPS devices for safe and independent ambulation. Vision loss also affects the patient's spouse and family. Referral to psychological counseling and support groups may be part of the rehabilitation team's approach to helping patients, and their families, cope and adapt. Social workers and other counselors may be called upon to contribute to this rehabilitation process. A model of a continuum of care encouraging referral from ophthalmologists to vision rehabilitation consultation and to other multidisciplinary services has been published (Fig 9-15). The goal of multidisciplinary vision rehabilitation is collaboration among services to best address patients' goals and achieve optimal clinical outcomes.

Binns AM, Bunce C, Dickinson C, et al. How effective is low vision service provision? A systematic review. *Surv Ophthalmol.* 2012;57(1):34–65.

Owsley C, McGwin G Jr, Lee PP, Wasserman N, Searcey K. Characteristics of low-vision reha- bilitation services in the United States. *Arch Ophthalmol.* 2009;127(5):681–689.

Pediatric Low Vision

Although vision loss is less frequent in the pediatric population, this cohort is an important group requiring the ophthalmologist's attention. Every child with loss of vision needs to be recognized, and the ophthalmologist's response should include recommending vision rehabilitation. Most adults with low vision have lost vision because of an ocular disease incurred later in life. Thus, they have already acquired many of the vision-aided skills (eg, reading, understanding social cues, cooking, self-care tasks) that are important for functioning in society. Children with low vision, however, need to learn these skills despite poor or no vision.

The most prevalent causes of visual impairment in children in the US are cortical visual impairment, retinopathy of prematurity, optic nerve hypoplasia, albinism, optic atrophy, and congenital infections. Many of these children have coexisting physical and/or cognitive disabilities that create further challenges to successful integration into society.

In addition, skill acquisition is developmentally linked to vision, thus requiring different interventions at different ages. It is important to be aware of the needs of each age group and tailor the assistance to those needs. Rehabilitation of infants and children requires a team approach, often involving occupational and physical therapists, special educators, and physicians working with the child and family from the earliest stages possible. Ophthalmologists may be one of the most consistent contacts over many years for the parents of a visually impaired child, and, as such, they need to be aware of and support the rehabilitation process. (See BCSC Section 6, *Pediatric Ophthalmology and Strabismus*, for a more detailed discussion of pediatric vision rehabilitation.)

其他服务

许多其他服务机构都提供了多学科联合的视觉康复治疗，比如验光检查、社会服务、退伍军人服务、驾驶康复服务、有声图书馆、交通服务、咨询和支援小组。一些国家（如某些欧洲国家）和机构（如美国退伍军人事务部）为视障者提供设备。一些机构提供定向和运动训练，指导患者使用视觉线索、望远镜、白色长手杖和 GPS 设备进行安全的独自步行。视觉缺失也会影响患者的配偶和家庭。将患者转诊到心理咨询和支援小组，这是视觉康复组织帮助患者及其家属应对和适应低视力所做工作的一部分。我们号召社会工作者和其他的指导顾问能加入进来，一起为患者的视觉康复做贡献。目前已经建立了一系列连贯的关怀鼓励转诊模式，即眼科医生推荐到视觉康复咨询中心以及其他多学科联合视觉康复治疗服务机构的模式（图 9–15）。多学科联合视觉康复的目标是实现各服务机构之间的最佳合作，尽最大可能解决患者的困难，达到最佳的临床效果。

Binns AM, Bunce C, Dickinson C, et al. How effective is low vision service provision? A systematic review. *Surv Ophthalmol.* 2012;57(1):34–65.

Owsley C, McGwin G Jr, Lee PP, Wasserman N, Searcey K. Characteristics of low-vision reha- bilitation services in the United States. *Arch Ophthalmol.* 2009;127(5):681–689.

小儿低视力

虽然与成人相比，儿童人群的全盲现象不太常见，但这个群体是一个特别需要眼科医生关注的重要群体。每一个失去视力的孩子都需要重视，眼科医生有向其建议视觉康复治疗方案的职责。大多数低视力成人是在生命的稍后期阶段患眼病而最终失去了视力。所以，在全盲之前他们已经掌握了许多与视觉保护方面相关的技能（例如阅读方式、理解社会现象、烹饪、照顾自己），这对他们融入社会非常重要。然而，视力低下的孩子需要在视力极差甚至是全盲的状态下学习这些技能，其难度将会大得多。

美国儿童视力障碍最常见的原因是大脑视皮层损伤、早产儿视网膜病变、视神经发育不全、白化病、视神经萎缩和先天性感染。这些儿童中有许多同时存在身体和（或）认知障碍，这将给他们成功地融入社会带来更多的挑战。

此外，从生长发育来看，儿童对相关技能的获得情况与其视力的好坏有关，因此需要在不同年龄段对其采取不同的干预措施。我们要清楚每个年龄段的需要，进而予以相应的帮助，这一点很重要。婴儿和儿童的视觉康复需要团队合作，这个团队包括职业治疗师、进行特殊教育的工作者和患者及其家属最先就诊的医生。在许多年中，眼科医生可能是视障儿童父母最持久的联系人之一，因此，他们需要了解并支持视觉康复过程。（见 BCSC 第 6 册《*小儿眼科与斜视*》，其中有更详细的与儿童视觉康复相关的内容。）

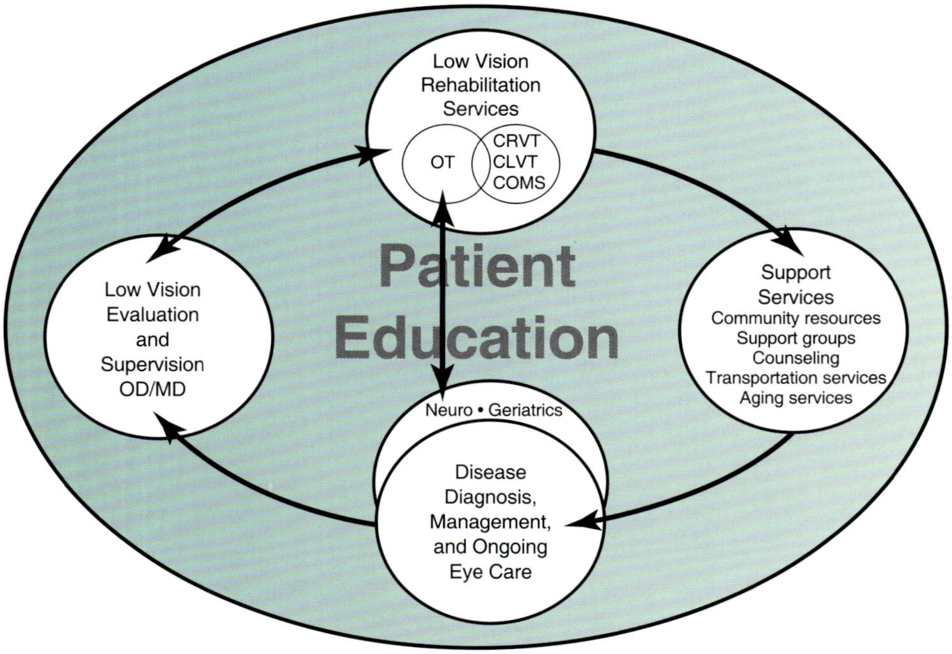

Figure 9-15 A model of vision rehabilitation developed by representatives of a range of collaborating vision rehabilitation professions. Vision rehabilitation can be part of the continuum of care for patients with vision loss when patients are diagnosed, referred for low vision evaluation, and then referred to other services, as indicated. CVRT = certified vision rehabilitation therapist; CLVT = certified low vision therapist; COMS = certified orientation and mobility specialist. *(From Jackson ML. Addressing core competencies in ophthalmology resident education: what the vision rehabilitation setting offers. J Acad Ophthalmol. 2010;3[1]:20.)*

Schwartz T. Causes of visual impairment: pathology and its implications. In: Corn AL, Erin JN, eds. *Foundations of Low Vision: Clinical and Functional Perspectives.* 2nd ed. New York: American Foundation for the Blind Press; 2010.

Ongoing Eye Care

Patients having vision rehabilitation should continue to see their ophthalmologist and to be monitored, including screening for glaucoma, diabetic retinopathy, or refractive changes. Treatment for disorders such as cataract and AMD should still be considered for patients with limited visual potential, even though normal or near-normal visual acuity may not be a potential outcome. The difference between 20/200 and 20/400 vision may substantially reduce the magnification required for reading and enhance the effectiveness of visual rehabilitation techniques.

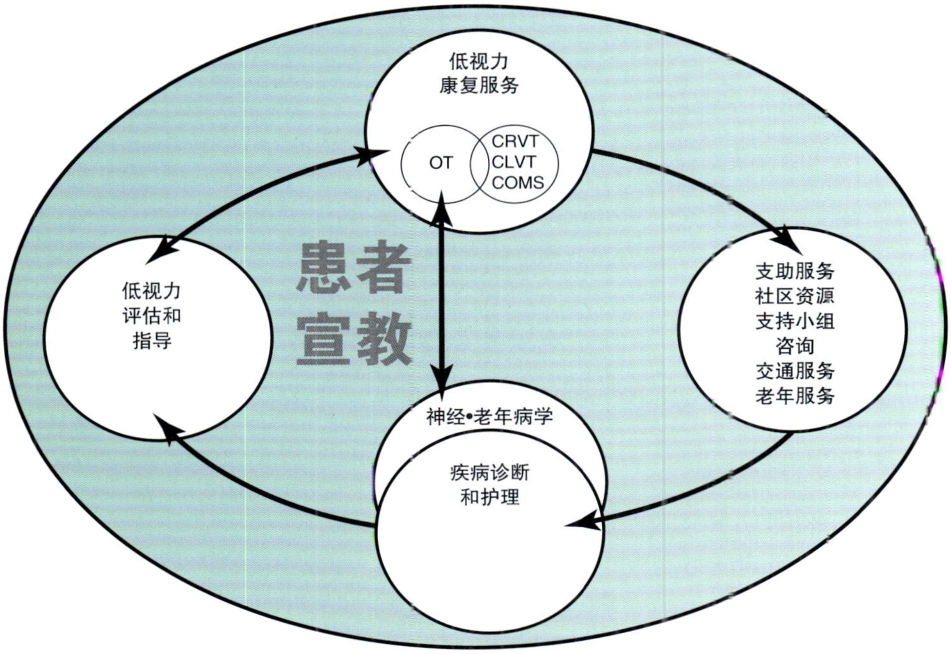

图 9-15　A 由视觉康复专家提出的视觉康复模型。当患者被诊断为低视力后，建议进行低视力评估，然后转诊到如图所示的相应的服务部门，视觉康复则是这一系列低视力患者管理流程中的一部分。图中的 CVRT 为 有执业许可证的视觉康复治疗师，CLVT 为有执业许可证的低视力治疗师，COMS 为有执业许可证的定向运动训练师。*（译者注：资料来源见前页原文。）*

Schwartz T. Causes of visual impairment: pathology and its implications. In: Corn AL, Erin JN, eds. *Foundations of Low Vision: Clinical and Functional Perspectives.* 2nd ed. New York: American Foundation for the Blind Press; 2010.

坚持眼保健运动

进行视觉康复治疗的患者应该定期找眼科医生复诊，进行眼部检查，包括筛查青光眼、糖尿病视网膜病变或屈光改变。某些低视力患者患有白内障和老年性黄斑变性（AMD）等常见眼病，视力提升的可能性很小，即使知道视力不能恢复正常或者接近正常，我们也要对其进行积极治疗。因为 20/200（0.1）和 20/400（0.05）的差异就可能会显著地减少阅读所需助视器的放大倍数，并增加视觉康复技术的作用。

Resources

Materials for patients

Resource materials and information about the many agencies and services should be provided to all patients. The American Academy of Ophthalmology's vision rehabilitation patient handout is available for download in English for ophthalmologists to give to patients (available at www.aao.org/low-vision-and-vision-rehab). It provides essential tips for making the most of remaining vision and offers a list of resources, including a website that allows patients to search for services in their community.

Materials for ophthalmologists

Information and materials for ophthalmologists include:

- American Academy of Ophthalmology. Vision Rehabilitation Committee. Preferred Practice Pattern Guidelines. *Vision Rehabilitation for Adults*. San Francisco: American Academy of Ophthalmology; 2017. Available at www.aao.org/ppp.
- American Academy of Ophthalmology. Vision rehabilitation web page updated with information about vision rehabilitation initiatives and education. Available at www.aao.org/low-vision-and-vision-rehab.
- Mishra A, Jackson ML, Mogk, LG. Comprehensive vision rehabilitation. *Focal Points: Clinical Practice Perspectives*. San Francisco: American Academy of Ophthalmology; 2017, module 4.

Chapter Exercises

Questions

9.1 What level of visual function has been designated as "legal blindness"?
  a. best-corrected visual acuity 20/200
  b. best-corrected visual acuity 20/70
  c. visual field extending 30° around fixation
  d. hemianopic visual field

9.2 What is the optimal prescription for a patient who requires +8.00 reading add?
  a. +8.00 OU with 10 prism diopters (Δ) base-in OU
  b. OD+8.00 with 8Δ base in; OS +8.00 with 8Δ base in
  c. +8.00 OU with 8Δ OU
  d. +8.00 OU with 10Δ OD

9.3 The American Academy of Ophthalmology's Preferred Practice Pattern regarding vision rehabilitation recommends referral to low vision consultation at what level of visual function?
  a. only when patients become legally blind
  b. when a patient's acuity is less than 20/40 or the patient has reduced contrast sensitivity, field loss, or a scotoma
  c. only if the patient asks for referral to vision rehabilitation
  d. when a patient cannot read fine print

资源

患者资料

患者能搜索到视觉康复服务机构的资料和信息。眼科医生可以在网站（www.aao.org/low-vision-and-vision-rehab）下载美国眼科学会的《视觉康复患者手册》英文版本并提供给患者。该手册提供了充分利用残存视力的基本技巧，也提供了一系列资源（如上面列出的网址），可以引导患者发现其所在社区的服务机构。

眼科医生资料

眼科医生的信息资料包括：

- American Academy of Ophthalmology. Vision Rehabilitation Committee. Preferred Practice Pattern Guidelines. *Vision Rehabilitation for Adults*. San Francisco: Ameri- can Academy of Ophthalmology; 2017. Available at www.aao.org/ppp.
- American Academy of Ophthalmology. Vision rehabilitation web page updated with information about vision rehabilitation initiatives and education. Available at www.aao.org/low-vision-and-vision-rehab.
- Mishra A, Jackson ML, Mogk, LG. Comprehensive vision rehabilitation. *Focal Points: Clinical Practice Perspectives*. San Francisco: American Academy of Ophthalmol- ogy; 2017, module 4.

章节练习

问题

9.1　“法定盲”指视力在什么水平？
　a. 最佳矫正视力低于 20/200
　b. 最佳矫正视力低于 20/70
　c. 视野范围在中心视力小于 30° 时
　d. 视野偏盲

9.2　如果患者需要配戴 +8.00D 的近附加，其配镜处方应该是什么？
　a. 双眼为 +8.00D 加 10 Δ BI 棱镜
　b. 右眼为 +8.00D 加 8 Δ BI 棱镜，左眼为 +8.00D 加 8 Δ BI 棱镜
　c. 双眼为 +8.00D 加 8 Δ 棱镜
　d. 双眼为 +8.00D，右眼加 10 Δ 棱镜

9.3　视功能在什么标准时，美国眼科学会的视觉康复最优训练模式组织会建议患者转诊去进行低视力咨询？
　a. 只有患者被诊断为法定盲时
　b. 当患者视力低于 20/40 或者患者存在进行性对比度视力下降、视野受损或中心暗点时
　c. 只要当患者要求转诊至视觉康复中心时
　d. 当患者不能阅读小字体读物时

Answers

9.1 **a.** The Social Security website states, "We consider you to be legally blind under Social Security rules if your vision cannot be corrected to better than 20/200 in your better eye, or if your visual field is 20 degrees or less, even with a corrective lens."

9.2 **a.** The rule of thumb for adding prism to high-add spectacles over 4.00 D is to incorporate base-in prism for each eye at a correction that is 2 D greater than the required add power.

9.3 **b.** The American Academy of Ophthalmology's Preferred Practice Pattern regarding vision rehabilitation recommends that patients with acuity less than 20/40, contrast sensitivity loss, peripheral field loss, or central field loss be referred for low vision evaluation.

答案

9.1　**a**。社保网站提出："按照社保规定，当你的优势眼最佳矫正视力低于 20/200 时，或者矫正后视野范围等于或小于 20° 时，诊断为法定盲。"

9.2　**a**。按照经验，遇到超过 +4.00 D 的高度数近附加配镜时，双眼需要同时给予 BI 棱镜，棱镜度数要参考矫正后的近附加度数来给，即按照比所需近附加多 2 D 的度数来给配镜处方。

9.3　**b**。患者视力低于 20/40，对比度视力下降，周边视野缺失，中心视野缺失时，美国眼科学会的视觉康复最优训练模式组织会建议患者转诊进行低视力评估。

（翻译　刘念　龚慧 // 审校　石一宁 // 章节审校　魏瑞华）

Basic Texts

Clinical Optics

Albert DM, Miller JW, Azar DT, Blodi BA, eds. *Albert & Jakobiec's Principles and Practice of Ophthalmology*. 4 vols. 3rd ed. Philadelphia: Elsevier/Saunders; 2008.

Corboy JM. *The* Retinoscopy *Book: An Introductory Manual for Eye Care Professionals*. 5th ed. Thorofare, NJ: Slack; 2003.

Duke-Elder S, Abrams D. *Ophthalmic Optics and Refraction*. St Louis: Mosby; 1970. *System of Ophthalmology*; vol 5.

Guyton DL, West CE, Miller JM, Wisnicki HJ. *Ophthalmic Optics and Clinical Refraction*. Baltimore: Prism Press; 1999.

Hunter DG, West CE. *Last-Minute Optics*. 2nd ed. Thorofare, NJ: Slack; 2010.

Lipson A, Lipson SG, Lipson H. *Optical Physics*. 4th ed. Cambridge: Cambridge University Press; 2011.

Milder B, Rubin ML. *The Fine Art of Prescribing Glasses Without Making a Spectacle of Yourself*. 3rd ed. Gainesville, FL: Triad Publishing Co; 2004.

Rubin ML. *Optics for Clinicians*. Gainesville, FL: Triad Publishing Co; 1993.

Stein HA, Slatt BJ, Stein RM, Freeman MI. *Fitting Guide for Rigid and Soft Contact Lenses*: A *Practical Approach*. 4th ed. St Louis: Mosby; 2002.

Tasman W, Jaeger EA, eds. *Duane's Ophthalmology on DVD-ROM*. Philadelphia: Lippincott Williams & Wilkins; 2013.

Yanoff M, Duker JS. *Ophthalmology: Expert Consult Premium Edition*. 4th ed. Philadelphia: Elsevier/Saunders; 2014.

参考内容

临床光学

Albert DM, Miller JW, Azar DT, Blodi BA, eds. *Albert & Jakobiec's Principles and Practice of Ophthalmology*. 4 vols. 3rd ed. Philadelphia: Elsevier/Saunders; 2008.

Corboy JM. *The* Retinoscopy *Book: An Introductory Manual for Eye Care Professionals*. 5th ed. Thorofare, NJ: Slack; 2003.

Duke-Elder S, Abrams D. *Ophthalmic Optics and Refraction*. St Louis: Mosby; 1970. *System of Ophthalmology*; vol 5.

Guyton DL, West CE, Miller JM, Wisnicki HJ. *Ophthalmic Optics and Clinical Refraction*. Baltimore: Prism Press; 1999.

Hunter DG, West CE. *Last-Minute Optics*. 2nd ed. Thorofare, NJ: Slack; 2010.

Lipson A, Lipson SG, Lipson H. *Optical Physics*. 4th ed. Cambridge: Cambridge University Press; 2011.

Milder B, Rubin ML. *The Fine Art of Prescribing Glasses Without Making a Spectacle of Yourself*. 3rd ed. Gainesville, FL: Triad Publishing Co; 2004.

Rubin ML. *Optics for Clinicians*. Gainesville, FL: Triad Publishing Co; 1993

Stein HA, Slatt BJ, Stein RM, Freeman MI. *Fitting Guide for Rigid and Soft Contact Lenses*: A *Practical Approach*. 4th ed. St Louis: Mosby; 2002.

Tasman W, Jaeger EA, eds. *Duane's Ophthalmology on DVD-ROM*. Philadelphia: Lippincott Williams & Wilkins; 2013.

Yanoff M, Duker JS. *Ophthalmology: Expert Consult Premium Edition*. 4th ed. Philadelphia: Elsevier/Saunders; 2014.

Related Academy Materials

The American Academy of Ophthalmology is dedicated to providing a wealth of high-quality clinical education resources for ophthalmologists.

Print Publications and Electronic Products

For a complete listing of Academy products related to topics covered in this BCSC Section, visit our online store at https://store.aao.org/clinical-education/topic/comprehensive-ophthalmology.html. Or call Customer Service at 866.561.8558 (toll free, US only) or+1 415.561.8540, Monday through Friday, between 8:00 AM and 5:00 PM (PST).

Online Resources

Visit the Ophthalmic News and Education (ONE®) Network at aao.org/onenetwork to find relevant videos, online courses, journal articles, practice guidelines, self-assessment quizzes, images, and more. The ONE Network is a free Academy-member benefit.

Access free, trusted articles and content with the Academy's collaborative online encyclopedia, EyeWiki, at aao.org/eyewiki.

相关学院资料

美国眼科学会致力于为眼科医生提供丰富的高质量的临床教育资源。

打印出版物和电子读物

如果想获得所有与本 BCSC 部分中的主题相关的学院读物清单，你可以访问我们的网店 https://store.aao.org/clinical-education/topic/comprehensive-ophthalmology.html。或者拨打电话 866.561.8558（在 US 通话免费）或者 +1 415.561.8540 咨询客服，客服工作时间为周一至周五的上午 8:00 到下午 5:00（PST）。

网络资源

访问眼科新闻和教育（ONE®）网站 aao.org/onenetwork 可以找到相关视频、网络资源、期刊报道、诊疗指南、自我评估测试、图片等等。ONE® 网站免费对会员开放。

我们与学院合作，打造令大家满意的在线百科全书平台，帮助大家在 aao.org/eyewiki 获取免费可信的文章和知识。

Study Questions

Please note that these questions are not part of your CME reporting process. They are provided here for your own educational use and identification of any professional practice gaps. The required CME posttest is available online (see "Requesting CME Credit"). Following the questions are a blank answer sheet and answers with discussions. Although a concerted effort has been made to avoid ambiguity and redundancy in these questions, the authors recognize that differences of opinion may occur regarding the "best" answer. The discussions are provided to demonstrate the rationale used to derive the answer. They may also be helpful in confirming that your approach to the problem was correct or, if necessary, in fixing the principle in your memory.

1. The simplest imaging system is a pinhole camera. What is a characteristic feature of this device?
   a. high magnification
   b. superb depth of field
   c. upright image formed at the image plane
   d. rapid exposure times

2. As it is unsafe to view a partial eclipse of the sun directly, observers are often advised to use a simple pinhole camera viewer to form an image of the eclipse. Of course, these pinhole images are small and dim. A better alternative is to use a +1.00 lens, held about waist-high, to project an image of the sun on the ground (see figure). How far should the lens be held from the ground to obtain a sharp image?

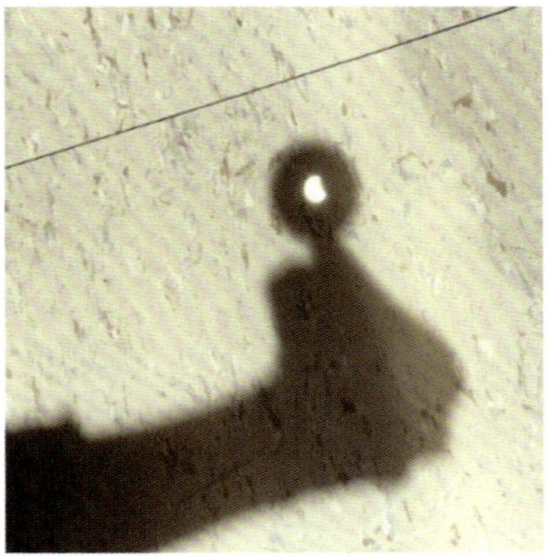

   a. 2.0 m
   b. 1.0 m
   c. 0.5 m
   d. It doesn't matter—any distance works well, just as in a pinhole camera.

学习的问题

以下问题不属于 CME 的讲述内容，仅供教学使用以及查缺补漏。CME 的学后测试可在网上查找（见 CME 学分需求），在问题后面的空白处写上答案和讨论。尽管我们已尽量避免产生歧义以及冗杂，但对于最佳答案仍可能有不一致的意见。讨论部分将演绎推导出答案的合理性，这些讨论有助于确认解决问题的方法是否正确，必要时应牢记这些原则。

1. 针孔照相机是最简单的成像系统，以下哪一项属于该设备的特点？
   a. 高倍放大率
   b. 极佳的景深
   c. 在像平面形成正像
   d. 曝光时间短

2. 在太阳下直接观察日偏食是不安全的，通常建议观察者观察针孔照相机所成日食的像。当然这些小孔像是比较小而且是暗淡的。更好一点的方法是使用一个 +1.00D 的透镜，拿在大约与腰部平齐的位置，将太阳的影像投射到地面上（如右图所示）。请问拿在距离地面多远的位置才能获得一个清晰的影像？

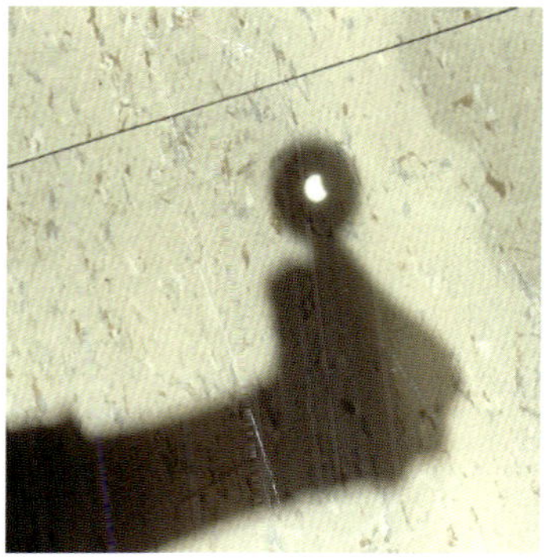

   a. 2 m
   b. 1 m
   c. 0.5 m
   d. 就像针孔照相机一样，任何距离都可以

3. Suppose a distant object is located to the left of a lens system, which focuses light from this object at +1.0 m to the right of the lens system. If a +3.00 lens is added adjacent to the lens system, where is the new image located?
   a. 25 cm to the right of the lenses
   b. 50 cm to the right of the lenses
   c. 75 cm to the right of the lenses
   d. 1.0 m to the right of the lenses

4. The power-cross description of a toric lens is +1.00 @ 25°, −2.00 @ 115°. What is the sphero-cylindrical specification of this lens, expressed in minus cylinder form?
   a. +1.00 ⊂ −2.00 × 115°
   b. −2.00 ⊂ +1.00 × 25°
   c. +1.00 ⊂ −3.00 × 25°
   d. −2.00 ⊂ +3.00 × 25°

5. When performing cross cylinder refinement of an astigmatic correction, it is necessary to adjust the spherical component of the correction to keep the circle of least confusion on the retina as cylinder power is varied. What is the proper rule for this compensation with a plus cylinder phoropter?
   a. Increase the plus sphere power by 1 click (0.25 D) for each 0.25 D increase in plus cylinder power.
   b. Increase the plus sphere power by 1 click (0.25 D) for each 0.25 D decrease in plus cylinder power.
   c. Increase the plus sphere power by 1 click (0.25 D) for each 0.50D increase in plus cylinder power.
   d. Increase the plus sphere power by 1 click (0.25 D) for each 0.50D decrease in plus cylinder power.

6. When a beam of monochromatic yellow light passes through a prism, how is its path altered?
   a. It is deflected toward the apex of the prism.
   b. It is deflected toward the base of the prism.
   c. It is displaced toward the base of the prism, but continues parallel to its original direction.
   d. It is dispersed into a spectrum of colors.

7. The radius of curvature of a convex passenger-side automobile rear-view mirror is typically about 1.0 m. Where does such a mirror form an image of an object 10.0 m behind the car?
   a. 10.0 m in front of the mirror (ie, on the opposite side of the mirror from the source object)
   b. 1.0 m in front of the mirror
   c. 0.47 m in front of the mirror
   d. 0.47 m behind the mirror (ie, on the same side of the mirror as the source object)

8. What is the concept of magnification appropriate for the discussion of astronomical telescopes?
   a. transverse magnification
   b. linear magnification
   c. longitudinal magnification
   d. angular magnification

3. 假设远处有一物体位于透镜左侧，1m 处的该物体成像在透镜系统的右侧。如果将 +3.00 D 的透镜附加于原有的透镜系统，此时新的像位于哪里？
   a. 透镜系统右侧 25 cm 处
   b. 透镜系统右侧 50 cm 处
   c. 透镜系统右侧 75 cm 处
   d. 透镜系统右侧 1.0 cm 处

4. 一复曲透镜的 2 条主子午线上的焦度分别为 +1.00 @ 25° 和 –2.00 @ 115° 。以负柱镜形式表示该透镜的球柱处方是？
   a. +1.00 ◯ –2.00 × 115°
   b. –2.00 ◯ +1.00 × 25°
   c. +1.00 ◯ –3.00 × 25°
   d. –2.00 ◯ +3.00 × 25°

5. 采用交叉圆柱镜精确散光时，当散光度数改变后，为了保证最小弥散圆始终位于视网膜上，需要调整球镜部分。对于一台具有正柱镜的综合验光仪来说，调整的原则是什么？
   a. 每增加 +0.25 D 散光需要增加 +0.25 D 球镜
   b. 每减少 +0.25 D 散光需要增加 +0.25 D 球镜
   c. 每增加 +0.50 D 散光需要增加 +0.25 D 球镜
   d. 每减少 +0.50 D 散光需要增加 +0.25 D 球镜

6. 当一束单色黄光通过棱镜时，它的传播路径会发生怎样的改变？
   a. 偏向棱镜顶
   b. 偏向棱镜底
   c. 偏向棱镜底，继续平行于原方向
   d. 散开成彩色光谱

7. 汽车后视镜是一凸面镜，其曲率半径通常为 1 m。车后 10 m 处的物体通过该后视镜后形成的像位于哪里？
   a. 后视镜前方 10 m 处（注：相对发光物，像在反射镜的另一侧）
   b. 后视镜前方 1 m 处
   c. 后视镜前方 0.47 m 处
   d. 后视镜后方 0.47 m 处（注：像与发光物在反射镜的同一侧）

8. 以下哪一项是天文望远镜的放大率概念？
   a. 横向放大率
   b. 线性放大率
   c. 纵向放大率
   d. 角放大率

Study Questions

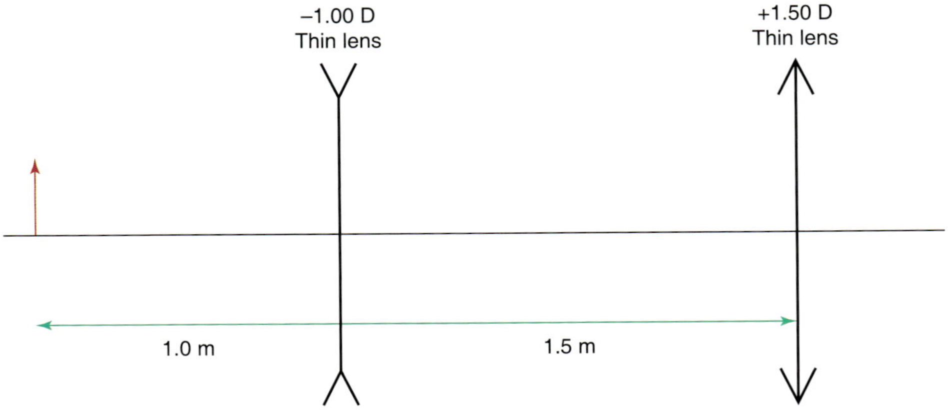

Questions 9 and 10 refer to the figure above. An object is 1.0 m to the left of a −1.00 D thin lens. The −1.00 D lens is, in turn, 1.5 m to the left of a 1.50 D thin lens.

9. Where is the (intermediate) image formed by the first lens?
   a. 2.0 m to the right of the lens
   b. 0.5 m to the right of the lens
   c. 0.5 m to the left of the lens
   d. 2.0 m to the left of the lens

10. What is the location of the final image?
   a. 1.0 m to the left of the second lens
   b. 1.0 m to the right of the second lens
   c. 4.0 m to the right of the second lens
   d. at optical infinity

11. Which laser–tissue interaction is the basis of photorefractive keratectomy?
   a. photochemical interaction
   b. photoablation
   c. plasma-induced ablation
   d. photodisruption

12. How do changes in wavelength, pupil size, focal length, or macular integrity affect the size of the Airy disc image on the retina?
   a. The Airy disc image on the retina is smaller when macular degeneration is present.
   b. The Airy disc image on the retina is smaller when the pupil size decreases.
   c. The Airy disc image on the retina is smaller when the wavelength of light is shortened.
   d. The Airy disc image on the retina is smaller when the focal length of the eye is shorter.

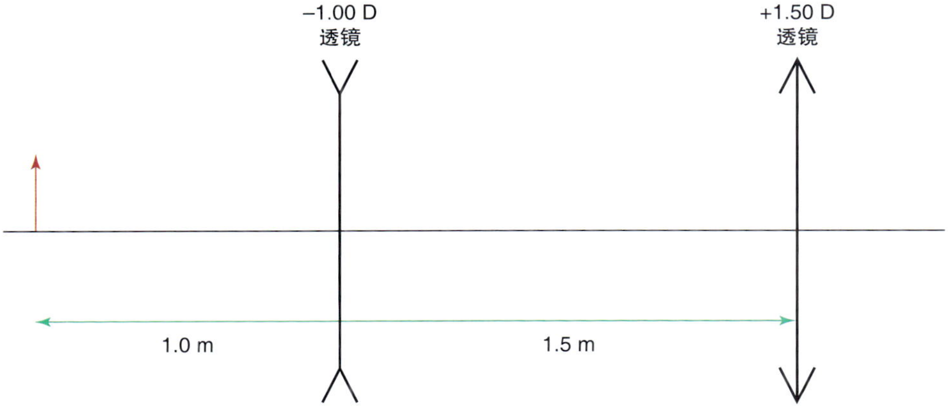

上图用于问题 9 和问题 10，物体位于 −1.00D 透镜左侧 1m 处，而该 −1.00 D 透镜位于 +1.50 D 透镜左侧 1.5 m 处。

9. 第一个透镜形成的像位于哪里?
   a. 第一个透镜右侧 2.0 m 处
   b. 第一个透镜右侧 0.5 m 处
   c. 第一个透镜左侧 0.5 m 处
   d. 第一个透镜左侧 2.0 m 处

10. 最终形成的像位于哪里?
   a. 第二个透镜左侧 1.0 m 处
   b. 第二个透镜右侧 1.0 m 处
   c. 第二个透镜右侧 4.0 m 处
   d. 光学无限远处

11. 下列哪项激光 – 生物组织作用是角膜屈光手术的基础?
   a. 光化学作用
   b. 光切削
   c. 等离子诱发切削
   d. 光致破裂

12. 以下关于波长、瞳孔、焦距以及黄斑完整性的改变对视网膜 Airy 斑大小的影响说法正确的是哪一项?
   a. 出现黄斑变性，视网膜上 Airy 斑较小
   b. 瞳孔变小，视网膜上 Airy 斑较小
   c. 光波长变短，视网膜上 Airy 斑较小
   d. 眼的焦距较短，视网膜上 Airy 斑较小

13. The radius of the bowl of the Goldmann perimeter is 333 mm. The diameter of the V_4 target is 9 mm. What is the diameter of the image of this target on the retina?
   a. 0.23 mm
   b. 0.46mm
   c. 0.9 mm
   d. 3.6 mm

14. LogMar notation (base-10 logarithm of the minimum angle of resolution) is frequently used to record visual acuity in clinical trials. What is the difference in LogMAR scores associated with a doubling of the minimum angle of resolution (such as the difference between a visual acuity of 20/40 and 20/80 or between 6/12 and 6/24)?
   a. 0.01 LogMAR
   b. 0.2 LogMAR
   c. 0.3 LogMAR
   d. 0.5 LogMAR

15. Where is the far point of a hyperopic eye?
   a. at optical infinity
   b. in front of the eye a finite distance away
   c. coincident with the nodal point
   d. behind the eye

16. A patient reports diplopia (double vision). With a simple occluder in front of the right eye, the diplopia goes away; with the occluder in front of the left eye, the diplopia persists. With the left eye occluded, placing a pinhole occluder over the right eye also resolves the diplopia. What is the most likely explanation of these findings?
   a. The patient has a cataract in the right eye.
   b. The patient has dry age-related macular degeneration with a subfoveal atrophic scar in the right eye.
   c. The patient has recently acquired strabismus.
   d. The patient has nonorganic visual loss—there is no physiologic explanation for monocular diplopia.

17. The definition of 20/20 vision is the ability to recognize Snellen letters and similar optotypes with features separated by 1 minute of arc. The typical 20/20 optotype subtends 5 minutes of arc, with features (such as the horizontal lines in the letter "E") separated by white spaces 1 minute of arc in width. How large should the 20/20 optotypes be on an eye chart to be viewed from 10 feet (304.8 cm)?
   a. 0.2 cm
   b. 0.44 cm
   c. 0.88 cm
   d. 1.27 cm

13. Goldmann 视野计碗形部分的曲率半径是 333 mm。V_4 目标的直径是 9 mm。该目标在视网膜上的像直径是多少？
   a. 0.23 mm
   b. 0.46 mm
   c. 0.9 mm
   d. 3.6 mm

14. LogMar 计录法（最小分辨角以 10 为底取对数）经常用于临床试验中的视力记录，当最小分辨角扩大 2 倍后，LogMar 计录值与原来的值相差多少？（比如视力为 20/40 和 20/80 之间，或者 6/12 和 6/14 之间的差异）
   a. 0.01 LogMAR
   b. 0.2 LogMAR
   c. 0.3 LogMAR
   d. 0.5 LogMAR

15. 远视眼的远点位于哪里？
   a. 光学无限远
   b. 眼前有限距离
   c. 节点处
   d. 眼球后方

16. 患者主诉复视（双影）。遮盖右眼后，复视消失；遮盖左眼后，复视仍存在。遮盖左眼，在右眼前放置小孔镜片，复视消失。这些检查结果最可能提示了什么？
   a. 右眼白内障
   b. 右眼发生年龄相关性的干性黄斑变性，伴有黄斑下萎缩灶
   c. 右眼新近发生获得性斜视
   d. 右眼视力下降是非器质性病变导致的——该单眼的复视无生理学原因可以解释

17. 20/20 的视力表示能够分辨以 1 弧分为细节特点的 Snellen 字母以及类似的字母。典型的 20/20 的视标对应的视角大小是 5 弧分，以 1 弧分的空白间距分开（比如 E 字母的水平线条之间），从 10 ft（304.8cm）的距离处看视力表上 20/20 的字母应该是多大？
   a. 0.2 cm
   b. 0.44 cm
   c. 0.88 cm
   d. 1.27 cm

18. What technique allows objective measurement of astigmatism?
    a. Jackson cross cylinder test
    b. astigmatic dial test
    c. retinoscopy
    d. stenopeic slit test

19. What is an example of a binocular balance test?
    a. method of spheres
    b. gradient method
    c. prism dissociation test
    d. heterophoria method

20. A patient sees well with a prescription for glasses of –8.00 sph in both eyes and a vertex distance of 15 mm. If new glasses are made with a vertex distance of 20 mm, what is the adjustment in the power of the lenses required to correct the refractive error?
    a. 1.12 D
    b. –0.67 D
    c. 0.37 D
    d. –0.33 D

21. At the beginning of the duochrome test, the patient is fogged with +0.75 D. The patient reports that the green side of the screen has the clearest letters. What is your next step in performing this test?
    a. Plus power is decreased or minus power is added until both sides of the duochrome chart are equally clear.
    b. The test is complete at this point.
    c. Additional fogging with more plus power must be added.
    d. The test cannot be performed.

22. The clinician is given a small examination room and will refract a patient. If the visual acuity screen is mounted on the wall 3 meters from the patient, what step will ensure that the refraction is correct?
    a. Add –0.33 D to the final prescription.
    b. Take no additional step. The refraction should be correct as measured.
    c. Perform a duochrome test.
    d. Refine the final sphere with a trial frame in a longer hallway (6 meters).

18. 以下哪种方法可以客观地测量散光?
    a. Jackson 交叉柱镜
    b. 散光盘
    c. 检影镜
    d. 裂隙片

19. 下列哪一项属于双眼平衡测试的方法?
    a. 球镜法
    b. 梯度法
    c. 棱镜分离测试
    d. 隐斜视法

20. 一患者双眼均配戴处方为 –8.00 D 的眼镜，顶点间距为 15 mm 时能清晰视物，如果定做一副顶点间距为 20 mm 的新眼镜，镜片度数应怎样调整才能矫正他的屈光不正?
    a. 1.12 D
    b.–0.67 D
    c. 0.37 D
    d.–0.33 D

21. 在红绿测试开始前，通常会先给患者使用 +0.75 D 的镜片进行雾视。如果患者报告绿色屏幕上的字母更清晰，下一步应该怎样调整?
    a. 减少正焦度或增加负焦度，直到两边不同颜色屏幕上的字母一样清晰
    b. 已经到达终点
    c. 继续增加正镜进行雾视
    d. 该测试不能继续进行

22. 临床医生在一个小检查室给患者验光，如果视力表距离患者 3 m，下列哪一项调整能保证验光准确?
    a. 在最终的处方上加上 –0.33 D
    b. 验光是准确的，不需要调整
    c. 进行红绿测试
    d. 在更远的距离（6 m）进行试镜，以精确地测出球镜度数

23. A 46-year-old patient with myopia has blurred distance vision wearing his 5-year-old pair of glasses, which have −4.00 D lenses for both eyes. He has no problem reading. We find the new distance spectacle power to be −5.50 D in both eyes. He expresses an interest in contact lenses. What is the likely effect on both reading and distance vision of changing the distance correction?
   a. He will be able to see well, far and near, with contact lenses corrected for distance vision.
   b. He will be able to see well, far and near, with single-vision spectacles, −5.50D OU.
   c. He will find it difficult to read with single-vision spectacles, −5.50 OU, and even more difficult to read with contact lenses that correct his distance vision.
   d. He will be able to see well, far and near, with contact lenses −4.00D for each eye.

24. What determines the choice of the curvature of the central rear surface of a contact lens,which we call the *base curve*?
   a. The reciprocal of the radius of curvature is the desired power of the lens.
   b. The base curvature determines the magnification of the image.
   c. The base curvature of a contact lens is chosen so that the lens fits well.
   d. The base curvature of the contact lens should be close to the base curve of the patient's glasses.

25. What is a consideration for intraocular lens calculation in the post–keratorefractive eye?
   a. Eyes that have undergone incisional refractive surgery like radial keratotomy are not susceptible to instrument errors.
   b. Employing standard keratometry in post-myopic LASIK eyes will result in a myopic postoperative refractive surprise.
   c. Employing standard intraocular lens formulas in the context of post-myopic LASIK eyes will result in a myopic refractive surprise.
   d. Standard keratometry will overestimate the refractive power of the cornea in postmyopic LASIK eyes.

26. How do dysphotopsias present, and what are their causes?
   a. Complaints of flashes in post-cataract surgery patients are referred to as positive dysphotopsias and generally improve with time.
   b. Complaints of a curtain impinging upon central vision are characteristic of negative dysphotopsias and may or may not improve with time.
   c. Positive dysphotopsias are speculated to be caused by internal reflections within the intraocular lens itself.
   d. Dysphotopsias do not occur when the intraocular lens is placed within the capsular bag.

27. For the modulation transfer function (MTF) of a novel intraocular lens (IOL), how do the curve's peaks and valleys relate to IOL performance?
   a. Monofocal IOLs demonstrate the highest MTF peaks.
   b. Extended-depth-of-focus (EDOF) lenses demonstrate greater depressions between peak focal lengths than conventional multifocal IOLs.
   c. Lower MTF values signify higher image quality.
   d. An IOL's modulation transfer function is unaffected by pupil size.

23. 一个 46 岁的近视患者戴镜检查时发现远视力下降，原来的眼镜已配戴 5 年，双眼原镜的处方均为 –4.00 D。主诉无近距离阅读困难症状，验光检查发现双眼近视均为 –5.50D。患者想配戴接触镜。如果更换远距矫正处方，患者的远视力会受到什么影响？
    a. 配戴矫正远视力的接触镜，看远、看近时的视力均良好
    b. 双眼均配戴处方为 –5.50 D 的单焦框架眼镜，看远、看近时的视力均良好
    c. 双眼均配戴处方为 –5.50 D 的单焦框架眼镜，近距离阅读困难；配戴矫正远视力的接触镜，近距离阅读更加困难
    d. 双眼均配戴处方为 –4.00 D 的接触镜，看远、看近时的视力均良好

24. 什么决定了接触镜中央后表面曲率的选择？什么是*基弧*？
    a. 曲率半径的倒数是透镜所需焦度
    b. 基本曲率决定了像的放大率
    c. 选择接触镜的基本曲率以便适配良好
    d. 接触镜的基本曲率与眼镜的基弧相近

25. 角膜屈光术后眼在植入人工晶体时需要考虑哪些情况？
    a. 放射状角膜切开术等切开屈光术后眼不受仪器误差的影响
    b. 标准角膜曲率计检查 LASIK 近视术后眼会引起意想不到的术后近视性屈光改变
    c. 标准人工晶体计算公式用于 LASIK 近视术后眼会引起近视性屈光改变
    d. 标准角膜曲率检查结果高估了 LASIK 近视术后眼的角膜屈光力

26. 失能性炫光的表现是什么？哪些原因会引起失能性炫光？
    a. *正失能性炫光*的现象通常发生在白内障术后的患者身上，他们会主诉眼前有闪光感，通常随时间而改善
    b. 负失能性炫光的特点是患者主诉中心视力有帘状遮挡，随时间的推移可能会改善，也可能不会改善
    c. 推测正失能性炫光可能是人工晶体自身的内部反射所造成
    d. 后囊植入人工晶体眼不会发生失能性炫光

27. 从人工晶体（IOL）的调制传递函数（MTF）上看，IOL 的性能对曲线的波峰和波谷的影响是什么？
    a. 单焦 IOL 的 MTF 峰值最高
    b. 扩展焦深（EDOF）晶体在 2 个峰焦距间比传统多焦 IOL 显示出更大的压抑
    c. MTF 数值小意味着更好的图像质量
    d. IOL 的调制传递函数不受瞳孔大小的影响

28. On postoperative examination, an appropriately powered toric intraocular lens (IOL) is found to be misoriented. What is the relevance of the degree and cause of the misalignment?
    a. Misalignment of a toric IOL by 90° will neither improve nor worsen the patient's preoperative astigmatism.
    b. Misalignment of a toric IOL lens by 10° will result in a clinically significant reduction in the efficacy of the astigmatism correction.
    c. Patients exhibit a reliable amount of excyclotorsion when recumbent, and this amount may be compensated for in preoperative calculation.
    d. Misalignment of an appropriately powered toric IOL will result in decreased efficacy but will not rotate the axis of the patient's postoperative astigmatic error.

29. What may sway an ophthalmologist's decision to implant a multifocal intraocular lens (IOL)?
    a. Approximately 20% of the light entering the pupil does not reach the retina because of dissipation in diffractive multifocal IOLs.
    b. Multifocal IOLs are especially beneficial in patients with maculopathies.
    c. Multifocal IOLs are more forgiving of decentration than conventional monofocal IOLs.
    d. Different IOL calculation formulas are required for multifocal lenses compared to monofocal lenses.

30. A patient presents for LASIK evaluation to eliminate the need for distance glasses correction of −10.00 D. What is the lowest keratometric reading treatable that will still avoid excessive corneal power?
    a. 40.0 D
    b. 41.0 D
    c. 42.0 D
    d. 43.0 D

31. Which refractive procedure minimizes optical aberrations?
    a. small-incision lenticule extraction
    b. photorefractive keratectomy
    c. phakic intraocular lens
    d. intracorneal ring segments

32. Which wavefront aberration is correctable with spectacles?
    a. spherical aberration
    b. trefoil
    c. positive defocus
    d. vertical coma

33. What property of light is used by the scanning laser polarimeter to measure thickness of the nerve fiber layer?
    a. focal spot size
    b. power level
    c. pulse duration
    d. polarization

28. 术后检查发现，正确度数的散光型人工晶体的轴位错置，错置的原因和程度之间有什么联系？
   a. 散光型人工晶体的轴位偏差 90° 对患者的原有散光没有影响
   b. 散光型人工晶体的轴位偏差 10° 会导致患者的散光矫正效果下降
   c. 患者躺下时眼球一定程度外旋，术前计算可能抵消这种旋转带来的影响
   d. 散光型人工晶体的轴位错置会引起散光矫正不足，但是不会影响患者术后的散光轴向

29. 眼科医生在选择多焦人工晶体时会考虑哪些因素？
   a. 由于多焦人工晶体的衍射损耗，大约有 20% 进入瞳孔的光线不会到达视网膜
   b. 有黄斑病变的患者选择多焦人工晶体更好
   c. 相对单焦人工晶体，多焦人工晶体更容易发生离心
   d. 相对单焦人工晶体，多焦人工晶体需要采用不同的人工晶体计算公式

30. 一患者有 -10.00 D 的近视，拟行 LASIK 近视手术，患者的角膜曲率最低是多少才能避免术后过多的角膜焦度？
   a. 40.0 D
   b. 41.0 D
   c. 42.0 D
   d. 43.0 D

31. 下列哪一项屈光性操作会减少像差的产生？
   a. 小切口微透镜取出
   b. 屈光手术
   c. 人工晶体植入
   d. 角膜基质环植入

32. 眼镜可以矫正以下哪种波前像差？
   a. 球差
   b. 三叶草
   c. 正离焦
   d. 垂直彗差

33. 扫描激光偏振计是运用光的哪种性质来测量视网膜神经纤维层的厚度的？
   a. 焦斑大小
   b. 能量级
   c. 脉冲宽度
   d. 偏振

34. What is the effect of common refractive errors on the apparent size of the optic disc as seen with a direct ophthalmoscope?
    a. The optic disc will appear smaller in a myopic eye than an emmetropic eye.
    b. The optic disc will appear larger in a hyperopic eye than an emmetropic eye.
    c. The optic disc will appear smaller in a myopic eye than a hyperopic eye.
    d. The optic disc will appear smaller in an aphakic eye than an emmetropic eye.

35. What 4 clinical features are part of the Charles Bonnet syndrome?
    a. vivid recurrent visual hallucinations, some degree of vision loss, no other neurological signs or symptoms, full insight that what is seen is not real
    b. seeing complex images such as colorful landscapes, a diagnosis of glaucoma, no other neurological signs or symptoms, no insight that what is seen is not real
    c. seeing hallucinations of people, no other neurological disease, no other ocular disease, full insight that what is seen is not real
    d. recurring images of people who talk to the patient and who the patient believes to be real, a diagnosis of macular degeneration, no neurological symptoms, no diagnosis

36. What level of visual field loss qualifies a patient for legal blindness concessions in the United States?
    a. hemianopic field loss
    b. foveal-sparing scotoma
    c. constriction to 20°
    d. severe glaucoma field loss with a mean defect of −19.00 on 30° field testing

37. What size of text would a patient with a foveal-sparing scotoma have difficulty reading?
    a. moderate-sized text, such as large-print books
    b. only small print, such as on medication labels
    c. both moderate-sized text and smaller text
    d. larger text, such as headlines

38. What 2 visual functions are displayed on a contrast sensitivity curve?
    a. spatial frequency and contrast threshold
    b. visual acuity and spatial frequency
    c. contrast threshold and contrast sensitivity
    d. visual acuity and critical print size

39. What is the reading distance for an adult patient, with a distance correction of −4.00 OU, who is reading with a pair of +6.00 D reading glasses?
    a. 10 cm
    b. 16.7 cm
    c. 25 cm
    d. 12.5 cm

34. 直接检眼镜可以看到屈光不正的视盘直径会发生什么样的改变？
   a. 相对正视眼，近视眼的视盘直径更小
   b. 相对正视眼，远视眼的视盘直径更大
   c. 近视眼的视盘直径小于远视眼
   d. 相对正视眼，无晶体眼的视盘直径更小

35. 哪 4 种临床表现属于 Charles Bonnet 综合征？
   a. 反复出现逼真的视幻觉，一定程度的视力下降，没有其他神经症状和体征，自觉所看到的不是真实的
   b. 看到复杂的影像如彩色的风景，会被诊断为青光眼，没有其他神经症状和体征，不知道自己所看到的不是真实的
   c. 看到的幻觉对象是人物，没有其他神经性疾病，没有其他的眼疾，自觉所看到的不是真实的
   d. 与患者交谈的人的图像反复出现，而患者确信还是真实的，则会被诊断为黄斑变性，若无其他神经症状，则没有诊断

36. 在美国，哪种程度的视野缺损会被视为法定盲？
   a. 半侧偏盲
   b. 黄斑回避暗点
   c. 收缩至 20°
   d. 视野测试显示平均缺损为 –19.00 的严重青光眼视野缺损

37. 有黄斑回避性暗点的患者阅读哪种大小的字体有困难？
   a. 中等大小的字体，如大字本
   b. 仅小号字体，如医学标签
   c. 中等大小以及小号字体
   d. 大号字体，如标题

38. 对比敏感度曲线可以体现哪 2 种视觉功能？
   a. 空间频率和对比度阈值
   b. 视力和空间频率
   c. 对比度阈值和对比敏感度
   d. 视力和临界的印刷字体大小

39. 一位成年患者，双眼看远用 –4.00 矫正，戴一副 +6.00 D 眼镜阅读，其阅读距离多少？
   a. 10 cm
   b. 16.7 cm
   c. 25 cm
   d. 12.5 cm

Answer Sheet for Section 3

Study Questions

Question	Answer	Question	Answer
1	a b c d	21	a b c d
2	a b c d	22	a b c d
3	a b c d	23	a b c d
4	a b c d	24	a b c d
5	a b c d	25	a b c d
6	a b c d	26	a b c d
7	a b c d	27	a b c d
8	a b c d	28	a b c d
9	a b c d	29	a b c d
10	a b c d	30	a b c d
11	a b c d	31	a b c d
12	a b c d	32	a b c d
13	a b c d	33	a b c d
14	a b c d	34	a b c d
15	a b c d	35	a b c d
16	a b c d	36	a b c d
17	a b c d	37	a b c d
18	a b c d	38	a b c d
19	a b c d	39	a b c d
20	a b c d		

第 3 册答题纸

学习的问题

问题	答案
1	a b c d
2	a b c d
3	a b c d
4	a b c d
5	a b c d
6	a b c d
7	a b c d
8	a b c d
9	a b c d
10	a b c d
11	a b c d
12	a b c d
13	a b c d
14	a b c d
15	a b c d
16	a b c d
17	a b c d
18	a b c d
19	a b c d
20	a b c d

问题	答案
21	a b c d
22	a b c d
23	a b c d
24	a b c d
25	a b c d
26	a b c d
27	a b c d
28	a b c d
29	a b c d
30	a b c d
31	a b c d
32	a b c d
33	a b c d
34	a b c d
35	a b c d
36	a b c d
37	a b c d
38	a b c d
39	a b c d

Answers

1. **b.** The magnification of a pinhole camera is limited by the distance from the pinhole to the image plane. The image formed by a pinhole camera is inverted, not upright. The small aperture limits the light available for image formation, requiring lengthy exposure times and poor sensitivity in dim light. The depth of field is nearly unlimited.
2. **b.** The sun is certainly a "distant object"! A +1.00 lens forms images of a distant object 1.0 m from the lens, on the opposite side of the lens from the object.
3. **a.** The power of the original lens system is given by the vergence equation: $U + P = V$. Here $0 + P = 1/1.00$, so $P = +1.00$ D. The net power of the new lens system is the sum of the original power plus the power of the added lens: $P_{new} = P_{old} + 3.00 = 4.00$ D. This new lens system forms an image according to the vergence equation: $0 + 4.00 = 1/v$, so $v = +0.25$ m.
4. **c.** The key to converting a power-cross description to a spherocylindrical specification is to determine the *difference* between the power in the 2 principal meridians. Here, the difference is 3.00 diopters (D). As we are asked for the answer in minus cylinder form, the spherical component is the power in the more positive meridian, here +1.00. The cylindrical component is thus −3.00D. This power is observed along the 115° meridian and is created by a minus cylinder lens component with axis 90° away; that is, axis 25°.
5. **d.** The compensation of the sphere power is always in the opposite direction from the change in cylinder power, in the ratio of a change in the sphere of one-half the change in cylinder.
6. **b.** A flat pane of glass displaces a beam of light, allowing it to continue in the original direction, as the deflection at each interface has an equal and opposite effect on the direction of the light beam. A prism may disperse white light into a spectrum, but in this case, the (yellow) light is monochromatic. The magnitude of the deflection of light by a prism depends on the orientation of the prism, but the deflection is always toward the base of the prism.
7. **c.** The power of the mirror $P = -2/r = -2.0$ D. Thus the vergence equation reads $-1/10.0 + (-2.0) = 1/v$ so $v = 1/(-2.1) = -0.47$ m; that is 0.47m away from the mirror on the side opposite the source object. This will be an erect, virtual image, minified by a factor of $0.47/10.0 = 0.047$. Such a small image is interpreted by the driver as an object farther away than the original source object—as the reminder printed on the mirror suggests: "OBJECTS IN MIRROR ARE CLOSER THAN THEY APPEAR."
8. **d.** Transverse magnification (sometimes also referred to as *linear magnification*) is the ratio of the size of the image to the size of the source object, as measured perpendicular to the optic axis. Longitudinal magnification (also known as *axial magnification*) is the ratio of the length of the image to the length of the source object, as measured along the optic axis. Neither concept is applicable to objects at astronomical distances. Angular magnification, the ratio of the apparent angle subtended by the image to that of the source object, is appropriate for afocal systems such as astronomical telescopes.
9. **c.** Vergence is the ratio of refractive index, n, divided by the distance from the object or to the image. Vergence (in diopters [D]) = n/distance (in meters). Vergence is negative for divergent light and positive for convergent light. In this case, the lenses are in air, for which the refractive index, n, is 1.000. Light diverges from the object so the vergence is negative. The object is 1.0 m from the lens and therefore has a vergence of −1.00 D = −1.000/1.0 m = −1.00 D. The first lens adds an additional −1.00 D of vergence. Light leaving the lens, therefore, has a vergence of −2.00 D. Light rays with a vergence of −2.00 D appear to be coming from a point 0.5 m to the left of the lens.

答案

1. **b** 。针孔相机的放大率受针孔到像平面距离的限制。针孔照相机所形成的像是倒立的，而不是正立的。小光圈限制了参与成像的光线，在昏暗的光线下，需要长时间的曝光和低光敏性。景深几乎是无限的。

2. **b**。太阳当然是一个"遥远的物体"！一个 +1.00 D 的镜片可以使一个无穷远的物体成像于镜片另一侧、距离镜片 1.0m 的地方。

3. **a**。根据聚散度方程，原透镜系统的焦度为 :$U + P = V$。这里，$0+P=1/1.00$，所以 $P=+1.00$ D。新透镜系统的纯焦度是原透镜系统焦度加上附加透镜的焦度：$P_{新}=P_{原}+3.00=4.00$ D 这个新透镜系统成像的像距依据聚散度方程计算为：$0+4.00=1/v$，所以 $v=0.25$ m。

4. **c** 。将焦度的十字交叉表示转换成球柱镜形式的关键关键是确定 2 条主子午线上的焦度之差。此处，焦度之差是 3.00 D。当我们被要求以负柱镜的形式给出配镜处方时，球镜度数为更为正度数子午线的焦度，这里是 +1.00 D。柱镜度数是 −3.00 D。这个焦度可沿 115° 子午线检测到，柱镜轴位与 115° 成 90° 角，即 25° 子午线。轴向为原轴向的正交轴向，即轴向转变为 25° 。

5. **d**。球镜焦度的补偿总是与柱镜焦度变换量符号相反，球镜的变化量与柱镜的变化量之比为 1/2。

6. **b**。光束穿过平板玻璃时，沿原方向继续传播，这是因为平板玻璃每个界面的偏转对光线的传播方向都有相等且相反的影响。棱镜可以将白光分解为彩色光带（光谱），但在这里，（黄色）光是单色光。棱镜偏转的大小取决于棱镜的方向。偏转总是朝向棱镜的底部。

7. **c**。球面镜的焦度为：$P =-2/r =-2.0$ D，因此，聚散度方程为 $-1/10.0+(-2.0)=1/v$，所以 $v=1/(-2.1)=-0.47$ m，即在镜前 0.47 m 处形成一正立的虚像，缩小倍数为 0.47/10.0=0.047。司机将这样的小像解读为比原物更远的物—就像镜子上的提示：**"镜中的物体比它看上去要近。"**

8. **d**。横向放大率（有时也称为*线性放大率*）是指像的大小与原物体大小的比值，即垂直于光轴的测量值。纵向放大率（也称为*轴向放大率*）是指沿光轴测量的像的长度与原物体的长度之比。这 2 个概念都不适用于天文距离上的物体。视角放大率，即像的视角与原物体的视角之比，适用于无焦系统，如天文望远镜。

9. **c**。聚散度是折射率 n 与物距或像距之比。聚散度（单位为：D）$=n/$距离（单位为：m）。将汇聚光束的聚散度定为正，发散光束定为负。在这种情况下，透镜在空气中（折射率 n 为 1.000），来自物体的光是发散的，所以聚散度为负。物体距透镜 1.0 m，因此物聚散度为 −1.00 D=−1.000/1.0 m = −1.00 D。第一个透镜附加 −1.00 D 的聚散度。因此，离开透镜的光，聚散度为 −2.00 D。−2.00 D 聚散度的光好像来自透镜左侧 0.5m 的点。

10. **b.** To answer questions 9 and 10, we treat the intermediate image as the object for the second lens. From this point on, the first lens can be ignored. The intermediate image is 2.0 m to the left of the second lens. The vergence of light entering the second lens is, therefore, –0.50 D. The lens adds +1.50 D of vergence. Therefore, the light exiting the lens has a vergence of +1.00 D. Light rays with a vergence of +1.00 D come to a focus 1.0 m to the right of the second lens.
11. **b.** Photorefractive keratectomy (PRK) and laser in situ keratomileusis (LASIK) are common refractive surgeries of the cornea. These procedures are based on photoablation using excimer lasers generating photons with wavelengths in the ultraviolet range that are absorbed within the corneal tissue.
12. **d.** The Airy disc is the central portion of a pattern of light and dark rings formed when light from a point source passes through a circular aperture and is diffracted. The formula for the diameter of the Airy disc is diameter = $2.44\lambda\ f/D$, where λ is the wavelength of the light, f is the focal length of the eye, and D is the diameter of the pupil. Thus, eyes with shorter focal lengths have a smaller Airy disc than eyes with longer focal lengths and therefore diffract less. Similarly, diffraction increases as the pupil size decreases and the wavelength of light increases. Retinal conditions such as macular degeneration have no effect on the size of the Airy disc.
13. **b.** Retinal image sizes are readily computed using the nodal point of the Gullstrand model eye, which is located 17 mm in front of the retina. By similar triangles, the diameter of the retinal image of an object located 333 mm from the eye, with a diameter of 9 mm, is 9 mm × (17/333) = 0.46 mm.
14. **c.** A change in acuity by a factor of 10 (such as a change from 20/20 to 20/200) corresponds to a difference of 1.0 LogMAR, since 1.0 is the common logarithm of 10. The common logarithm of 2 is 0.301, which we round to 0.30 for clinical purposes. This is "built-in" to the common ETDRS eye charts, which feature proportional steps of 0.10 LogMAR between lines, so that a 3-line change in acuity corresponds to a change of 0.30 LogMAR (ie, a doubling [or halving] of the visual angle).
15. **d.** The far point is the point conjugate to the fovea, with relaxed accommodation. In an emmetropic eye, this is at optical infinity. The hyperopic eye has a refractive apparatus with less optical power than that which produces emmetropia, so rays originating at the fovea emerge as diverging rays from the eye, and thus produce a virtual image *behind* the eye. A suitable plus sphere lens images distant objects at the far point, correcting this refractive error
16. **a.** Inhomogeneous cataracts frequently split the incident light into 2 or more divergent paths, resulting in monocular diplopia. Dry age-related macular degeneration may reduce retinal sensitivity to the diminished retinal illumination seen through a pinhole, but does not cause double vision. (Macular edema may cause monocular diplopia, however.) Recently acquired strabismus frequently causes binocular diplopia, but this resolves if either eye is covered. As these examples illustrate, the notion that monocular diplopia cannot be physiologic in origin is clearly incorrect.
17. **b.** A 20/20 optotype is 5 minutes of arc in height, or 1/12 of a degree. To convert from degrees to radian measure, multiply by $\pi/180$, since there are 180° in a half-circle. So our 20/20 optotype must subtend $\pi/(180 \times 12) = 0.00145$ radians. At 304.8 cm, this spans a height of 0.44 cm.
18. **c.** Jackson cross cylinder, astigmatic dial, and stenopeic slit tests are all subjective measures of astigmatism.Retinoscopy is a means of objectively determining the refractive status of an eye, including the astigmatism.

10. **b**。为了回答问题 9 和问题 10，我们将中间像作为第二个透镜的物。从这一点上，忽略第一个透镜。中间的像位于第二透镜左侧 2.0m 处。因此，进入第二透镜的物的聚散度为 –0.50D。该透镜加 1.50D 的聚散度。因此，离开透镜的光有 +1.00D 的聚散度。+1.00D 聚散度的光聚焦在第二个透镜右侧 1.0m 处。

11. **b**。屈光性角膜切削术（PRK）和准分子激光原位角膜磨镶术（LASIK）是角膜屈光性手术。这种术式是基于准分子激光产生波长在紫外线范围内的光子，这些光子在角膜组织中被吸收的光消融原理。

12. **d**。Airy 斑是由暗环包围的中央圆光斑构成的图样，它是由来自点光源的光经圆孔发生衍射而成。Airy 斑直径的计算公式为：直径 =2.44 λ *f*/*D*，其中 λ 是光的波长，*f* 是眼睛的焦距，*D* 是瞳孔的直径。因此，焦距较短的眼睛比焦距较长的眼睛有较小的 Airy 斑，因此，衍射较小。同样，随着瞳孔尺寸的减小和光波长的增加，衍射增加。黄斑变性等视网膜疾病不影响爱里斑大小。

13. **b**。视网膜像的大小可以很容易地用 Gullstred 模型眼的节点来计算，节点位于视网膜前 17 mm 处。通过相似三角形，距离眼睛 333 mm、直径 9 mm 的物体的视网膜像直径为 9 mm ×（17/333）= 0.46 mm。

14. **c**。视力的变化是 10 倍（例如从 20/20 到 20/200 之间的变化），相当于 1.0 LogMAR，因为 1.0 是 10 的常用对数。2 的常用对数为 0.301，为了方便临床，我们把它定为 0.30。这是常用 ETDRS 视力表的“内置”，它的特点是行间隔为 0.10 LogMAR，因此，三行视力变化对应 0.30 LogMAR，即视角的双倍（或一半）变化。

15. **d**。远点是调节松弛时的黄斑凹共轭点。在正视眼中，它为无限远处的一点。远视眼的屈光力能力比正视眼的弱，因此，从中央凹发出的光线以发散的形式从眼睛中射出，从而在眼睛*后面*形成一个虚像。一个合适的正球面透镜使远处的物体成像在远点处，来矫正这一屈光不正。

16. **a**。非均匀性白内障经常将入射光分裂成 2 个或更多的发散路径，导致单眼复视。干性老年性黄斑变性可能会导致小瞳下视网膜对照明减弱的敏感性降低，但不会造成复视。（黄斑水肿可能导致单眼复视）。最近几天发生的斜视通常会导致双眼复视，但如果遮盖其中任何一只眼的话，这个问题就会解决。正如这些例子所示，单眼复视不是起源于生理性因素的概念显然是不正确的。

17. **b**。20/20 的视标高度为 5 弧分，或者说是 1/12°。要将度数（°）转换为弧度 rad，需乘以 π/180，因为半圆是 180°。因此，我们的 20/20 视标必须对应 π/（180×12）= 0.00145 rad。在 304.8 cm 处，需要 0.44 cm 的高度。

18. **c**。Jackson 交叉柱镜、散光表盘和裂隙片检查都是散光的主观测量方法。视网膜检影镜是客观地确定眼睛屈光状态包括散光的一种手段。

19. **c.** The method of spheres is a measurement of the amplitude of accommodation. The gradient and heterophoria methods are ways to determine the accommodative convergence/accommodation (AC/A) ratio. The prism dissociation test allows direct comparison of the eyes and confirmation of equal fogging to be performed prior to determining the final sphere refinement.
20. **d.** The far point of the eye and the focal point of the original glasses coincide at this location: −0.125 −0.015 m = −0.140 m (in front of the eye). The same calculation with a 20-mm vertex distance requires a lens with a focal length of −0.120 m (since −0.120 −0.020 also equals −0.140). Thus, the required lens has a power of 1/(−0.120) = −8.33 D, a difference of −0.33 D.
21. **c.** If the green side is still clearer after the initially fogging, the eye was probably overminused prior to the test. Additional fogging (plus lens power) should be added until the 2 sides of the duochrome chart are equally clear, or the red side is clearer.
22. **d.** Refracting in a short room is inherently inaccurate because normal fogging techniques to relax accommodation will not be effective. One method to relax the accommodation would be to move the patient to a longer hallway to complete the refraction in a trial frame. Another option would be to install mirrors to optically extend the room length to 6 meters.
23. **c.** The old glasses do not give clear vision for distance, and now function almost as reading glasses. New spectacles, fully correcting the distance vision about 12 mm from the eye,have the advantage of "near effectivity," which reduces accommodative demand, compared to an emmetropic eye or one corrected by a contact lens. In this age range (eg, 46 years of age), people with myopia who are still able to read with their correct distance glasses are likely to find it more difficult to read with contact lenses. The presbyopic myopic patient wearing glasses can also read more easily by pushing the glasses farther away from the eyes.
24. **c.** To achieve a good fit with contact lenses, the rear surface's curvature is chosen according to the shape of the cornea. The central rear surface is usually spherical, but can be toric in shape to fit a cornea with astigmatism. Peripheral curvatures of both the cornea and the rear surface of the contact lens are flatter. A "tear lens" fills in space between the cornea and lens, especially with rigid contact lenses. The desired power of the contact lens is then achieved by adjusting the shape of the front surface of the contact lens. Spectacle lenses are manufactured with various base curvatures, which can be measured with a "lens clock." The lens manufacturer uses a standard series of base curves for various lens powers, chosen to minimize aberrations associated with off-axis viewing through theglasses. Exceptions from a standard series of base curves are made, for example, to match the patient's previous glasses, or to deal with aniseikonia—changing the magnification by changing the base curve.
25. **d.** Standard keratometry misses the flattest part of the cornea of eyes that have undergone myopic keratorefractive correction. This results in an overestimation of corneal power by keratometry and, if these values are employed in intraocular lens calculation, a hyperopic refractive surprise. Radial keratotomy corneas are also steeper in the mid-periphery than they are in the central cornea and are susceptible to instrument errors from keratometry as well. Misjudgment of the effective lens position occurs when employing standard IOL formulas to myopic keratorefractive eyes and this too results in hyperopic refractive surprise.
26. **c.** Positive dysphotopsias are speculated to be caused by internal reflections within the intraocular lens. Flashes and complaints of a curtain impinging upon central vision are both suggestive of retinal detachment and should not be ascribed to dysphotopsias. Dysphotopsias do indeed occur even when the intraocular lens is appropriately positioned within the capsular bag.

19. **c**。球镜法是一种调节幅度的测量方法。梯度和隐斜的测量方法是确定：调节性集合 / 调节（AC / A）比率的方法。棱镜分离法可直接进行双眼的比较，在测定最终球镜之前确定双眼等量雾视。

20. **d**。眼睛的远点和原始眼镜的焦点在此位置重合: –0.125 m –0.015 m = –0.140 m（眼前）。20mm 顶点距离需要焦距为 –0.120 m 的透镜（因为 –0.120–0.020 也等于 –0.140）。因此，所需透镜的焦度为 1 /（– 0.120 m）= –8.33 D，相差 –0.33 D。

21. **c**。如果在最初雾视后绿色仍然很清晰，则在测试之前眼睛可能是过矫。应加大雾视（加球镜），直到双色图表的两侧同样清晰，或红色一侧更清晰。

22. **d**。在小空间内完成验光，本质上是不准确的，因为放松调节的功能不起作用。放松调节的一种方法是将患者带到较长的走廊，在框架眼镜上完成验光。另一种方法是利用镜子，通过光学原理将房间长度延长到 6 m。

23. **c**。旧眼镜不能达到远距离的清晰视力，此时的功能几乎就和阅读眼镜一样。新眼镜是在距离眼睛 12 mm 处的距离，达到了远距离的清晰视力，它与正视眼或通过隐形眼镜矫正的眼睛相比，具有“视近有效性”优点，因为它降低了调节需求。在这个年龄段（例如 46 岁）的近视人群，他们仍然能够通过足矫的眼镜完成近距离阅读，但是他们戴接触镜阅读时会感到更困难。戴眼镜的老视近视患者也可以通过将眼镜拿远看的方法使视物更清楚。

24. **c**。为了适应接触镜，可以根据角膜的形态选择后表面的曲率。中央后表面通常是球形的，但可以是复杂的曲面，以适应具有散光的角膜。角膜和接触镜后表面周边曲率更平坦。在角膜与接触镜之间形成一个“泪液镜”，尤其是硬性接触镜。然后通过调节接触镜前表面的形状来实现接触镜的所需曲率。眼镜镜片可制造成不同曲率，并且可以测量。镜片制造使用标准系列的基弧来得到各种镜片的度数，选择基弧是为了减少通过眼镜周边注视时产生的像差。也有一系列标准基弧之外的使用，例如，匹配患者先前的眼镜，或者通过改变基弧改变眼镜放大率来处理双眼不等像。

25. **d**。标准角膜曲率测定法忽略了经过近视角膜屈光矫正的角膜中最平坦的部分。这导致通过角膜测量法高估了角膜屈光力，并且如果在人工晶体计算中采用这些值，出现意外的远视屈光不正。放射状角膜切开术的角膜在旁周边比在中央更陡，而且也容易受角膜测量仪器误差的影响。当对近视性角膜屈光眼使用标准 IOL 公式时，会发生对有效晶状体位置的误判，这也会导致远视屈光不正。

26. **c**。正失能性炫光是由人工晶状体内的内部反射引起的。闪光和中央视觉遮挡抱怨都提示视网膜脱离，不属于失能性炫光。即使人工晶状体在囊袋内时，失能性炫光也不会发生。

27. **a.** Monofocal intraocular lenses demonstrate the highest modulation transfer function (MTF) peaks.Extended-depth-of-focus (EDOF) lenses have lower amplitude depressions between peaks than conventional multifocal intraocular lenses. Higher MTF values signify higher image quality. In examination of an intraocular lens's modulation transfer function, the pupil size and the spatial frequency of the object are always specified. Alterations of either of these will affect the MTF curve.
28. **b.** Misalignment of a toric intraocular lens by as little as 10° will result in a substantial reduction in the efficacy of the astigmatism correction. Misalignment by 90°, rather than merely negating the benefit of the toric lens, will double the patient's resultant astigmatism. Excyclotorsion may be observed when the patient lies down. However, the degree of cyclotorsion is variable and unpredictable. Any misalignment of a toric intraocular lens (other than a misalignment of exactly 90°) will also rotate the patient's postoperative astigmatic axis.
29. **a.** Diffractive multifocal lenses dissipate about 20% of the light entering the pupil. This light does not find its way to the retina. Patients with maculopathy are poor candidates for multifocal intraocular lenses (IOLs). These lenses are highly sensitive to decentration.Although many clinical parameters are important in the decision to insert a multifocal IOL, the IOL formulas employed are the same as those for conventional Monofocal IOLs.
30. **b.** A 0.8 D change in keratometry value (K) corresponds to approximately a 1.00 D change of refraction. The following equation is often used to predict corneal curvature after keratorefractive surgery: $K_{postop} = K_{preop} + (0.8 \times RE)$, where K_{preop} and K_{postop} are preoperative and postoperative *K* readings, respectively, and *RE* is the refractive error to be corrected at the corneal plane. When myopic corrections are performed, the minimum corneal power tolerable is 33.0 D. Therefore, the formula becomes $33.0 = K_{preop} + (0.8 \times -10.00)$ where K_{preop} equals 41.0.
31. **c.** All forms of keratorefractive surgical procedures produce some form of unwanted optical aberrations.Small-incision lenticule extraction and photorefractive keratectomy act as surgical removal procedures. Intracorneal ring segments act as surgical additionprocedures, changing the relationship between the anterior and posterior curvature of the cornea. Aphakic intraocular lens adds an intraocular lens into the system and, after the healing of the surgical incisions, causes minimal change in the higher-order aberrations of the eye.
32. **c.** Positive defocus, also known as *myopia*, is a lower-order aberration that is correctable with spectacles. All other aberrations are higher order, such as vertical coma and trefoil, which are fourth-order aberrations, and secondary astigmatism and spherical aberration, which are fifth-order aberrations. These higher-order aberrations can be correctable with rigid gas-permeable lenses and wavefront-guided keratorefractive surgery, but not with spectacles.
33. **d.** The retinal nerve fiber layer is birefringent, meaning it polarizes light or changes the polarization of incident light that passes through it. The scanning laser polarimeter uses this property to measure nerve fiber layer thickness. The cornea is also birefringent, so a corneal compensator is necessary to eliminate the cornea's polarization effects.

27. **a**。单焦点人工晶体显示出最高的调制传递函数（MTF）峰值。与传统的多焦点人工晶体相比，扩展焦深（EDOF）晶状体在峰值上具有较低幅度的下降。较高的 MTF 值表示较高的像质。在测量人工晶状体的调制传递函数时，都是在特定的瞳孔大小和空间频率下进行的，其中任何一个值的改变都会影响到 MTF 曲线。

28. **b**。复曲面人工晶体偏位 10° 将导致散光矫正作用显著降低。偏位 90° ，而不是仅仅否定复曲面镜片的好处，将使患者的散光加倍。当患者躺下时可以观察到外旋转。然而，旋转的程度是可变的以及不可预测的。复曲面人工晶体的任何偏位（除了精确的 90° 偏位）也将使患者的术后散光轴旋转。

29. **a**。衍射多焦点晶体可消散约 20% 的瞳孔的光的，这种光线不能到达视网膜。黄斑病变患者是多焦点人工晶状体（IOL）的不良适应者，这些人的晶体对偏心非常敏感。尽管在决定植入多焦点 IOL 时有许多临床参数都很重要，但所采用的 IOL 公式与常规单焦点 IOL 的公式相同。

30. **b**。角膜曲率测量值（K）的 0.8 D 变化对应于大约 1.00 D 的屈光变化。以下等式通常用于预测角膜屈光手术后的角膜曲率：$K_{postop} = K_{preop} + (0.8 \times RE)$，其中 K_{preop} 和 K_{postop} 分别是术前和术后的 K 值，RE 是要在角膜平面矫正的屈光不正。当进行近视矫正时，可容忍的最小角膜焦度允许值为 33.0D。因此，公式变为 $33.0 = K_{preop} + (0.8 \times -10.00)$，其中 K_{preop} 等于 41.0。

31. **c**。所有形式的角膜屈光手术都会产生某些不想要的光学像差。小切口晶状体摘除术和光性屈光性角膜切削术都是去除性手术。角膜内基质环填充术属于添加性手术，改变了角膜的前表面和后表面之间的曲率。无晶状体眼人工晶体植入术是将人工晶体植入眼中，并且能在手术切口愈合之后，引起最小的高阶像差的变化。

32. **c**。正离焦，也称为*近视*，是一种可以用眼镜矫正的低阶像差。所有其他像差都是高阶像差，例如垂直彗差和三叶草差，它们是四阶像差，像散和球差是五阶像差。这些高阶像差可以通过 RGP 和波前像差引导的角膜屈光手术来矫正，但不能用眼镜矫正。

33. **d**。视网膜神经纤维层是双重折射的，这意味着它能使光线偏振或改变穿过视神经纤维层的入射光的偏振方向。扫描激光偏振计利用该特性来测量神经纤维层的厚度。角膜也是双折射的，因此需要角膜补偿器来消除角膜的偏振效应。

34. **d.** With direct ophthalmoscopy, the examiner uses the optics of the patient's eye as a simple magnifier to look at the retina. The optics of the normal eye are approximately +60D, so using the formula for a simple magnifier, the magnification is 60/4, or 15×. If the patient's eye is myopic, a minus lens is dialed in, to overcome the extra plus power "error lens" inside the patient's eye. Those 2 lenses create a Galilean telescope effect, increasing magnification and decreasing the field of view. Similarly, the retina of a hyperopic eye will be magnified less than 15× because of the reverse Galilean telescope created by the minus power error lens inside the patient's eye and the plus lens of the direct ophthalmoscope.Thus, the size of the optic disc will appear smaller in a hyperopic eye—f which aphakia is an extreme example—han in an emmetropic eye or a myopic eye.
35. **a.** Vivid recurrent hallucinations, some degree of vision loss, no other neurological signs or symptoms, and full insight that what is seen is not real are all required to make a diagnosis of Charles Bonnet syndrome. A diagnosis other than Charles Bonnet syndrome should be considered when patients do not have full insight that what they are seeing is not real.
36. **c.** Legal blindness (due to visual field constriction) in the United Sates is determined as a visual field of equal to or less than 20° around central fixation measured with a Goldmann Ⅲ4e target. A point seen at 10 dB or higher on a static automated threshold field test is considered to be seen with a 4e stimulus. A mean defect of 22 dB or greater on an automated 30° static threshold perimetry test is also considered legal blindness by the Social Security Administration in the United States.
37. **d.** Patients with foveal-sparing scotomas have difficulty seeing large targets, such as larger letters on a visual acuity chart or larger text such as headlines of a newspaper, depending on the size of the remaining central visual field.
38. **a.** Contrast sensitivity varies with spatial frequency or target size. The contrast sensitivity curve represents the relationship between contrast threshold and spatial frequency.
39. **a.** Higher reading adds require a closer working distance at the focal point of the lens.This patient has uncorrected myopia of 4.00 D in addition to the +6.00 D of reading add,therefore an effective reading add of +10.00 D. This requires a reading distance at the focal point of the lens, which will be 1/10 m (ie, 10 cm, or 4 in).

34. **d**。通过直接检影镜检查，检查者使用患者眼睛的光学系统作为简单的放大镜来观察视网膜。正常眼球的光学系统的焦度约为 + 60.00D，因此使用简单放大镜的公式，放大倍率为 60/4（15 倍）。如果患者的眼睛是近视眼，则需增加一个负球镜，来抵消患者眼额外的正焦度“误差透镜”。这 2 个镜头形成了 Galileo 望远镜效果，增加了放大并减少了视野。类似地，远视眼的视网膜的放大倍率小于 15 倍，这是由于患者眼内的负焦度误差透镜和直接检眼镜的正透镜产生的反 Galileo 望远镜效果造成的。因此，视盘的大小在远视眼中看起来比正视眼或近视眼更小，其中无晶体眼是最极端的例子。

35. **a**。活性周期性视幻觉，一定程度的视力丧失，没有其他神经系统体征或症状，以及不充分自知所看到的不真实都是诊断 Charles Bonnet 综合征所必需的。当患者不能完全知道他们所看到的不真实时，应考虑除 Charles Bonnet 综合征以外的诊断。

36. **c**。在美国，定义法定盲（由于视野缩小）为用 Goldmann Ⅲ4e 靶标测量的中心注视范围等于或小于 20° 的视野。在静态环境测试中在 10 dB 或更高处看到的点被认为是用 4e 刺激看到的。在自动 30° 静态视野检查中，平均缺陷为 22 dB 或更大，也被美国社会保障局定为法定盲。

37. **d**。患有黄斑回避性暗点的患者很难看到大的视标，例如视力表上的较大字母或较大的文本（例如报纸的标题），这取决于剩余的中心视野的大小。

38. **a**。对比灵敏度随空间频率或视标大小而变化。对比敏感度曲线表示对比度阈值和空间频率之间的关系。

39. **a**。更高的阅读附加需要将工作距离靠近透镜的焦点。该患者在未矫正 4.00 D 近视下，还要用 +6.00 D 的阅读附加，因此，有效的阅读附加应为 +1.00 D。这就需要阅读距离在透镜的焦点处，也就是 1/10 m（10 cm 或 4 in）。

（翻译 刘凤阳 许军 // 审校 石一宁 李易）

“2018–2019 基础与临床科学教程”《临床光学》

译后感

回想起来已经是 30 年前的事了。

那是 1987 年，有幸被国家公派赴美进修眼科，参加了美国眼科学会 AAO 年会，正是在这次会上，我遇到这套 13 册的眼科“基础与临床科学教程”（Basic and Clinical Science Course）。我的美国导师李英尧（King Y Lee），也就是美中眼科协会（COAS）和中华眼科学会金苹果奖的创始人将这一套书借给了我。

1990 年，中国的眼科精英立志将其引入中国，与美国眼科学会商谈获得了免费版权，但只是草草摘要出版了其中的几本，因为 AAO 的 BCSC 教程每一册每 3 年必须更新 1 次，而我们的资金和翻译、出版速度无法跟进。我常常将带回的复印本作为临床教学的基本教材，其教材的内容层次、逻辑、照片、图表、表格、参考文献等都是精心设计的，使得枯燥的医学学习过程成为一种享受，轻松而愉悦。

二

我入门眼科时，我的母亲石广礼先生说，中国老一代眼科人口口相传“一部眼科学，半部屈光史”。我的主任也是将我们第一批改革开放后的大学本科五年毕业生的第一年眼科住院医师培训放在了验光室，检影、处方、磨片、装镜，我们一干就是 6 个月。

可是，任何一部眼科学，都是将屈光学或视光学放在教材的最后一部分，似是可有可无。而冗长繁重的学习过程，使我们常常将书的尾部省略了。

眼科教材的屈光学一章，经典的有几大块：屈光不正分类（近视、远视和散光）与老视、屈光不正的矫正。不知道眼球屈光发育为何意，更是不知何谓“眼球的正视化”，没有屈光成分的概念，更无法理解验光的屈光度是 4 个主要的屈光成分相互匹配、补偿和代偿的结果。眼科医生不知道幼儿、学龄前儿童、青少年在 15 岁之前的视觉发育过程就好比身高、智力，是需要一个过程的，也就是视力是逐步从 0.02 发育到成人的 1.0，屈光度也是从远视 +3.00D 逐步匹配、补偿发育到成人的 +/–0.50D 的，这一基础教育的空白与缺陷，导致了长达 30 年的对儿童视力的误判和儿童远视的误治，一直延续至今，其所产生的浩浩荡荡的近视人流，直逼中国国防、中华民族健康底线！

三

我们在 2000 年对附近的全日制小学、中学和大学、幼儿园人群进行横断面眼健康调查，结果震惊了沉浸于后节手术鼎盛期的我，近视检出率，小学一年级为 48%，初一为 84%，初三、高三 95%，这正与 2000 年我国台湾地区大学生的入校发病率 94.5% 接近！由于是对城市重点中小学学生的屈光度进行非睫状肌麻痹的自动验光，我们还为以后的纵断面进行了设计，并立志倾力连续追踪 3 年、6 年、9 年、12 年、15 年。我们曾寄希望于获得一些科研经费，完成 15 年的宏伟蓝图，可是当我们将汇总的流调论文投向杂志社，编辑老师说，没有散瞳不能发表，没有人口基数分层筛选没有代表性。尽管我们将 20 世纪 90 年代国外数篇非睫状肌麻痹下的儿童屈光度改变的论文也予以提交，尽管流行病学中某一人群的全体人员的数据是有效的……但是由于 19 年前的人们还没有时间关注健康，更不要说关注未来 3 ~ 50 年后是否能看见，又怎么能够将经费拨给未来的课题：我们全科人背着设备折旧费，牺牲自己的休息时间，加班加点地完成任务，但是难于支撑，更不被理解，在苦苦挣扎了 6 年，汇总了 3 年纵断面数据后，压垮骆驼的最后一根稻草逼停了我们的计划。

怎么办？按照 1945 年美国海军部的近视研究所的报告，高中时期为 0.8 的视力依然会有 10% 的人会在大学期间发展为近视，1974 年日本海军部的高度近视研究所报告，30 年后日本将会出现病理性近视爆发流行，当年日本的近视发病率仅为 35%，2000 年的我国台湾、香港和大陆的高中学生近视已达 95%，试想 30 年后的 2030 年，我们的病理性近视会爆发流行吗？令人不寒而栗……不幸被我言中的是，2000 年幼儿园小班的孩子现在已经 23 岁，当年 18 岁的高三学生已步入了 35 岁，当年 25 岁的大学生已经是 44 岁的中年人，我常常会想，当年被忽视了眼部健康的孩子们目前的近视患病率是多少？又有多少是病理性近视？他们在未来的五六十年的生命长河中，什么时候会突发视网膜脱离？什么时候会因正常眼压性青光眼而逐步失明？什么时候会因近视性黄斑病变而导致视力永无 0.3 ?

四

难道医者一定要变为弃医从文的周树人、弃医从政的孙逸仙？尽管 10 年前人们视书为粪土，我还是拾起笔墨，选取最直白的语言，开始了医学写作之路。

2010 年，我们出版《近视防治三岁抓起》。

2012 年，我和方严教授的《中国儿童青少年近视形成机制和预测与防控》一书出版，书中总结了 20 多年研究成果，主要包含以下内容：①系统观察描述我国儿童青少年近视的形成、发展等发病规律，寻找出近视防控的关键年龄点；②根据眼球发育与大脑发育、身体发育的关系，提出“二次发育”理论，阐述儿童青少年近视的病因；③分析儿童青少年近视防治的盲区，针对眼球光学－生物特性，提出眼球屈光发育的预测公式；④分析眼球的生物力学在儿童青少年近视形成中的关键作用，提出“眼球过度发育的内动力”理论，建立以增强巩人眼球负荷能力、减少眼球过度生长的内动力预防治疗体系；⑤通过眼底形态学变化规律与病理学改变的对应关系，量化描述近视常见眼底改变，建立临床简易可行的眼底观察指标与进展预测体系。

2013年，方严教授和我将收集的13年的高度近视，以及因近视而患视网膜脱离病人的玻璃体切除术后的眼底照片分类，编辑出版了《病理性近视眼眼底改变》一书，并提出近视防控的目标是防止出现高度近视，是关乎“国民素质、国防安全”的大事。

2017年，我们出版了《拒绝近视——石一宁大夫有话说》，面对近视人群洪流，首先在国家民族层面，提出了系统性框架战略和可实施可操作可持续具体战术。

2014年及2017年，方严教授和我在《临床眼科杂志》和陕西科学技术出版社率先出版了《中国儿童青少年近视防控流程的建议——近视防控的共识》，为2018年国家顶层战略项目“共同呵护好孩子的眼睛，让他们拥有一个光明的未来”提供了可实施的一揽子方案。

2018年，我们出版了中英文双语对照的《近视手册2017》，将200多年来的人类近视防控研究一览无余地展现在国人眼前，无论是医学基础研究的人员、眼科医生，还是眼镜界、眼保健行业的人员，乃至于苦苦寻觅的家长，对他们来说，这本书无异于一部有关近视的“百科全书”。就“近视” 这一知识门类来讲，本书从目录的安排上，几乎涉及了有关近视的解剖、生理、遗传、环境、生物工程、验光配镜、营养物质基础、神经调节、心理与物理因素、免疫、微量元素、分子生物学、近视类型、运动与生活等所有的内容，远远超过了手册的界限。这本书的读者范围很广，只要是对近视感兴趣的各行各业人士，它都是一本有用的工具书。面对“越治越多”的儿童青少年近视，有人窃喜“眼健康事业将成为价值万亿的大产业”，有人开始新一轮的“短平快”。面对这一现状，有人开启了“快餐”服务，原本应回报社会百姓巨额社会财富的技术又成为吸金噱头，这些都让我的心流血，我们只能眼睁睁看着11年后的中国病理性近视流行爆发，面对病理性近视的三大不可逆双目失明并发症而束手无策！

时至今日，人们仍然误将中国的近视防控设计成为快餐，60年的代价仅仅只是在单纯远视力检查的基础上加上了电脑验光，而将几个亿未来的失明和低视力灾难转化为上万亿的医疗健康产业！

而另一方面，中国的“眼视光医生”在消减了大量基础与临床医学教育的情况下，转入了临床眼科，眼看中国已无视光学博士，中国的眼镜业、中国初级眼保健业实现高等化教育的普及变得遥遥无期。

五

上述现象究其根本，是由于缺少一本国际通用的视光学教科书！

机缘巧合，2008年在“中华健康快车”项目进入陕西时，我们有幸争取到了国际眼科联盟（International Council of Ophthalmology，ICO）的国际眼科医师考试在西北地区设立的唯一考点。

国际眼科联盟是一个世界性的眼科专业协会，源于1857年，正式成立于1927年。光学、屈光与器械（Optics, Refraction and Instruments）作为 ICO 考试三部分的 A（视觉科学 Visual Sciences）、C（临床眼科 Clinical Ophthalmology）必过项目的 B 部分，横亘在进入临床眼科考试的入口，考试规定，不通过 B 部分，后面的临床部分不能进行，也就是说，不具备光学、屈光和器械知识，没有资格当眼科医生。

美国眼科学会（AAO）的“基础与临床科学教程”BCSC 的第 3 册《临床光学》（原书名为 *Clinical Optics*），被指定为国家医学考试的 ICO 考试点的第二步必考科目的必考书。

没有中文版教材的现状一直困扰着中国考生，成为中国考生系统学习视光知识、理解考题、通过考试的巨大障碍，大量的中国眼科医生被挡在临床眼科考试的门外，多数人放弃了继续深造的机会。

六

我想如果有机会将美国眼科学会的考试用书翻译成中英文双语，既可以供中国考生学习专业，又可以提高他们的专业英语水平。这对于完善西北地区乃至全国眼科专业医生全面的规范化理论水平培训将会有极大的帮助。同时也加强了临床和基础医学、专科和相关学科的横向纵向联系，促进了西北地区眼科医生与全国先进地区的业务交流，更增加了中国眼科医生国际化的融入能力，加快了与世界接轨的步伐，对提升眼科医生的专业技术奠定了基础。也为我们视光学专业学生找到了视光学教科书。

我在 2012 年以 AAO 会员价买进了网络版，转化出文档，组织了 10 人小组，3 个月翻译成稿，但到想要出版时才发现没有版权，无法出版和发行，只好束之高阁达 8 年之久。

七

当几本与近视相关的著作相继顺利出版发行后，我心底的这个夙愿又开始浮动了。与我的老同学朱壮涌总编和付琨编辑提出了奢侈的要求：购买版权，出双语翻译版！他们顶着压力答应了，立即联系 AAO 出版商签订了合同，最新一版“2018–2019 基础与临床科学教程”《临床光学》于 2018 年 11 月 19 日发到我的信箱，用“激动”一词来描述此刻心情一点都不为过。

我立即邀请有共识的同道者 40 人组成翻译组，并邀请 10 名教授组成审校组开始分章节审校，特别是视光教育家高祥璐教授为总审校。我心里知道，这不是一件容易的事情：需要在最短的 3 年版权时间内，最准确地保留原著风格、原汁原味地翻译出国际通用视光教材，同时还要有原文做对照、又需要符合中国出版总局的要求，还需要统一专业用语和翻译词汇。

好事多磨，翻译稿上交，返回，再审校，再返回，拉锯战式的 3 审 3 校，终于画上了句号：在多雨而漫长的 2019 年之夏开印了！

我又邀请了 8 位教授为中英文双语版“2018–2019 基础与临床科学教程”《临床光学》作序，包括组织 ICO 国际考试的 David Taylor 教授和引进 ICO 考试的中华健康快车创会主席方黄吉雯女士；邀请了与我一起奋斗在大西北的兰州大学的张文芳院长分享 10 年的点点滴滴；还有在教育界辛勤耕耘视光专业数十载的刘陇黔教授、魏瑞华教授和何伟教授；当然还包括老搭档方严教授！

付印之际，我如愿以偿地邀请到我心目中的偶像——王宁利教授为本书作序！

期待此书能为中国视光领域添砖加瓦，以承载起解救几亿近视中国人、90% 以上的未来高度近视的中国人之重任！

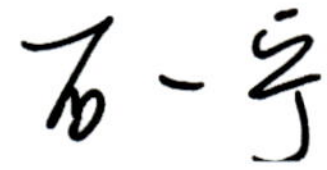

2019 年 7 月 15 日耳顺之年于西安